ORTHOPAEDIC SURGERY ESSENTIALS

TRAUMA

ORTHOPAEDIC SURGERY ESSENTIALS
TRAUMA

ORTHOPAEDIC SURGERY ESSENTIALS

Adult Reconstruction
Daniel J. Berry, MD
Scott P. Steinmann, MD

Foot and Ankle
David B. Thordarson, MD

Hand and Wrist
James R. Doyle, MD

Oncology and Basic Science
Timothy A. Damron, MD
Carol D. Morris, MD

Sports Medicine
Anthony A. Schepsis, MD
Brian D. Busconi, MD

Pediatrics
Kathryn E. Cramer, MD
Susan A. Scherl, MD

Spine
Christopher M. Bono, MD
Steven R. Garfin, MD

Trauma
Charles Court-Brown, MD
Margaret McQueen, MD
Paul Tornetta III, MD

ORTHOPAEDIC SURGERY ESSENTIALS

TRAUMA

Series Editors

PAUL TORNETTA III, MD
Professor
Department of Orthopaedic Surgery
Boston University School of Medicine;
Director of Orthopaedic Trauma
Boston University Medical Center
Boston, Massachusetts

THOMAS A. EINHORN, MD
Professor and Chairman
Department of Orthopaedic Surgery
Boston University School of Medicine
Boston, Massachusetts

Authors

CHARLES COURT-BROWN, MD, FRCS ED (ORTH)
Consultant Orthopaedic Trauma Surgeon
Edinburgh Orthopaedic Trauma Unit
Royal Infirmary of Edinburgh
Edinburgh, United Kingdom;
Professor of Orthopaedic Trauma
University of Edinburgh

MARGARET MCQUEEN, MD, FRCS ED (ORTH)
Consultant Orthopaedic Trauma Surgeon
Edinburgh Orthopaedic Trauma Unit
Royal Infirmary of Edinburgh
Edinburgh, United Kingdom;
Senior Lecturer
University of Edinburgh

PAUL TORNETTA III, MD
Professor
Department of Orthopaedic Surgery
Boston University School of Medicine;
Director of Orthopaedic Trauma
Boston University Medical Center
Boston, Massachusetts

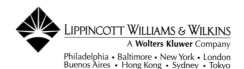

LIPPINCOTT WILLIAMS & WILKINS
A **Wolters Kluwer** Company

Philadelphia • Baltimore • New York • London
Buenos Aires • Hong Kong • Sydney • Tokyo

Acquisitions Editor: Robert Hurley
Managing Editor: Jenny Kim
Developmental Editor: Grace Caputo, Dovetail Content Solutions
Production Manager: Bridgett Dougherty
Senior Manufacturing Manager: Benjamin Rivera
Marketing Director: Sharon Zinner
Design Coordinator: Holly McLaughlin
Production Services: Nesbitt Graphics, Inc.
Printer: Courier

Library of Congress Cataloging-in-Publication Data
Court-Brown, Charles M.
  Trauma / Charles Court-Brown, Margaret McQueen, Paul Tornetta
III. -- 1st ed.
    p. ; cm. -- (Orthopaedic surgery essentials)
  Includes bibliographical references and index.
  ISBN 0-7817-5096-2
  1. Fractures--Treatment. 2. Orthopedic surgery.   I. McQueen,
Margaret M. II. Tornetta, Paul. III. Title. IV. Series.
  [DNLM: 1. Fractures--surgery. 2. Multiple Trauma--surgery.
3. Orthopedic Procedures--methods.   WE 175 C862t 2006]
  RD101.C833 2006
  614'.315--dc22

                                            2005019954

Care has been taken to confirm the accuracy of the information presented and to describe generally accepted practices. However, the authors, editors, and publisher are not responsible for errors
or omissions or for any consequences from application of the information in this book and make
no warranty, expressed or implied, with respect to the currency, completeness, or accuracy of the
contents of the publication. Application of this information in a particular situation remains the
professional responsibility of the practitioner.

        The authors, editors, and publisher have exerted every effort to ensure that drug selec-
tion and dosage set forth in this text are in accordance with current recommendations and practice at the time of publication. However, in view of ongoing research, changes in government reg-
ulations, and the constant flow of information relating to drug therapy and drug reactions, the
reader is urged to check the package insert for each drug for any change in indications and dosage
and for added warnings and precautions. This is particularly important when the recommended
agent is a new or infrequently employed drug.

        Some drugs and medical devices presented in this publication have Food and Drug Ad-
ministration (FDA) clearance for limited use in restricted research settings. It is the responsibility
of the health care provider to ascertain the FDA status of each drug or device planned for use in
their clinical practice.

        To purchase additional copies of this book, call our customer service department at
(800) 639-3030 or fax orders to (301) 824-7390. International customers should call
(301) 714-2324.

        Visit Lippincott Williams & Wilkins on the Internet: at LWW.com. Lippincott Williams
& Wilkins customer service representatives are available from 8:30 am to 6 pm, EST.

                                            10 9 8 7 6 5 4 3 2 1

To our families, without whom this book would have been written in half the time!

CONTENTS

Contributing Authors   ix
Series Preface   xi
Foreword   xiii
Preface   xv

SECTION I: GENERAL PRINCIPLES

1. Epidemiology   1
2. Fracture Healing and Biomechanics   7
3. The Multiply Injured Patient   12
4. Open Fractures   19
5. Gunshot Injuries   27
6. Stress Fractures   32
7. Periprosthetic Fractures   43
8. Osteoporotic Fractures   53
9. Pathological Fractures   59

SECTION II: UPPER LIMB

10. Shoulder Girdle   68
11. Proximal Humeral Fractures   89
12. Humeral Diaphyseal Fractures   103
13. Distal Humeral Fractures   115
14. Proximal Forearm Fractures and Elbow Dislocations   124
15. Fractures of the Forearm Diaphysis   141
16. Fractures of the Distal Radius and Ulna   153
17. Hand Fractures and Dislocations   170
    17.1 Carpal Injuries   174
    17.2 Metacarpal Injuries   187
    17.3 Phalangeal Injuries   196
    17.4 Finger Dislocations   204

SECTION III: SPINE AND PELVIS

18. Cervical Spine Fractures   208
19. Thoracolumbar Fractures and Dislocations   226
20. Pelvic and Acetabular Fractures   238

SECTION IV: LOWER LIMB

21. **Proximal Femoral Fractures and Hip Dislocations** 259
    21.1 Hip Dislocation 259
    21.2 Proximal Femoral Fractures 264
22. **Subtrochanteric Fractures** 284
23. **Femoral Diaphyseal Fractures** 290
24. **Distal Femoral Fractures** 303

25. **Patellar Fractures** 313
26. **Proximal Tibial Fractures and Knee Dislocations** 322
27. **Tibia and Fibula Diaphyseal Fractures** 339
28. **Tibial Plafond Fractures** 354
29. **Ankle Fractures** 366
30. **Foot Fractures and Dislocations** 383

SECTION V: TECHNIQUES OF FRACTURE MANAGEMENT

31. **Nonoperative Management** 412
32. **Plating** 427
33. **Intramedullary Nailing** 440
34. **Other Internal Fixation Techniques** 452

35. **External Fixation** 467
36. **Arthroplasty** 475
37. **Amputations** 482

SECTION VI: COMPLICATIONS

38. **Acute Compartment Syndrome** 492
39. **Nonunions and Bone Defects** 503

40. **Infection** 520
41. **Other Complications** 528

Index 539

CONTRIBUTING AUTHORS

Christopher M. Bono, MD
Assistant Professor
Department of Orthopaedic Surgery
Boston University School of Medicine
Attending Spine Surgeon
Boston University Medical Center
Boston, MA

Marie D. Rinaldi, BA
Robert Wood Johnson Medical School
University of Medicine and Dentistry, New Jersey
Newark, NJ

SERIES PREFACE

Most of the available resources in orthopaedic surgery are very good, but they either present information exhaustively—so the reader has to wade through too many details to find what he or she seeks—or they assume too much knowledge, making the information difficult to understand. Moreover, as residency training has advanced, it has become more focused on the individual subspecialties. Our goal was to create a series at the basic level that residents could read completely during a subspecialty rotation to obtain the essential information necessary for a general understanding of the field. Once they have survived those trials, we hope that the *Orthopaedic Surgery Essentials* books will serve as a touchstone for future learning and review.

Each volume is to be a manageable size that can be read during a resident's tour. As a series, they will have a consistent style and template, with the authors' voices heard throughout. Content will be presented more visually than in most books on orthopaedic surgery, with a liberal use of tables, boxes, bulleted lists, and algorithms to aid in quick review. Each topic will be covered by one or more authorities, and each volume will be edited by experts in the broader field.

But most importantly, each volume—*Pediatrics, Spine, Sports Medicine,* and so on—will focus on the requisite knowledge in orthopaedics. Having the essential information presented in one user-friendly source will provide the reader with easy access to the basic knowledge needed in the field, and mastering this content will give him or her an excellent foundation for additional information from comprehensive references, atlases, journals, and on-line resources.

We would like to thank the editors and contributors who have generously shared their knowledge. We hope that the reader will take the opportunity of telling us what works and does not work.

—Paul Tornetta III, MD
—Thomas A. Einhorn, MD

FOREWORD

Orthopaedic Surgery Essentials: Trauma represents a collaborative effort by three world-renowned experts in orthopaedic traumatology from both sides of the Atlantic Ocean. It presents up-to-date information for the treatment of musculoskeletal injuries from both a European perspective and a United States perspective. The reader learns what to expect and what to do for the unexpected.

The book is based on evidence-based medicine combined with the authors vast personal experience. *OSE: Trauma* is a perfect state-of-the-art reference book with guiding principles for fracture diagnosis and treatment. The basic science of fracture repair and biomechanics is presented, and special challenges in fracture management are addressed, including increased velocity of injuries, poor bone quality in the osteoporotic, and periprosthetic fractures. Changes in treatment–with less invasive approaches and improved technology are also covered. It embraces both surgical and nonsurgical management of patients.

The book clearly and logically supplies a single source for fracture care, including

> Epidemiology
> Anatomy
> Fracture classification
> Radiologic assessment
> Treatment methods
> Associated injuries
> Complications

The bullet-style format offers an efficient method for the reader to gather information quickly on any particular fracture or on all fractures. In addition, excellent charts, diagrams, and x-ray photos further enhance the text. *OSE: Trauma* is extremely helpful for medical students, orthopaedic residents, orthopaedic nurses, emergency room physicians, primary care physicians, general orthopaedic surgeons, and academic orthopaedic surgeons.

I am thankful that Charles Court-Brown, Margaret McQueen, and Paul Tornetta were willing to share their time and knowledge with all of us.

Robert A. Winquist, M.D.
Clinical Professor of Orthopedic Surgery
University of Washington
Seattle, Washington

PREFACE

There has been an explosion of interest in the management of orthopaedic trauma in the past two decades. As a result, the larger textbooks have become reference books. We believe that there is a need for a more concise text that summarizes modern fracture management. Thus, *Orthopaedic Surgery Essentials: Trauma, 1/e* has been designed to complement the larger texts. In writing the book we were guided by two objectives: the need for brevity in a rapidly expanding field and the requirement for evidence-based surgery. The former has been addressed by the bullet-point format of the book and the latter by the use of tables that present the current results of the different treatment methods of virtually all fractures. We have also analyzed the epidemiology of fractures so that surgeons can see which fractures are common, how they are caused, and which other musculoskeletal injuries are associated with them.

The book is divided into six sections. Section I discusses fracture epidemiology and healing and the management of the multiply injured patient. It also contains chapter-length overviews of open fractures, gunshot injuries, stress fractures, periprosthetic fractures, osteoporotic fractures, and pathological fractures. Most of the *OSE: Trauma* discusses individual fractures, detailing the classification, surgical anatomy, epidemiology, assessment, treatment, and complications of each. This approach is found in Sections II, III, and IV, which cover the upper limb, the spine and pelvis, and the lower limb, respectively. The last portion of the book, Sections V and VI, deal with surgical techniques and complications.

The book is not a multiauthor compilation but has been written by the three of us, although we are very grateful to Chris Bono and Marie Rinaldi for the excellent chapters on spinal fractures. Multiauthor books often lack consistency, and we hope that we have avoided that. We also believe that the fusion of European and North American expertise is beneficial.

We would also like to express our thanks to Paul Appleton, Stuart Anderson, Ian Beggs, Gary Keenan, John Keating, Mike Robinson, Robin Mitchell, and David Ring who generously donated images from their collections and to Bob Winquist for his foreword. We are hopeful that this book will be of interest to all surgeons interested in trauma.

Charles Court-Brown
Margaret McQueen
Paul Tornetta III
August, 2005

EPIDEMIOLOGY

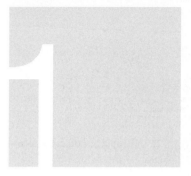

The treatment of fractures has always been important in orthopaedic surgery, but the types of fractures being treated are changing quickly in many parts of the world in response to a progressively aging population and improved motor vehicle safety, road and workplace legislation, and gun control laws. Surgeons often assume the fractures typically discussed and written about are in fact the common fractures, but this is not always the case. Much of the literature concerns the management of complex fractures such as severe open fractures and fractures of the acetabulum, pelvis, and spine. However it is important to understand the epidemiology of all fractures to know which are the common fractures, how they are caused, and which members of society present with them. This knowledge facilitates medical treatment and appropriate planning of health care systems.

The data in this chapter come from one orthopaedic trauma unit that takes all orthopaedic trauma from a well-defined population. In this study all outpatient and inpatient fractures in patients 12 years and older during the year 2000 were analyzed. All patients from out of the study area were excluded. The data have been used to document the precise epidemiology of fractures. It is accepted that it will not represent the populations treated by particular hospitals such as level 1 trauma centers in the United States and parts of Europe, but it is likely to be representative of the overall population of many countries. The overall data regarding fracture epidemiology are presented in this chapter, and more specific data for each fracture type are given in the appropriate chapters.

FRACTURE INCIDENCE

In the year 2000, 5,953 fractures were treated in the Orthopaedic Trauma Unit in Edinburgh, Scotland. The unit served a local population of 534,715 adults in the year 2000. Patients from outside the area were not included in the analysis. The overall fracture incidence is therefore 11.13/1,000 per year with 11.16/1,000 per year in men and 10.64/1,000 per year in women. The age- and sex-specific incidence of the overall population is shown in Figure 1-1. This shows that fractures have a bimodal distribution in

men and a unimodal distribution in women with the rise in female incidence around the time of the menopause. In men there is a high incidence in young men, and the later second rise in incidence starts about the age of 60 years.

Distribution

Despite the overall age and sex distribution curves shown in Figure 1-1, different fractures actually have different curves. Analysis of the data of all inpatient and outpatient fractures has allowed the construction of age and sex-distribution curves for each fracture. There are in fact eight different distribution curves, which are shown in Figure 1-2. The types of fracture that correspond to each curve are listed in Table 1-1. Note that the curves are diagrammatic and the height of the curves varies between fractures.

Type A

Type A is the most common fracture distribution curve with fractures commonly presenting in young men and older women. A number of fairly common fractures such as those of the tibial diaphysis and radial neck and distal radius present with this type of curve. If all ankle fractures are combined, they have a type A distribution, but in Table 1-1

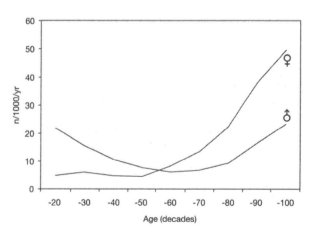

Figure 1-1 The age- and gender-specific incidence of fractures.

A. Unimodal young male. Unimodal older female

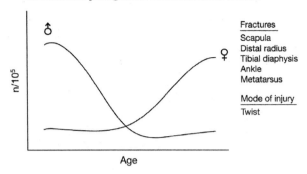

Fractures
Scapula
Distal radius
Tibial diaphysis
Ankle
Metatarsus

Mode of injury
Twist

B. Unimodal young male

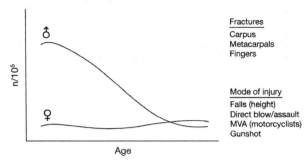

Fractures
Carpus
Metacarpals
Fingers

Mode of injury
Falls (height)
Direct blow/assault
MVA (motorcyclists)
Gunshot

C. Unimodal young male. Unimodal young female

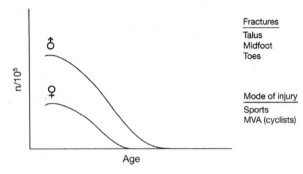

Fractures
Talus
Midfoot
Toes

Mode of injury
Sports
MVA (cyclists)

D. Unimodal young male. Bimodal female

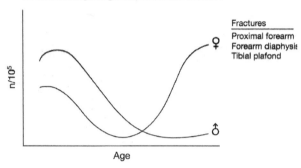

Fractures
Proximal forearm
Forearm diaphysis
Tibial plafond

E. Unimodal older female

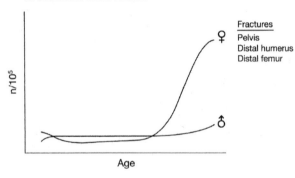

Fractures
Pelvis
Distal humerus
Distal femur

F. Unimodal older male. Unimodal older female

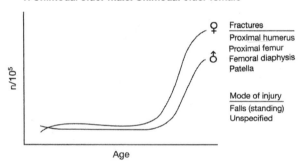

Fractures
Proximal humerus
Proximal femur
Femoral diaphysis
Patella

Mode of injury
Falls (standing)
Unspecified

G. Bimodal male. Unimodal older female

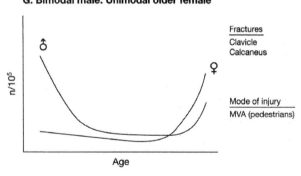

Fractures
Clavicle
Calcaneus

Mode of injury
MVA (pedestrians)

H. Bimodal male. Bimodal female

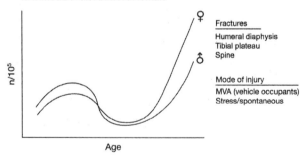

Fractures
Humeral diaphysis
Tibial plateau
Spine

Mode of injury
MVA (vehicle occupants)
Stress/spontaneous

I. Unimodal older male. Linear female

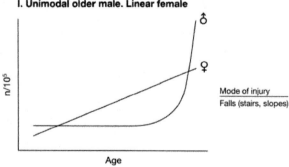

Mode of injury
Falls (stairs, slopes)

Figure 1-2 The distribution curves for different fractures and causes of fracture.

TABLE 1-1 DISTRIBUTION CURVES FOR DIFFERENT FRACTURES*

Fracture	Type	Fracture	Type
Clavicle		Proximal femur	
Medial	A	Head	B
Diaphyseal	G	Neck	F
Lateral	A	Intertrochanteric	F
Scapula		Subtrochanteric	F
Intra-articular	A	Femoral diaphysis	A
Extra-articular	A	Distal femur	E
Proximal humerus	F	Patella	F
Humeral diaphysis	H	Tibial plateau	H
Distal humerus	E	Tibial diaphysis	A
Proximal forearm		Tibial plafond	D
Radial head	H	Ankle	
Radial neck	A	Medial malleolus	D
Olecranon	F	Lateral malleolus	A
Radius and ulna	F	Bimalleolar	E
Forearm diaphysis		Trimalleolar	E
Radius	A	Suprasyndesmotic	C
Ulna	H	Talus	
Radius and ulna	B	Neck	C
Distal radius	A	Body	C
Carpus		Calcaneus	
Scaphoid	B	Intra-articular	G
Nonscaphoid	A	Extra-articular	B
Metacarpus	B	Midfoot	C
Hand phalanges	B	Metatarsus	A
		Toe phalanges	C

*See Figure 1-2.

it can be seen that different types of ankle fracture actually have different curves, and only lateral malleolar fractures have a type A curve.

Type B

Type B curves show a unimodal distribution in young men with a fairly even distribution in women throughout the decades. These fractures mainly occur in the hand and affect the carpus, metacarpals, and digits. Extra-articular calcaneal fractures and fractures of the forearm diaphyses also have a type B distribution as do nonosteoporotic thoracolumbar spine fractures (Table 1-1). Overall, carpal fractures have a type B distribution, but further analysis shows that the carpal scaphoid has a type B distribution, whereas the other carpal bones have a type A distribution.

Type C

Type C fractures affect young men and women. Table 1-1 shows that these occur in the foot and ankle affecting the talus, midfoot, and toes. Suprasyndesmotic ankle fractures also have this distribution.

Type D

Type D fractures are unusual. They occur in younger men but show a bimodal distribution in women. Fractures of the tibial plafond and the medial malleolus show this type of curve.

Type E

Type E fractures occur mainly in older women and are usually osteopenic or osteoporotic. Bimalleolar and trimalleolar ankle fractures show this type of curve as do fractures of the distal humerus, pelvis, and distal femur. Distal femoral fractures are often thought of as high-energy intra-articular fractures presenting in younger patients, but in the overall population they are very much more common in older patients. The same is true of fractures of the distal humerus.

Type F

This fracture type is relatively common. Like type E fractures, the type F curve should be thought of as representing an osteoporotic or osteopenic fracture distribution. Type F fracture curves are seen in older men and women. The most common examples of type F fractures are seen in the proximal humerus and proximal femur, but analysis shows that olecranon fractures, combined proximal radius and ulnar fractures, and patellar fractures have a similar distribution.

Type G

Type G fractures show a bimodal male distribution and a unimodal female distribution in older women. This distribution is mainly seen in the clavicle diaphysis, although intra-articular calcaneal fractures also show the same distribution, as do fractures of the acetabulum.

Type H

Type H fractures are comparatively uncommon. They have a bimodal distribution in both men and women and are seen in the tibial plateau, radial head, and isolated fractures of the ulnar diaphysis. This distribution is also seen in cervical spine fractures and humeral diaphyseal fractures.

Frequency

It is well established that some fractures such as distal radial fractures are very common and many surgeons will treat them. Other fractures such as fractures of the femoral head are extremely rare, and the majority of surgeons never see a case. The incidence of different fractures is often misquoted in the literature because the information regarding incidence is only taken from inpatient data. When both inpatient and outpatient data are analyzed, accurate figures for the incidence of different fractures can be obtained. A list of fractures and order of their frequency is shown in Table 1-2, which shows that about 60% of fractures comprise fractures of the distal radius, metacarpals, proximal femur, finger phalanges, and ankle. Some fractures, such as those of the scapula and talus, are very rare and mainly seen in level 1 trauma centers, usually following high-energy injuries.

OSTEOPOROTIC FRACTURES

In recent years there has been a particular interest in fractures in osteoporotic bone (Chapter 8). It is commonly believed that osteoporotic fractures occur in the vertebrae, proximal humerus, distal radius, and proximal femur, but

TABLE 1-2 FRACTURES ARRANGED IN ORDER OF DECREASING INCIDENCE

	No.	%	n/10^{5a}	Men/Women
Distal radius	1,044	17.5	195.2	31/69
Metacarpal	697	11.7	130.3	85/15
Proximal femur	692	11.6	129.4	26/74
Finger phalanx	574	9.6	107.3	68/32
Ankle	539	9.0	100.8	47/53
Metatarsal	403	6.8	75.4	43/57
Proximal humerus	337	5.7	63.0	30/70
Proximal forearm	297	5.0	55.5	46/54
Toe phalanx	212	3.6	39.6	66/34
Clavicle	195	3.3	36.5	70/30
Carpus	159	2.7	29.7	72/28
Tibial diaphysis	115	1.9	21.5	61/39
Pelvis	91	1.5	17.0	30/70
Forearm	74	1.2	13.8	64/36
Calcaneus	73	1.2	13.7	78/22
Proximal tibia	71	1.2	13.3	54/46
Humeral diaphysis	69	1.2	12.9	42/58
Patella	57	1.0	10.7	44/56
Femoral diaphysis	55	0.9	10.3	36/64
Distal tibia	42	0.7	7.9	57/43
Spine	40	0.7	7.5	62/38
Distal humerus	31	0.5	5.8	29/71
Midfoot	27	0.4	5.0	48/52
Distal femur	24	0.4	4.5	33/67
Scapula	17	0.3	3.2	59/41
Talus	17	0.3	3.2	82/18
Sesamoid	1	0.01	0.2	100/0
	5,953	**100**	**1113.3**	**50/50**

[a]Incidence per 100,000 population.

with an increasingly aging population the epidemiology of osteoporotic fractures is unquestionably changing. Table 1-3 shows the incidence of fractures analyzed by age, together with the percentage of patients older than 65 and 75 years. If one accepts that the distal radius is predominantly an osteoporotic fracture, it is clear that fractures of the pelvis, femoral diaphysis, distal femur, patella, and distal humerus are also likely to be mainly osteoporotic. Obviously many pelvic fractures presenting to level 1 trauma centers occur in young patients, but the overwhelming majority of pelvic fractures are in fact ramus fractures occurring in the elderly.

A review of Figure 1-2 and Table 1-1 shows that if the overall fracture areas shown in Table 1-3 are subdivided according to their exact anatomical location, there are yet more fractures that are osteoporotic. The type E and F fracture curves listed in Table 1-1 represent osteoporotic fractures. Thus whereas ankle fractures as a whole are not considered osteoporotic, bimalleolar and trimalleolar fractures are. So are combined fractures of the proximal radius and ulna and olecranon fractures.

The most interesting osteoporotic fracture is that of the femoral diaphysis. This was the index fracture that caused orthopaedic surgeons to adopt more aggressive management techniques in multiply injured patients in the 1970s and 1980s, and it was associated with young adults injured in motor vehicle accidents. Improved road safety programs and

vehicle design, together with an increasingly elderly population and a large increase in periprosthetic fractures (Chapter 7), has resulted in a massive change in the epidemiology of femoral diaphyseal fractures in a very short period. This is emphasized by comparing the femoral fractures treated in the Edinburgh Orthopaedic Trauma Unit in 1990 and 2000. The average age of patients with femoral diaphyseal fractures in 1990 was 44 years, and 27.6% were older than 65 years. This compares with an average age of 68 years and 69.1% older than 65 years of age in 2000. The femur is probably the bone in which the epidemiological change that has resulted from a rapidly aging population is most obvious. Osteoporotic fractures are discussed further in Chapter 8.

CAUSES OF FRACTURE

There are many causes of fracture and they differ in different age groups. It is possible to group causes into basic categories, however, and to construct distribution curves in the same way as has been done for the different fracture types. Nine basic curves cover all causes of fracture. These are shown in Figure 1-2. The curves tend to be fairly obvious in that type B and C curves are associated with high-energy injuries, gunshot injuries, and sporting injuries and affect younger patients. Standing falls have a

TABLE 1-3 FRACTURES ARRANGED IN ORDER OF DECREASING PATIENT AGE

	No.	Average age (y)	>65 y (%)	>75 y (%)
Proximal femur	692	80.5	91.2	78.9
Pelvis	91	69.6	72.5	57.1
Femoral diaphysis	55	68.0	69.1	58.2
Proximal humerus	337	64.8	57.0	36.2
Distal femur	24	61.0	50.0	41.7
Sesamoid	1	58.0	0	0
Patella	57	56.5	49.1	22.8
Distal humerus	31	56.4	45.2	29.0
Distal radius	1044	55.5	45.8	28.2
Humeral diaphysis	69	54.8	40.5	17.4
Scapula	17	50.5	41.2	29.4
Proximal tibia	71	48.9	23.9	12.7
Ankle	539	45.9	20.8	10.2
Proximal forearm	297	45.7	24.2	13.5
Spine	40	43.5	17.5	12.5
Metatarsal	403	42.8	14.2	5.7
Calcaneus	73	40.4	12.3	4.1
Tibial diaphysis	115	40.0	17.4	11.3
Distal tibia	42	39.1	14.3	7.1
Clavicle	195	38.3	17.4	12.3
Finger phalanges	574	36.2	10.6	5.1
Midfoot	27	36.0	0	0
Toe phalanges	212	35.3	6.5	4.6
Forearm	74	34.6	13.5	12.2
Carpus	159	33.6	7.5	2.5
Talus	17	30.5	0	0
Metacarpals	697	29.9	5.5	3.6
****	**5,953**	**49.1**	**33.0**	**22.6**

type F distribution, which also accounts for the unspecified group of patients in whom there was no history of the cause of fracture. Most of these patients were elderly and confused. The type I distribution is unique to falls down stairs or slopes and shows a unimodal distribution affecting older men and a linear distribution affecting women.

The incidences of the different causes of fracture are shown in Table 1-4. About 45% of all fractures are caused by falls from a standing height, with direct blows, assaults, or crush injuries accounting for about 14% and sports injuries for about 13%. It is interesting to note that motor vehicle accidents only account for about 7% of all fractures.

TABLE 1-4 AVERAGE AGE, INCIDENCE, AND GENDER RATIO FOR EACH MODE OF INJURY

	Average age (y)	Incidence (%)	Men/women (%)
Twist	45.0	6.5	36/64
Fall			
From standing height	64.6	45.3	29/71
Down stairs or slope	49.1	4.1	40/60
From height	38.2	5.8	72/28
Direct blow/assault/crush	32.3	14.1	79/21
Sport	25.6	12.8	83/17
Motor vehicle accident			
Vehicle occupant	37.5	1.8	49/51
Pedestrian	48.3	1.7	52/48
Motorcyclist	31.2	1.4	89/11
Cyclist	29.5	2.3	76/24
Stress/spontaneous	58.9	0.5	30/70
Others	56.9	3.7	46/54

SUGGESTED READING

Buhr AJ, Cooke AM. Fracture patterns. Lancet 1959;14:531–536.

Chang KP, Center GR, Nguyen TV, et al. Incidence of hip and other osteoporotic fractures in elderly men and women: Dubbo osteoporosis epidemiology study. J Bone Miner Res 2004; 19:532–536.

Court-Brown CM, Garg A, McQueen MM. The epidemiology of proximal humeral fractures. Acta Orthop Scand 2001;72:365–371.

Court-Brown CM, McBirnie J. The epidemiology of tibial fractures. J Bone Joint Surg (Br) 1995;77:417–421.

Court-Brown CM, McBirnie J, Wilson G. Adult ankle fractures: an increasing problem? Acta Orthop Scand 1998;69:43–47.

Johnell O, Kanis J. Epidemiology of osteoporotic fractures. Osteoporos Int 2004, E-pub.

Melton LJ, Atkinson EJ, Madhok R. Downturn in hip fracture incidence. Public Health Rep 1996;111:146–150.

Shinoda-Tagawa T, Clark DE. Trends in hospitalization after injury: older women are displacing younger men. Inj Prev 2003;9: 214–219.

Thorngren KG, Hommel A, Norman PO, et al. Epidemiology of femoral neck fractures. Injury 2002;33:(Suppl 3):C1–C7.

FRACTURE HEALING AND BIOMECHANICS

FRACTURE HEALING

The process of fracture healing has evolved over a considerable period and has only recently been altered by surgeons using fracture fixation techniques. Until about 150 years ago, all fractures were treated nonoperatively, and callus formation was the most important feature of bone union. Fracture fixation started about 150 years ago but was popularized by the work of the AO group 40 to 50 years ago. They promoted rigid fracture fixation and demonstrated how this altered callus formation. For a period, callus was regarded as undesirable and thought to represent inadequate surgical technique. In the past 20 to 25 years, however, renewed interest in intramedullary nailing of long-bone fractures and less rigid fracture fixation has meant that surgeons have again appreciated the value of callus in fracture union.

Bone Tissue

Bone consists of mesenchymal cells imbedded in an extracellular matrix that contains mineral, which gives bone strength and stiffness in compression and bending. It has a good vascular supply but also contains nerves and lymphatics. The two types of bone are distinguished by their mechanical and biological properties: woven or immature bone and lamellar or mature bone. Their characteristics are listed in Table 2-1.

TABLE 2-1 CHARACTERISTICS OF WOVEN AND LAMELLAR BONE

Occurrence	Immature bones[a]	Mature bones
	Forms de novo	Forms only on or in existing matrix
	Healing bone	
	Metabolic and neoplastic disease	
Rate of deposition and turnover	Rapid	Slower
Collagen fibrils		
Diameter	Irregular	Regular
Orientation	No consistent orientation	Parallel fibrils form distinct lamellae
		Organized in response to loads
Osteocytes		
Size	Variable	Regular
Number	Greater	
Orientation	Variable	Between lamellae
Mineral density	Variable	Regular
Mechanical properties	Easily deformed	Stiffer

[a]Rare after 4 years of age.
From Buckwalter JA, Einhorn TA, Marsh JL. Bone and joint healing. In: Bucholtz RW, Heckman JD, eds. *Rockwood and Green's fractures in adults.* Vol 1, ed 5. Philadelphia: Lippincott Williams & Wilkins, 2001:246.

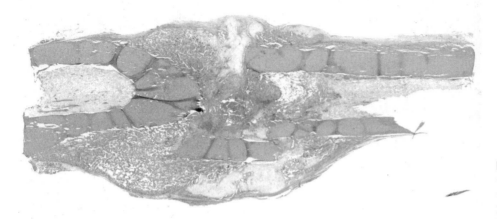

Figure 2-1   An osteotomy in a rabbit tibia treated with a cast. Note the malunion and the considerable periosteal callus formation, which has resulted in fracture union.

Fracture Repair

Fractures initiate a sequence of inflammatory repair and remodeling. Fractures damage the cells, blood vessels, bone matrix, and the surrounding soft tissues such as periosteum and muscles. A hematoma forms in and around the fracture site, and the vascular damage associated with the fracture deprives the osteocytes of nutrition, ensuring that the bone ends die as far back as the collateral circulation permits. Damaged periosteum and muscle also contributes necrotic tissue to the fracture site.

Inflammatory mediators released from dead and dying tissue cause local vascular dilation leading to plasma exudation and local edema. Polymorphs, macrophages, and lymphocytes migrate to the fracture. These cells release cytokines, which stimulate angiogenesis. The hematoma, necrotic tissue, and exudates are resorbed, and fibroblasts and chondrocytes appear and form callus.

Fracture callus is initially composed of fibrous tissue and cartilage. It rapidly fills the space between the bone ends being stimulated, mainly by movement and hypoxia. Initially callus is separated into hard and soft callus (Fig. 2-1). Hard callus forms by intramembranous ossification at the periphery of the callus mass with soft callus forming centrally. The soft callus is converted to bone through the process of endochondral ossification, and the process continues until new bone bridges the fracture site. Increasing callus progressively improves fracture stability.

There is a close correlation between the activation of genes for blood vessel, cartilage, and bone-specific proteins in the cells and the development of granulation tissue, cartilage, and bone, demonstrating that fracture repair depends on the regulation of gene expression in the cells. Because chondrogenesis, endochondral ossification, and intramembranous ossification occur at the same time in different parts of the forming callus (see Fig. 2-1), it is clear that local mediators, including mechanical stresses, determine gene expression and the type of tissue formed. Local factors also include growth factors such as transforming growth factor β (TGFβ) released from cells and platelets, and oxygen tension.

Mineralization of fracture callus is initiated by the cells synthesizing a matrix with a high concentration of type I collagen fibrils. Calcium hydroxyapatite crystals are then deposited in the matrix. As mineralization proceeds, the bone ends gradually become enveloped in callus and the fracture unites. The fracture repair process continues with replacement of woven bone by lamellar bone and absorption of unnecessary callus. This process, known as remodeling, may take a considerable time.

Stabilized Fractures

Surgical stabilization alters the process of fracture healing (Fig. 2-2). The most significant alteration to fracture

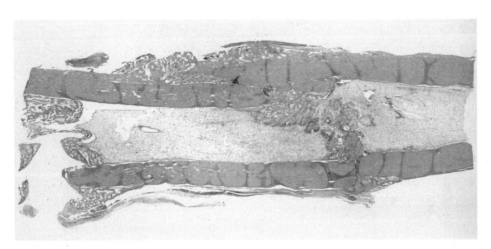

Figure 2-2   An osteotomy in an externally fixed rabbit tibia. There is less periosteal callus but considerably more intramedullary ossification.

healing was the widespread introduction of rigid plating. Animal studies showed that if an osteotomy was made in a long bone using a thin saw blade, direct bone union could be achieved if the bone ends were compressed and held rigidly. Under these circumstances, lamellar bone forms directly across the fracture by direct extension of osteones. Osteoclasts cut across the fracture line, osteoblasts deposit new bone, and blood vessels follow the osteoblasts. This is known as direct bone union or contact healing. As the gap between the bones widens, a greater degree of remodeling is required.

There is some debate about just how clinically applicable direct bone union actually is. It can be argued that the use of a thin saw blade to undertake an osteotomy in a laboratory experiment, in which there is minimal soft tissue damage associated with the osteotomy, does not duplicate the clinical situation where there is often fairly extensive damage to the muscle, periosteum, and local blood supply. In the clinical situation, necrosis of the bone ends often prevents the degree of fracture compression that can be achieved in a laboratory experiment. It is in fact likely that although direct bone union can theoretically occur in the clinical situation, it is rare, and most fractures treated by rigid plating actually unite using the fracture healing process already described, with the proviso that the rigid fixation imparted by the plate reduces callus formation and therefore prolongs the time at which clinical union is achieved. This explains the refracture rate if plates are removed from long bones too early.

Intramedullary Nailing

There has always been concern that intramedullary nailing of long bones will damage the intramedullary circulation of the bone, and when this is combined with the inevitable periosteal damage produced by the fracture, the result will be impaired union or even nonunion. Early experiments showed that intramedullary nailing of dog ulnar osteotomies resulted in the inner one half to two thirds of the cortex showing reduced vascularity. This argument was later extended to cover intramedullary reaming when it was shown that reaming of the canine tibia resulted in a 70% reduction of cortical blood supply compared with 31% if an unreamed nail was used. It was also clear that the intramedullary blood supply returned very quickly, however, and that reaming, or indeed any intramedullary stimulation, caused an increase in periosteal blood supply and therefore in periosteal callus formation. This, combined with the less rigid fracture fixation imparted by intramedullary nailing, ensures rapid healing with good callus formation. This is a feature of intramedullary nailing of long bones.

Factors That Affect Fracture Union

Union does not always occur in an equivalent time in apparently equivalent fractures, for several reasons. A number of the factors that affect union are listed in Box 39-1 in Chapter 39. The main factor that affects the rate of union is the soft tissue damage associated with the fracture. This is often difficult to assess in the clinical situation where the criteria used to estimate muscle or periosteal damage are very imprecise. Impaired fracture union is often described as delayed or nonunion. *Delayed union* is a poor term often used because surgeons feel that all fractures should unite in a specific time. But it is clear that fracture union will vary often as a result of some of the factors listed in Box 39-1. Nonunion, or the failure of a fracture to unite at all, is discussed in Chapter 39. However a number of factors have recently been shown to have a major influence on fracture union.

Age

Age alters the rate of fracture healing. Healing is most rapid in infants and declines with increasing age up to skeletal maturity. After the cessation of growth, the adult union times detailed in this book become the norm. Evidence indicates, however, that union times in long bones slowly increase in adulthood with increasing age, particularly in less severe fractures when the union time is less affected by the severity of the soft tissue injury. There is also some evidence that the rate of nonunion is higher in older patients. Indeed it is perhaps surprising that the association between age and union is not more obvious, given the poor periosteum, increased medical comorbidities, and increased effects of smoking and peripheral vascular disease seen in the elderly.

Nutrition

Diseases such as vitamin C deficiency affect bone union, but these are rare in most parts of the world. Malnutrition in the elderly is not, however, and evidence indicates that the increased metabolic demands associated with a fracture may not be met in the elderly, resulting in a number of surgical complications including infection, wound dehiscence, and impaired union.

Smoking

In recent years it has become clear that smoking has a significant effect on fracture union. Interestingly, it also has an important effect on the risk of fracture. A recent meta-analysis of smoking and fracture risk has shown that current smokers are at a significantly greater risk of fracture than both previous smokers and nonsmokers, and the risk for previous smokers is higher than for nonsmokers. It has been estimated that reduced bone mineral density only accounts for 23% of the increased smoking-related risk of hip fracture. Studies of the management of tibial fractures in smokers and nonsmokers have clearly shown that smoking decreases union, slows healing, and increases complications.

Bone Diseases

Osteoporosis (see Chapter 8) does not impair bone healing, although other diseases (Box 39.1) may. Pathological fractures caused by tumor (see Chapter 9) may show impaired union.

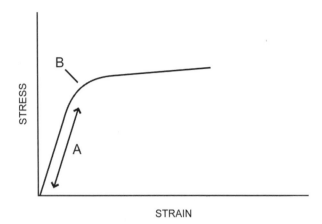

Figure 2-3 A typical stress-strain curve for human cortical bone. The elastic modulus is calculated from the slope of the line A. B is the yield point.

BIOMECHANICS OF INTACT BONE

Cortical Bone

The mechanical properties of cortical bone are represented by the stress-strain curve shown in Figure 2-3. Stress is the force applied to a bone divided by its cross-sectional area. Strain is the percentage change in bone length in response to an applied force. As increased stress is applied to a bone it will eventually give, and the point at which the stress-strain curve decreases is known as the yield point. The maximum recorded stress is the ultimate strength of bone, and the elastic modulus of bone is determined from the slope of the initial-linear part of the curve.

Bone is loaded cyclically during normal activities, and the load required to cause bone to fail is lower if the load is applied repeatedly. The material properties of bone also depend on the rate at which the load is applied and the direction of the applied load with respect to the orientation of the bone microstructure. Cortical bone is stiffer and

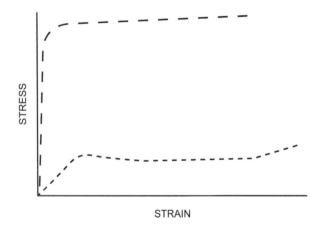

Figure 2-4 Stress-strain curves for cortical (lower curve) and cancellous (upper curve) bone. The yield points vary considerably.

stronger longitudinally than transversely, and it is particularly susceptible to shearing forces.

Cancellous Bone

Cancellous bone is less dense than cortical bone. Its porosity is much greater, and the stress-strain curve for cancellous bone differs from that of cortical bone (Fig. 2-4) with the yield point occurring at a much lower stress value. This is of importance because the classical osteoporotic fractures are cancellous, and the effect of age is to reduce the yield point so fractures occur with minimum force.

BIOMECHANICS OF HEALING

Healing associated with callus formation is clearly biomechanically superior to direct bone union or minimal callus formation associated with the use of a rigid plate. The bending rigidity of a long bone varies with the fourth power of its radius, and the wide callus seen with intramedullary nailing of long bones will therefore stabilize the fracture more quickly than if a plate or a very rigid external fixator is used. External fixation provides the possibility of altering the biomechanics of healing, and fracture rigidity can be lessened by widening the space between the external fixator and the bone or by placing the pins close together and further away from the fracture site.

Stages of Fracture Healing

The biomechanical stages of fracture healing were described by White and his coworkers (1977) using an externally fixed rabbit tibial osteotomy model. They found four stages of fracture healing (Table 2-2). They assessed the angular displacement of bone for a given torque at different times after commencement of the healing process

TABLE 2-2 FOUR STAGES OF FRACTURE HEALING PROPOSED BY WHITE ET AL. (1977)

Stage	Description
I	Bone fails through the original fracture site Low stiffness, rubbery pattern Torque-angle curve like day 21 in Figure 2-5
II	Bone fails through the original fracture site High-stiffness, hard-tissue pattern Torque-angle curve like day 27 in Figure 2-5
III	Bone fails partially through original fracture and intact bone High-stiffness, hard-tissue pattern Torque-angle curve like day 49 in Figure 2-5
IV	Bone fails through intact bone High-stiffness, hard-tissue pattern Torque-angle curve like day 56 in Figure 2-5

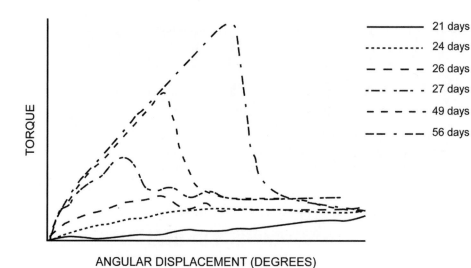

ANGULAR DISPLACEMENT (DEGREES)

Figure 2-5 Angular displacement of healing osteotomies in rabbit femurs as a function of applied torque. See Table 2-2 for description of different stages of bone healing. Data from White et al. (1977).

(Fig. 2-5). The days refer to rabbit tibiae and clearly the process will be longer in humans, but Figure 2-5 correlates biomechanics and fracture healing, indicating the increasing stiffness of healing bone as the fracture unites.

SUGGESTED READING

Akeson WH, Woo SLY, Rutherford L. The effects of rigidity of internal fixation plates on long bone remodelling: a biomechanical and quantitative histological study. Acta Orthop Scand 1976;47:241–249.

Aro H, Chao E. Bone-healing patterns affected by loading, fracture fragment stability, fracture type and fracture site compression. Clin Orthop 1993;293:11–15.

Buckwalter JA, Einhorn TA, Marsh JL. Bone and joint healing. In Bucholz RW, Heckman JD, eds. *Rockwood and Green's fractures in adults*. Vol 1, ed 5. Philadelphia, Lippincott Williams & Wilkins 2001:245–272.

Einhorn TA. The cell and molecular biology of fracture healing. Clin Orthop 1998;335S:S7–S21.

Goodship AE, Kenwright J. The influence of induced micromovement upon the healing of experimental tibial fractures. J Bone Joint Surg (Br) 1985;67:650–655.

Grundnes O, Reikeras O. The role of the haematoma and periosteal sealing for fracture healing in rats. Acta Orthop Scand 1993;64:47–49.

Hipp JA, Hayes WC. Biomechanics of fractures. In Browner BD, Jupiter JF, Levine AM, et al., eds. Skeletal trauma. Ed 3. Philadelphia, WB Saunders, 2003:90–119.

Rahn BA, Gallinaro P, Baltensperger A, et al. Primary bone healing: an experimental study in the rabbit. J Bone Joint Surg (Am) 1971;53:783–786.

Tencer AF. Biomechanics of fractures and fixation. In Bucholz RW, Heckman JD, eds. *Rockwood and Green's fractures in adults*. Vol 1, ed 5. Philadelphia, Lippincott Williams & Wilkins 2001:3–36.

White AA, Panjabi MM, Southwick WO. The four biomechanical stages of fracture repair. J Bone Joint Surg (Am) 1977;59:188–192.

THE MULTIPLY INJURED PATIENT

The treatment of patients who present with multiple injuries changed considerably in the 1970s and 1980s with the introduction of early fracture fixation. Prior to that, many surgeons believed it was harmful to operate unnecessarily on patients who were already significantly injured. A number of studies showed the value of early femoral fracture fixation in particular, however, and surgeons quickly adopted the philosophy of early total care, fixing all major fractures as soon as possible after admission. This philosophy was challenged in the 1990s by surgeons who pointed out that early time-consuming surgery was not appropriate for all patients, particularly those who were very seriously injured or who presented with severe chest or head trauma. Thus the concept of damage control surgery was initiated, and this philosophy is widely followed today.

It is important to remember that although early fracture stabilization is unquestionably important, there have been major advances in intensive care and in the understanding of the problems of systemic inflammatory response syndrome (SIRS), adult respiratory distress syndrome (ARDS), and multiple organ failure (MOF). Thus advances in the management of the multiply injured patient have been made collectively by surgeons, anaesthetists, and intensivists. In addition there has also been a greater appreciation of the importance of rapid patient transport to an appropriate hospital, prehospital care, and rehabilitation programs for the multiply injured patient.

EPIDEMIOLOGY

Multiple injuries have a number of different causes including gunshot injuries, explosions, airplane and train crashes, earthquakes, and other natural disasters. But surgeons usually see polytrauma victims who have been injured in falls from a height or, more commonly, motor vehicle accidents. It has been estimated that 10 to 15 million people are injured and about 800,000 die on the world's roads annually. However underreporting is common, and the figures are probably significantly higher. Table 3-1 shows the list of the top 12 killers as published by the World Health Organization in 2002, and it can be seen that road traffic accidents are the 11th most common cause of death. This situation is clearly changing, however, and it has been estimated that road traffic accidents will be the third commonest cause of death after heart disease and unipolar major depression by 2020. By that time it is forecast that wars will be eighth and HIV tenth.

The problem of motor vehicle accidents varies from country to country, and it is interesting to note that the countries with the best medical systems do not necessarily have the lowest mortality. Figure 3-1 shows the fatality rates in the OECD (Organization for Economic Cooperation and Development) countries, which clearly demonstrates that the countries with aggressive injury prevention campaigns have the lowest fatality rates. Thus although all countries should have advanced trauma retrieval and treatment systems, the key to minimizing the morbidity and mortality related to motor vehicle accidents is prevention.

TABLE 3-1 TOP 12 "KILLERS" AS PUBLISHED BY THE WORLD HEALTH ORGANIZATION IN 2002	
Cause of Death	**Percentage**
Heart disease	12.6
Stroke	9.6
Lower respiratory infection	6.6
HIV/AIDS	4.9
Lung disease	4.8
Perinatal conditions	4.3
Diarrhea	3.1
Tuberculosis	2.8
Trachea/lung cancers	2.2
Malaria	2.1
Road traffic accidents	2.1
Diabetes	1.7

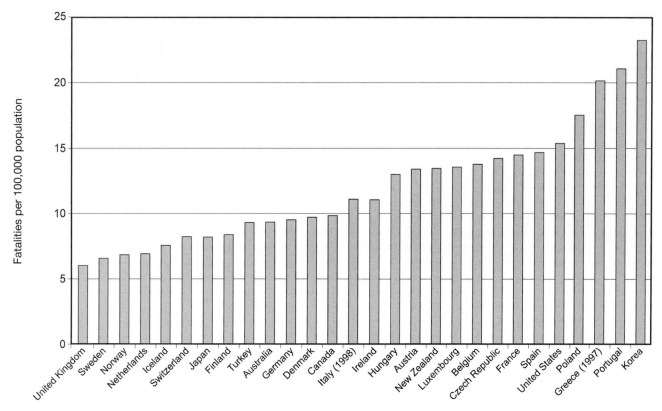

Figure 3-1   Recent fatality rates in motor accidents in 28 OECD countries. (Data from Safety on Roads, OECD, 2002.)

ASSESSMENT

Many systems have been derived to assess, classify, and apply a numerical value to polytrauma patients and their injuries. These have proved most helpful in predicting outcome and in permitting comparisons among different countries and institutions. They have also, however, encouraged surgeons to review patients more systematically. The best known injury scoring systems are the Glasgow Coma Scale (GCS) and the Injury Severity Score (ISS). The Glasgow Coma Scale is shown in Table 3-2. It ranges from 3 to 15, with 15 being normal. There are three sections: eye opening, verbal response, and motor response, with increasing scores based on increasing patient response.

The Injury Severity Score is based on the Abbreviated Injury Scale (AIS). The AIS gives a score of 1 to 6 for each body system: external, head and face, neck, thorax, abdomen and pelvic contents, spine and extremities, and bony pelvis. Score 1 represents a minor injury; 2, a moderate injury; 3, a severe but not life-threatening injury; 4, a severe life-threatening injury; 5, an injury where survival is uncertain; and 6, an unsurvivable injury. The AIS scores for a number of different musculoskeletal injuries are shown in Table 3-3. The ISS is computed by squaring the scores of the three most severely injured body systems and adding them together. Thus a polytrauma patient with an incomplete cervical cord lesion (score 4 squared = 16), a sternal fracture (score 2 squared = 4), and a crushed pelvis (score 4 squared = 16) would have an ISS of 36. Any patient with an individual AIS of 6 is given

an ISS of 75. The definition of a seriously injured patient was always taken as an ISS more than 16, the injury level associated with more than a 10% mortality, although with improved retrieval and treatment methods, patients with much higher ISS values now regularly survive.

TABLE 3-2 GLASGOW COMA SCALE

Parameter	Score
Eye opening	
Spontaneous	4
To voice	3
To pain	2
None	1
Verbal response	
Oriented	5
Confused	4
Inappropriate words	3
Incomprehensible sounds	2
None	1
Motor response	
Obeys command	6
Localized pain	5
Withdraws to pain	4
Flexion to pain	3
Extension to pain	2
None	1

TABLE 3-3 EXAMPLES OF THE MUSCULO-SKELETAL ABBREVIATED INJURY SCORE (AIS)

Injury	Score
Contusions/sprains	1
Interphalangeal dislocation	1
Digital fracture	1
Hind- or midfoot dislocation	1
Patellar tendon laceration	2
Hip dislocation	2
Calcaneus fracture	2
Medial malleolus fracture	2
Closed humeral fracture	2
Clavicle fracture	2
Open humeral fracture	3
Crushed elbow or shoulder	3
Severe degloving injury	3
Femoral fracture	3
Open tibial fracture	3
Above knee amputation	4
Severe pelvic fracture with blood loss ≤20% by volume	4
Severe pelvic fracture with blood loss ≥20% by volume	5

The Revised Trauma Score (RTS) is based on the Glasgow Coma Scale, the respiratory rate, and the systolic blood pressure. It is shown in Table 3-4. The most sophisticated scoring system is the TRISS score, used to predict the probability of survival. This is calculated from the Revised Trauma Score and the Injury Severity Score but also

TABLE 3-4 REVISED TRAUMA SCORE

Result	Score
Respiratory rate (breaths/min)	
10–29	4
>29	3
6–9	2
1–5	1
0	0
Systolic blood pressure (mm/Hg)	
>89	4
76–89	3
50–75	2
1–49	1
0	0
Glasgow Coma Scale score	
13–15	4
9–12	3
6–8	2
4–5	1
3	0
RTS = 0.9368 GCS + 0.7326 SBP + 0.2908 RR	

From Champion HR, Copes WS, Sacco WJ, et al. The major outcome trauma study: establishing national norms for trauma care. J Trauma 1990;30:1356–1365.

TABLE 3-5 FORMULAS AND AGE INDEXES USED TO CALCULATE THE TRISS SCORE

Probability of survival (P_s) = $1/(1+e^{-b})$
$b = b0 + b1$ (RTS) $+ b2$ (ISS) $+ b3$ (age index)
Age index = 0 if patient <55 years
                    1 if patient ≥55 years

	Blunt	Penetrating
b0	−0.4499	−2.5355
b1	0.8185	0.9934
b2	−0.0835	−0.0651
b3	−1.7430	−1.1360

incorporates a number of coefficients (b0-b3) derived from multiple regression analysis of the Major Trauma Outcome Study (MTOS). The coefficients and formulas used to calculate the TRISS score are shown in Table 3-5.

As with all scoring systems, a number of concerns have been raised about the usefulness of the different injury scores. Probably the most important criticism from the point of view of musculoskeletal injury is that the effect of multiple fractures is underestimated. This is particularly true of bilateral femoral or tibial diaphyseal fractures, which are associated with a mortality that is undoubtedly higher than would be predicted from the ISS. New variations of these scoring systems are frequent, but the basic scores listed in this chapter are widely used.

RESUSCITATION

There has been debate about the merits of extensive prehospital resuscitation, and there is no doubt that it varies markedly in different parts of the world. Most systems employ the principle of "scoop and run" by delivering the patient as quickly as possible to an appropriate hospital. Basic resuscitation with maintenance of the airway, breathing, and circulation is undertaken, but it is usually counterproductive to attempt more until the patient is in an appropriate hospital. Under certain circumstances a trained medical team may attend a trauma situation, but few countries can afford to divide their expensive medical resources between the trauma scene and the admitting hospital.

Hospital resuscitation should be undertaken according to the basic principles laid down by the American College of Surgeons and demonstrated in their Advanced Trauma Life Support (ATLS) courses. In many countries attendance at one of these courses, or an equivalent course, is mandatory during orthopaedic training. The ATLS protocols involve the systematic examination and resuscitation of multiply injured patients. The basic components of a resuscitation protocol are shown in Box 3-1.

■ The important initial steps are to check that the airway is clear and maintained using an oropharyngeal airway, nasopharyngeal airway, endotracheal tube, or a cricothyroidotomy as indicated.
■ Breathing and oxygenation are maintained by examining for and treating a blocked airway, pneumothorax, tension

BOX 3-1 RESUSCITATION/TREATMENT PROTOCOL BASED ON ATLS GUIDELINES

1. **Primary survey and resuscitation (patient stabilization)**
   - **A** Airway and cervical spine
   - **B** Breathing and oxygenation
   - **C** Circulation and hemorrhage
   - **D** Dysfunction of the CNS
   - **E** Exposure and environmental
2. **Consider transfer to more appropriate hospital if indicated**
3. **Secondary survey**
   - **A** Allergies
   - **M** Medicines
   - **P** Previous medical history/Pregnancy
   - **L** Last meal
   - **E** Events leading to trauma
4. **Definitive care**
   - Early total care
   - Damage central surgery
5. **Tertiary survey**
   - Missed injuries

pneumothorax, hemothorax, flail chest, or pericardial tamponade.

- It is vital to control hemorrhage and maintain circulation, remembering that bilateral femoral fractures and pelvic fractures may be associated with significant occult blood loss.
- Fluid resuscitation is achieved through two large-bore intravenous cannulas, one in each cubital fossa.
- An immediate cross match is undertaken, although O+ or type-specific blood may be required.
- A thorough examination of the abdomen, pelvis, and limbs is essential, looking for signs of abdominal and pelvic bleeding, pelvic instability, and hemorrhage and limb damage, particularly open fractures.
- A complete CNS examination is undertaken to check the patient's responsiveness and score on the Glasgow

Coma Scale. In conscious patients a neurological examination of the limbs is important.

- Radiographical examination of the chest and pelvis is mandatory, and radiographs of the head, neck, and spine are undertaken if clinically required.
- Once the patient is adequately stabilized, a secondary survey and appropriate investigations such as MRI scans are obtained.
- A management plan for definitive treatment is then decided, with life-threatening injuries treated first.
- It is important to carry out a tertiary survey within 24 hours of admission after the initial treatment has been carried out.
- Studies have indicated that up to 65% of injuries are initially missed, although these injuries are rarely life threatening.
  - The literature suggests that the number of missed injuries correlates with the ISS of the patient, and over 50% of missed injuries are musculoskeletal.
  - Analyses suggest that over 50% of missed injuries are potentially avoidable.

FRACTURE TREATMENT

Early Total Care

- In the early 1980s, the concept of early total care of major skeletal injuries had become accepted.
- Studies had shown that early femoral fracture fixation was associated with decreased pulmonary complications and reduced hospital stay.
- The concept of early fracture fixation was broadened to include virtually all fractures, and it seems likely that surgeons often strove primarily to fix too many fractures in patients who may have benefited from early fixation of the long bones and later fixation of other fractures.
- Table 3-6 shows the results of an analysis of 17 papers comparing early and late long-bone fixation.

TABLE 3-6 AN ANALYSIS OF 1,227 PATIENTS WHO HAD EARLY OR LATE LONG-BONE FIXATION (USUALLY FEMORAL)

	Improved results with early fixation (%)	No difference between early and late fixation (%)
Mortality	0	100
Multiple organ failure	0	100
Hospital costs	0	100
ARDS[a]	46.1	53.9
Pulmonary complications[a]	67.0	33.0
Pneumonia[a]	19.8	80.2
Ventilator days[a]	13.6	86.4
ICU days[a]	49.0	51.0
Hospital days[a]	42.6	57.4
Systemic infection[a]	52.9	47.1

[a]Showed improvement with early fixation.
Data from Dunham CM, Bosse MJ, Clancy TV, et al. Practice management guidelines for the optimal timing of long-bone fracture stabilization in polytrauma patients: The EAST practice management guidelines work group. J Trauma 2001;50:958–967.

- Early fracture fixation reduces morbidity but not mortality, the incidence of multiple organ failure, or overall hospital costs.
- The problem with early total care involving early fracture fixation of all patients was that the philosophy was applied to all patients regardless of the severity of injury and whether or not there was severe coexisting pulmonary damage.
  - A number of articles suggested that reamed nailing caused ARDS in a small subset of patients, but it became clear it was not the method of femoral fracture management that caused the problem but the early extensive surgery performed on this small number of severely injured patients.
  - This led to the concept of damage control surgery.

Damage Control Surgery

- The principle behind damage control surgery is that the clinical course after severe blunt trauma is determined by three main factors: the initial degree of injury (the "first hit"), the patient's biological response, and the type of treatment (the "second hit").
- Evidence indicates that early reamed femoral nailing is associated with significantly higher levels of interleukin-6 and elastase, and clinical work has shown that primary external fixation and secondary nailing is associated with less blood loss, shorter operating times, and a lower incidence of multiple organ failure (MOF) and adult respiratory distress syndrome (ARDS) than primary intramedullary nailing.
  - Thus in selected patients there is logic in delaying definitive surgery until the condition of the patient improves.
- MOF and ARDS are discussed in more detail in Chapter 41.
- The question is determining which patients are suitable for early total care and which for damage control surgery.
  - Most patients will be fit enough for early total care, but a number of parameters have been shown to be

---

BOX 3-3 CONDITIONS IN WHICH DAMAGE CONTROL SURGERY SHOULD BE CONSIDERED

Polytrauma + ISS >20 and thoracic trauma (AIS >2)
Polytrauma with severe abdominal/pelvic trauma and
  hemodynamic shock (BP <90 mm Hg)
ISS ⩾40
Bilateral lung contusions
Initial mean pulmonary arterial pressure >24 mm Hg
Pulmonary artery pressure increase >6 mm Hg
  during long-bone intramedullary nailing

Adapted from Pape HC, Giannoudis P, Krettek C. The timing of fracture treatment in polytrauma patients: relevance of damage control orthopedic surgery. Am J Surg 2002;183:622–629.

---

associated with an adverse outcome in multiply injured patients (Box 3-2).
- Box 3-3 lists a number of conditions where damage control surgery should be considered.

Suggested Treatment

- Most polytrauma patients will be stable after resuscitation and can be treated by early total care involving primary fracture fixation.
  - In these patients definitive long-bone stabilization can be carried out, but it may be wise to delay the definitive treatment of coexisting metaphyseal or intra-articular fractures until a later date.
- Patients in whom the parameters listed in Box 3-2 or the conditions listed in Box 3-3 exist are best treated by damage control surgery utilizing primary external fixation and secondary definitive management for long-bone fractures.
- The problem arises with those patients in whom the clinical situation is less clear.
  - In these patients the clinical situation should be reevaluated after volume resuscitation and the control of hemorrhage has been established.
- If the clinical condition is satisfactory, early total care is reasonable, but damage control surgery can be undertaken if the patient's condition deteriorates.
- An algorithm for the management of polytraumatized patients is given in Algorithm 3-1.

Head Injury

- Head trauma is the leading cause of death in young adults in the Western world.
- There has been considerable debate about whether early fracture fixation worsens the prognosis in patients who have a co-existing head injury and musculoskeletal injuries.
- There is no evidence that it does, however, and studies have shown that patients with mild, moderate, or severe head injuries have similar mortality rates, ICU days, total hospital days, CNS outcome, adverse CNS events,

---

BOX 3-2 PARAMETERS ASSOCIATED WITH ADVERSE OUTCOME IN MULTIPLY INJURED PATIENTS

Unstable condition or difficult resuscitation
Coagulopathy (platelet count <90,000)
Hypothermia (<32°C)
Shock and >25 units of blood
Bilateral lung contusions or initial chest radiographs
Multiple long bones plus truncal injury AIS ⩾2
Probable operating time >6 hr
Arterial injury and hemodynamic instability (RR <90)
Exaggerated inflammatory response (I1-6 >800 pg/mL)

From Pape HC, Giannoudis P, Krettek C. The timing of fracture treatment in polytrauma patients: relevance of damage control orthopedic surgery. Am J Surg 2002;183:622–629.

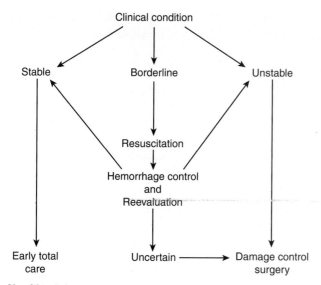

Clinical condition

Stable ← Borderline → Unstable

Resuscitation

Hemorrhage control
and
Reevaluation

Early total
care ← Uncertain → Damage control
surgery

Algorithm 3-1   The treatment of polytrauma patients. (Adapted from Pape HC, Giannoudis P, Krettek C. The timing of fracture treatment in polytrauma patients: relevance of damage control orthopedic surgery. Am J Surg 2002;183:622–629.)

TABLE 3-7 RESULTS OF THE MANAGEMENT OF POLYTRAUMA PATIENTS

Patients	1,495
GCS	11.4
ISS	27.8
Mortality rate	18.5%
Causes	
Head trauma	11.4%
Cardiovascular failure	32.7%
ARDS	35.3%
MOF	20.6%
Complications	
ARDS	28.4%
MOF	16.4%
Renal failure	1.6%
Pneumonia	7.4%
Sepsis	4.2%

From Pape HC, Remmers D, Rice J, et al. Appraisal of early evaluation of blunt chest trauma: development of a standardized scoring system for initial clinical decision making. J Trauma 2000;49:496–504.

ARDS and other pulmonary complications whether or not they have early long-bone fixation.
- The severity of the head injury is the strongest predictor of mortality, but it has been shown that extracranial injuries will increase mortality in patients who have a moderate or severe head injury.

Spinal Fractures
- The philosophy of early internal fixation of spinal fractures in polytraumatized patients has lagged behind the early treatment of long-bone injuries, but good evidence indicates that early spinal fracture fixation in polytraumatized patients is advantageous.
- Patients with operatively treated spinal fractures have significantly less pulmonary complications and a shorter length of hospital stay than those treated nonoperatively.
  - They also have less kyphotic deformity and late pain.
- Studies that have compared early and late spinal fracture fixation have also shown significantly less pulmonary complications, ICU days, total hospital days, and hospital costs compared with patients treated with late fixation.
- The treatment of spinal fractures is discussed further in Chapters 18 and 19.

Outcome
- The outcome of polytraumatized patients varies considerably among different centers and among different hospitals and obviously depends on many variables.
- Table 3-7 gives the mortality and complications for 1,495 patients treated according to the principles outlined in this chapter in Hanover, Germany.
  - Clearly these results reflect excellent surgical practice and represent the results that many hospitals will aspire to, given modern treatment methods.

Multiple Injuries in the Elderly
- In patients over 65 years of age, trauma is the fifth most common cause of death, and as the population ages, the problems of dealing with the polytraumatized elderly will increase.
- Elderly patients are five times more likely to die after trauma than younger patients, with multiple organ failure and sepsis the most common cause of death.
- The basic treatment for elderly patients with polytrauma is the same as for younger patients, although there is sometimes debate about how aggressive treatment should be, particularly when patients have a number of significant medical co-morbidities.
- The arguments relating to the management of the polytraumatized elderly patient are well summarized by Jacobs et al. (2003) in the Practice Management Guidelines for Geriatric Trauma produced by the EAST Practice Management Guidelines Work Group.
  - They have summarized the problems related to the management of polytraumatized elderly patients and have analyzed the literature in detail (Box 3-4).
- The EAST Group has shown that older patients should be treated identically to younger patients.
- Box 3-4 indicates that a number of parameters predict a poor outcome, but the authors of the EAST report are clear that surgeons should not withdraw treatment based on these initial parameters.
- The mortality in severely injured geriatric patients is higher than in younger patients, and a sensible approach to treatment withdrawal should be discussed with the family based on the patient's continuing progress.
  - Treatment should not be denied on the basis of age.
  - The protocols discussed earlier in this chapter should be followed.

BOX 3-4 CONCLUSIONS OF THE EAST GERIATRIC TRAUMA GUIDELINES GROUP

1. Advanced patient age, by itself, is not predictive of a poor outcome after trauma and should not be used as the sole criteria for denying or limiting care.
2. Preexisting comorbidities adversely affect outcome in elderly patients, but their effect is progressively less pronounced with advancing age.
3. In patients ≥65 years, a GCS of ≤8 is associated with a very poor prognosis.
4. Postinjury complications have a greater effect on survival and hospital stay than in younger patients. They should be appropriately treated.
5. Unless moribund on admission, an aggressive approach should be pursued in the elderly because the majority will return home, and up to 85% will return to independent function.
6. In patients ≥55 years, a base deficit of ≤−6 is associated with 66% mortality.
7. In patients ≥65 years, a Trauma Score <7 is associated with 100% mortality.
8. In patients ≥65 years, an admission respiratory rate of <10 is associated with 100% mortality.
9. Patients ≥55 years are often undertriaged to inappropriate trauma centers.

From Jacobs DG, Plaisier BR, Barie PS, et al., for EAST Practice Management Guidelines Work Group. Practice management guidelines for geriatric trauma. J Trauma 2003;56:391–416.

SUGGESTED READING

Baker SP, O'Neill B, Haddon W, et al. The injury severity score: a method for describing patients with multiple injuries and evaluating emergency care. J Trauma 1974;14:187–196.

Boyd CR, Tolson MA, Copes WS. Evaluating trauma care: the TRISS method. Trauma score and the Injury Severity Score. J Trauma 1987;27:370–378.

Champion HR, Copes WS, Sacco WJ, et al. The Major Outcome Trauma Study: establishing national norms for trauma care. J Trauma 1990;30:1356–1365.

Dunham CM, Bosse MJ, Clancy TV, et al. Practice management guidelines for the optimal timing of long-bone fracture stabilization in polytrauma patients: the EAST practice Management Guidelines Work Group. J Trauma 2001;50:958–967.

Ertel W, Keel M, Eid K, et al. Control of severe hemorrhage using C-clamp and pelvic packing in multiply injured patients with pelvic ring disruption. J Orthop Trauma 2001;15:468–474.

Gabbe BJ, Cameron PA, Wolfe R. TRISS: does it get better than this? Acad Emerg Med 2004;11:181–186.

Giannoudis PV. Current concepts of the inflammatory response after major trauma: an update. Injury 2003;34:397–404.

Giannoudis PV, Vevsi VT, Pape HC, et al. When should we operate on major fractures in patients with severe head injuries? Am J Surg 2002;183:261–267.

Jacobs DG, Jacobs DO, Kudsk KA, et al., for EAST Practice Management Guidelines Work Group. Practice management guidelines for nutritional support of the trauma patient. J Trauma 2004; 57:660–678.

Jacobs DG, Plaisier BR, Barie PS, et al., for EAST Practice Management Guidelines Work Group. Practice management guidelines for geriatric trauma. J Trauma 2003;56:391–416.

Johnson KD, Cadambi A, Seibert GB. Incidence of adult respiratory distress syndrome in patients with multiple musculoskeletal injuries; effect of early operative stabilization of fractures. J Trauma 1985;25:375–384.

Pape HC, Giannoudis P, Krettek C. The timing of fracture treatment in polytrauma patients: relevance of damage control orthopedic surgery. Am J Surg 2002;183:622–629.

Pape HC, Grimme K, van Grievesen M, et al. Impact of intramedullary instrumentation versus damage control for femoral fractures on immunoinflammatory parameters: Prospective randomized analysis by the EPOFF study group. J Trauma 2003;55:7–13.

Pape HC, Remmers D, Rice J, et al. Appraisal of early evaluation of blunt chest trauma: development of a standardized scoring system for initial clinical decision making. J Trauma 2000;49: 496–504.

Riska EB, Myllynen P. Fat embolism in patients with multiple injuries. J Trauma 1982;22:891–894.

Swiontkowski M. The multiply injured patient with musculoskeletal injuries. In: Bucholz RW, Heckman JD, eds. Rockwood and Green's fractures in adults, 5th ed., Vol 1. Philadelphia: Lippincott Williams & Wilkins, 2001.

Teasdale G, Jennett B. Assessment of coma and impaired consciousness: a practical scale. Lancet 1974;2:81–84.

OPEN FRACTURES

Open fractures are associated with a soft tissue defect that permits contamination by the outside environment (Fig. 4-1). Historically the difficulty of managing soft tissue and bone defects often meant the incidence of infection was considerable and the requirement for amputation was high. With the advent of improved plastic surgery and fracture fixation techniques, however, complications related to open fractures have diminished, although they still remain a challenge to orthopaedic surgeons.

CLASSIFICATION

Although there are other classifications of open fractures, the Gustilo classification has now been adopted worldwide. It is based on the size of the wound, the amount of soft tissue damage or contamination, and the type of fracture. There are three fracture types, with the Gustilo type III fractures divided into three subtypes based on the extent of the periosteal damage, the presence of contamination, and the extent of arterial injury. The classification is shown in Table 4-1.

The Gustilo classification has been shown to be prognostic in terms of time of union and the incidence of nonunion and infection, particularly with respect to open fractures of the tibia. However, as with all classification systems, surgeons should be aware of a number of drawbacks. The Gustilo classification was formulated with diaphyseal, rather than metaphyseal or intra-articular, fractures in mind. It was also designed to be used in long bones such as the femur and tibia rather than in smaller bones such as the metacarpals or metatarsals. As with all classifications, it inevitably contains a number of subjective terms such as "significant periosteal stripping" and refers to the length of skin wounds, which will vary considerably with age. It is impossible to avoid these problems in any classification system that is practical to use, and the Gustilo classification has become accepted as the main classification of open fractures.

EPIDEMIOLOGY

Very little is known about the epidemiology of open fractures. The incidence of open fractures varies in different places and in different institutions depending on many factors, including the incidence of road traffic accidents and gunshot injuries. Level 1 trauma centers obviously see more open fractures than smaller peripheral hospitals, but the overall incidence of open fractures is probably similar in many parts of the world. Table 4-2 shows the epidemiology of 960 consecutive open fractures seen in Edinburgh, Scotland, over a 6-year period. It is likely this information is applicable to many parts of the world. The overall incidence of open fractures was 3.2%, with 3.3% in the upper limb, 3.7% in the lower limb, and 0.3% in the limb girdles. Table 4-2 shows the wide variation in the incidence of open fractures. The highest incidence is in tibial diaphyseal fractures, where about 21% are open. Fractures of the femoral diaphysis, hand and foot phalanges, forearm diaphyses, tibial plafond,

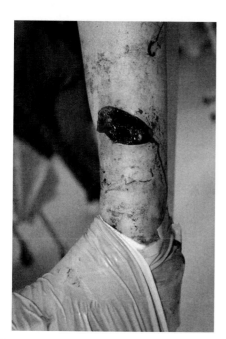

Figure 4-1 A Gustilo IIIa open tibial fracture.

TABLE 4-1 GUSTILO CLASSIFICATION OF OPEN FRACTURES

Type	Definition
I	Open fracture with a clean wound <1cm in length
II	Open fracture with a laceration of >1 cm long and without extensive soft-tissue damage, flaps, or avulsions
III	Either an open fracture with extensive soft-tissue laceration, damage, or loss; an open segmental fracture; or a traumatic amputation. Also: High-velocity gunshot injuries Open fractures caused by farm injuries Open fractures requiring vascular repair Open fractures older than 8 hours
IIIa	Adequate periosteal cover of a fractured bone despite extensive soft-tissue laceration or damage High-energy trauma irrespective of size of wound
IIIb	Extensive soft-tissue loss with significant periosteal stripping and bone damage Usually associated with massive contamination
IIIc	Association with arterial injury requiring repair, irrespective of degree of soft-tissue injury

From Gustilo RB, Mendoza RM, Williams DM. Problems in the management of type III (severe) open fractures. A new classification of type III open fractures. J Trauma 1984;24:742–746.

TABLE 4-2 INCIDENCE OF OPEN FRACTURES: AN ANALYSIS OF 960 FRACTURES OVER A 6-YEAR PERIOD

Fracture location	Open Fractures (%)	Gustilo Type (%)					Average Age (y)
		I	II	IIIa	IIIb	IIIc	
Tibial diaphysis	21.2	23.5	19.6	23	29.6	4.3	43
Femoral diaphysis	12.3	20.3	16.9	23.7	30.5	8.5	32
Hand phalanges	10.1	32	52.9	5.7	1	8.4	39
Foot phalanges	9.0	28.6	52.2	11.9	—	7.1	38
Forearm diaphysis	8.0	48.8	21.9	9.8	17.1	2.4	35
Tibial plafond	6.1	18.2	9.1	45.4	27.3	—	46
Patella	5.7	18.5	48.1	29.6	3.7	—	41
Distal femur	5.6	30	20	—	50	—	43
Distal humerus	5.4	35.7	50	7.1	7.1	—	41
Humeral diaphysis	5.3	68.7	18.7	6.2	6.2	—	48
Tarsus	3.2	—	30	36.6	23.3	10	35
Tibial plateau	2.4	30	40	20	10	—	44
Distal forearm	2.1	62.3	26.1	10.1	1.4	—	62
Carpus	2.0	13.3	6.7	66.6	13.3	—	33
Ankle	1.4	17.5	42.5	35	5	—	49
Proximal forearm	1.0	37.5	50	12.5	—	—	48
Metatarsus	0.9	27.2	36.4	18.2	18.2	—	38
Scapula	0.7	100	—	—	—	—	28
Pelvis	0.6	—	—	80	20	—	29
Metacarpus	0.4	43.7	56.3	—	—	—	43
Proximal humerus	0.3	—	60	40	—	—	32
Clavicle	0.2	50	—	50	—	—	33
Proximal femur	0.02	100	—	—	—	—	40
Fibula	0	—	—	—	—	—	—
Spine	0	—	—	—	—	—	—

patella, distal femur, distal humerus, and humeral diaphysis are all associated with incidences of more than 5%. In fractures of the metatarsus, scapula, pelvis, metacarpus, proximal humerus, and proximal femur, however, the incidence is very low. If an open fracture does occur in these areas, the injury tends to be very severe. The incidence of open spinal fractures is so low that effectively they are unsurvivable. The only exception to this is gunshot spinal fractures, which are relatively uncommon in civilian practice. Table 4-2 also shows that the age of the patient varies, with younger patients tending to have open fractures of the pelvis, femoral diaphysis, proximal humerus, carpus, and forearm diaphyses as a result of road traffic accidents or other high-energy injuries, with open fractures of the humeral diaphysis, proximal forearm, ankle, and distal forearm occurring in older patients as a result of low-energy injuries.

Table 4-2 also shows the incidences of the different Gustilo types for each fracture. The highest incidence of Gustilo type III fractures occurs in the pelvis, carpus, and lower limb. With the exception of open carpal fractures, open upper limb fractures tend to be less severe. In the lower limb there is a high incidence of Gustilo type III fractures in the femoral diaphysis, around the knee, in the tibial diaphysis and plafond, and in the tarsus. Gustilo IIIc fractures are rare but are most commonly seen in high-energy injuries to the tarsus, femoral diaphysis, and tibial diaphysis. They also occur in the fingers and toes, where they are often treated by amputation (see Chapter 37).

PREOPERATIVE ASSESSMENT

- A complete history and physical examination is essential.
  - Some of the main factors that should be obtained in the history are shown in Box 4-1.
- Age does not affect patient management, but older patients tend to be osteopenic and the fractures may be associated with greater comminution.
- Information about general health is important because conditions such as diabetes mellitus, metabolic bone diseases, or neuromuscular conditions may alter the type of operative treatment, and cardiovascular, pulmonary, and other medical comorbidities may affect anesthesia and later intensive care.
- The preaccident mental and physical state of the patient is important because, for example, a Gustilo type IIIb open tibial fracture in a demented nonambulator with medical comorbidities might well be successfully treated by primary amputation rather than by attempted bone reconstruction.
- The mode of injury should be carefully established to determine whether the open fracture has occurred as a result of a high- or low-energy injury and whether there is potential for significant fracture contamination.
  - High-energy injuries are associated with significantly greater bone and soft tissue damage, and therefore open fractures following road traffic accidents, falls from a height, crushing injuries, or gunshot injuries, are often more difficult to manage and associated with a worse prognosis than those that occur after a simple fall, a fall downstairs, or a sports injury.
- The physical examination must include an assessment of other injuries using ATLS principles.
  - Examination of the limb should include a careful assessment of the vasculature with palpation of the pulses and determination of limb color and distal capillary return. The surgeon should be aware that if the patient is hypotensive or peripherally shut down, an incorrect preoperative assessment of the vascular status of a limb may be made.
  - If there is any doubt about the vascular supply, a Doppler examination or angiogram should be obtained.
- Examination of the neurological status of the limb is also important.
  - Abnormal sensation or motor power may suggest intracranial, spinal, or peripheral nerve damage.
  - A peripheral nerve lesion associated with a limb fracture suggests considerable soft tissue injury and probably a poor prognosis for the limb.

Examination of the Open Wound

- Ideally the open wound should not be examined by every member of the medical and nursing staff prior to surgery!
  - If possible, a digital image of the wound should be obtained soon after the patient is admitted to the hospital, so that it, rather than the wound, can be repeatedly examined. This policy has been shown to be associated with a lower infection rate.
- It is important, however, that the surgeon examine the wound carefully.
  - The location and extent of the wound may allow a preoperative determination of the need for plastic surgery, particularly if it is obvious there will be exposed subcutaneous bone after debridement. The presence of skin degloving should be noted.
  - The length of the wound is used in the Gustilo classification, and a loose relationship exists between wound

---

BOX 4-1 IMPORTANT FEATURES OF THE CLINICAL HISTORY AND PHYSICAL EXAMINATION

History	Previous injuries
Age	**Physical Examination**
General health	Other injuries
Specific comorbidities	Limb vascularity
Previous disability	Peripheral pulses
Alcohol and drugs	Capillary refill
Ambulatory status	Hypotension
Residence	Neurological status
Cause of injury	Skin and soft tissue
High or low energy	damage
Potential for infection	
Other injuries	

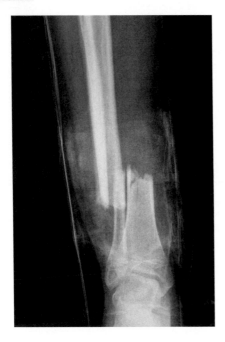
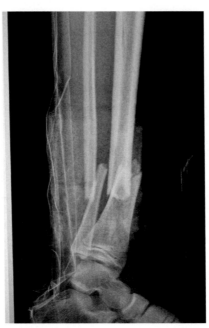

Figure 4-2 Anteroposterior and lateral radiographs of the fracture shown in Figure 4-1. Radiographs taken after intramedullary nailing are shown in Figure 33-7 in Chapter 33.

length and prognosis, but it should never be assumed a small wound necessarily carries a good prognosis because there may be significant associated contamination and tissue damage.

■ The number of skin wounds should be determined. Two or three small wounds placed close together strongly indicates a high-energy injury and degloving in the area.

■ The degree of wound and skin contamination should be assessed, as should the presence of bone fragments in the wound.

■ The apparently intact tissues of the limb should also be examined because there may be other injuries or evidence of skin tattooing from the road or from a vehicle wheel having passed over the limb.

Radiologic Examination

■ Usually, only anteroposterior and lateral radiographs are required (Fig. 4-2).
  ■ They should include adjacent joints and any associated injuries.

■ There are a number of features that the surgeon should look for when examining the radiographs (Box 4-2).

■ MRI and CT scans are rarely required in the acute situation but may be helpful in open pelvic, intra-articular, carpal, and tarsal fractures.

■ Angiography may be required in Gustilo IIIb or IIIc fractures. In the polytraumatized patient, the surgeon must decide if a delay for further imaging is appropriate.

TREATMENT

Surgeons tend to concentrate on the method of fracture treatment when treating open fractures, but a number of procedures are involved if their treatment is to be successful (Box 4-3).

BOX 4-2 IMPORTANT RADIOLOGIC FEATURES IN OPEN FRACTURES

The location and morphology of the fracture
The presence of comminution signifying a high-energy injury
■ Secondary fracture lines that may displace on treatment
■ The distance the bone fragments have traveled from their normal location. Wide displacement suggests bone avascularity
■ Bone defects suggesting missing bone
■ Gas in the tissues

BOX 4-3 PROCEDURES INVOLVED IN THE TREATMENT OF OPEN FRACTURES

Debridement
    Skin
    Fat and fascia
    Muscle
    Bone
Wound closure
Antibiotics
    Intravenous
    Bead pouch technique
Fracture stabilization
Secondary debridement
Soft tissue cover

Debridement

- The most important procedure in the treatment of open fractures is debridement, or wound excision.
  - All devitalized or contaminated tissue must be removed.
- Until relatively recently, it was difficult to reconstruct large soft tissue and bone defects, and surgeons tended to be conservative with tissue resection.
- With the introduction of improved surgical fixation and bone reconstruction techniques, and particularly with the development of free flaps and distally based fasciocutaneous flaps, it is now much easier to reconstruct tissue defects. Therefore the primary surgical debridement should be aggressive when required.
- The literature suggests that debridement should be performed within 6 hours of the injury.
  - No clinical evidence indicates the results of debridement after 6 hours are worse than the results prior to 6 hours, but logic dictates that debridement should be done as soon as possible after injury and there should be no unnecessary delay.
- The basic rules of debridement are given in Box 4-4.

Skin

- Skin is very resistant to direct trauma but susceptible to shearing forces, the plane of cleavage being outside the deep fascia.
- Shearing forces may produce extensive degloving injuries, which particularly affect the lower limb and may be circumferential.
- Elderly patients are particularly at risk of degloving, and circumferential degloving in an elderly multiply injured patient may require amputation (Fig. 4-3).
- Isolated skin wounds caused by direct trauma can be treated by local excision of the contaminated wound edges.
- If there are several wounds in close proximity, they should be excised en bloc, as there will be extensive associated soft tissue damage.
- After the initial skin excision, it is important to examine for skin degloving. All degloved skin should be resected until dermal bleeding is encountered.

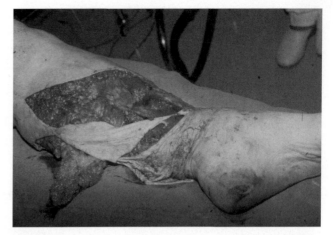

Figure 4-3 Degloving associated with a Gustilo IIIb fracture. The degloving was circumferential.

- If a large area of degloved skin is excised, split skin graft can be harvested from the excised skin for later use.
- After the initial skin excision, the surgeon should extend the open wound to allow adequate exposure of the underlying bone and soft tissues.
  - There are no indications not to do this. Even small skin incisions may be associated with considerable contamination.
- The direction and length of the skin extensions will depend on the location and size of the open wound, but ideally extensions should be longitudinal and, where possible, follow normal surgical approaches.

Fat and Fascia

- All devitalized fat must be removed.
- The extent of fat necrosis may well be greater than was apparent preoperatively, and extensive fat resection with excision of the overlying skin may be required in some cases.
- Fascial resection rarely presents a problem, but it should be borne in mind that foreign material may spread between the deep fascia and the underlying muscles.

Muscle

- All devitalized muscle should be removed.
- It can be difficult to assess muscle viability fully at the initial debridement, particularly if the patient is hypotensive.
  - The classic signs of muscle viability are color, consistency, contractility to mechanical stimulation, and bleeding.
  - Muscle bleeding is probably the best test of viability, but the surgeon should be guided by the appearance and consistency of the muscle.
  - Muscles that are shredded or disintegrate on touch should be excised.
  - It is often easier to determine muscle viability at a relook debridement 36 to 48 hours after the initial exploration. By this time the patient's condition has stabilized and muscle vascularity is easier to determine.

BOX 4-4 SURGICAL PRINCIPLES OF DEBRIDEMENT

- With the exception of low-velocity gunshot wounds, which can be treated with antibiotics and local wound care, all open fractures require surgical debridement. Failure to do this constitutes inadequate treatment.
- All affected tissue planes should be explored.
- The bone ends must be exposed and carefully examined for contamination and soft tissue stripping.
- All devitalized and contaminated tissue should be excised and all devitalized bone fragments removed.
- The wound should not be closed primarily.

Bone

- Resection of bone should be dealt with in the same way as soft tissue resection.
- All devitalized separate bone fragments should be removed regardless of their size.
- As with muscle, it may be difficult to determine bone vascularity, and if the surgeon is concerned about the viability of periosteal or muscle attachment to a bone, it may be advantageous to reexamine the bone fragments during the re-look procedure.

Lavage

- Lavage with fluids such as normal isotonic saline or antibiotic solutions is an essential part of the debridement procedure.
- Ten to 15 liters of lavage fluid should be used to remove bone clots and other devitalized debris and ideally reduce the level of bacterial contamination.
- Some experimental evidence indicates that the addition of antibiotics is associated with a lower infection rate, but there is no clinical evidence of the usefulness of antibiotic solutions.

Wound Closure

- Open wounds should not be closed primarily.
  - There is no logical reason to do so because all wounds that have been adequately debrided can be closed only under tension.
- If wound closure is possible, it should be undertaken at the re-look procedure 36 to 48 hours after the initial surgery.
- Primary wound extensions can be closed, but there is no practical advantage if the main wound is being left open.
  - Even closure of the wound extensions may cause tissue tension.
- The only exception to the rule about closing wounds primarily is if a primary flap is undertaken.
  - This is not always logistically possible, and if it is done, it deprives the surgeon of the opportunity to reexamine the soft tissues at a re-look procedure.
  - In expert hands, primary flap cover can be associated with good results, although it is unlikely the results will be better than those associated with a re-look procedure and wound closure within 48 hours of the injury.
  - Vacuum-assisted closure (VAC) systems have been used for a number of years to close skin defects with good results. At the moment, they cannot be recommended for the closure of open wounds related to fractures in view of the time taken for the soft tissues to close and the consequent risk of infection.

Antibiotic Prophylaxis

- Some 60% to 70% of open wounds are associated with positive cultures in the emergency department.

- Most of the contaminating bacteria are normal skin flora, although more virulent bacteria also gain entry to the wound.
- Although 7% of bacteria isolated in the initial culture cause later infection, where gram-negative bacteria are recovered from the initial culture, 50% cause later infection.
- Early antibiotic administration has been useful in both animal and clinical studies, and animal work has shown that the sooner the antibiotics are administered, the lower the infection rate.
- Most surgeons use a first- or second-generation cephalosporin as prophylaxis for Gustilo type I and II open fractures.
  - The initial dose should be given as soon as possible after diagnosis with a three-dose intravenous regimen being used.
- In Gustilo type III open fractures, surgeons may use a three-dose intravenous regimen of a third-generation cephalosporin or a combination of a second-generation cephalosporin and an aminoglycoside.
  - If there is any chance of clostridial contamination, intravenous penicillin should be given. If the patient is allergic to penicillin, clindamycin or metronidazole should be used.
  - This is important in open pelvic fractures where the open fracture may have entered the rectum or vagina.
- A bead pouch technique has recently been introduced to reduce the incidence of late infection.
  - Antibiotic-impregnated polymethylmethacrylate beads can be placed into the wound after debridement has been undertaken.
  - These beads usually contain gentamycin or tobramycin.
  - Evidence indicates that the incidence of infection in open tibial fractures treated by intramedullary nailing decreases from 16% to 4% with the use of a bead pouch technique.
  - The technique is not a substitute for either a thorough debridement or prophylactic intravenous antibiotics, however.

Fracture Stabilization

- Open fractures should be treated by surgical stabilization.
- The main exception to this rule is open fractures of the terminal phalanges of the hand and foot.
  - In severe open distal phalangeal fractures, K-wire fixation may be used to stabilize the distal phalanx, but generally these fractures are treated by debridement, antibiotic cover, and nonoperative management. The outcome is usually favorable because the blood supply to the terminal phalanges of the hand in particular is good.
- Cast management is associated with poorer results than operative management in open long-bone fractures.
- Surgical stabilization minimizes later soft tissue injury and promotes capillary ingrowth.

- There is also good evidence it is associated with a decreased infection rate.
- If plastic surgery is required, fracture stabilization is mandatory.
- Traction should not be employed for open fractures.
- The surgical treatment of different fractures is discussed in Chapters 10 through 30.

Secondary Debridement

- It is suggested that all open long-bone and pelvic fractures be reexplored 36 to 48 hours after the initial debridement.
- Primary flap cover can be undertaken, but the advantages of a secondary debridement are considerable.
  - Residual contamination can be excised and the vascularity of the soft tissues and bone fragments reassessed once the patient has been stabilized.
  - It is also an excellent time to carry out definitive soft tissue closure because in the majority of cases there will be no residual contamination or devascularized tissue.
- If the wound does require further debridement, this should be undertaken, and the patient returned to the operating room 36 to 48 hours later for a further debridement.
  - This is a particular problem in crush injuries, in which progressive myonecrosis can occur.
- The wound should not be closed until all devitalized or contaminated tissue has been removed.

Soft Tissue Cover

- Most open wounds do not require plastic surgery.
- Increasingly, however, plastic surgery techniques are being used in open fractures.
- The most frequently used plastic procedures involve split skin grafting (Fig. 4-4), local muscle flaps such as the gastrocnemius flap, local flaps such as the proximal or distal fasciocutaneous flap (Fig. 4-5), or free flaps (Fig. 4-6).
- The commonest free flaps are the latissimus dorsi, rectus femoris, and radial forearm flap.

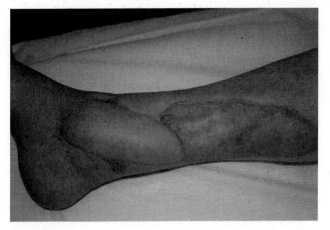

Figure 4-5   A distally based fasciocutaneous flap use to cover a defect on the leg.

Obviously, there is wide variation in the types of soft tissue treatment used, but an analysis of soft tissue surgery used in the 960 open fractures detailed in Table 4-2 does allow an appreciation of the need for the different types of soft tissue cover (Table 4-3). Of the open fractures, 716 (74.5%) did not need plastic surgery in their management. A number of these patients were very seriously injured and either died or had a primary amputation. The vast majority of patients had their fractures treated successfully without plastic surgery, however. One hundred and forty-one (14.7%) of the open fractures were treated by split skin grafting, 12 (1.2%) by muscle flaps, 76 (7.9%) by local flaps, and 15 (1.6%) by free flap cover. Table 4-3 shows the distribution of the different types of soft tissue cover in different body areas. It shows that the requirement for plastic surgery is highest in the tibia and hindfoot, with about 55% of patients requiring some form of plastic surgery. Open fractures of the tibial diaphysis, plateau, and plafond are associated with the greatest requirement for flap cover. In this series, patients with open distal humerus, metatarsus, proximal femur, clavicle, proximal humerus, and pelvis did not need plastic surgery, although obviously split skin grafting and flap cover will occasionally be required in these fractures.

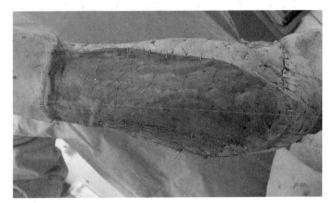

Figure 4-4   A split skin graft used on the leg.

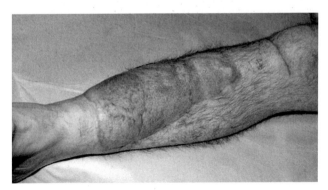

Figure 4-6   A latissimus dorsi free flap used to cover a defect on the leg. The cosmetic effect is generally better than with a fasciocutaneous flap (see Fig. 4-5).

TABLE 4-3 REQUIREMENT FOR PLASTIC SURGERY AND THE TYPE OF SURGERY IN OPEN FRACTURES

Fracture location	Plastic surgery (%)	Split skin graft (%)	Muscle flap (%)	Local flap (%)	Free flap (%)
Tibial diaphysis	55.2	40.1	7.9	44.1	7.9
Ankle	55.0	68.2	—	27.3	4.5
Tibial plafond	54.5	16.7	—	83.3	—
Carpus	46.6	57.1	—	14.3	28.6
Tarsus	40.0	83.3	—	8.3	8.3
Forearm diaphysis	38.2	71.5	—	9.5	19.0
Tibial plateau	30.0	—	66.6	33.3	—
Distal femur	30.0	100	—	—	—
Femoral diaphysis	28.8	100	—	—	—
Patella	18.5	100	—	—	—
Metacarpus	12.5	100	—	—	—
Distal forearm	8.7	100	—	—	—
Proximal forearm	6.2	100	—	—	—
Humeral diaphysis	6.2	100	—	—	—
Hand phalanges	2.7	62.5	—	37.5	—
Foot phalanges	2.5	100	—	—	—

SUGGESTED READING

Court-Brown CM, McQueen MM, Quaba AA, eds. Management of open fractures. London: Martin Dunitz, 1996.

Court-Brown CM, Rimmer S, Prakash U, et al. The epidemiology of open long bone fractures. Injury 1998;29:529–534.

Erdmann MW, Court-Brown CM, Quaba MM. A five year review of islanded distally based fasciocutaneous flaps on the lower limb. Br J Plast Surg 1997;50:421–427.

Gopal S, Giannoudis P, Murray A, et al. The functional outcome of severe, open tibial fractures managed with early fixation and flap coverage. J Bone Joint Surg (Br) 2004;86:861–867.

Gustilo RB, Anderson JT. Prevention of infection in the treatment of 1035 open fractures of long bones: retrospective and prospective analysis. J Bone Joint Surg (Am) 1976;58:453–458.

Gustilo RB, Mendoza RM, Williams DM. Problems in the management of type III (severe) open fractures. A new classification of type III open fractures. J Trauma 1984;24:742–746.

Hammert WC, Minarchek J, Trzeciak MA. Free-flap reconstruction of traumatic lower extremity wounds. Am J Orthop 2000; 29(Suppl 9):22–26.

Haury B, Rodeheaver G, Vensito I, et al. Debridement: an essential component of traumatic wound care. Am J Surg 1978;135:238–242.

Herscovici D, Sanders RW, Scaduto JM, et al. Vacuum-assisted wound closure (VAC therapy) for the management of patients with high-energy soft tissue injuries. J Orthop Trauma 2003;17:683–688.

Nieminen H, Kuokkanen H, Tukianinen E, et al. Free flap reconstructions of 100 tibial fractures. J Trauma 1999;46:1031–1035.

Olson SA, Finkemeier CG, Moehring HD. Open fractures. In: Bucholz RW, Heckman JD, eds. Rockwood and Green's fractures in adults, 5th ed. Philadelphia: Lippincott Williams & Wilkins, 2001.

Pollak AN, McCarthy ML, Burgess AR. Short-term wound complications after application of flaps for coverage of traumatic soft-tissue defects about the tibia. The Lower Extremity Assessment Project (LEAP) Study Group. J Bone Joint Surg (Am) 2000; 82:1681–1691.

Yaremchuk MJ. Acute management of severe soft tissue damage accompanying open fractures of the lower extremity. Clin Plast Surg 1986;13:621–632.

Zalavras CG, Patzakis MJ. Open fractures: evaluation and management. J Am Acad Orthop Surg 2003;11:212–219.

Zalavras CG, Patzakis MJ, Holtom P. Local antibiotic therapy in the treatment of open fractures and osteomyelitis. Clin Orthop 2004;427:86–93.

GUNSHOT INJURIES

Gunshot injuries are an increasing problem in many countries. With the continuation of warfare in many parts of the world, together with a very large number of guns in circulation, there has been an increase in the number of gunshot injuries and fatalities since the 1970s. Although warfare contributes significantly to mortality from gunshot injury, since 1933 over a million American civilians have been killed by guns, more than the total number of Americans killed in all wars! The homicide rate from gunshot injuries in males aged 15 to 24 in the United States is about 20 times higher than in other industrialized nations, but the problem is worsening worldwide, and as the incidence of gunshot injuries increases, so does the incidence of gunshot fractures.

BALLISTICS

Gunshot injuries are classified as low velocity if the bullets traveled at less than 1,000 feet per second and high velocity if the bullets traveled at more than 2,000 feet per second. This is an arbitrary definition and varies among different authorities. Clearly the inference is that high-velocity wounds are more serious, and there is no doubt that bullet velocity is an important determinant of wound severity. The kinetic energy transferred to the target is defined as mass multiplied by velocity to the second power ($KE = MV^2$). A number of factors determine the severity of injury, however (Box 5-1).

The mass, velocity, shape, and composition of the bullet all help determine the degree of injury. Larger bullets traveling at lower velocities may cause more damage than

BOX 5-1 FACTORS ALTERING THE SEVERITY OF GUNSHOT INJURIES

Bullet Characteristics	Tissue Characteristics
Velocity	Distance and path within body
Mass	
Shape	Biological characteristics of tissues
Design and composition	
Yaw	Mechanism of tissue disruption
Range	

smaller high-velocity bullets. Shotgun pellets or bullets that fragment on impact cause significant damage, and yaw, or the tendency of a bullet to deviate from the longitudinal axis, will alter the degree of injury. Yaw is minimized by causing the bullet to spin by rifling the barrel of the firearm and placing helical grooves in it.

Tissue characteristics are also important. As a bullet passes through the tissues, they offer resistance, which depends on their elasticity, cohesiveness, and density. Thus, although liver and muscle absorb about the same amount of energy per centimeter of tissue, their different structural characteristics mean that the liver is more severely traumatized by bullet wounds.

The three components of a bullet's effect on tissues are the sonic pressure wave, the permanent cavity, and the temporary cavity. A sonic pressure wave precedes the bullet and can produce up to 117 atmospheres of pressure. The wave is of very short duration, however, and usually causes no significant tissue damage. The permanent cavity refers to the tissue directly destroyed by the bullet during its passage through the body. This may result from tissue laceration or crushing, and the bone may be damaged by direct impact. The size of the permanent cavity varies with the characteristics listed in Box 5-1. It is possible to have a relatively small entry wound but a large underlying permanent cavity.

The temporary cavity refers to the transient expansion of the tissues that follows behind the bullet as a result of the release of kinetic energy. The temporary cavity can be as much as 30 times the size of the bullet. Tissue characteristics will determine the damage caused by the temporary cavity, with elastic tissues such as lungs sustaining less damage than inelastic tissues such as bone. The temporary cavity size is related to contamination. As the bullet enters, it creates the temporary cavity and negative pressure, which pulls contaminated residue from the outside environment into the defect.

BONE DAMAGE

Bone damage from a bullet may follow direct contact and be part of the permanent cavity caused by the bullet, or the damage may be caused indirectly by the temporary cavity.

The damage varies considerably depending on the factors listed in Box 5-1. The kinetic energy of the bullet may be insufficient to cause a fracture, and unicortical splintering or a bone divot may result. In cancellous bone it is possible for a bullet to traverse the bone without causing a complete fracture. In high-energy bullet injuries, significant bone comminution is common, and even the temporary cavity may cause considerable bone damage.

VASCULAR DAMAGE

Vascular injury can be caused directly by the bullet or may be associated with cavitation effects. In high-energy injuries, both mechanisms may cause considerable vascular damage. The extent of the vascular injuries may vary from intimal disruption to extensive arterial damage. Partial laceration of the arterial wall is a particular problem because vascular constriction will not occur and the hemorrhage may be considerable. Because extensive vascular damage may be associated with a small bullet entry hole, there may be significant hemorrhage into a limb with increased tissue pressure necessitating fasciotomy.

The incidence of vascular injury depends on the factors listed in Box 5-1, but it also varies with the location of the wound. Table 5-1 gives a list of the incidence of vascular injury in different body areas. Injuries to the calf or leg and forearm or antecubital fossa are associated with the highest incidences of vascular injury.

There is debate as to how potential vascular injury should be investigated. Patients may present with obvious signs of an avascular limb with absent pulses and the classical signs of ischemia. In these patients urgent surgical exploration is required, although an on-table angiogram may be helpful. Patients who present with no signs of ischemia with normal pulses do not require urgent angiography, although Doppler pressures can be measured to exclude occult vascular damage, which has been shown to be present in about 10% of limbs with a normal vascular examination. Both angiography and color-flow duplex imaging have been used to investigate vascular damage. Both are effective, but angiography remains the gold standard. The investigation of vascular injuries is outlined in Algorithm 5-1, adapted from Bartlett et al. (2000).

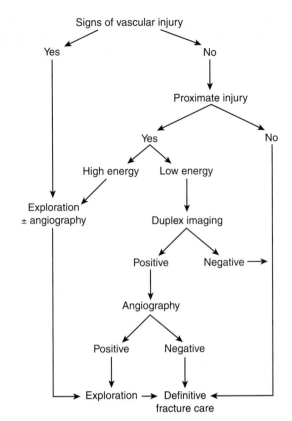

Algorithm 5-1 Algorithm for the investigation of vascular injury in gunshot fractures. (Adapted from Bartlett et al., 2000.)

It makes use of the concept of a proximate injury, an injury in which the missile track passes within 1 inch of the known anatomical path of a major vessel.

Treatment of vascular damage must be undertaken as an emergency. More than 6 hours of ischemia usually results in permanent tissue damage, even if revascularization is successful. Fasciotomy should be undertaken following revascularization. The success rate of expeditious vascular reconstruction is variable and depends on the location of the vascular injury as well as the extent of the associated muscle and bony injury.

NEUROLOGICAL DAMAGE

It is reported that the incidence of nerve damage following gunshot injuries varies between 2% and 100%, the difference presumably relating mainly to the type of weapon used. Results from both World War II and the Vietnam War suggest that about 70% of nerve injuries recover spontaneously without surgery, with 90% of them recovering after 3 to 9 months. Clearly the prognosis for different nerve lesions varies, and Box 5-2 lists the factors associated with a poorer prognosis after gunshot injuries. Proximal nerve lesions resolve more slowly than distal lesions, and multiple or dense nerve lesions have a poorer prognosis than isolated lesions. Nerve repair is successful in about 25% of neurotmeses. Based on these findings, it is reasonable to treat neuropraxias and axonotmeses nonoperatively with primary surgery

TABLE 5-1 INCIDENCE OF VASCULAR INJURY IN DIFFERENT BODY AREAS

Location of wound	Incidence (%)
Lateral thigh	<1
Medial or posterior thigh	7–9
Popliteal fossa	9–10
Calf or leg	18–22
Upper arm or shoulder	9–10
Medial or posterior upper arm	6–8
Forearm or antecubital fossa	17–22

Data from Ordog GJ, Balasubramanium S, Wasserberger J, et al. Extremity gunshot wounds: I. Identification and treatment of patients at high risk of gunshot injuries. J Trauma 1994;36:358–368.

BOX 5-2 FACTORS ASSOCIATED WITH A WORSE PROGNOSIS AFTER NERVE DAMAGE

Neurotmesis
Proximal nerve damage
Multiple nerve lesions
Reflex sympathetic dystrophy

reserved for neurotmeses. Surgeons can wait for 3 to 4 months to see if nerve function will recover. Reflex sympathetic dystrophy can be a particular problem after gunshot injuries, which is discussed in more detail in Chapter 41.

TREATMENT

The treatment of open fractures due to gunshot injuries is essentially similar to treatment of open fractures caused by other means and is discussed in Chapter 4. There are a number of issues that are debated by orthopaedic surgeons, however.

Debridement of Low-Energy Wounds

- Unlike low-energy wounds caused by blunt trauma, most low-energy gunshot wounds can be safely treated with simple local wound care with superficial irrigation (Fig. 5-1).
  - Many can be treated on an outpatient basis in the same way as a similar closed fracture of the same bone would be treated.
  - Using this method of management, infection rates of between 0% and 5% have been reported, although Ordog et al. (1994) in a series of over 16,000 patients reported an infection rate of only 1.8%, all of which responded to oral antibiotics without the need for hospital admissions.
  - The infection rate varies in different anatomical areas. For instance, low-velocity gunshot fractures of the femoral shaft have an infection rate similar to crush injuries; gunshot tibia fractures have an infection rate

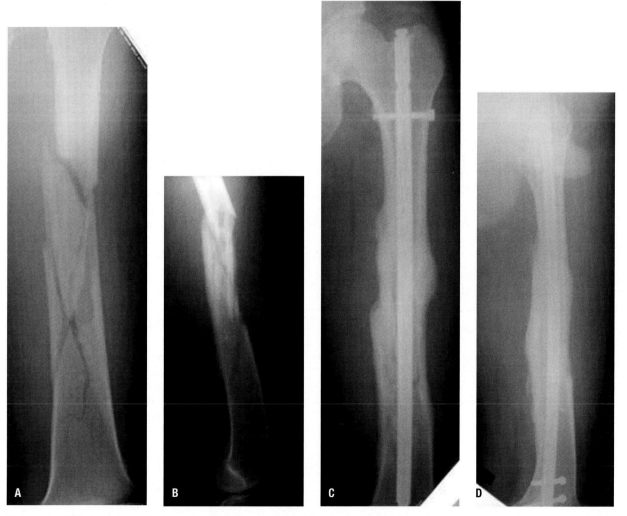

Figure 5-1 (A,B) AP and lateral radiographs of a C3-3 open femoral fracture caused by a low velocity gunshot injury. Note the lack of displacement of the fracture fragments suggesting less soft tissue damage. This was treated successfully with an intramedullary nail.

similar to that of Gustilo IIIb injuries if the entrance is over the medial subcutaneous border of the bone.

- High-energy wounds should be treated in the same way as open fractures caused by blunt trauma: a thorough tissue debridement with removal of all dubious and devitalized soft tissue and bone (Fig. 5-2).
  - Shotgun wounds in particular may contain wadding, which can cause bacterial contamination in a wound in which there is major soft tissue injury.
  - The presence of shotgun wadding is unusual if the gun was fired at a distance of more than 6 feet.
  - It may be difficult to know if a wound is associated with a low-energy or high-energy injury, and if there is any debate it is wise to undertake a formal surgical debridement.
  - High-velocity gunshot wounds should always be left open to facilitate drainage.

Role of Antibiotics

- There is also debate about the role of antibiotics in low-energy gunshot wounds.
- A number of studies have indicated no apparent benefit from the routine administration of antibiotics, but many surgeons feel that because the assessment of contamination is often very difficult, it is wise to administer an antibiotic, usually a first- or second-generation cephalosporin, for 48 to 72 hours.

- High-energy gunshot wounds should be treated with antibiotics in the same way as high-energy open fractures that follow blunt trauma (see Chapter 4).

Fractures

- Low-velocity gunshot fractures can be treated in the same manner as the equivalent closed fracture.
- Thus a number of low-velocity gunshot injuries are treated nonoperatively according to the principles outlined elsewhere in this book.
- High-velocity gunshot fractures should be treated in the same way as the equivalent fracture produced by blunt trauma.
- Thus surgical fixation is indicated using internal or external fixation techniques.
- There are a number of absolute indications for surgical stabilization of gunshot fractures (Box 5-3).

Joint Injuries

- A gunshot injury to a joint may be suggested by an entry wound close to the joint, by a joint effusion or hemarthrosis, by painful or restricted joint movement, or through imaging using plain radiographs or CT scanning.
  - It is important to remove intra-articular bullets or metallic debris to minimize later mechanical wear, lead synovitis, and arthropathy.

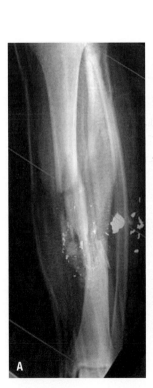
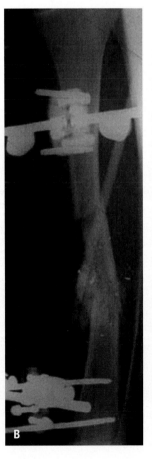
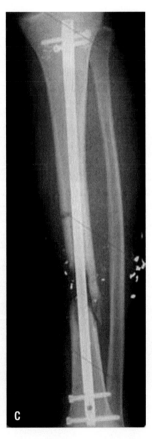

Figure 5-2   (A) A-P radiographs of a C3-3 open tibial fracture caused by a high velocity gunshot injury (B). A temporary external fixator was used (C) followed by definitive intramedullary nailing. Note the bone loss associated with major soft tissue damage.

BOX 5-3 INDICATIONS FOR FIXATION OF GUNSHOT FRACTURES

High-energy fractures
Fractures associated with vascular reconstruction
Fractures associated with nerve repair
Significant contamination (e.g., shotgun wadding)
Compartment syndrome
Multiple fractures

- Lead is twice as soluble in synovial fluid as in serum, and systemic lead toxicity has been reported as early as 2 days after injury.
- Arthrotomy is often required to ensure adequate debridement, but increasingly this is being performed arthoscopically, particularly in the knee joint.
- A 3-day course of a broad-spectrum antibiotic should be used.
- Gunshot injuries to the hip joint have been demonstrated to be associated with intra-abdominal injuries in 10% to 30% of cases.
  - Visceral contamination may cause septic arthritis and a poor outcome. If a gunshot injury to the hip joint is suspected, careful assessment of any intra-abdominal wound is mandatory.
  - Gunshot wounds to the shoulder joint may cause a pneumothorax and lung damage as well as considerable damage to the major vessels and brachial plexus.
- The knee is a common area for gunshot wounds.
  - Bullets passing through the knee without fracture may cause infection, but arthroscopic debridement and a short course of antibiotics is sufficient treatment.
  - Intra-articular damage is common, and 42% meniscal damage and 15% chondral damage has been noted after low-velocity gunshot injuries to the knee.
  - Intra-articular fractures can be devastating and femoral condylar fractures caused by bullets may be unreconstructable.

Spinal Gunshot Wounds

- As with all gunshot injuries, the spinal column and spinal cord can be injured directly or indirectly by the effects of cavitation.
- The direction of the bullet is important because if it passes through bowel there may be visceral contamination and infection.
- In the majority of cases, the bullet passes through the spinal canal or remains in the canal.
- It has been estimated that 20% of spinal gunshot injuries are cervical, 50% are thoracic, and 30% are lumbar in location.
- It is important to determine the extent of spinal cord injury.

- More than 50% of gunshot injuries result in complete cord injury.
- In 70% of injuries, the neurological level is at least one level higher than the vertebral level.
- In 20% of injuries, the neurological and vertebral levels are the same, and in the remaining 10%, the vertebral level is higher than the neurological level.
- About 25% of patients with a complete cord lesion will recover one level at 1 year after injury.
- About 33% of patients with incomplete lesions will improve with recovery varying from one level to full recovery by 1 year.
- There is debate about the role of bullet removal from the spinal canal, but there is little good evidence that it facilitates neurological recovery, and the only indication is in patients with incomplete spinal cord lesions who are showing signs of progressive neurological deterioration. Some studies have reported better neurological recovery after bullet removal from the lumbar spine, but, as yet, the evidence for this is weak, and laminectomy for bullet removal can further destabilize the spine.
- Treatment of the spinal fracture should be according to the general principles outlined in Chapters 18 and 19.
- If the bullet has passed through the abdomen, a 2-week course of a broad-spectrum antibiotic has been shown to reduce the incidence of later infection or osteomyelitis significantly.

SUGGESTED READING

Bartlett CS, Helfet DL, Hausman MR, et al. Ballistics and gunshot wounds: Effects on musculosketetal tissues. J Am Acad Orthop Surg 2000;8:21–36.
Bono CM, Heary RF. Gunshot wounds to the spine. Spine J 2004;4:230–240.
Eismont FJ, Lattuga S. Gunshot wounds of the spine. In: Browner BD, Jupiter JB, Levine AM, et al., eds. Skeletal trauma, 3rd ed. Philadelphia: Saunders 2003.
Fackler ML. Wound ballistics and soft tissue treatment. Tech Orthop 1995;10:163–170.
Johnson EC, Strauss E. Recent advances in the treatment of gunshot fractures of the humeral shaft. Clin Orthop 2003;408:126–132.
Molinari RW, Yang EC, Strauss E, et al. Timing of internal fixation in low-velocity extremity gunshot fractures. Contemp Orthop 1994;29:335–339.
Nowatarski P, Brumback RJ. Immediate interlocking nailing of fractures of the femur caused by low- to mid-velocity gunshots. J Orthop Trauma 1994;8:134–141.
Ordog GJ, Balasubramanium S, Wasserberger J, et al. Extremity gunshot wounds: I. Identification and treatment of patients at high risk of gunshot injuries. J Trauma 1994;36:358–368.
Ordog GJ, Wasserberger J, Balasubramanium S, et al. Civilian gunshot wounds: outpatient management. J Trauma 1994;36:106–111.
Rose RC, Kujisaki CK, Moore EE. Incomplete fractures associated with penetrating trauma: etiology, appearance and natural history. J Trauma 1988;28:106–109.
Tornetta P, Hui RC. Intraarticular findings after gunshot wounds through the knee. J Orthop Trauma 1997;11:422–424.
Wright DG, Levin JS, Esterhai JL, et al. Immediate internal fixation of low-velocity gunshot-related femoral fractures. J Trauma 1993;35:678–682.

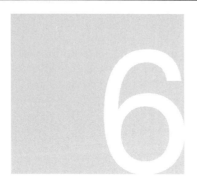

STRESS FRACTURES

Stress fractures were first cited by Breihaupt in 1855. He described fatigue fractures of the metatarsals in Russian army recruits. Prior to the 1960s, most descriptions of stress fractures came from the military, but since then there has been increasing awareness of the problems of stress fractures in athletes. Stress fractures occur as a result of overuse, usually in patients who give no history of specific trauma to account for the fracture. There are two types: fatigue fractures and insufficiency fractures. Fatigue fractures (Fig. 6-1) occur in normal bone as a result of repetitive loading, and insufficiency fractures (Fig. 6-2) occur in abnormally weak bone subjected to normal loads. Fatigue fractures usually occur in young patients and are most commonly seen in athletes and military recruits, although they are also seen in patients who pursue activities that involve repetitive loading such as ballet dancers. Insufficiency fractures are usually seen in the elderly and in patients who have diseases associated with abnormally weak bone.

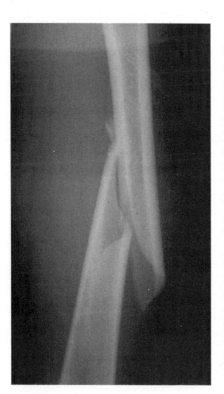

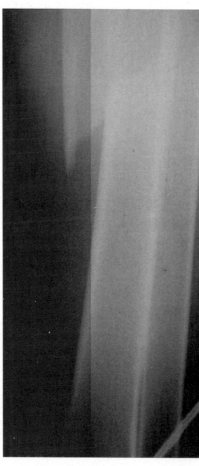

Figure 6-1 A-P and lateral radiographs of a fatigue fracture of the femoral diaphysis in a young military recruit.

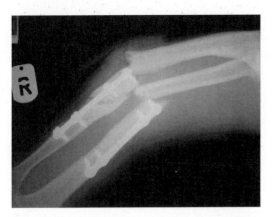

Figure 6-2   An unusual insufficiency in a forearm plated 42 years earlier. The fracture has occurred through screw holes. Note the long-standing ulnar nonunion.

ETIOLOGY

Fatigue Fractures

The etiology of fatigue fractures is multifactorial. The literature is somewhat contradictory, but this is probably because the two populations that are almost invariably studied are military recruits and high-performance athletes, and these groups are physically and psychologically very different. A review of the literature shows that many causes of fatigue fracture have been suggested, but good evidence indicates that a number of factors are in fact implicated. Box 6-1 lists the factors that have been shown to have some association with fatigue fractures as well as those with a possible association and those that have been suggested but for which there is little or no proof.

Gender

There is no doubt that women have a higher incidence of fatigue fractures than men, but the reason for this is complex. In military recruits the gender difference relating to fatigue fractures has been estimated to be as much as 12:1 in favor of female recruits. In athletes the difference is much less marked, with most studies suggesting that about 55% of sports-related fatigue fractures occur in

BOX 6-1 FACTORS ASSOCIATED WITH FATIGUE FRACTURES

Probable	Possible
Gender	Shoe wear
Height	Foot type
Weight	Dietary calcium intake
Bone diameter	Joint mobility
Muscle size	**No evidence**
Physical conditioning	Type of terrain
Training regime	Sleep pattern
Inadequate nutrition	Ethnic origin
Delayed menarche	Educational level
Reduced bone mineral density	Residence

women. There is also evidence that female athletes have a higher incidence of femoral, metatarsal, and pelvic fatigue fractures.

The increased incidence of fatigue fractures in women is mainly related to body size. There is good evidence that increased height and lean weight is associated with a lower incidence of fatigue fractures. This applies both to men and women, but obviously women are usually of smaller build. Comparison of similarly sized men and women shows no significant difference in the incidence of fatigue fractures. Studies have also shown there is a positive correlation between the incidence of fatigue fracture and diaphyseal diameter, indicating that bone size is probably the most important factor associated with gender variation.

In addition to bone size there is also good evidence that muscle size affects the incidence of fatigue fractures. Muscles would seem to have a protective role in resisting the mechanical forces that cause fatigue fractures. It has been suggested that the muscles attached to the ends of long bones convert tensile and shear forces into compression forces in much the same way as a tension band does in the management of olecranon or patellar fractures (see Fig. 34-11 in Chapter 34).

Nutrition

The literature regarding the role of dietary calcium in preventing fatigue fractures is contradictory. The bone mineral density of children between 2 and 16 years of age has been found to correlate with dietary calcium intake, but studies investigating the relationship between calcium intake and the incidence of fatigue fractures have shown inconsistent results, possibly because most of the patients studied were not actually calcium deficient. Eating disorders are definitely associated with an increased risk of fatigue fractures in female athletes, and the interrelationship among eating disorders, amenorrhea, and osteoporosis is well known. Inadequate dietary intake is likely responsible for the amenorrhea and the low bone mineral density. There is evidence that improved nutrition and consequent weight gain reduces the incidence of fatigue fractures in female athletes. The relationship between decreased bone mineral density and fatigue fractures in women is such that DXA scans (see Chapter 8) should be obtained in women who present with stress fractures, particularly if they are athletes and give a history of eating disorders or menstrual irregularity.

Delayed Menarche

Studies have shown that delayed menarche in women is associated with osteopenia and stress fractures. This has been shown in both female athletes and ballet dancers.

Physical Conditioning

The protective role of muscles has already been discussed, but there is evidence that the conditioning of muscles is also important. Fatigue compromises muscle function, and fatigued muscles do not protect against fatigue fractures as well as nonfatigued muscles. This explains why fatigue fractures tend to occur in military recruits who are suddenly subjected to an intensive exercise regimen. The same phenomenon is seen in athletes who suddenly increase their training schedules.

Exercise Regimens

The classic study of Milgrom et al. (1985) of 295 male Israeli military recruits showed that 31% developed stress fractures and 80% were in the femoral or tibial diaphysis. They showed that 53% developed symptoms in weeks 1 through 4 of basic training, and 22% developed symptoms in weeks 5 through 8. More recently the intensive exercise that relatively unconditioned military recruits are exposed to has been altered in a number of the armed forces around the world, and good evidence now indicates that a more gentle introduction to exercise is associated with a dramatic reduction in the incidence of stress fractures, presumably because of the effect of muscle conditioning previously discussed. In athletes it has been shown that 30% of high-performance runners may develop fatigue fractures within 1 to 2 weeks of increasing their training distance. This can occur even in extremely fit individuals averaging 115 km per week.

Shoe Wear

Different shoe wear does seem to have an effect on fatigue fractures, in that it has been shown the incidence of calcaneal fatigue fracture in military recruits diminishes if training shoes rather than combat boots are used for walking. There is no indication that different types of training shoes or different combat boots are associated with a lower incidence of fatigue fractures, however. An Israeli study has shown that the use of an orthotic device inside the combat boot reduces the incidence of fatigue fractures in military recruits.

Foot Type

There is some evidence that varus alignment of the lower limb, a cavus, or a pronated foot are all associated with an increased incidence of stress fractures, but in a condition that is clearly multifactorial there is little evidence that foot type plays a major part in determining the incidence of fatigue fractures.

Joint Mobility

There is some evidence that military recruits with less than 60 degrees passive external rotation of the hip have a higher incidence of tibial stress fractures, but, as with foot type, the evidence is weak and more studies are required.

BOX 6-2 COMMON CAUSES OF INSUFFICIENCY FRACTURES

Osteoporosis	Osteopetrosis
Inflammatory joint disease	Hyperparathyroidism
Rheumatoid arthritis	Scurvy
Juvenile chronic arthritis	Irradiation
Psoriatic arthritis	Drugs (e.g., corticosteroids, biophosphonates, methotrexate)
Ankylosing spondylitis	
Osteomalacia or rickets	
Diabetes mellitus	Previous arthroplasty and other limb surgery
Fibrous dysplasia	Previous fractures
Paget's disease	Vascularized fibular bone grafts
Pyrophosphate arthropathy	
Osteogenesis imperfecta	

Insufficiency Fractures

There are many causes of insufficiency fractures, of which osteoporosis is the most common. However, any disease or treatment associated with bone weakness may be associated with an insufficiency fracture. The most common associated conditions are shown in Box 6-2.

EPIDEMIOLOGY

Fatigue Fractures

Fatigue fractures usually occur in young adults. The average age for athletes and military recruits is 20 to 27 years. Women are more commonly affected than men. Analysis of the distribution of fatigue fractures shows differences among military recruits, athletes, and ballet dancers (Table 6-1). The information contained in Table 6-1 comes from a number of different studies, and obviously fatigue fractures of other areas have been reported.

Table 6-1 shows that the essential difference between military recruits and ballet dancers compared with athletes is that in military recruits and ballet dancers the fatigue fractures occur in the lower limb as a result of marching or

TABLE 6-1 RELATIVE FREQUENCIES OF DIFFERENT STRESS FRACTURES IN ATHLETES, MILITARY RECRUITS, AND BALLET DANCERS

Fracture location	Frequency (%)		
	Athletes	Military recruits	Ballet dancers
Tibia	42.9	53.4	22.0
Tarsus	19.8	2.9	—
Femur	9.0	31.6	—
Metatarsus	8.2	9.2	63.0
Fibula	8.0	1.5	—
Ribs	3.9	—	—
Spine	3.9	—	7.0
Pelvis	2.4	1.5	—
Ulna	1.0	—	—
Radius	0.6	—	—
Medial malleolus	0.2	—	—
Patella	0.2	—	—

prolonged dancing. The distribution of fatigue fractures in athletes depends on their sport, although runners have a similar distribution to military recruits, complaining of fatigue fractures of the femur, tibia, tarsus, and metatarsus in particular. The types of sport associated with fatigue fractures obviously vary in different countries, but in addition to running, sports such as basketball, volleyball, and football are associated with fatigue fractures mainly of the lower limb, whereas weight lifting, rowing, tennis, diving, and throwing sports are associated with upper limb fatigue fractures. In sports such as gymnastics, fatigue fractures of the upper and lower limbs may occur.

Insufficiency Fractures

There are no studies of the epidemiology of insufficiency fractures. Indeed, it would be almost impossible to undertake such a study. It is likely that the incidence of insufficiency fractures is rising given the fact that a greater number of patients with osteopenia and osteoporosis are in the community (see Chapter 8).

DIAGNOSIS

- The presenting complaint of fatigue fractures is gradually increasing pain in the area of the fracture exacerbated by exercise and particularly by the repetitive action that has caused the fracture. For example, runners complain of increasing pain on running, and rowers complain of increasing pain in the shoulder or base of the cervical spine on rowing as they exacerbate a fatigue fracture of an upper rib.
  - The pain tends to be relieved by rest.
  - There is usually no history of a particular traumatic event.
- Patients with insufficiency fractures may present in a similar way but complain of pain on walking rather than running.
  - In older patients, however, symptoms may be relatively mild and nonspecific, and pain may not be such a prominent feature as it is in younger patients.
  - In young female athletes, the clinical history should include information about menstrual irregularity and diet.
  - In older patients, it is important to see if there is an underlying cause for insufficiency fracture, and a careful systematic history should be taken, bearing in mind the conditions listed in Box 6-2.
- Physical examination may indicate the site of the stress fracture, but locating the point of maximum tenderness can be difficult, particularly if the stress fracture is in the proximal femur, pelvis, or spine.
- Many other musculoskeletal tissue lesions can mimic stress fractures. The diagnosis is therefore usually made radiologically.

Radiologic Examination

- Most fatigue and insufficiency fractures are diagnosed using standard anteroposterior and lateral radiographs.

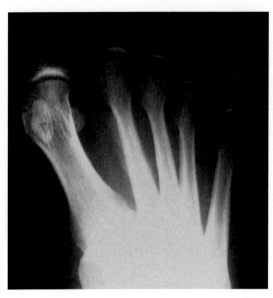

Figure 6-3 A stress fracture of the 2nd metatarsal. Initial radiographs were negative. Note the callus formation indicating fracture healing.

- The findings vary considerably, depending on the age of the fracture.
  - In the very early stage, radiographs may not show evidence of a fracture, and it is not unusual to diagnose a fracture at a later stage during the healing process (Fig. 6-3). Thus the radiologic findings may vary from failure to identify a fracture to significant callus formation.
- If there is doubt about the presence of a stress fracture, scintigraphy (Fig. 6-4) or MRI scanning can be used.
- Both are effective in diagnosing occult stress fractures, and studies have shown that both investigative methods are highly successful in diagnosing stress fractures associated with negative radiographs.
- MRI scanning is advantageous in that it shows the fracture line and associated periosteal edema, although this degree of visualization is rarely needed for treatment.

TYPES OF STRESS FRACTURE

Lower Limb

Table 6-1 shows that stress fractures of the lower limb are more common than those of the upper limb.

Femur
- Table 6-1 shows that stress fractures of the femur are relatively common, particularly in military recruits (see Fig. 6-1).
- Studies have shown that in military recruits about 34% of femoral fatigue fractures are in the neck, 27% occur in the mid-diaphyseal area, 27% in the lower diaphysis, and 11% in the medial femoral condyle.
- This distribution is somewhat different from athletes, where about 55% have been reported to occur in the distal diaphysis and about 24% in the femoral neck, the rest being mid-diaphyseal or condylar in location.

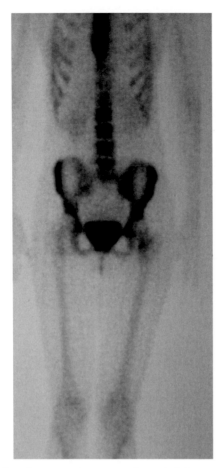

Figure 6-4   A bone scan showing uptake in the left proximal femur indicating a stress fracture.

Femoral Head

- Femoral head stress fractures have been described in military recruits.
- The presenting symptom is hip pain during prolonged marching.
- Treatment is symptomatic with the patient being rested and weight bearing restricted until the symptoms settle.

- Only about 10% of patients become pain free after treatment, with 20% of patients reporting marked pain and 70% reporting mild pain.

Femoral Neck

- Femoral neck stress fractures classically occur in long-distance runners and military recruits.
- They present as hip pain in younger patients who have undertaken recent unaccustomed long-distance running or walking (Fig. 6-5).
- The assumption is often made that proximal femoral stress fractures only occur in the femoral neck, but studies have shown they can also affect the greater and lesser trochanters.
- Fullerton and Snowdy (1988) classified femoral neck stress fractures into tension, compression, and displaced fractures depending on the position of the fracture in the femoral neck (Fig. 6-6).
- Treatment depends on the type of fracture.
  - Tension-type fractures should be treated surgically (see Fig. 6-5) with cannulated screws (see Chapters 21 and 34) because of the potential for late displacement.
  - Compression-type stress fractures can be treated nonoperatively by avoiding physical exercise and undergoing a regimen of protected weight bearing until union has occurred.
  - If union does not occur or there is evidence of displacement, cancellous screw fixation should be undertaken.
  - Displaced femoral neck stress fractures should be treated surgically.
  - Displaced fatigue femoral neck fractures in young patients should be treated with cannulated screws, but displaced insufficiency fractures in the elderly are better treated by hemiarthroplasty or arthroplasty (see Chapters 21 and 36).
  - Internally fixed fatigue fractures should be protected by nonweight bearing for about 3 months.

Femoral Diaphysis

- Stress fractures of the femoral diaphysis can either be fatigue (see Fig. 6-1) or insufficiency fractures (see Figs. 7-1 and 7-2).

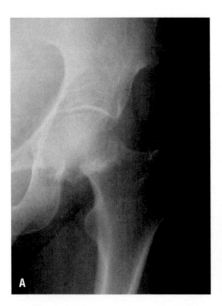
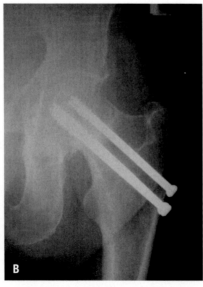

Figure 6-5   A-P radiographs of a 37-year-old patient who presented with hip pain after a half marathon. (**A**) The femoral neck stress fracture (**B**) was treated with cancellous screw fixation.

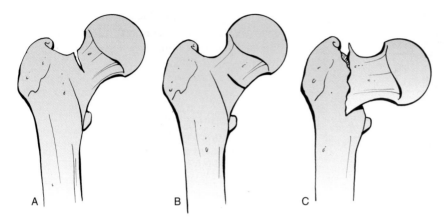

Figure 6-6 The Fullerton and Snowdy classification of femoral neck stress fractures. They are divided into tension (**A**), compression (**B**), and displaced (**C**) fractures.

- With an increasing incidence of elderly in the population, insufficiency fractures are becoming more common, and it is likely they will be encountered more frequently by orthopaedic surgeons.
- They are often periprosthetic fractures. Their treatment is discussed in Chapter 7.
- As with other stress fractures, fatigue fractures of the proximal diaphysis often occur after unaccustomed exercise.
- They are best treated by reamed intramedullary nailing (see Chapter 33), and union rates are almost 100%.
- Intramedullary nailing is recommended even if the fracture is undisplaced because nonoperative management is time consuming, painful, and frequently unsuccessful.

Distal Femur
- Distal diaphyseal fractures present in the same way as mid-diaphyseal fractures and should be similarly treated by intramedullary nailing.
- Undisplaced fatigue and insufficiency fractures of the femoral condyles can be treated nonoperatively by restriction of activity and nonweight bearing.
- Displaced condylar fractures should be treated by open reduction and internal fixation using conventional plating techniques (see Chapter 32).

Patella
- Stress fractures of the patellar are very unusual.
- Table 6-1 does show that they do occur in athletes, although cases have been described in basketball players.
- They usually occur in adolescent athletes.
- An insufficiency fracture has also been described in a cerebral palsy patient.
- The treatment of stress fractures of the patellar is normally nonoperative with restriction of activities until union.
- Partial patellectomy for a longitudinal stress fracture of the patella has been described.

Tibial Diaphysis
- Tibial stress fractures are usually transverse, although longitudinal fractures have been described.
- These have also been described in the femoral and fibular diaphysis, although very rarely.
- It is likely that longitudinal fractures of the tibia are in fact long insufficiency spiral fractures, which are difficult to visualize on a uniplanar radiograph.
- Most tibial fatigue fractures are usually seen in the proximal and middle thirds, whereas transverse insufficiency fractures occurring in older patients usually present in the distal third of the tibia usually close to the ankle joint (Fig. 6-7).

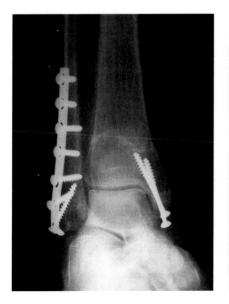
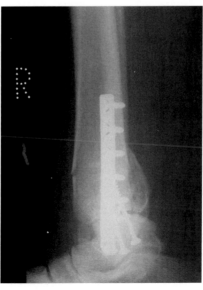

Figure 6-7 A-P and lateral radiographs of a distal tibial insufficiency fracture that occurred after an earlier ankle fracture.

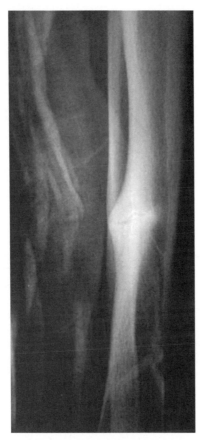

Figure 6-8   A posterior unicortical tibial stress fracture. This was successfully treated by intramedullary nailing.

- Because of the numbers of both cemented and uncemented knee arthroplasties being undertaken, however, proximal tibial insufficiency fractures are becoming more common.
- Most tibial fatigue fractures are treated nonoperatively with the use of a below-knee cast or patellar tendon bearing cast.

- Insufficiency fractures of the proximal tibia related to the presence of the cemented or uncemented arthroplasty can be treated nonoperatively if there is no evidence of any loosening of the implant.
  - If the implant is loose, revision arthroplasty is required.
- Tibial stress fractures may be complete or unicortical usually involving the anterior cortex but occasionally the posterior cortex (Fig. 6-8).
- These stress fractures may become chronic, with nonoperative management proving unsuccessful.
  - If this occurs, the fracture should be treated by intramedullary nailing (see Chapter 33). Good results have been reported.

Fibula
- Fibular fatigue fractures occur more commonly in athletes (Table 6-1).
- About 55% occur in the proximal fibula, with the rest being evenly distributed between the middle and distal thirds.
- There are case reports of longitudinal and bilateral fibular fractures in athletes.
- It is likely that longitudinal fibular fractures are insufficiency fractures.
- Most insufficiency fibular fractures occur distally in the fibula around the tibiofibular syndesmosis and are usually transverse (Fig. 6-9).
- Treatment is symptomatic with restriction of activity.
  - A cast may be used for symptomatic relief.
- An unusual cause of fibular stress fracture is following the use of a vascularized fibular graft to reconstruct tibial or femoral defects.
- A transplanted fibular graft takes a considerable time to hypertrophy and is therefore relatively weak for a prolonged period.
- Stress fractures have been documented to occur in these grafts.
- Treatment is symptomatic and surgery is rarely required.

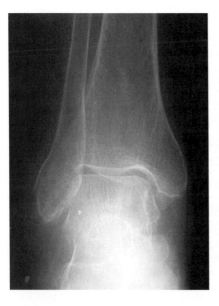
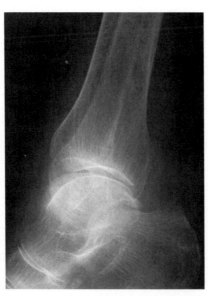

Figure 6-9   A stress fracture of the distal fibula.

Medial Malleolus

- Stress fractures of the medial malleolus are very rare.
- It is interesting that they differ from most stress fractures in that they are more common in men and virtually all are fatigue fractures occurring in younger patients.
- Most of these fractures have been associated with basketball or running, although a medial malleolar fatigue fracture has been recorded in a young gymnast.
- Patients complain of ankle pain, particularly on exercise.
- The treatment is usually symptomatic with rest until the symptoms settle, but internal fixation with two 3.5-mm cancellous screws (see Chapters 29 and 34) is advised if there is any evidence of displacement.

Tarsus

- Talar fatigue fractures are rare but have been reported in runners.
- They usually occur in the talar neck, but a stress fracture of the talar dome has been reported.
- Treatment is usually symptomatic, but if MRI imaging shows displacement it is advisable to fix the talar neck fracture with two 3.5-mm cancellous screws (see Chapters 30 and 34).
- A case of talar stress fracture following resection of a talocalcaneal coalition has been reported in an adolescent.

Calcaneus

- Calcaneal stress fractures are extremely rare with only a few being reported.
- They most commonly occur in military recruits, and it has been shown that alteration of shoe wear reduces their incidence.
- Treatment is nonoperative with restriction of activities until the fracture unites.

Midfoot

- Stress fractures of the navicular and cuboid bones are much more common in athletes than in military recruits.
- Navicular fractures are more commonly seen than cuboid fractures and have been reported to account for up to 80% of tarsal fatigue fractures in athletes.

- Cuboid fatigue fractures have been reported to be associated with plantar fascia disruption.
- Treatment is symptomatic with surgery being reserved for displaced fractures (see Chapter 30) or nonunions.

Metatarsus

- Table 6-1 indicates that metatarsal fatigue fractures are relatively common, particularly in ballet dancers.
- Even in athletes and military recruits, they account for about 9% of all fatigue fractures.
- Most surgeons are familiar with the classic march fracture of the second or third metatarsal diaphysis with the patient presenting with midfoot pain after a prolonged walk (see Fig. 6-3).
- The other relatively common location of metatarsal fatigue fracture is in the proximal third of the fifth metatarsal, and again these often occur in athletes or after walking (Fig. 6-10). They are also common in basketball players.
- Fractures of the proximal fourth metatarsal have also been reported in athletes.
- The relationship between foot shape and the incidence of stress fractures has been examined, and there appears to be a higher incidence of fatigue fracture of the lateral metatarsals in feet with a metatarsus adductus deformity.
- Again, the fifth metatarsal is most commonly involved followed by the fourth and third metatarsals.
- Fifth metatarsal stress fractures have also been reported after calcaneal osteotomy.

Upper Limb

- Fatigue and insufficiency fractures of the upper limb are much less common than those of the lower limb (Table 6-1).
- They are caused by repetitive movements and normally encountered in athletes, although occupation-related upper limb stress fractures have been reported.

Shoulder Girdle

- Fatigue fractures of the shoulder girdle are very rare.

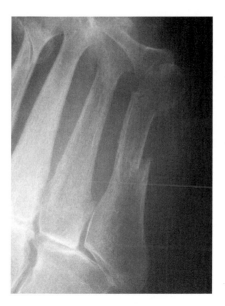
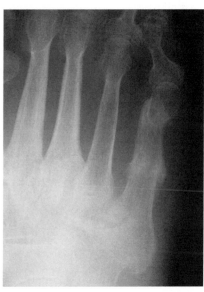

Figure 6-10 An insufficiency fracture of the 5th metatarsal. This is unusual in that it was segmental. It occurred in an 63-year-old patient with no history of injury.

- The most common examples of these are fatigue fractures of the clavicle, which occur mainly in rowers or in athletes involved in throwing events such as baseball.
- They have also been described in gymnasts and divers who take weight on their upper limbs.
- Acromial fatigue fractures have been described in weight lifters, a golfer, a car mechanic, and following the repetitive use of a screwdriver! An insufficiency acromion fracture has also been described.
- Treatment of fatigue and insufficiency fractures of the shoulder girdle is symptomatic and involves rest until the fracture heals.

Humerus

- Stress fractures of the humerus are relatively uncommon.
- As with shoulder girdle stress fractures, fatigue fractures of the humerus are more common in weight lifters and in throwing sports such as baseball.
- A proximal humeral fatigue fracture has been described, but most proximal humeral stress fractures are insufficiency fractures that occur in women treated many years earlier with radiation for breast carcinoma (see Fig. 12-7 in Chapter 12).
- In the early days of radiation treatment, the doses tended to be higher and less focused than they are now, and insufficiency fractures followed by nonunion are still encountered.
- Most humeral fatigue fractures are diaphyseal, and many have been documented in baseball pitchers, although they have been diagnosed in a swimmer and a badminton player.
- As with other upper limb stress fractures, treatment is normally nonoperative with restriction of activities until union occurs.

Ulna

- Stress fractures of the ulna are unusual, but when they occur they tend to be seen in weight lifters and throwers.
- As with humeral diaphyseal stress fractures, most ulnar fractures have been recorded in baseball players, although a number have occurred in different Japanese martial arts.
- They have also been described in tennis players, polo players, and baton twirlers, and they can be associated with the use of crutches.
- Treatment is nonoperative with cessation of activities until union.

Radius

- Stress fractures of the radius are less common than those of the ulnar.
- Distal radial fatigue fractures have been described in sports in which athletes bear weight such as gymnastics or diving.
- Radial diaphyseal fractures may also occur in gymnasts or in similar sports, but they can also be associated with racquet sports or golf.
- Again treatment is essentially symptomatic with restriction of activities until union of the fracture.

Hand

- Stress fractures of the hand are extremely rare.
- Hand fractures have been described in hockey and tennis players.
- Scaphoid fractures have been described in sports where athletes bear weight such as gymnastics.
- As with other upper limb fractures, the treatment is almost invariably symptomatic with restriction of activities until union occurs.

Ribs

- Table 6-1 indicates stress fractures of the ribs are surprisingly common.
- They are mainly associated with rowing, and it has been stated that they occur in 6% to 12% of high-level rowers.
- Upper rib fractures have also been reported in weight lifters and baseball pitchers, with lower rib stress fractures occurring in golfers and tennis players.
- The treatment is invariably nonoperative with cessation of activities until union occurs.

Sternum

- Sternal stress fractures are rare and most present as insufficiency fractures in the elderly.
- There is an association between increasing thoracic kyphosis and sternal insufficiency fracture.
- Fatigue fractures have been described in two military recruits doing triceps dips, and the condition has also been described in a wrestler.

Spine

Lumbar Spine

- Most spinal stress fractures occur in the sacrum.
- Both fatigue and insufficiency fractures occur, although the latter are more common.
- Fatigue fractures of the sacrum usually occur in long-distance runners, although they have been reported in volleyball and basketball players and in military recruits.
- Their importance is that the athlete will present with pain that mimics degenerative disc disease, which they may also have.
- Sacral stress fracture should be considered in athletes who present with low back pain, particularly if there is a history of eating disorders or menstrual irregularity.
- Treatment is by restriction of activity until union occurs.
- Insufficiency fractures of the sacrum are probably more common than was previously thought.
- With the increasing incidence of the elderly in society, it is likely that osteoporotic insufficiency sacral fractures account for some of the low back pain in the elderly.
- Osteomalacia is now less common in many countries but is still responsible for insufficiency fractures of the sacrum and pelvis.
- Sacral insufficiency fractures have also been reported after radiation, and it has been suggested that about 20% of patients have occult sacral insufficiency fractures after pelvic radiation for primary neoplasia.
- They have also been reported after the use of lumbosacral fixation in osteopenic women, and the condition

has even been reported after sexual intercourse in a 64-year-old woman with rheumatoid arthritis who was taking prednisolone! The treatment of sacral insufficiency fractures is obviously nonoperative with restriction of activities until union occurs.

■ Other spinal insufficiency fractures have been documented.

■ They occur in severe ankylosing spondylitis, and it is theorized that congenital spondylolisthesis may be caused by a stress fracture of the pars interarticularis.

■ Insufficiency thoracic fractures have also been diagnosed after spinal instrumentation for Scheurmanns disease and after lumbosacral arthrodesis.

Cervical Spine

■ Stress fractures of the cervical and upper thoracic spinous processes used to be relatively common in manual workers. The condition was known as clay shoveler's fracture.

■ It occurred mainly in laborers who performed activities involving lifting asymmetrically distributed weights with their arms extended, although it has also been reported in athletes and cricketers.

■ The condition is now rare because of the introduction of mechanical lifting aids.

Pelvis

■ As with sacral stress fractures, it is likely that most stress fractures of the pelvis are insufficiency fractures related to osteoporosis and occur in advanced old age.

■ They are probably one of the causes of pelvic or hip pain in elderly patients who fail to mobilize and in whom radiographs show no sign of a proximal femoral or pubic ramus fracture.

■ Fatigue pelvic fractures also occur, however, and, as with sacral fatigue fractures, they are usually seen in runners or military recruits.

■ The fractures usually occur in the pubic rami and present with localized groin pain.

■ Treatment is symptomatic and involves restriction of activities until union occurs.

■ Both fatigue and insufficiency acetabular fractures can occur.

■ An analysis of acetabular fractures in athletes and military recruits who presented with hip pain indicates that about 6% had fatigue fractures of the acetabulum.

　■ About 60% had acetabular roof fractures and 40% had anterior column fractures, with most of the latter patients presenting also with fatigue fractures of the pubic rami.

■ Insufficiency acetabular fractures are associated with acetabular prostheses and are an unusual cause of prosthetic loosening.

PAGET'S DISEASE

■ As Box 6-2 indicates, a number of diseases are associated with insufficiency fractures, but the classic metabolic bone disease in which insufficiency fractures occur is Paget's disease.

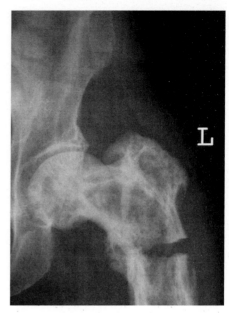

Figure 6-11 Paget's disease in a femur. The stress fractures start as microfractures on the tension (convex) side of the bone.

■ Paget's disease commonly presents in the skull, spine, pelvis, femur, and tibia, but insufficiency fractures usually occur in the femur.

■ It is more common in men, but the incidence of insufficiency fractures is higher in women, presumably due to their smaller bone mass and their increased susceptibility to osteoporosis (see Chapter 8).

■ Analysis of the most common sites of femoral insufficiency fractures in Paget's disease shows that about 21% occur in the femoral neck or trochanteric area, 29% occur in the subtrochanteric area, 21% in the proximal third of the femur, and 19% in the middle third and 11% in the distal third of the femur.

■ Pagetic fractures are usually related to the deformity that occurs in pagetic bone.

■ They usually start as transverse pseudofractures that start on the tension side of a bowed long bone (Fig. 6-11).

■ These may heal or extend to become a complete insufficiency fracture.

■ Treatment is symptomatic depending on the age, health, and functional status of the patient, but complete fractures are usually treated by intramedullary nailing with one or more femoral osteotomies being undertaken if the femur is significantly bowed.

■ Tibial diaphyseal fractures present in much the same way, and the treatment is similar.

SUGGESTED READING

Cook SD, Harding AF, Thomas KA, et al. Trabecular bone density and menstrual function in women runners. Am J Sports Med 1987;15:503–507.

Devas MB. Stress fractures. Edinburgh: Churchill Livingstone, 1975.

Egol KA, Koval KJ, Kummer F, et al. Stress fractures of the femoral neck. Clin Orthop 1998;348:72–78.

Fullerton LR, Snowdy HA. Femoral neck stress fractures. Am J Sports Med 1988;16:365–377.

Grundy M. Fractures of femur in Paget's disease of bone. J Bone Joint Surg (Br) 1970;52:252–263.

Kiuru MJ, Pihlajamaki HK, Ahovuo JA. Bone stress injuries. Acta Radiol 2004;45:317–326.

Lloyd-Smith DR, Clement DB, McKenzie DC, et al. A survey of overuse and traumatic hip and pelvic injuries in athletes. Sports Med 1985;13:8–10.

Matheson GO, Clement DB, McKenzie DC, et al. Stress fractures in athletes. A study of 320 cases. Am J Sports Med 1987;15:46–58.

Milgrom C, Giladi M, Stein H, et al. Stress fractures in military recruits. A prospective study showing an unusually high incidence. J Bone Joint Surg (Br) 1985;67:732–735.

Orava S, Puranen J, Aka-Ketola L. Stress fractures caused by physical exercise. Acta Orthop Scand 1978;49:19–27.

Zahger D, Abramovitz A, Zelikovsky L, et al. Stress fractures in female soldiers: an epidemiological investigation of an outbreak. Mil Med 1988;153:448–450.

PERIPROSTHETIC FRACTURES

Periprosthetic fractures occur in two circumstances: either around total joint prostheses used to treat arthritis (Fig. 7-1) or around the implants used to treat fractures, most of the latter occurring in the femur following the treatment of proximal femoral fractures in the elderly (Fig. 7-2). Although the incidence of periprosthetic fractures is relatively low, the large numbers of total joint prostheses being inserted combined with the increasing age and improved health of the population, together with the greater requirement for revision joint surgery, means that surgeons will encounter an increasing number of these difficult fractures.

EPIDEMIOLOGY

There are two types of periprosthetic fractures: intraoperative and postoperative.

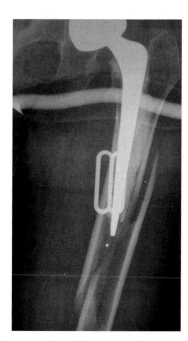

Figure 7-1   A periprosthetic fracture around a cemented bipolar arthroplasty.

Intraoperative Fractures

The incidence of intraoperative femoral fractures during cemented hip arthroplasty has been reported as between 0.4% and 27%, although most studies using cemented hip prostheses report an incidence of about 1%. The incidence of periprosthetic fracture during uncemented hip arthroplasty has been reported to be as high as 17.6%, but most series report an incidence of between 2.6% and 4%. In total knee replacement, the intraoperative fracture incidence is lower, about 0.1% for primary arthroplasty and 0.8% for revision arthroplasty. Intraoperative fractures of the acetabulum and glenoid are extremely rare, but the incidence of humeral periprosthetic fractures during total shoulder replacement has been reported to be as high as 3%. Intraoperative periprosthetic fractures around the elbow have been reported to occur in up to 12% of cases, although the incidence in most series is between 3% and 5%. Both the distal humerus and proximal ulna are affected.

Postoperative Fractures

The incidence of postoperative or late periprosthetic fractures is shown in Table 7-1. The incidence of postoperative femoral periprosthetic fracture in revision hip surgery is about three to four times higher than that associated with primary arthroplasty. In revision knee arthroplasty, the incidence is about double that of primary arthroplasty. Information about the incidence of periprosthetic fractures following shoulder and elbow revision surgery is sparse, but there is evidence that the incidence of periprosthetic fractures after elbow arthroplasty is lower if an unconstrained rather than a semiconstrained or constrained device is used.

Information about the incidence of periprosthetic fractures after proximal femoral fracture fixation is shown in Table 7-2. The data in Table 7-2 are taken from a study of 6,696 consecutive hip fractures from one center. Patients who present with proximal femoral fractures are at risk of subsequent periprosthetic fractures because of their age, bone quality, medical comorbidities, and susceptibility to further lower energy trauma. Table 7-2 shows that the incidence of late periprosthetic fracture is

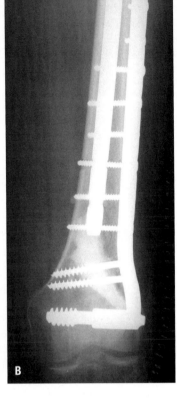
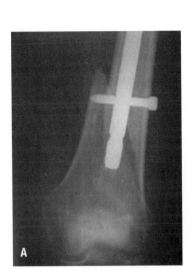

Figure 7-2 (**A**) A late fracture around the tip of a long reconstruction nail. (**B**) This was fixed with a dynamic condylar screw (DCS) system.

higher following the use of a proximal femoral nail or uncemented hemiarthroplasty, although, as with the use of arthroplasty for arthritis, it is revision surgery that is associated with the highest incidence of periprosthetic fracture.

RISK FACTORS

A number of risk factors are associated with an increased incidence of periprosthetic fractures (Box 7-1). Obviously,

TABLE 7-1 INCIDENCE OF DIFFERENT PERIPROSTHETIC FRACTURES

Fracture location	Range (%)	Average (%)
Hip replacement		
Acetabulum	0.02–0.8	Very rare
Femur		
Primary	0.8–2.3	1
Revision	2.8–4.2	3
Knee replacement		
Femur	0.9–2	1
Tibia	0–0.4	0.4
Shoulder replacement		
Humerus	0–2	<1
Elbow replacement		
Humerus and ulna		
Constrained	3.3–21	>10
Semiconstrained	3–17	5–10
Unconstrained	2.5–4.3	3–4
Ankle replacement		
Tibia and talus	0–22	3–5

BOX 7-1 RISK FACTORS FOR PERIPROSTHETIC FRACTURES

Osteopenia
Osteoporosis
  Primary
  Secondary
Bone disease
  Rheumatoid arthritis
  Osteomalacia
  Paget's disease
  Osteopetrosis
  Osteogenesis imperfecta
Neuromuscular disease
  Parkinson disease
  Neuropathic arthropathy
  Poliomyelitis
  Cerebral palsy
  Myasthenia gravis
  Ataxia
Revision arthroplasty
Uncemented implants
Narrow intramedullary canal
Previous surgery (e.g., osteotomy)

TABLE 7-2 PERIPROSTHETIC FRACTURES FOLLOWING DIFFERENT TYPES OF PROXIMAL FEMORAL FRACTURE FIXATION

Fixation technique	Hip fractures (n)	Implant-related fractures		Median time to fracture (wk)[a]
		(n)	(%)	
Compression hip screw	1734	34	1.2	78
Proximal femoral nail	254	10	3.9	30
Cancellous screws	939	15	1.6	4
Uncemented hemiarthroplasty	1953	54	2.8	9
Primary cemented arthroplasty	600	12	2.0	84
Revision cemented arthroplasty	210	16	7.6	9
Others	6	0	0	—

[a]The median time that elapsed before fracture is shown.
Data from Robinson CM, Adams CI, Craig M, et al. Implant-related fractures of the femur following hip fracture surgery. J Bone Joint Surg (Am) 2002;84:1116–1122.

many other bone and neuromuscular disorders could be associated with periprosthetic fractures, but these are the more common conditions. The most common risk factor is increasing age with its associated osteopenia, osteoporosis, and increased incidence of medical comorbidities. Revision arthroplasty is associated with diaphyseal damage caused by cortical thinning, cortical penetration by broaches, or the use of cortical windows to remove prostheses. Increasingly, patients have more than one implant in the femur. The combination of hip hemiarthroplasty or arthroplasty with a knee replacement, supracondylar nail, or condylar screw plate system leaves a stress riser between the implants, and insufficiency fractures in this area are relatively common.

There are specific risk factors related to each long bone. The risk factors associated with hip and knee arthroplasty are shown in Box 7-2. This shows that femoral periprosthetic fractures are more common in patients with hip dysplasias and abnormal femora, particularly if the intramedullary canal is narrow. Supracondylar femoral fractures are associated with distal femoral notching, caused by excessive removal of the anterior distal femoral cortex such that load transmission is transferred from cortical to cancellous

bone. This has been said to be responsible for up to 45% of supracondylar periprosthetic fractures. The principal problem with elbow arthroplasty is that about 95% of elbow arthroplasties are performed because of advanced rheumatoid arthritis, and a high incidence of periprosthetic fractures can therefore be expected.

HIP REPLACEMENT

The majority of periprosthetic fractures encountered by surgeons are in the femur and follow hip arthroplasty. There are a number of femoral classification systems relating to the location of the fracture with regard to the femoral prosthesis. Most classifications separate periprosthetic fractures according to whether the fracture is proximal, around the tip of the prosthesis, or distal to the prosthesis. The other important factor to be aware of is whether the prosthesis is stable or unstable. The Vancouver classification combines fracture location and prosthetic stability (Fig. 7-3). In this classification, periprosthetic fractures are divided into three types based on their location (Table 7-3).

Treatment

The treatment of periprosthetic fractures related to hip prostheses depends on whether the fracture is intraoperative or postoperative, its location, and whether the prosthesis is stable.

Type A Fractures

- Fractures involving the trochanters are usually intraoperative and caused by the attempted passage of a large prosthesis such as an uncemented hemiarthroplasty or an uncemented total arthroplasty.
- If an intraoperative fracture occurs around an uncemented press fit total arthroplasty, the treatment depends on the surgeon's assessment of implant stability.

BOX 7-2 RISK FACTORS FOR HIP AND KNEE ARTHROPLASTY

Hip replacement
Cortical stress risers (e.g., supracondylar nail)
Screw holes
Plates
Hip dysplasia
Proximal femoral focal deficiency
Knee replacement
Distal femoral notching

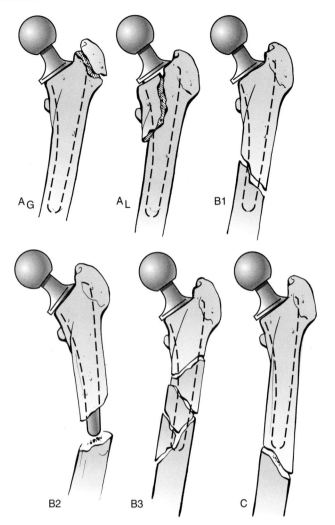

Figure 7-3   The Vancouver classification of periprosthetic femoral fractures.

■ If the implant is stable, the fracture can be wired, but if the fracture has rendered the implant unstable, it should be replaced with a cemented prosthesis after wiring of the fracture.

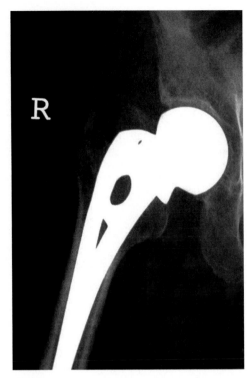

Figure 7-4   A type A fracture around an uncemented hemiarthroplasty.

■ Postoperative type A fractures (Fig. 7-4) can usually be treated nonoperatively unless the implant is unstable, in which case revision arthroplasty is required.

Type B Fractures
■ Most type B fractures occur postoperatively.
■ In B1 fractures with a stable prosthesis, the treatment is plating using a conventional plate or a plate designed to use a combination of screws and cable fixation (Fig. 7-5).
  ■ If a conventional plate is used, the screws must be placed around the implant.
  ■ This is usually possible with a cemented implant, but not if the implant is an uncemented press fit device.

TABLE 7-3 VANCOUVER CLASSIFICATION OF PERIPROSTHETIC FEMORAL FRACTURES[a]

		Incidence (%)	
Type	**Location**	**Intraoperative**	**Postoperative**
A	Proximal to prosthesis	80	5
B	Around or just below prosthesis	15	85
C	Below tip of prosthesis	5	10
Subtypes			
A_g	Greater trochanter fracture		
A_l	Lesser trochanter fracture		
B_1	Implant stable		
B_2	Implant loose		
B_3	Implant loose and bone stock inadequate		

[a]See also Figure 7-3.

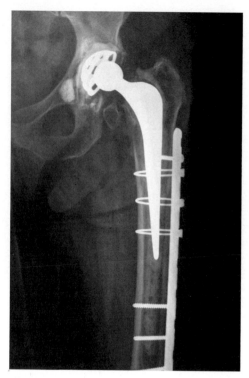

Figure 7-5   A stable type B fracture treated with a plate using screws and cables.

Under these circumstances, plate and cable fixation is useful.

■ An alternative is the use of a femoral or tibial cortical onlay allograft. The allograft is bivalved and wired around the fracture with an interface of morselized allograft.

■ Even if plate fixation is used, supplementary bone graft is useful in B_1 fractures. The literature suggests that 80% of B_1 fractures treated with plates will unite successfully.

■ The treatment of B_2 fractures is revision arthroplasty using a long-stem device supplemented by bone graft. Both cemented and uncemented prostheses can be used.

■ B_3 fractures are similarly treated with a long-stem prosthesis supplemented by onlay allograft.

   ■ If the bone defect associated with the B_3 fracture is large, a segmental allograft replacement may be used.

   ■ Alternatively, a tumor prosthesis can be used in elderly patients.

Type C Fractures

■ In type C fractures (Fig. 7-6), the prosthesis will usually be stable and the fracture can be treated with a conventional or locking plate or a retrograde supracondylar nail, depending on the exact location of the fracture and the presence of a coexisting knee replacement.

■ If the prosthesis is loose, the treatment is as for a B_2 periprosthetic fracture.

■ Type B and C intraoperative fractures are less common. They can occur during dislocation of a hemiarthroplasty or total arthroplasty prosthesis in revision surgery and are usually avoidable if adequate periacetabular soft tissue dissection is undertaken prior to attempted dislocation.

■ If they occur, they should be treated by the insertion of a long-stem arthroplasty.

Acetabular Fractures

■ Periprosthetic acetabular fractures are rare. They can occur intraoperatively and postoperatively.

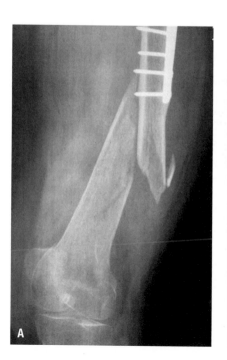

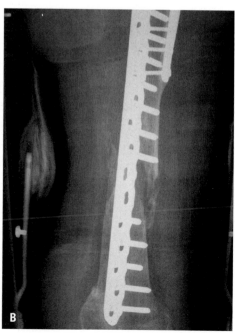

Figure 7-6   (A) Type C fracture in a 84-year-old patient who had had a McLaughlin pin and plate inserted 20 years earlier. (B) A locking compression plate was used to treat the fracture, which successfully united.

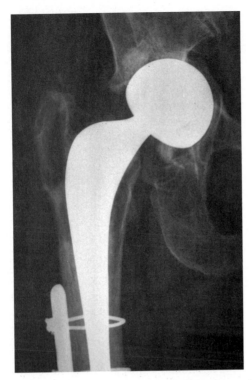

Figure 7-7   An acetabular fracture created by the insertion of a bipolar acetabular prosthesis.

- Intraoperative periprosthetic acetabular fractures are usually due to overreaming of the acetabulum or to the attempted insertion of a press fit cementless acetabular prosthesis into an underreamed acetabulum.
- They may also be caused by the attempted insertion of an overlarge hemiarthroplasty prosthesis (Fig. 7-7).
- Treatment can be nonoperative if the fracture is minor or by plate fixation, with or without grafting if the fracture is extensive.
- The prosthetic acetabulum can be inserted, but the patient should remain non–weight bearing for 3 months.
- Postoperative periprosthetic acetabular fractures are associated with pelvic osteolysis and with excessive acetabular reaming, causing hoop stresses in the acetabulum.

- These should be treated operatively with reconstruction of the acetabulum using internal fixation and grafting as required.

Proximal Femoral Fracture Fixation

The distribution of late periprosthetic fractures after proximal femoral fracture fixation is shown in Table 7-4. This shows that, like any prosthetic fracture, with hip arthroplasty there are relatively few type A fractures except following the insertion of an uncemented hemiarthroplasty when almost 20% of the periprosthetic fractures can be expected to be in the trochanteric area. Most periprosthetic fractures after proximal femoral fracture fixation are type B fractures, although the overall incidence of type B fractures is not as high as following total hip arthroplasty (Table 7-3). Between 13% and 47% of periprosthetic fractures after proximal femoral fracture fixation are type C fractures, the highest incidence occurring after the use of a compression hip screw.

- The treatment of periprosthetic fractures around implants used to treat proximal femoral fractures depends on the type of implant used and whether the fracture has united.
- Table 7-2 indicates that proximal femoral fractures associated with a compression hip screw or a proximal femoral nail will probably have united by the time the periprosthetic fracture occurs.
- This contrasts with proximal femoral fractures associated with the use of cancellous screws. These fractures tend to occur early because the three cancellous screws inserted into the femoral head and neck to treat the subcapital fracture are placed too close together.
  - A fracture occurs at the stress riser between the proximal ends of the screws, and an intertrochanteric or subtrochanteric fracture occurs close to the ununited subcapital fracture (Fig. 7-8).
  - This is best treated by removal of one of the cancellous screws and the placement of a dynamic hip screw up or close to the track of the removed cancellous screw. This will stabilize both fractures.
- If the proximal femoral fracture has united prior to the periprosthetic fracture, it is advisable to remove the

TABLE 7-4 DISTRIBUTION OF PERIPROSTHETIC FRACTURES AFTER PROXIMAL FEMORAL FRACTURE FIXATION

	Distribution (%)		
	Type A	Type B	Type C
Compression hip screw	2.9	50	47
Proximal femoral nail	—	80	20
Cancellous screws	—	86.7	13.3
Uncemented hemiarthroplasty	18.5	63	18.5
Primary cemented arthroplasty	—	75	25
Revision cemented arthroplasty	7.8	66.7	25.5

Data from Robinson CM, Adams CI, Craig M, et al. Implant-related fractures of the femur following hip fracture surgery. J Bone Joint Surg (Am) 2002;84:1116–1122.

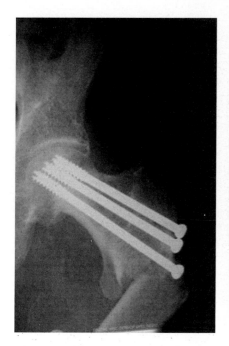
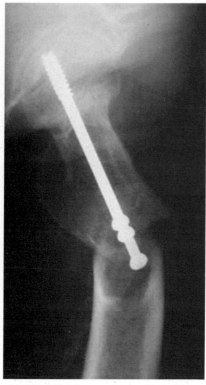

Figure 7-8 A-P and lateral radiographs of a fracture secondary to cancellous screw fixation of a femoral neck fracture. Note the incorrect location of the screws (see Chapter 21).

proximal femoral nail or dynamic hip screw and use a locked intramedullary nail or long reconstruction nail to stabilize the periprosthetic fracture.

■ Either will suffice, but in view of the age of these patients and their inevitable osteopenia, a reconstruction nail is preferred.

■ Periprosthetic femoral fractures following uncemented or cemented hemiarthroplasty, cemented bipolar arthroplasty, or cemented or uncemented total hip arthroplasty undertaken to treat proximal femoral fracture are treated in the same way as detailed for elective arthroplasty.

KNEE REPLACEMENT

Periprosthetic fractures of the distal femur are best classified using the Lewis and Rorabeck classification, which defines the displacement of the fracture and the stability of the prosthesis (Table 7-5).

■ Type 1 fractures are undisplaced supracondylar fractures associated with a stable prosthesis.

■ They can be treated nonoperatively or operatively with nonoperative management associated with a 1% complication rate compared with 5% for operative management.

■ Nonoperative management is preferred unless the patient cannot manage non-weight-bearing mobilization.

■ Any late displacement of a type 1 fracture should be managed operatively.

■ Type 2 fractures are displaced fractures with a stable prosthesis.

■ These should be managed operatively.

■ Operative management for type 1 and 2 fractures is best undertaken with a locked LISS plate (Fig. 7-9) or with a retrograde supracondylar nail if the design of the implant permits it.

■ Bone grafting can be used as required.

■ Successful operative treatment usually allows the patients to return to prefracture function at about 3 months.

■ Type 3 fractures are supracondylar fractures where the prosthesis is loose.

TABLE 7-5 LEWIS AND RORABECK CLASSIFICATION OF SUPRACONDYLAR PERIPROSTHETIC FRACTURES ASSOCIATED WITH KNEE ARTHROPLASTY

Fracture type	Fracture quality	Prosthesis
I	Undisplaced	Intact
II	Displaced	Intact
III	Undisplaced or displaced	Loose or failing (significant wear)

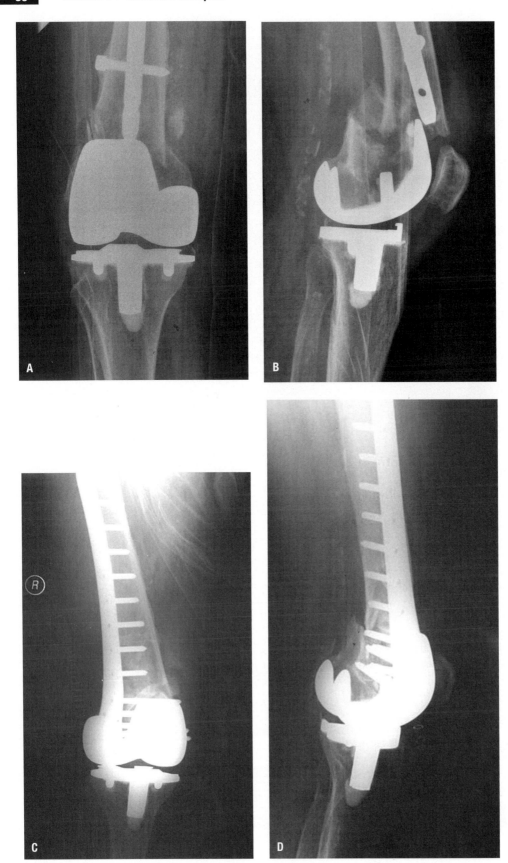

Figure 7-9   (A,B) A periprosthetic fracture between a reconstruction nail and a knee prosthesis. (C,D) This was successfully treated with a LISS plate.

■ These are treated by revision arthroplasty using a stemmed femoral component or, if the bone stock is poor, by the use of a segmental allograft to facilitate bone reconstruction prior to revision arthroplasty.

■ Alternatively, a tumor prosthesis can be used in elderly patients.

Proximal Tibia

■ Proximal tibial periprosthetic fractures are very rare.
■ They can involve one condyle, the metaphysis, or the tibial tubercle.
■ They are usually intraoperative, although postoperative insufficiency fractures of the metaphysis can occur.
■ Intraoperative condylar fractures are treated by screw fixation prior to insertion of the tibial component.
■ Metaphyseal fractures are best treated by the use of a cemented stemmed tibial component.
■ Tibial tubercle fractures should be repaired.
■ Postoperative proximal tibial metaphyseal periprosthetic fractures should be treated nonoperatively if the implant is stable and by revision if it is unstable.

Patellar Fractures

■ The incidence of periprosthetic patellar fractures is unknown. They are, however, relatively uncommon but can occur both intraoperatively and postoperatively.
■ Most intraoperative patellar fractures are caused by excessive resection of the patella during resurfacing. There is a higher incidence during revision surgery if the patella is recut.
  ■ They should be treated by tension banding and the later insertion of a patellar prosthesis once the periprosthetic fracture has united.
■ Most postoperative periprosthetic patellar fractures are vertical in orientation and do not disrupt the extensor mechanism.
  ■ Their treatment depends on the stability of the prosthesis.
  ■ If stable the fracture can be treated nonoperatively.
  ■ Unfortunately, many of these fractures are associated with an unstable prosthesis and should be treated by tension banding of the fracture and later insertion of a patellar prosthesis.
  ■ Alternatively, the patellar prosthesis can be discarded.

SHOULDER REPLACEMENT

Humeral Fractures

■ The classification of humeral fractures following the insertion of a total shoulder replacement or hemiarthroplasty is essentially the same as for the femur (see Fig. 7-3).
■ Type A intraoperative undisplaced greater tuberosity fractures can be treated by wiring or by suturing.
  ■ If they occur postoperatively they can be treated nonoperatively.

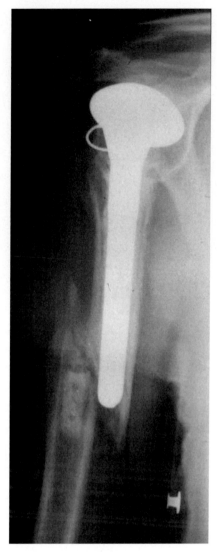

Figure 7-10   A type B postoperative humeral periprosthetic fracture.

  ■ Displaced postoperative greater tuberosity fractures should be treated operatively because of the alteration of shoulder function secondary to rotator cuff retraction.
■ Type B fractures associated with a stable humeral prosthesis (Fig. 7-10) should be treated by plate fixation, the unstable prosthesis being treated by revision arthroplasty.
■ Type C fractures distal to the prosthesis are treated similarly, using plates for stable prostheses and revision arthroplasty for unstable prostheses.

Glenoid Fractures

■ Periprosthetic fractures of the glenoid are extremely rare and intraoperative.
■ They should be treated by glenoid reconstruction prior to the insertion of the prosthesis.

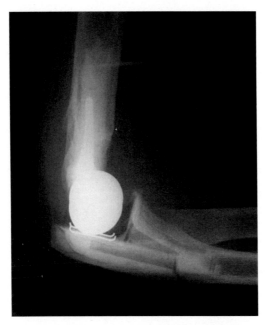

Figure 7-11   A periprosthetic elbow fracture involving the ulna.

ELBOW REPLACEMENT

■ Periprosthetic elbow fractures may involve the humerus or ulna (Fig. 7-11), and occasionally the stem of the implant may fracture.

■ Because most elbow replacements are carried out in patients with advanced rheumatoid arthritis, intraoperative fractures are relatively common.

■ These should be treated by fixation of the humerus or ulna or by the use of a long-stemmed implant that acts as an intramedullary device.

■ Treatment of postoperative fractures depends on the stability of the implant and the quality of the bone.

■ Undisplaced postoperative fractures around the humeral or ulnar stem of the prosthesis can be treated nonoperatively if the prosthesis is stable or by revision surgery if it is unstable.

■ The same basic approach is used for fractures proximal to the humeral component or distal to the ulnar component.

ANKLE REPLACEMENT

■ Total ankle arthroplasty is still a relatively uncommon procedure, but periprosthetic fractures can occur in the lateral or medial malleolus or in the talus.

■ There is little documentation about the treatment of such fractures, and it is suggested that basic surgical principles be followed.

■ If the prosthesis is stable, nonoperative management may be appropriate.

■ If the prosthesis is unstable, either revision arthroplasty or ankle fusion is appropriate.

■ Conversion of failed total ankle arthroplasty to ankle fusion using external fixation and bone graft can have a success rate of 90%.

SUGGESTED READING

Bourne RB. Fractures of the patella after total knee replacement. Orthop Clin North Am 1999;30:287–291.

Brady OH, Kerry R, Masri BA, et al. The Vancouver classification of periprosthetic fractures of the hip: a rational approach to treatment. Tech Orthop 1999;14:107–114.

Campbell JT, Moore RS, Iannotti JP, et al. Periprosthetic humeral fractures: mechanisms of fracture and treatment options. J Shoulder Elbow Surg 1998;7:406–413.

Ewald FC, Simmons ED, Sullivan JA, et al. Capitellocondylar total elbow replacement in rheumatoid arthritis: long-term results. J Bone Joint Surg (Am) 1993;75:498–507.

Howell JR, Masri BA, Garbuz DS, et al. Cable plates and onlay allografts in periprosthetic femoral fractures after hip replacement: laboratory and clinical observations. Instr Course Lect 2004;53:99–110.

Kumar S, Sperling JW, Haidukewych GH, et al. Periprosthetic humeral fractures after shoulder arthroplasty. J Bone Joint Surg (Am) 2004;86:680–689.

Lewallen DFG, Berry DJ. Periprosthetic fracture of the femur after total hip arthroplasty: treatment and results to date. Instr Course Lect 1998;47:243–249.

Lewis PL, Rorabeck CH. Periprosthetic fractures. In: Engh GA, Rorabeck CH, eds. Revision total knee arthroplasty. Baltimore: Williams & Wilkins, 1997.

Mabrey JD, Wirth MA. Periprosthetic fractures. In: Bucholz RW, Heckman JD, eds. Rockwood and Green's fractures in adults, 5th ed. Philadelphia: Lippincott Williams & Wilkins, 2001.

Morrey BF, Adams RA. Semiconstrained arthroplasty for the treatment of rheumatoid arthritis of the elbow. J Bone Joint Surg (Am) 1992;74:479–490.

Robinson CM, Adams CI, Craig M, et al. Implant-related fractures of the femur following hip fracture surgery. J Bone Joint Surg (Am) 2002;84:1116–1122.

Rorabeck CH, Taylor JW. Periprosthetic fractures of the femur complicating total knee arthroplasty. Orthop Clin North Am 1999;30:265–277.

Sarvilinna R, Huhtala HS, Puolakka TJ, et al. Periprosthetic fractures in total hip arthroplasty: an epidemiologic study. Int Orthop 2003;27:359–361.

Stuart MJ, Hanssen AD. Total knee arthroplasty: periprosthetic tibial fractures. Orthop Clin North Am 1999;30:279–286.

Tsiridid E. Dall-Miles plates for periprosthetic femoral fractures a critical review of 16 cases. Injury 2004;35:440–441.

OSTEOPOROTIC FRACTURES

With a rapidly aging population, osteoporosis has become a very important and expensive medical problem. Improved medical care in an increasingly affluent society has caused massive changes in population dynamics over a relatively short period. Osteoporotic fractures were always assumed to involve the vertebrae, proximal humerus, proximal femur, and distal radius, but in recent years improvements in road safety and workplace legislation in particular have led to a reduction in fractures in younger people, which, combined with an increase in fractures in the elderly, has led to major changes in fracture epidemiology. This is highlighted in Table 8-1, which shows information about the incidences of different fractures at different ages. The information is taken from the population discussed in Chapter 1. If the age characteristics of distal radial fractures are accepted as indicating an osteopenic fracture, then fractures of the pelvis, femoral diaphysis, distal femur, patella, and distal humerus are all probably usually secondary to osteopenia, with humeral diaphyseal and scapula fractures also showing similar age characteristics.

TABLE 8-1 AGE CHARACTERISTICS OF DIFFERENT FRACTURES

Fracture location	No.	Average age (y)	>65 y (%)	>75 y (%)	Osteopenic fracture?[a]
Proximal femur	692	80.5	91.2	78.9	Yes
Pelvis	91	69.6	72.5	57.1	Yes
Femoral diaphysis	55	68.0	69.1	58.2	Yes
Proximal humerus	337	64.8	57.0	36.2	Yes
Distal femur	24	61.0	50.0	41.7	Yes
Sesamoid	1	58.0	0	0	No
Patella	57	56.5	49.1	22.8	Yes
Distal humerus	31	56.4	45.2	29.0	Yes
Distal radius	1,044	55.5	45.8	28.2	Yes
Humeral diaphysis	69	54.8	40.5	17.4	Yes
Scapula	17	50.5	41.2	29.4	No
Proximal tibia	71	48.9	23.9	12.7	No
Ankle	539	45.9	20.8	10.2	No
Proximal forearm	297	45.7	24.2	13.5	No
Spine	40	43.5	17.5	12.5	No
Metatarsal	403	42.8	14.2	5.7	No
Calcaneus	73	40.4	12.3	4.1	No
Tibial diaphysis	115	40.0	17.4	11.3	No
Distal tibia	42	39.1	14.3	7.1	No
Clavicle	195	38.3	17.4	12.3	No
Finger phalanges	574	36.2	10.6	5.1	No
Midfoot	27	36.0	0	0	No
Toe phalanges	212	35.3	6.5	4.6	No
Forearm	74	34.6	13.5	12.2	No
Talus	17	30.5	0	0	No
Metacarpals	697	29.9	5.5	3.6	No
Total	**5,953**	**49.1**	**33.0**	**22.6**	

[a]Suggests whether they are osteopenic or osteoporotic.

Unfortunately, the data on spinal fractures is inaccurate because at most only 33% to 40% of people with osteoporotic vertebral fractures are admitted to the hospital. In addition to the information presented in Table 8-1, a review of the fracture distributions presented in Table 1-2 shows that types E and F mainly affect older patients. As fractures of the olecranon and proximal radius and ulna and bi- and tri-malleolar ankle fractures show these distributions, it seems likely they are also related to osteopenia or osteoporosis.

The scope of the problem is considerable. It has been estimated that 15% of postmenopausal white women and 35% of women above 65 years of age in the United States are osteoporotic. Thirty-two percent of women and 17% of men who reach 90 years of age sustain a proximal femoral fracture, and although patients with proximal femoral fractures account for only 7% of fractures in the United States, they account for 52% of hospital bed days. There is also good evidence that the incidence of proximal femoral fractures continues to rise, particularly in men.

The cost of treating osteoporotic fractures has been estimated as $13.8 billion per year in the United States and 1.7 billion pounds ($2.7 billion) in the UK. There seems little doubt that the problems and expense associated with osteoporotic fractures will continue to increase and will probably assume a dominant role in the health care systems of many countries over the next 20 to 30 years.

DEFINITION

Osteoporosis is an age-related skeletal disorder characterized by reduction of bone mass that increases the risk of fracture. There is confusion about the relationship between age-related *osteopenia* and *osteoporosis,* with both terms often used synonymously. The World Health Organization definition of osteoporosis is that it exists when the bone mass is at least 2.5 standard deviations below the ideal peak bone mass. If the bone mass is within 1 standard deviation of the ideal peak bone mass, the patient is considered to have normal bone. If the bone mass is between 1 and 2.5 standard deviations below peak bone mass, the patient is osteopenic. It must be understood that the definition is arbitrary. The U.S. Food and Drug Administration has taken 2 standard deviations below peak bone mass as a level at which treatment for osteoporosis should be instituted, and there is evidence that even if the bone mass is 1 standard deviation below peak bone mass, the incidence of fractures rises. It has been shown that for each increase of 1 standard deviation below peak bone mass, there is a 1.7 to 1.8 times increase in incidence of distal radial fractures and a 2.6 times increase in proximal femoral fractures. Osteopenia and osteoporosis should be thought of as an age-related reduction of bone mass associated with an increasing incidence of fracture, with treatment recommended at 2 to 2.5 standard deviations below peak bone mass.

It is also important to realize that osteoporosis is only one factor in the etiology of age-related fractures. A number of the factors associated with age-related fractures are shown in Box 8-1. Many patients with a low bone mass do not have other additional risk factors and therefore are at a low risk of sustaining an osteoporotic fracture.

BOX 8-1 RISK FACTORS FOR OSTEOPENIC OR OSTEOPOROTIC FRACTURES

Bone mass
Rate of current bone loss
History of previous low-energy fracture
History of low-energy fracture in parent or sibling
Body weight <85% of ideal weight
Recent weight loss
Falls
Causes of primary osteoporosis (see Box 8-2)
Causes of secondary osteoporosis (see Box 8-2)

BONE MASS

Peak bone mass is determined by a number of factors listed in Box 8-2. Most racial studies have been undertaken in the United States, where it has been demonstrated that the white population has a significantly higher incidence of osteoporotic fractures than the black population. Genetic factors account for much of the variation in bone mass, but hormonal factors play a significant role. Both men and women show a dramatic increase in bone mass during puberty, and it seems likely that diet and physical exercise may play an important role at this time. Male puberty ends later than female puberty, and consequently peak bone mass in males is achieved later. The age of pubertal onset is important, with delayed puberty associated with a lower bone mass. Once peak bone mass has been achieved, studies indicate that bone mass steadily deteriorates throughout life. This is true of both cortical and cancellous bone. In women the loss of bone mass accelerates after the menopause with an increase of about 2% bone loss per year, the increase greater in cancellous than in cortical bone. The increase in bone loss tends to level off between 5 and 10 years after menopause.

Studies of the effect of age-related changes in both cortical and cancellous bone have been undertaken. These

---

BOX 8-2 CAUSES OF OSTEOPOROSIS

Primary factors
Race
Genetic factors
Hormonal factors
Diet
Physical activity
Secondary factors
High alcohol consumption
Smoking
Drugs: corticosteroids, chemotherapy, benzodiazepines, anticonvulsants
Hypogonadism
Decreased renal function
Vitamin D deficiency
Hyperparathyroidism
Thyrotoxicosis
Gastrointestinal disorders
Organ transplantation
Immobility

have shown that in cortical bone the ultimate stress, ultimate strain, and energy absorption decreases by 5%, 9%, and 12% per decade and that changes in bone porosity account for 76% of the reduction in bone strength. An equivalent study in cancellous bone showed that the compressive strength decreased by 8.5% per decade, and bone density also decreased significantly with age. It was found that changes in bone density accounted for 92% of the reduction in the mechanical strength of cancellous bone. These and other studies have shown that osteoporosis is essentially a mechanical problem relating to thinning of bone trabeculae and bone cortices, associated with an increased degree of porosity. In cortical bone this is partially compensated by an increase in bone diameter during aging. The rapid bone loss after menopause in females is due to increased osteoclasis and consequent trabecular damage.

CAUSES OF OSTEOPOROSIS

Age-related bone loss may be affected by any of the secondary factors detailed in Box 8-2. Studies indicate that about 35% of women and 50% of men who present with symptomatic vertebral fractures have a secondary cause of osteoporosis in addition to primary bone loss. One of the most common causes of osteopenia is the use of corticosteroids, and even low-dose oral or inhaled cortical steroids have been reported to increase the rate of bone loss in the calcaneus and distal and proximal radius by two to three times in patients compared with controls. It can be difficult to separate the effects of corticosteroids from underlying diseases such as rheumatoid arthritis, which are associated with osteoporosis, and the combination of both disease and treatment greatly increases the risk of fracture.

Hypogonadism in males can be a particular problem if puberty is delayed. Androgens increase cortical thickness through both periosteal and endosteal growth as well as by increasing trabecular bone formation at the epiphyses. Prepubertal hypogonadism can be treated successfully by testosterone, with the bone mineral density increased by up to 26%. The effects of long-standing adult hypogonadism can also be similarly treated. Other diseases associated with osteoporosis are listed in Box 8-2.

There is evidence that moderate alcohol consumption may be associated with an increase in bone mineral density, but that alcohol abuse is associated with osteoporosis and in particular with an increased fracture risk. Excessive alcohol intake lowers the bone mineral density, but there are a number of other factors to take into consideration because the excessive use of alcohol is also associated with falls, poor nutrition, increased renal excretion of calcium and magnesium, malabsorption of calcium, and secondary hypogonadism. Alcoholism has been shown to be associated with a 2.8 times increase in the risk of proximal femoral fractures, with cirrhosis associated with a 3.5 times increase.

In recent years it has become clear that organ transplantation is associated with osteoporosis. It is said to affect cancellous more than cortical bone. Most of the information has come from patients undergoing cardiac transplantation, although there is good evidence of moderate to severe osteoporosis after renal and liver transplantation as well. It seems likely that the patients undergoing transplantation have a diminished bone mass prior to surgery, but that the use of immunosuppressive therapy in particular causes postoperative osteoporosis.

DIAGNOSIS

Radiologic Examination

■ The radiologic features of osteoporosis are diffuse demineralization and cortical thinning (Fig. 8-1) with

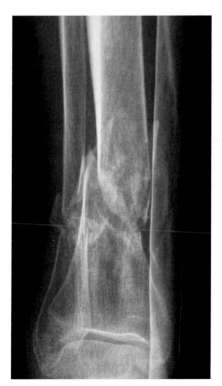
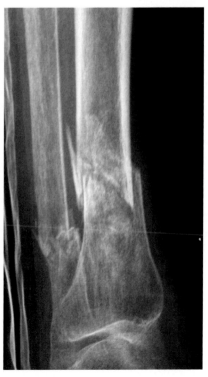

Figure 8-1 A-P and lateral radiographs illustrating cortical osteoporosis. Note the cortical thinning and diffuse demineralization.

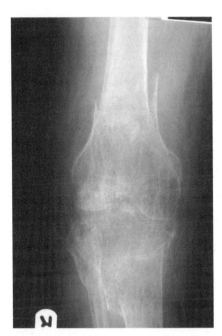
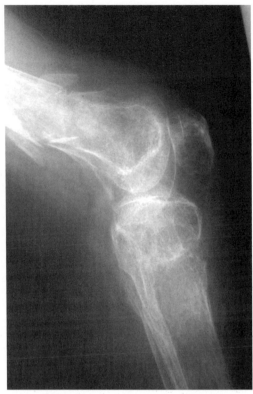

Figure 8-2   A-P and lateral radiographs illustrating cancellous osteoporosis. There is significant demineralization and increased space between the trabeculae. The patient had had a previous insufficiency fracture of the proximal tibia.

increased space between trabeculae seen in cancellous bone (Fig. 8-2).

- There has to be a considerable loss of bone mass, however, before osteoporosis is obvious on plain radiographs.
- A 15% to 20% reduction of anterior, posterior, or central vertebral height is accepted as a radiologic definition of osteoporosis, but the best way of assessing osteoporosis is with dual X-ray absorptiometry (DXA).
- DXA scanning is associated with low radiation (5 mrad) and a precision of 1% in the spine and 3% to 4% in the proximal femur.
- It is also associated with an accuracy of between 4% and 6%.
- There are four main indications for assessing bone mass with a DXA scan (Box 8-3).

BOX 8-3 INDICATIONS FOR ASSESSMENT OF BONE MASS WITH DXA SCAN

- Diagnosis of osteopenia or osteoporosis
- Confirmation of suspected radiographical demineralization
- Documentation of disease processes associated with osteopenia (see Box 8-2)
- Assessment of the effect of the disease processes or treatment

Risk Assessment

Assessment of fracture risk may be global or site specific. Spine and femoral neck DXA scans are equally good predictors of global fracture risk. This is most likely to be used by orthopaedic surgeons. Site-specific assessment can be used, but it has in fact been shown that the risk of spinal fracture is as well predicted by proximal femoral scanning as by spinal scanning. Site-specific scanning may be used if a particular body area is of interest, however.

- Bone mass is expressed as either a T score or a Z score.
  - The T score expresses bone mineral density as the number of standard deviations by which the given value differs from the mean peak bone mass. The T score provides an indication of the risk of developing fractures, and this risk increases with decreasing T scores.
  - The Z score expresses bone mineral density as the number of standard deviations by which the given value differs from the bone mineral density of an age-matched and sex-matched reference group.

PREVENTION

- The most important aspect of minimizing osteoporotic fractures is preventing osteoporosis.
- There are two main principles.

- First, the peak bone mass should be as high as possible, and this is largely determined during adolescent growth.
- Second, the excessive loss of bone mass in post-menopausal women should be minimized.

- Box 8-2 shows the primary factors associated with osteoporosis.
- Peak bone mass is improved by adequate diet, normal hormonal status, and physical activity.
- Calcium and vitamin D levels must be appropriate for the patient's age, and although osteomalacia is now relatively unusual in the developed world, dietary calcium intake is often deficient, particularly in adolescents, and calcium supplements, particularly in adolescent girls, are useful.
  - There is evidence that patients who take supplementary dietary calcium have a lower rate of bone loss.
  - Supplementary vitamin D is useful in patients who are deficient in vitamin D, but there is less evidence that the administration of vitamin D to vitamin D–competent patients is indicated.
- Calorific intake should be monitored, as should the ideal body weight. Inappropriately low body weight is associated with osteoporosis.
- Amenorrhea and oligomenorrhea should be investigated and treated in women as should hypogonadism in males.
- Smoking and excessive alcohol intake obviously should be avoided, and the diseases listed in Box 8-2 should be treated.

Fall Prevention and Protection

- Table 1-4 shows that falls from a standing height are responsible for almost half of all fractures in a Western population.
- Prevention of falls is clearly important (Box 8-4).
- The use of hip protectors and exercise regimens in the elderly have been shown to be somewhat advantageous, but the problem of falls is multifactorial and more research is required.

Estrogen

- Estrogen levels in women start to decline in their late 30s and early 40s.

BOX 8-4 IMPORTANT FACTS ABOUT FALLS FROM A STANDING HEIGHT

- Falls from a standing height cause 45% to 50% of all fractures.
- 33% of all patients >65 years, living in the community, fall each year.
- 50% to 60% of patients in nursing and residential care fall each year.
- 3% to 12% of falls result in fractures.
- <1% of individual falls cause hip fractures, but the annual incidence of hip fractures in frequent fallers is about 15%.
- 23% of injury-related falls in patients >65 years cause death.

- Studies have indicated that the administration of estrogen to perimenopausal women minimizes bone loss in 80% of patients.
- It has been demonstrated to reduce the rate of vertebral and proximal femoral fractures by 50% and 25%, respectively.
- Potential complications are an increase in the incidence of endometrial and breast carcinoma.
- Estrogen replacement therapy is an effective method of maintaining bone mass and preventing fractures, but it is contraindicated in women with a family history of breast carcinoma, thrombophlebitis, or stroke.
- The benefits of estrogens cease within 5 years of discontinuing its use.
- It is interesting to note that the risk of intracapsular fracture reverts to normal more quickly than the risk of extracapsular fracture.

Testosterone

- About 16% of males with hypogonadism have vertebral crush fractures.
- Testosterone improves calcium balance and increases bone mass, the effect being more obvious in adolescent males with open epiphyses.
- Thus testosterone should be used to treat young males with hypogonadism.
- Some evidence indicates that testosterone increases bone mass in normal males, but little evidence shows an associated reduction in fractures in older males who take testosterone.
- Currently it is not in use as a general treatment for male osteoporosis.

Bisphosphonates

- Bisphosphonates have become important drugs in the treatment of osteoporosis.
- Etidronate is a first-generation bisphosphonate used for the treatment of Paget's disease but has been reportedly effective in osteoporosis.
- Today third-generation bisphosphonates are widely used.
- Alendronate has been shown to increase bone mass in the vertebral column by 2% to 4% and in the proximal femur by 1% to 2% per year depending on the dose.
- Risedronate has also been shown to increase bone mass and to reduce the incidence of vertebral fractures by up to 65%.
- The key to the success of these medications will be if they reduce the incidence of other fractures associated with falls, and there is less evidence of this at the moment.
- Thus for the drugs to be effective, the patients' tendency to fall must be reduced.
- The principal complications are esophageal irritation and gastrointestinal upset, although some patients report bone pain.

Other Agents

- Calcitonin binds to osteoblasts and decreases their activity and numbers. Studies suggest it is effective in stabilizing and increasing spinal bone mass in early and late menopausal women, and its use is associated with a decrease in vertebral fractures but not proximal femoral fractures.

- It has been used successfully in treating localized regional osteoporosis.
- It is usually admitted as a nasal spray, and rhinitis appears to be the main side effect.

- Estrogens, bisphosphonates, and calcitonin work mainly by preventing bone resorption.
- If the main problem is lack of osteoblastic bone, agents that stimulate osteoblast function are required.
- Sodium fluoride has been found to increase spinal bone density and to decrease the incidence of vertebral fractures.

  - It is not a first-line agent for the treatment of osteoporosis.

SUGGESTED READING

Ahlborg HG, Johnell O, Karlsson MK. An age-related medullary expansion can have implications for the long-term fixation of hip prostheses. Acta Orthop Scand 2004;75:154–159.

Ahlborg HG, Johnell O, Nilsson BE, et al. Bone loss in relation to menopause: a prospective study during 16 years. Bone 2001; 28:327–331.

Bates DW, Black DM, Cumming SR. Clinical use of bone densitometry: clinical applications. JAMA 2002;288:1898–1900.

Cummings SR, Black DM, Thompson DE. Effect of alendronate on risk of fracture in women with a low bone density but without vertebral fracture: results from the Fracture Intervention Trial. JAMA 1998;280:2077–2082.

Findlay SC, Eastell R, Ingle BM. Measurement of bone adjacent to tibial shaft fracture. Osteoporos Int 2002;13:980–989.

Hasserius R, Karlsson MK, Nilsson BE, et al. Prevalent vertebral deformities predict increased mortality and increased fracture rate in both men and women: a 10-year population-based study of 598 individuals from the Swedish cohort in the European Vertebral Osteoporosis Study. Osteoporos Int 2003;14:61–68.

Ingle BM, Hay SM, Bottjer HM, et al. Changes in bone mass and bone turnover following ankle fracture. Osteoporos Int 1999; 10:408–415.

Johnell O, Kanis J. Epidemiology of osteoporotic fractures. Osteoporos Int 2004, E-pub.

Johnell O, Kanis JA, Oden A, et al. Mortality after osteoporotic fractures. Osteoporos Int 2004;15:38–42.

Karlsson M. Is exercise of value in the prevention of fragility fractures in men? Scand J Med Sci Sports 2002;12:197–210.

Lane JM, Nydick M. Osteoporosis: current modes of prevention and treatment. J Am Acad Surg 1999;7:19–31.

Lane JM, Russell L, Kahn SN. Osteoporosis. Clin Orthop 2000; 373:139–150.

Lucas TS, Einhorn TA. Osteoporosis: the role of the orthopedist. J Am Acad Orthop Surg 1993;1:48–56.

PATHOLOGICAL FRACTURES

The term *pathological fracture* is usually applied to a fracture that occurs through an area of weakness in the bone caused by a primary benign or malignant tumor or, more commonly, by a metastatic deposit (Fig. 9-1) or multiple myeloma (Fig. 9-2). It is these conditions that are discussed in this chapter. The term *pathological fracture* can also refer to stress or osteoporotic fractures, discussed in Chapters 6 and 8.

ETIOLOGY

Most pathological fractures occur as a result of metastatic spread or multiple myeloma. Primary bone tumors are very rare, and only about 10% of patients who present with primary bone tumors have an associated fracture. Box 9-1 lists a number of the more common primary and secondary malignant tumors and benign tumors that may present with fractures. Remember, however, that virtually any tumor can be associated with a fracture.

Metastases

Metastases account for most of the pathological fractures seen by orthopaedic surgeons. Fractures are a relatively uncommon complication of metastases, with only 4% of patients who have metastases presenting with a fracture. The incidence varies with the type of tumor and location

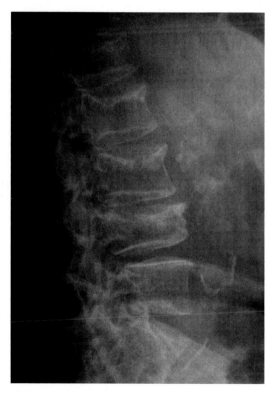

Figure 9-1 A metastatic deposit from breast carcinoma that has caused a pathological fracture.

Figure 9-2 Pathological lumbar fractures caused by multiple myeloma.

of the metastatic deposit. The skeleton is the third most common site of involvement by metastatic disease after the lung and liver. Data from autopsies have shown that about 70% of patients with solid tumors have skeletal metastases, although only about 20% are symptomatic. All solid tumors may metastasize to the skeleton, but about 75% of metastases are secondary to breast, prostate, lung, and kidney tumors. The other tumor commonly to metastasize to bone is thyroid. Autopsy studies have indicated that 80% of patients with breast cancer may have skeletal metastases compared with 85% of patients with prostatic carcinoma, 50% with thyroid carcinoma, 44% with lung carcinoma, and 30% with renal cell carcinoma.

Metastatic fractures may be the initial sign of the presence of a tumor or may be the first sign of recurrent disease. If this is the case, the period between the detection of the primary tumor and the later metastases may vary considerably, and in patients with breast or thyroid tumors there may be a period of 10 to 15 years before skeletal metastases become apparent.

Survival rates for patients with skeletal metastases vary, but in general the prognosis is poor (Table 9-1), with the median survival for patients with bone metastases from thyroid carcinoma 48 months compared with 40 months for prostate carcinoma, 24 months for breast carcinoma, and 6 months for lung carcinoma and melanoma. If both skeletal and visceral metastases are present, the prognosis is worse. Renal cell metastases are often solitary, and if successfully treated with wide excision the prognosis is often favorable. If there is a fracture associated with a renal cell metastasis, however, the prognosis is worse.

Tumor Spread

Three interrelated processes are important in the development of skeletal metastases. The ability of tumor cells to travel to a distant site varies and depends on the loss of cell contact inhibition and the production of tumor angiogenesis factor and angiogenin. Cell contact inhibition is regulated by cell adhesion molecules, and the expression of these molecules has to be altered to permit metastatic spread.

The spread of metastases is clearly impossible without a vascular or lymphatic channel through which the deregulated cells can spread. Neovascularization is facilitated by the production of tumor angiogenesis factor and angiogenin by the tumor cells. They are able to cross the vascular basement membrane and enter the venous and lymphatic systems. Once in the venous system, metastases tend to occur in sites that are rich in vascular sinuses and hemopoietic marrow (e.g., in the spine, pelvis, proximal femur, and proximal humerus), although other locations are possible (see Table 9-1). There are also regional variations presumably related to blood supply, with breast carcinoma metastasizing to the thoracic spine and prostatic carcinoma to the lumbar spine. There is an imbalance between metastatic spread and the osseous circulation, however. Bone receives about 10% of cardiac output but has a higher metastatic tumor prevalence than other sites that have a greater blood flow. There would therefore seem to be a third factor that influences metastatic spread. Tumor cells leave the vasculature and enter bone by producing proteolytic enzymes. Osteocalcin is thought to act on tumor cells as a chemotactic agent. Tumor infiltration of bone is a multifactorial process that has yet to be fully defined.

TABLE 9-1 THE INCIDENCE, COMMON SITES, TYPE, AND MEDIAN SURVIVAL OF THE COMMON METASTATIC TUMORS

Primary tumor	Incidence of metastases (%)	Common metastatic sites	Median survival[a] (mo)	Type of metastases
Breast	80	Spine, pelvis, femur, skull, ribs, humerus	24	80%–90% osteolytic
Prostate	85	Spine, femur, skull, ribs, sternum	20	Osteoblastic
Kidney	30	Humerus, spine, femur, pelvis, ribs, foot, skull, sternum	?	<50% solitary
Thyroid	50	Skull, ribs, sternum, spine, humerus	48	Osteolytic; may be solitary
Lung	44	Spine, ribs	6	Osteolytic

[a]Median survival of renal cell carcinoma is longer, but depends on whether it is solitary.

Classification

Bone metastases may be osteolytic, osteoblastic, or mixed (see Table 9-1). Osteolytic metastases are associated with a high incidence of fractures. New bone formation can occur in response to metastases, but this varies with different tumors. Some tumors, such as prostatic carcinoma, form new bone in response to humeral factors that stimulate osteoblasts. In other tumors there may be reactive bone laid down in response to bone damage caused by the tumors. Tumors such as breast and lung carcinoma directly resorb bone, providing significant osteolysis and increasing the risk of fracture.

DIAGNOSIS

History and Physical Examination

■ Patients may present with a history of known carcinoma and recent onset of pain from an occult metastasis, or alternatively the metastasis may be the initial presentation of an unknown primary tumor.

 ▪ In any patient with a history of previous carcinoma, the possibility of metastatic spread must be considered in all patients older than 40 years who present with pain, and a radiologically destructive lesion should be assumed to be metastatic spread until proved otherwise.

■ A complete history must be taken.

 ▪ Patients may well consider that a previous cancer has been cured and not volunteer the appropriate information. Alternatively, they may not be sure why previous surgery was undertaken and unaware of the diagnosis.

 ▪ Questions regarding general health, weight loss, fevers, night sweats, and fatigue are important, and a thorough history of social or occupational factors such as smoking or previous exposure to asbestos or radiation must be undertaken.

■ Physical examination should include a careful examination of breasts, thyroid, and prostate and palpation for lymphadenopathy.

 ▪ Investigations include the standard hematological tests including serum calcium estimation because hypocalcaemia may also occur.

 ▪ Serum electrophoresis should be undertaken to look for multiple myeloma, and prostatic specific antigen should be analyzed to check for prostatic carcinoma.

 ▪ Other tumor makers may be useful, but the investigation of an occult primary usually employs different imaging techniques and biopsy of the metastasis.

Radiologic Examination

■ The initial imaging of metastases and metastatic fractures is with good quality plain anteroposterior and lateral radiographs (Fig. 9-3).

■ It is important not to miss a metastasis on the periphery of a radiograph, and all of the appropriate area must be X-rayed.

■ Investigation of hip pain should include radiography of the pelvis, and investigation of knee pain should always include X-rays of the proximal femur.

■ If a lesion is detected, radiographs of the whole bone must be obtained because the metastasis may be multifocal.

 ▪ Radiographs of the whole bone are particularly important if internal fixation of a metastatic fracture is required because the presence of distal metastases in the humerus or femur may alter the type of surgery or implant used.

■ In spinal metastases, anteroposterior and lateral radiographs should also be obtained.

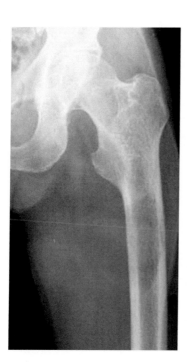 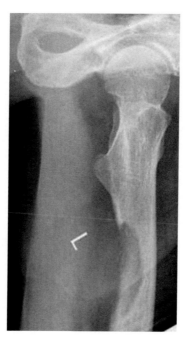

Figure 9-3 A-P and lateral radiographs of a bronchial carcinoma metastasis in the femur.

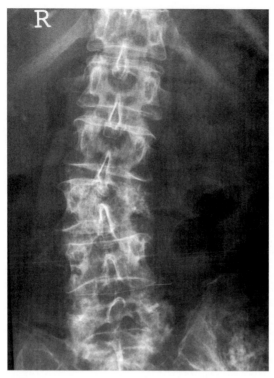

Figure 9-4 An A-P radiograph showing an absent left L3 pedicle: the "winking owl sign."

■ The characteristic early radiologic appearance is of an absent pedicle, the so-called winking owl sign (Fig. 9-4).
■ Radiography may indicate whether the lesion is benign or malignant (Fig. 9-5).
■ Metastatic deposits are usually eccentrically located and involve the cortex. They are often associated with an acute periosteal reaction and a poorly developed zone of transition between normal bone and the tumor. There may be irregular intraosseous calcification, and extraosseous calcification may also be seen.
■ In benign tumors, there tends to be no periosteal reaction and a clear zone of transition between normal and abnormal bone. Intraosseous calcification tends to be regular, and extraosseous calcification is rare.
■ If a metastasis is found, it is essential to X-ray other possible common metastatic sites: the spine, ribs, pelvis, femora, and humeri.
■ X-rays should be taken of any bone that has been painful or is tender on palpation.
■ It requires about 50% of destruction of normal cancellous bone for a tumor to become apparent on plain radiographs, and further imaging may be needed to visualize the extent of metastatic spread.
■ A whole-body technetium 99m bone scan is useful for detecting metastases (Fig. 9-6).
■ The technique has a 95% to 97% sensitivity for detecting metastases but may give false-positive results in non-neoplastic conditions such as Paget's disease or osteoarthritis.
■ Some lytic tumors may not exhibit the reparative processes detected by bone scanning and therefore a scan may appear negative, although gallium scanning may be useful under these circumstances.
■ CT and MRI scans are very useful for detecting both primary and secondary tumors, particularly if they are in the pelvis or spine where plain radiography is more difficult. An MRI scan may produce false-positive results because of bone marrow changes from previous radiotherapy or chemotherapy, but it is particularly useful for delineating the extent of the soft tissue component of a tumor (Fig. 9-7).

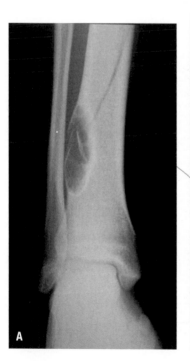

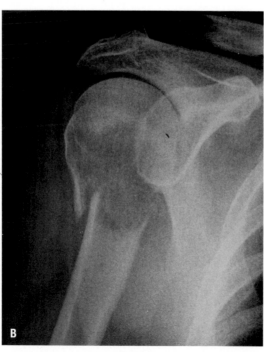

Figure 9-5 (A) A benign bone cyst with an associated fracture. (B) A malignant lesion.

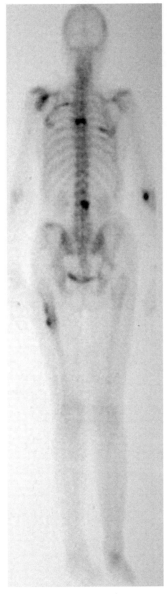

Figure 9-6   A bone scan showing multiple metastases.

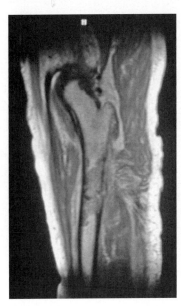

Figure 9-7   MRI scan of a malignant lesion. Note the cortical and soft tissue involvement.

the location of the metastasis, the degree of pain, the radiologic appearance of the lesion, and the size of the lesion. By scoring between 1 and 3 for each variable, he arrived at a maximum of 12 points and showed that a score of 9 or more is an indication for prophylactic fixation. This system is useful, but as with all scoring systems it only provides an indication of outcome. Prophylactic fixation should be considered in patients who experience more bone pain on weight bearing than at rest or in those patients where a tumor occupies more than 50% of the bone. As surgical treatments improve, it is likely prophylactic surgery will become more common, although the use of bisphosphonates has been shown to reduce the incidence of pathological fractures.

TREATMENT

Nonoperative Treatment

■ Patients who have skeletal metastases without a fracture are treated by chemotherapy, hormonal therapy, or

Prediction of Fracture

Surgeons may be asked to predict whether a radiologically apparent skeletal metastasis is going to fracture. Obviously prophylactic fixation is preferable to internal fixation carried out after fracture, but only about 4% of skeletal metastases are associated with a fracture. Prediction of impending fracture is often difficult, but a history of increasing pain is important, particularly if the pain is induced by weight bearing and relieved by rest. Prophylactic internal fixation relieves pain in patients who display up to 50% to 75% of cortical involvement. It is commonly stated that the indication for prophylactic fixation of an impending fracture is the presence of a destructive lesion of at least 2.5 cm in diameter or the loss of at least 50% of the cortex of a long bone. These statements have not been rigorously tested, but they do indicate a requirement for prophylactic surgery.

Mirel (1989) derived a scoring system to predict the risk of fracture (Table 9-2). He defined four predictive variables:

TABLE 9-2 SCORING SYSTEM TO PREDICT FRACTURES

Variable	Score		
	1	**2**	**3**
Site	Upper arm	Lower extremity	Peritrochanteric
Pain	Mild	Moderate	Severe
Lesion	Blastic	Mixed	Lytic
Size	<1/3 diameter	1/3–2/3 diameter	>2/3 diameter

From Mirel H. Metastatic disease in long bones: A proposed scoring system for diagnosing impending pathologic fractures. Clin Orthop 1989;249:256–264.

radiotherapy with internal fixation used if it is felt a fracture is impending.

- Approximately 4% of patients who have skeletal metastases fracture, with most of the fractures occurring in the spine, pelvis, femur, and humerus.

- Nonoperative management of pathological fractures is associated with nonunion rates of between 16% and 35% but varies with the type of tumor and the location of the fractures.

- Studies have shown 67% union in fractures associated with multiple myeloma compared with 44% in renal cell carcinoma, 37% in breast carcinoma, and less than 10% in lung carcinoma.

- The requirement for radiation also increases the incidence of nonunion, and doses of radiation as low as 2,000 rad will significantly inhibit bone union in the absence of rigid fixation.

- Nonoperative management frequently means a patient is in pain and nonambulant for a considerable portion of his or her remaining life.

- The introduction of humeral nailing, reconstruction femoral nailing, and modular joint replacement has revolutionized the surgery of metastatic fractures, and few pathological fractures are treated nonoperatively, although the medical condition of the patient may justify a nonoperative approach.

- The projected life expectancy of the patient may influence the decision of whether surgery is indicated.

- Unless life expectancy is very short, surgery should be considered because it will diminish pain and improve the quality of the patient's remaining life.

Surgical Treatment

- The type of surgery required to treat metastatic fractures may be different from the surgery used for non-neoplastic fractures.

- Table 9-1 indicates the average life expectancy of patients who present with the common metastatic fractures, and it is important that whatever technique is used allows immediate full weight bearing in the lower limb and maximal function in the upper limb.

- Polymethylmethacrylate (PMMA) may be used to augment internal fracture fixation if there is a large bone defect, but with closed intramedullary nailing now preferred to plating for most fractures, the requirement for supplementary PMMA has lessened.

- Surgeons may also have to use supplementary bone grafting if curettage of a tumor deposit is required and a bone defect left as a result.

Upper Limb

- About 20% of all metastases occur in the upper limb, with few occurring outside the humerus (Fig. 9-8).

- Most humeral metastases occur in the proximal third of the diaphysis, and nowadays the treatment of choice is closed locked intramedullary nailing. Both antegrade and retrograde approaches can be used (see Chapter 33).

- Retrograde nailing is particularly useful in metastatic surgery, given the proximal location of many of the metastases in the humerus. Good pain relief and adequate postoperative function has been reported in about 90% of patients treated by closed humeral nailing (see Fig. 9-8).

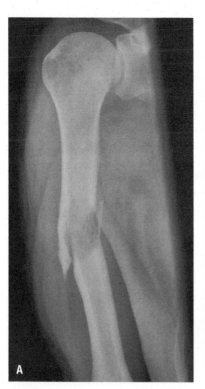
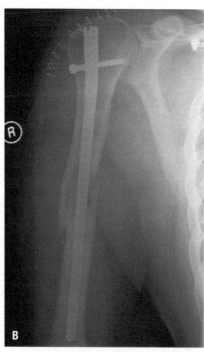

Figure 9-8   (A) A pathological fracture caused by a renal carcinoma metastasis. (B) This was treated with antegrade nailing.

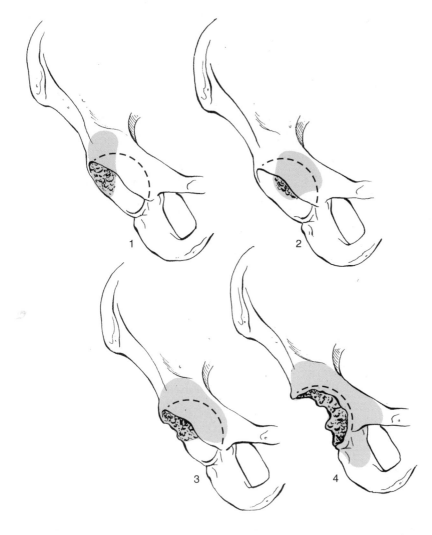

Figure 9-9   Harrington (1981) classification of periacetabular metastases (see Table 9-3).

- If the metastasis is very proximal or very distal, nailing may not be possible. Under these circumstances, the best treatment is a proximal modular hemiarthroplasty or an elbow replacement.

Pelvis

- Most pelvic metastases do not present with fractures. Patients usually complain of local pain frequently caused by periacetabular tumor deposits.
- These were classified by Harrington (1981) according to the area and extent of tumor infiltration (Fig. 9-9 and Table 9-3).

Femur

- About 25% of all metastasis are in the femur.
- They commonly involve the proximal femur with diaphyseal and distal lesions less frequent.
- Breast carcinoma is the most common tumor to metastasize to the proximal femur, and an estimated 10% of all patients with disseminated breast carcinoma and 1.4% of all patients with breast carcinoma have a proximal femoral fracture.
- Overall, about 85% of femoral metastatic fractures are associated with breast, kidney, or lung neoplasia or multiple myeloma.

- Lesser trochanter fractures (Fig. 9-10) are rare and should always be assumed malignant, although Figure 21.2-16 in Chapter 21 shows this is not always the case.
- The treatment of femoral pathological fractures depends on their location.

TABLE 9-3 CLASSIFICATION OF PERIACETABULAR METASTASES BY HARRINGTON[a]

Type	Description
I	Involves the acetabulum but leaves sufficient bone stock to use a conventional hip replacement
II	Loss of structural continuity of a medial acetabular wall necessitates the use of a protrusio acetabuli shell
III	Loss of structural continuity of the medial acetabular wall, roof and rim. Threaded pins are cemented into the superior acetabulum prior to arthroplasty
IV	An en-bloc resection of the acetabulum may be required

[a]See also Figure 9-9.

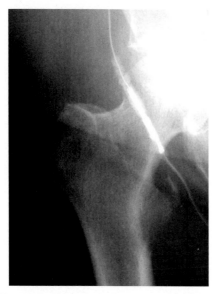

Figure 9-10   A pathological fracture of the lesser trochanter.

- Both impending and actual fractures of the femoral head and neck should be treated by arthroplasty. The success rate of internal fixation is too low to justify its routine use, and the speed of fracture union is slow in patients with reduced life expectancy.
- Usually a cemented bipolar arthroplasty or a total hip replacement (see Chapter 36) is used. Uncemented prostheses are not recommended.
- If there is contiguous acetabular involvement, total hip replacement should be used using Harrington's principles, discussed in the section on pelvic metastases.
- It is important to image the entire femur prior to hip arthroplasty. If there is any suggestion of distal

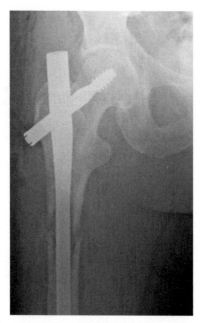

Figure 9-11   The use of a long reconstruction nail to stabilize a pathological subtrochanteric fracture.

metastases, a long-stem implant should be used to bypass metastases that might fracture later.
- Intertrochanteric and subtrochanteric fractures should be treated by reconstruction nailing (Fig. 9-11) using the techniques outlined in Chapter 33.
- Hip screw/plate systems can be used, but the results of using reconstruction nails are superior.
  - Studies indicate that 90% to 95% of patients become mobile and have either no pain or minimal pain after treatment using a reamed or unreamed reconstruction nail.
  - Because the treatment of intertrochanteric and subtrochanteric fractures is closed if a reconstruction nail is used, PMMA is not generally required to enhance the stabilization as it is if a screw/plate system is used. In view of the possibility of distal metastases and later fractures, long-stem reconstructive nails should always be used.
- Femoral diaphyseal fractures can be treated by the use of a conventional statically locked nail.
- Distal femoral pathological fractures can be treated by retrograde nailing (see Chapter 33). If there is extensive metaphyseal or intra-articular involvement, the use of a modular knee prosthesis is advised.
- The significant complication associated with the use of conventional intramedullary or reconstruction nails is embolization leading to acute oxygen desaturation and death.
  - This has been reported in 4% to 10% of patients and probably relates to the fact that the patients are in poor physical condition at the time of nailing.
  - Despite this complication, intramedullary nailing remains the best treatment of metastatic fractures of the femur.

Spine

- Spinal metastases are relatively common, occurring in up to 70% of patients with metastases.
- Only a relatively small number of patients, however, experience symptoms, and only about 5% have neurological symptoms.
- About 15% of spinal metastatic lesions occur in the cervical spine, 50% in the thoracic spine, and about 30% in the lumbar spine.
- Neurological compression occurs anteriorly in 70% of patients, laterally in 20%, and posteriorly in the remaining 10%.
- The treatment of spinal metastases depends on the mode of presentation, the degree of spinal involvement, and the presence of neurological symptoms.
- If the patient is asymptomatic and the metastasis is detected on a radiograph or scan, treatment is nonsurgical with maintenance of appropriate cancer therapy and symptomatic treatment for the fracture, unless there is extensive vertebral destruction, in which case spinal stabilization may be undertaken.
- Patients with extensive destruction are usually symptomatic, however, complaining of pain or neurological involvement.
- The indication for surgery in patients with pain but no neurological involvement is more than 50% vertebral destruction or significant canal compromise as shown on an MRI scan.

TABLE 9-4 EVALUATION SYSTEM FOR SPINAL METASTASES

Symptom	Score		
	0	1	2
General condition (performance status)	Poor (10%–40%)	Moderate (50%–70%)	Good (80%–100%)
Number of extraspinal skeletal metastases	>3	1–2	0
Metastases to internal organs	Irresectable	Resectable	No metastases
Primary tumor	Lung, stomach	Kidney, lung, uterus, unknown	Thyroid, prostate, breast, rectum
Number of spinal metastases	>3	2	1
Spinal cord palsy	Complete	Incomplete	None

From Tokuhashi Y, Matsuzaki H, Toriyama S, et al. Scoring system for the preoperative evaluation of metastatic spine tumor prognosis. Spine 1990;15:1110–1113.

- If neurological compromise is present, the indication for surgery is generally the involvement of one vertebra, good adjacent bone for fixation, and a life expectancy of more than 3 months.
- The surgical treatment of spinal metastases involves posterior stabilization techniques and vertebroplasty (see Chapter 19), which has been shown to give up to 83% pain relief in metastatic vertebral fractures.
- When required, surgical treatment tends to be either posterolateral transpedicular fixation if spinal decompression is not required or anterior corporectomy and fixation if spinal decompression is required.
- The prognostic evaluation system drawn up by Tokuhashi et al. (1990) is shown in Table 9-4.
- A score of 5 or fewer points to survival of less than 3 months, whereas a score of 9 to 12 indicates a survival of more than 12 months.

Primary Tumors

- Fractures occurring in association with primary bone tumors are treated in the same way as a primary tumor would be treated if the fracture had not occurred.
- This is usually en bloc resection and bone reconstruction.

Benign Tumors

- Fractures associated with benign tumors are usually relatively easy to treat. They usually occur in small bones or in the metaphyses of long bones.
- In a number of benign tumors, such as unicameral bone cysts or nonossifying fibromas, the fracture initiates abolition of the tumor, although this may be a slow process.
- The fracture commonly heals quickly, however, and a supplementary cast may be all that is required.
- If the fracture does not heal or if it recurs, curettage and bone grafting of the tumor may be undertaken. Rarely is internal fixation and grafting required.

SUGGESTED READING

Chan D, Carter SR, Grimer RJ, et al. Endoprosthetic replacement for bony metastases. Ann R Coll Surg Engl 1992;74:13–18.

Diel IJ, Solomayer EF, Bastert G. Bisphosphonates and the prevention of metastasis: first evidences from clinical and preclinical studies: review. Cancer 2000;88:3080–3088.

Eftekhar NS, Thurston CW. Effect of irradiation on acrylic cement with special reference to fixation of pathological fractures. J Biomech 1975;8:53–56.

Flinkkila T, Hyvonen P, Lakovaara M, et al. Intramedullary nailing of humeral shaft fractures. A retrospective study of 126 cases. Acta Orthop Scand 1999;70:133–136.

Galasko CSB. Skeletal metastases. London: Butterworths, 1986.

Harrington KD. The management of acetabular insufficiency secondary to metastatic malignant disease. J Bone Joint Surg (Am) 1981;63:653–664.

Harrington KD. Metastatic disease of the spine. J Bone Joint Surg (Am) 1986;68:1110–1115.

Hipp JA, Springfield DS, Hayes WC. Predicting pathologic fracture risk in the management of metastatic bone defects. Clin Orthop 1995;312:120–135.

Jacofsky DJ, Haidukewych GJ. Management of pathologic fractures of the proximal femur: state of the art. J Orthop Trauma 2004;18:459–469.

Levine AM, Aboulafia AJ. Pathologic fractures. In: Browner BD, Jupiter JB, Levine AM, et al., eds. Skeletal trauma, 3rd ed. Philadelphia: WB Saunders, 2003.

Mirel H. Metastatic disease in long bones. A proposed scoring system for diagnosing impending pathologic fractures. Clin Orthop 1989;249:256–264.

Schneiderbauer MM, Von Knoch M, Schleck CD, et al. Patient survival after hip arthroplasty for metastatic disease of the hip. J Bone Joint Surg (Am) 2004;86:1684–1689.

Taneichi H, Kaneda K, Takeda N, et al. Risk factors and probability of vertebral body collapse in metastases of the thoracic and lumbar spine. Spine 1997:22:239–245.

Tokuhashi Y, Matsuzaki H, Toriyama S, et al. Scoring system for the preoperative evaluation of metastatic spine tumor prognosis. Spine 1990;15:1110–1113.

10 SHOULDER GIRDLE

Fractures and dislocations of the shoulder girdle are common, particularly fractures of the clavicle and subluxations or dislocations of the acromioclavicular and glenohumeral joints. In the 1960s, two large series of clavicle fractures gave the incidence of nonunion as 0.1% to 0.8%. These series included both children and adults, and it is now apparent that their results underestimated the incidence of clavicular nonunion and some of the problems associated with clavicle fractures. In the last few years, considerable interest has been expressed in clavicle fractures, and recent studies have detailed nonunion rates of up to 20%. Some studies have suggested that clavicular shortening is associated with a high incidence of complications. There has also been renewed interest in the problems of treating distal clavicle fractures associated with disruption of the coracoacromial ligaments.

Fractures of the scapula are much less common and often associated with high-energy injuries. There has been an increasing awareness of the problems of treating so-called floating shoulders, in which there are ipsilateral clavicle and scapular fractures, and scapulothoracic dissociation, where the whole scapulothoracic articulation is disrupted. A number of the current controversies associated with shoulder girdle injuries and their treatment are listed in Box 10-1.

BOX 10-1 CURRENT CONTROVERSIES IN THE TREATMENT OF CLAVICLE FRACTURES

What is the incidence of nonunion of middle third clavicle fractures?
Which midshaft clavicle fracture should be treated operatively?
Do Neer II lateral clavicle fractures require surgery?
If so which treatment is best?
How should clavicle nonunions be treated?
Which scapular fractures should be treated surgically?
Does floating shoulder require operative treatment?
Do type III acromioclavicular dislocations need surgery?
What are the indications for surgical treatment of glenohumeral dislocation?
Which factors predict glenohumeral redislocation?

SURGICAL ANATOMY

The shoulder girdle consists of the clavicle and scapula, which are joined to each other by the acromioclavicular joint and the coracoclavicular ligaments (Fig. 10-1). The clavicle articulates with the sternum at the sternoclavicular joint, and the scapula is attached to the chest wall and spine by serratus anterior, rhomboids major and minor, levator scapulae, and trapezius muscles.

The sternoclavicular joint is a synovial joint supported by a fibrous capsule. The joint has no inherent stability, which is provided by strong anterior and posterior sternoclavicular ligaments. The interclavicular ligament joins the two clavicles, and a costoclavicular ligament joins each clavicle to the first rib. On the right side, the sternoclavicular joint lies

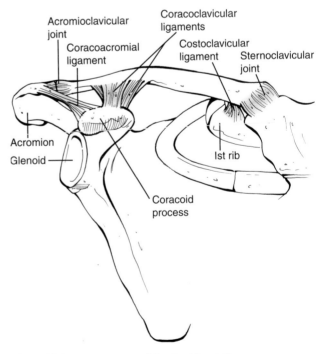

Figure 10-1 The anatomy of the shoulder girdle.

in front of the innominate artery and the right subclavian vein, and the left sternoclavicular joint lies in front of the common carotid artery and the left subclavian vein. These relations are important in posterior sternoclavicular dislocations and if sternoclavicular surgery is planned.

The clavicle has a sigmoid shape and is flattened from above downward in its lateral quarter. It is stabilized by the sternoclavicular joint and interclavicular and costoclavicular ligaments medially and by the acromioclavicular joint and coracoclavicular ligaments laterally. Medially, it gives rise to the pectoralis major, sternohyoid, and sternocleidomastoid muscles, the latter tending to elevate the medial fragment in midshaft fractures. The subclavius muscle attaches to the undersurface of the clavicle. Laterally, the deltoid muscle originates from the clavicle anteriorly and trapezius inserts posteriorly. The trapezius is responsible for the posterior displacement of lateral clavicle fractures associated with coracoclavicular ligament damage. The subclavian artery and vein lie behind the proximal third of the clavicle, and the brachial plexus passes behind the middle third of the bone. Both are at risk from fractures and during surgery.

The acromioclavicular joint is a synovial joint surrounded by a fibrous capsule, the upper part of which is thickened to form the acromioclavicular ligament. There is no inherent instability, and the supporting soft tissues are weaker than in the sternoclavicular joints. Thus dislocation is more common.

The scapula is a complex bone that is only attached by muscles, the acromioclavicular joint, and the coracoclavicular ligaments. It is flat, with costal and dorsal surfaces, and has two processes, the coracoid and the spine, which curves upward to end as the acromion. The glenoid forms part of the shoulder joint. The muscles that hold the scapula to the chest wall and spine have already been detailed. A number of muscles originate from the scapula to insert into the humerus: supraspinatus, infraspinatus, teres major and minor, and deltoid. The long head of triceps originates from below the glenoid, and the long head of biceps arises from above the glenoid. The short head of biceps and coracobrachialis originate from, and pectoralis minor inserts into, the coracoid process. The suprascapular nerve and vessels run in the suprascapular notch on the upper border of the scapula and may be at risk in fractures of the scapula.

CLAVICLE FRACTURES

CLASSIFICATION

A number of simple classifications have been proposed that divide the clavicle into thirds and define the location of the fracture. Distal clavicle fractures were classified by Neer, with type I being stable extra-articular fractures. Type II fractures were unstable fractures associated with damage to the coracoacromial ligaments, and type III fractures were intra-articular fractures. Craig introduced a better

classification, but Robinson has devised the most comprehensive classification (Fig. 10-2). In this classification are three basic types depending on the location of the fracture. Type 1 fractures are in the medial third, type 2 fractures are in the middle third, and type 3 fractures are in the distal third of the clavicle. All fractures are divided into types A and B according to the degree of displacement. Type A fractures show less than 100% translation and type B fractures more than 100% translation. Types 1 and 3 fractures are further subdivided depending on the presence of an intra-articular fracture. Thus a 1A2 fracture is an intra-articular medial third fracture with less than 100% displacement, and a type 3B1 fracture is an extra-articular lateral third fracture with displacement.

Type 2 fractures are further subdivided according to angulation or comminution. Type 2A2 fractures are not translated but angulated. Type 2B1 fractures are displaced simple wedge fractures, and type 2B2 fractures are displaced comminuted or segmental fractures. This classification is straightforward, clinically relevant, and has been shown to be reproducible.

EPIDEMIOLOGY AND ETIOLOGY

The epidemiology of clavicle fractures is shown in Table 10-1. They are usually isolated and occur in younger patients, more commonly in men. Open fractures are very rare, with an incidence of 0.2% in a large series. Almost 70% of the fractures are in the middle third, with 28% being lateral third fractures. Medial third fractures are very rare. Table 10-2 shows the distribution of clavicle fractures according to the mode of injury.

TABLE 10-1 EPIDEMIOLOGY OF FRACTURES OF THE CLAVICLE

Proportion of all fractures	3.3%
Average age	38.3 y
Men/women	70%/30%
Distribution	Type G
Incidence	$36.5/10^5$/y
Open fractures	0%
Most common causes	
Fall	30.9%
Sport	23.4%
Motor vehicle accident	27.2%
Robinson classification	
Type 1	2.8%
Type 2	69.2%
Type 3	28.0%
Most common subgroups	
2B1	37.5%
3A1	16.2%
2A2	13.5%
2B2	12.8%

Data on causes, fracture types, and subgroups from Robinson CM. Fractures of the clavicle in the adult. Epidemiology and classification. J Bone Joint Surg Br 1998;80B:476–484.

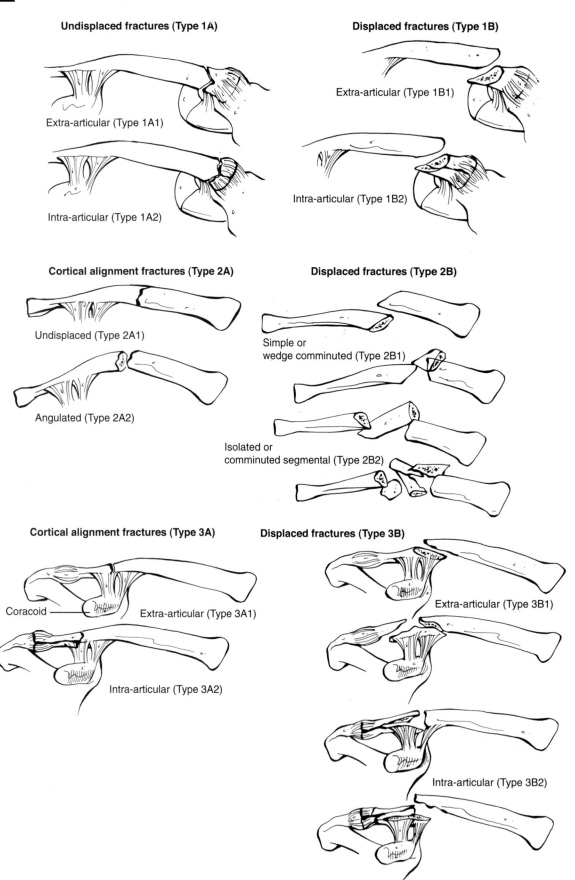

Figure 10-2   The Robinson classification of clavicle fractures.

TABLE 10-2 EPIDEMIOLOGY OF CLAVICLE FRACTURES ACCORDING TO THE MODE OF INJURY

Mode of injury	Prevalence (%)	Age (y)	Robinson Type		
			1	2	3
Fall	30.9	46.3	2.6	51.1	46.3
Sport	23.4	21.2	1.3	88.9	9.8
Motor vehicle accident	27.2	30.1	2.2	75.7	22.1

Data from Robinson CM, Court-Brown CM, McQueen MM, et al. Estimating the risk of nonunion following nonoperative treatment of a clavicular fracture. J Bone Joint Surg Am 2004;86A:1359–1365.

Most clavicle injuries are low-energy injuries, with over 50% occurring in falls or sports injuries and about 27% in motor vehicle accidents (MVA). About 50% of MVA clavicle fractures occur in cyclists. The prevalence of type 1 injury is consistently low, but Table 10-2 shows that in older patients the prevalence of type 2 midshaft and type 3 lateral fractures is very similar. In younger patients the prevalence of type 2 fractures is higher. The most common subgroups are shown in Table 10-1, which indicates that displaced simple or wedge midshaft fractures account for 37.5% of clavicle fractures, with angulated midshaft fractures and comminuted or segmental midshaft fractures accounting for 13.5% and 12.8%, respectively. Lateral clavicular fractures are usually undisplaced extra-articular fractures (16.2%), with 8.5% being displaced fractures associated with coracoclavicular ligament damage (Neer type II).

Associated Injuries

Most clavicle fractures are isolated injuries, but there may be further local damage. Patients may present with an ipsilateral glenoid neck fracture, a floating shoulder, or damage to the acromioclavicular joint. In severe high-energy injuries, there may be major damage to the scapular attachments, causing a scapulothoracic dissociation (Fig. 10-3). Pneumothorax has been reported to occur in 3% of patients with clavicle fractures, and rarely adolescent patients may present with a combination of an atlantoaxial rotatory displacement in combination with the clavicle fracture. This is more common in children, however.

DIAGNOSIS

Clinical History and Examination

- Most clavicle fractures are isolated, and the patients present with a painful shoulder, often associated with a local prominence.
- Neurovascular involvement is extremely rare but can occur.
  - If there is evidence of a brachial plexus lesion or vascular damage, it is more likely the patient has a scapulothoracic dissociation (see Fig. 10-3) and may have significant damage to the local soft tissues, ribs, and lungs.
- Patients who present with an apparently isolated clavicle fracture following high-energy injuries should be examined for associated injuries to the scapula, ribs, or lung, and a thorough examination according to ATLS principles should be undertaken.

Radiologic Examination

- The diagnosis of a clavicle fracture is usually made on an anteroposterior radiograph.
- If there has been high-energy trauma, a chest X-ray should be taken to look for associated rib or lung injury.
- If there is tenderness around the scapula or shoulder, scapular views should be obtained.
- A chest X-ray should be examined to see if there is lateral displacement of the scapular suggestive of a scapulothoracic dissociation.
- To visualize the clavicle, an oblique radiograph may be obtained.
- Sternoclavicular fractures and dislocations and medial third (type 1) fractures are often difficult to diagnose on plain radiographs, and CT scans are helpful.

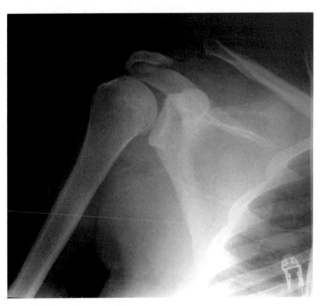

Figure 10-3 A scapulothoracic dissociation with disruption of the acromioclavicular joint. Note the lateral displacement of the scapula. There was avulsion of the vascular pedicle and the brachial plexus. The arm was amputated.

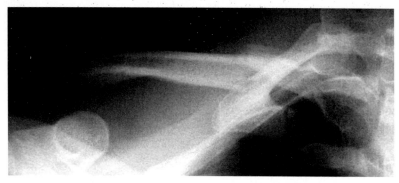

Figure 10-4 A fracture of the medial third of the clavicle. These are often undisplaced, and displacement, as shown here, suggests a high-energy injury.

■ Lateral clavicle (type 3) fractures with coracoclavicular ligament damage may be diagnosed by a stress view with the patient holding a weight in the ipsilateral arm.

■ This X-ray also helps diagnose acromioclavicular subluxation or dislocation.

TREATMENT

Medial Third Fractures

■ Medial third clavicle fractures are very rare (see Table 10-1 and Fig. 10-4).

■ There are two common types: a fracture of the medial clavicular physis and an undisplaced fracture of the medial clavicular diaphysis.

■ The medial clavicular physis may not close until about 25 years of age, and it is likely a number of sternoclavicular dislocations reported in the past were actually physeal fractures with anterior or posterior displacement of the clavicular metaphysis.

■ If the clavicular metaphysis displaces anteriorly, the treatment options are nonoperative management or open reduction and suturing of the displaced epiphysis using an absorbable suture.

■ In young patients, nonoperative management may result in remodeling, but in older patients open reduction and suturing is straightforward.

■ K-wires should not be used because penetration of the great vessels has been reported.

■ Posterior displacement of the clavicular metaphysis should be treated by closed reduction using a towel clip to pull up the clavicle.

■ If the reduced position is unstable, interosseous suturing should be used.

■ Posterior displacement may rarely give rise to acute vascular or laryngeal compromise.

■ Under these circumstances, reduction should be undertaken with the assistance of a thoracic surgeon.

■ Medial diaphyseal fractures of the clavicle are usually undisplaced or minimally displaced and treated nonoperatively.

■ Nonunion is extremely rare, and a good functional outcome can be expected.

Middle Third Fractures

■ Table 10-1 shows that about 70% of clavicle fractures are in the middle third (Fig. 10-5).

■ They are usually treated nonoperatively, although plating and intramedullary pinning are also used.

Nonoperative Treatment

■ At first sight it is difficult to understand why there is a wide variation (0.1% to 15% in different series) in the incidence of nonunion in nonoperatively managed fractures.

■ Many clavicle fractures have an excellent prognosis when managed nonoperatively.

■ Fractures in adolescents and young adults heal well as do undisplaced (2A1) and angulated (2A2) fractures in older patients.

■ The incidence of nonunion varies with the case mix of the series.

■ The higher rates of nonunion come from series dealing with 2B1 and particularly 2B2 fractures where a large series has shown an incidence of 9.4%.

■ Table 10-3 shows the results of nonoperative management, plating, and intramedullary pinning in displaced middle third fractures.

■ The overall rate of nonunion is relatively low, but the articles covered in Table 10-4 do not correlate outcome with the degree of clavicular displacement or shortening.

■ There is considerable disagreement about the effect of shortening, but evidence indicates that shortening of

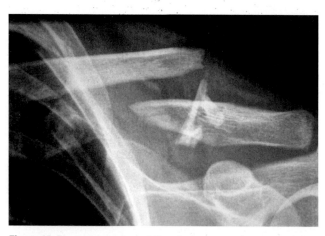

Figure 10-5 A mid-diaphyseal clavicle fracture with an intermediate fragment. This is a Robinson 2B2 fracture.

TABLE 10-3 COMPARATIVE RESULTS OF THE TREATMENT OF DISPLACED (2B1 AND 2B2) CLAVICLE FRACTURES

Result/complication	Nonoperative (%)		Plates (%)		IM Pins (%)	
	Range	Average	Range	Average	Range	Average
Excellent/good	69.2–86.4	78.1	91.8–100	93.9	—	—
Good range of motion	84.6–87.5	85.9	95	95	89.7–100	94.1
Nonunion	4.6–15.4	6.5	0–4.1	3.1	1.7–6.4	4.4
Malunion	17.5–37.2	30.8	0–11.6	5.8	—	—
Refracture	—	—	0–1.6	1.1	0	0
Infection	—	—	0.4–5.2	2.1	0	0

more than 20 mm results in a higher incidence of nonunion and thoracic outlet syndrome.
■ A prospective study of 581 middle third clavicle fractures has shown that increased age, female gender, displacement, and comminution are all independent predictors of nonunion.
■ If nonoperative management is to be used, the arm should be supported in a sling for 10 to 14 days, and afterward a physical therapy program can be instituted.
■ Some surgeons still favor a figure-eight bandage, but studies have clearly shown this method of management confers no benefit, and indeed its use has been associated with nerve palsies.

Surgical Treatment

Plating
■ The series that comprise the data shown in Table 10-3 all dealt with selected high-energy injuries and therefore differ from the series using nonoperative management.
■ The results of plating are good, but nonunion does occur, and bone grafting must be used to fill any bone defects.
■ AO principles must be followed and six cortices secured on each side of the fracture (Fig. 10-6). Thus, in comminuted fractures, an eight- or ten-hole plate may be required.
■ Where possible, prebent clavicular plates should be used because bending straight reconstruction or locking compression plates can be difficult.

■ The plate is usually placed on the superior surface of the clavicle, but good results have been reported with anteroinferior plating.

Intramedullary Pinning
■ Intramedullary pinning has been used since the early 1970s.
■ Kirschner wires have been used, but migration into the subclavian vessels and mediastinum has occurred, and it is preferable to use a thicker threaded pin.
■ The fracture can be reduced closed and the pins inserted either medially or laterally.
■ Care must be taken not to damage the underlying vessels.
■ Because the clavicle is sigmoid in shape, the end of the pin will penetrate the bone and may cause skin irritation.
■ Table 10-3 shows that good results can be obtained, but the technique should not be used if the fracture is irreducible or if there is evidence of vascular or neurological involvement. Thus it is more suitable for fractures that can also be treated nonoperatively.

Suggested Treatment
■ Nonoperative management should be used for the majority of clavicle fractures.
■ Further studies are required to define the role of operative treatment in displaced and comminuted fractures, but given the low incidence of nonunion in most fracture types, it is suggested that primary clavicle fixation be restricted to the indications listed in Box 10-2 and that plating be used.

TABLE 10-4 RESULTS OF THE TREATMENT OF NEER II (ROBINSON 3B1 AND 3B2) FRACTURES

Result/complication	Nonoperative (%)		K-wires (%)		Coracoclavicular stabilization (%)		Hook plate (%)	
	Range	Average	Range	Average	Range	Average	Range	Average
Excellent/good	78.2–87.5	81.6	52.6–95.6	68.8	90.1–100	97.2	72.2–100	76.2
Nonunion	13.6–43.7	21.8	4.3–46.1	14.3	0	0	0–11.1	9.5
Infection	—	—	0–38.5	8.6	0–9.1	2	0	0
Wire migration	—	—	0–54.5	27.3	—	—	—	—

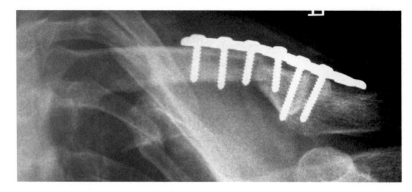

Figure 10-6   A clavicle fracture treated with a plate.

Lateral Fractures

- Neer first pointed out the importance of coracoclavicular integrity in the prognosis of lateral clavicle fractures (Fig. 10-7).
- There is good evidence that his type I and III fractures (Robinson 3A1 and 3A2) heal with minimal functional loss and should be treated nonoperatively.
- The debate concerns Neer type II (3B1 and 3B2) fractures.
    - As the stabilizing effect of the coracoclavicular ligaments is lost, the medial clavicle displaces superiorly and posteriorly.
    - Nonoperative management results in a high incidence of nonunion, and various operative methods have been used.
    - The most common methods are transacromial K-wires (see Fig. 34-13 in Chapter 34) with or without a tension band, coracoclavicular stabilization using a screw or a synthetic ligament, or a hook plate that passes under the acromion (Fig. 10-8).
    - The results of these methods are given in Table 10-4.

Nonsurgical Treatment

- Table 10-4 shows there is a high incidence of nonunion, and thus many surgeons now favor operative treatment.
- As with midshaft clavicle fractures, nonoperative management involves 10 to 14 days in a sling followed by physical therapy.
- It is routinely used for Neer type I and III fractures and for Neer type II fractures in the elderly where physical demands are less.

BOX 10-2 INDICATIONS FOR SURGICAL TREATMENT OF CLAVICLE DIAPHYSEAL FRACTURES

Open fractures
Floating shoulder
Multiple trauma
Scapulothoracic dissociation
Vascular damage
Progressive neurological deficit
Impending skin disruption
Shortening of >2 cm
Severe B2 fractures

Surgical Treatment

Kirschner Wires

- The results of using transacromial K-wires are clearly not as good as other methods of operative management, even if a tension band is used.
- K-wire migration is at best a nuisance (see Fig. 34-13 in Chapter 34) and has occasionally proved fatal.
- They provide less secure fixation than other operative methods, hence the high nonunion rate.

Coracoclavicular Stabilization

- Coracoclavicular stabilization can be done by placing a 3.5-mm screw through the clavicle into the coracoid.
- This can be done closed theoretically, but it is very difficult, and open screw insertion is suggested.
- Screw fixation should be supplemented by the use of a synthetic ligament made of Dacron or mersilene.
- This is passed under the coracoid and tightened over the clavicle to secure the fracture. Table 10-4 shows that this method gives the best results.

Hook Plate

- The hook plate (see Fig. 10-8) was designed for the management of acromioclavicular dislocation, but it is useful for distal clavicle fractures.

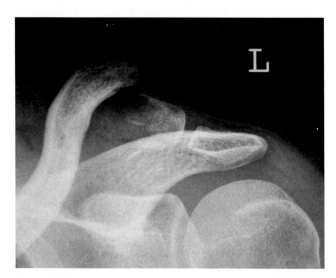

Figure 10-7   A Neer II (Robinson 3B1) lateral clavicle fracture. The coracoclavicular ligaments are ruptured and the clavicle is displaced upward and posteriorly.

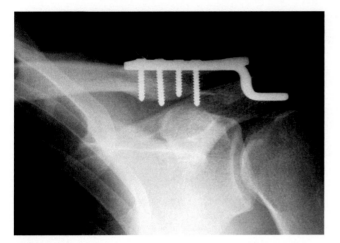

Figure 10-8 The fracture shown in Figure 10-6 treated with a hook plate.

- As with all plates, correct application is essential, and good results can be achieved. Figure 10-7 suggests a high nonunion rate, but with attention to surgical technique this can be minimized.
- The problem is shoulder stiffness from the subacromial location of the plate. These plates usually need to be removed.

Suggested Treatment

- Neer type I and III fractures (3A1 and 3A2) should be managed nonoperatively with a sling followed by physical therapy.
- Neer II (3B1 and 3B2) fractures should be treated operatively using a hook plate or by using a prosthetic ligament to reconstruct the coracoclavicular ligaments.
- In elderly patients with low functional demands, Neer type II fractures can be treated nonoperatively.

Distal Physeal Fractures

- These are usually seen in children but have been reported up to age 15.
- They resemble a Neer type II fracture in that the distal metaphysis separates from the physis and displaces upward, leaving the coracoclavicular ligaments attached to the undersurface of the periosteal sleeve of the clavicle.
- If this occurs in an adolescent, reduction and internal fixation should be undertaken because remodeling will not occur.
- Union is rapid, and transacromial Kirschner wires can be used. These should be removed at 3 to 4 weeks.

COMPLICATIONS

- Box 10-3 lists complications associated with clavicle fractures.

Nonunion

- The overall incidence of nonunion is shown in Tables 10-3 and 10-4.

BOX 10-3 COMPLICATIONS OF CLAVICLE FRACTURES AND THEIR TREATMENT

Nonunion
Malunion
Thoracic outlet syndrome
Brachial plexopathy
Vascular damage
Pneumothorax
Reflex sympathetic dystrophy

- Many nonunions are asymptomatic and do not require surgery.
  - This is particularly true of the elderly where the demands on the shoulder are much less than in younger patients.
- It is universally accepted that the best treatment method is internal fixation and bone grafting (Fig. 10-9).
- It is sometimes possible merely to resect the ends of the nonunion and apply a plate under compression.
- However, because most nonunions follow 2B1 or 2B2 fractures, bone grafting is usually required.
- Plate fixation is preferred by most surgeons, but intramedullary pins can be used. A comparative analysis of the two techniques is shown in Table 10-5. This shows that the results are very similar, and there is a high union rate with good function.
- Open reduction and plating of clavicular nonunions requires care.
  - It can be difficult to mobilize the ends of the bone and any ununited fragments.
  - Damage to the subclavian vein and brachial plexus has been reported.
  - As with primary plating, six cortices must be secured in each side of the nonunion, and an eight- or ten-hole plate may be required if extensive bone grafting is needed.
- Most plate failure follows the use of too short plates.
- Partial or total claviculectomy has been used for the treatment of nonunion.

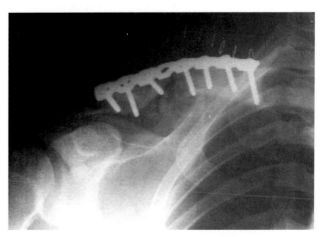

Figure 10-9 A clavicular nonunion treated by plating and grafting. There is a bone defect following reduction and plating, and bone grafting is therefore required.

TABLE 10-5 THE RESULTS OF TREATING CLAVICLE NONUNIONS[a]

Result/complication	Plates (%)		IM Pins (%)	
	Range	Average	Range	Average
Excellent/good	83.3–100	91.6	78.6–85.7	82.3
Persistent nonunion	0–18.2	8.1	0–11.1	5.6
Pain free	68.2–100	81.9	71.4–85.7	81.6
Infection	0–9.1	2.4	0	0

[a]Supplementary bone graft used in most cases.

■ Partial resection is stated to be useful in jockeys who require a short convalescent period and is said to have few short-term complications, but the long-term complications are unknown.

· ■ Total claviculectomy should be reserved for the management of severe thoracic outlet syndrome.

Malunion

■ Table 10-3 shows that the incidence of malunion in nonoperatively managed clavicle fractures is relatively high.

■ Most are asymptomatic or merely cosmetically unattractive.

■ Some patients present with shoulder fatigue and weakness, numbness, and paraesthesia in the hand and forearm and a drooped shoulder.

■ Examination shows shoulder asymmetry and may show evidence of a brachial plexopathy.

■ If this is the case, nerve conduction studies should be obtained.

■ The treatment is osteotomy, straightening and plating of the clavicle utilizing bone graft as required. Studies indicate that good results can be obtained following this procedure.

Thoracic Outlet Syndrome

■ This is usually caused by the presence of cervical ribs, scalenus muscle hypertrophy, or fibrous bands, but it may also be caused by clavicular nonunion.

■ Treatment is by osteotomy and restoration of the normal cervicoaxillary anatomy.

■ This is usually successful, but in severe cases excision of the clavicle or the first rib is required.

■ Thoracic outlet syndrome can also be caused by chronic posterior sternoclavicular dislocation.

Brachial Plexus Lesion

■ This may follow a clavicular malunion and be part of a thoracic outlet syndrome, or it may be caused by excessive callus formation, subclavian pseudoaneurysm, or direct damage to the plexus from fracture fragments or during surgery.

■ Usually the medial and posterior cords are involved.

■ Neuropraxia of the musculocutaneous nerve following a clavicle fracture has been reported.

Other Complications

■ Vascular damage following clavicle fracture is surprisingly rare given the proximity of the subclavian vein to the medial half of the clavicle.

■ The subclavian vein is in fact more commonly damaged during nonunion surgery. Damage to the axillary and subclavian arteries has been reported.

■ Reflex sympathetic dystrophy has also been reported but is very rare.

SCAPULAR FRACTURES

Scapular fractures are rare, although they have been documented in 7% of multiply injured patients. They may involve the body, neck, spine, glenoid, acromion, or coracoid process and may be associated with shoulder dislocation or occasionally with acromioclavicular dislocation. They are frequently caused by high-energy injuries, and the incidence of injuries to local structures such as the clavicle, ribs, brachial plexus, and lungs is relatively high.

CLASSIFICATION

Ideberg and colleagues developed the current classification of glenoid fractures (Fig. 10-10). Type I fractures are glenoid rim fractures with 1A fractures having a fragment of 5 mm or less and 1B fractures having larger rim fragments. Type II fractures are inferior, involving part of the neck. Type III fractures are superior fractures, extending to the base of the coracoid process. Type IV fractures are horizontal fractures, involving the neck and body with the fracture line inferior to the scapular spine, and type V fractures are type IV fractures with an additional neck fracture.

Acromial fractures have been subdivided into three types (Fig. 10-11). Type I acromial fractures are undisplaced, with 1A fractures being avulsion fractures and 1B fractures involving the body of the acromion. Type II fractures are displaced fractures that do not narrow the subacromial space. In type III fractures, the subacromial

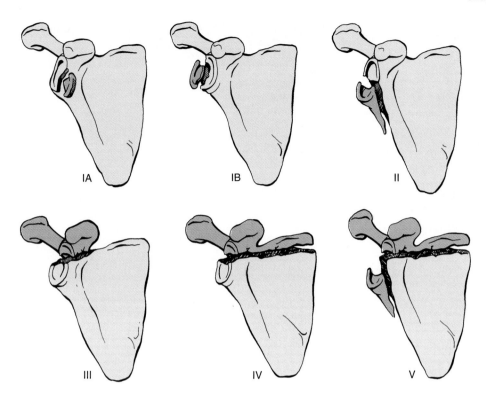

Figure 10-10 The Ideberg classification of scapular fractures.

space is narrowed. Undisplaced acromial fractures associated with superior migration of a glenoid neck fracture are included as type III fractures. The classification of coracoid fractures is straightforward, with type I fractures behind the coracoclavicular ligaments and type II fractures in front of them (Fig. 10-12).

EPIDEMIOLOGY

The basic epidemiology of scapular fractures is shown in Table 10-6. They are type A fractures (see Chapter 1) usually presenting in young men after high-energy injuries and

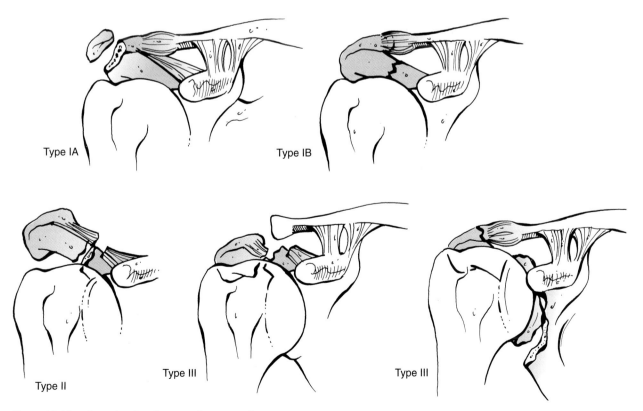

Figure 10-11 The Kuhn classification of acromion fractures.

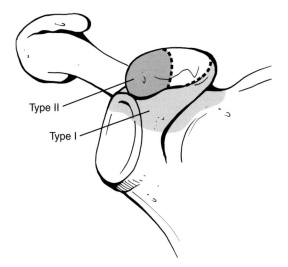

Figure 10-12   The Ogawa classification of coracoid fractures.

TABLE 10-6 EPIDEMIOLOGY OF SCAPULAR FRACTURES

Proportion of all fractures	0.3%
Average age	50.5 y
Men/women	59%/41%
Distribution	Type A
Incidence	$3.2/10^5/y$
Most common causes	
Fall	23.5%
Sport	23.5%
Motor vehicle accident	17.6%

TABLE 10-7 INCIDENCE OF SCAPULAR FRACTURES BASED ON LOCATION

	Incidence (%)	
Fracture location	**Range**	**Average**
Body	23.1–73.2	41.1
Neck	19.5–61.5	31.5
Glenoid	3.8–29.6	27.1
Spine	3.8–11.5	9.2
Coracoid	0–9.8	4.4
Acromion	5.9–12.1	9.9
Associated injuries	80.5–92.3	86.2

in older women after low-energy injuries. Because of the rarity of scapular fractures, the epidemiological data relating to the location of different fractures in the glenoid presented in Table 10-7 has been taken from the literature. It can be seen that the fractures of the body, neck, and glenoid are much more common than fractures of the spine, coracoid, and acromion. Little worthwhile information is available about the precise distribution of scapular body fractures, and further classification is not likely to alter treatment. The distribution of the different types of glenoid fractures was documented by Ideberg and colleagues, however (Table 10-8). This indicates that most scapular fractures are glenoid rim fractures and other fractures are very rare, but when they occur they are the result of high-energy injuries and associated with a significant number of other injuries. Glenoid fractures tend to occur in older patients.

The epidemiology of acromion fractures is shown in Table 10-9. Acromion fractures tend to occur in younger patients than glenoid fractures. Most acromion fractures are undisplaced or avulsion fractures with only 45% displaced. Avulsion fractures are isolated injuries, but other fractures tend to occur in multiply injured patients. The distribution of coracoid fractures has been documented by Ogawa and colleagues. They have shown that 83% of coracoid fractures occur behind the coracoclavicular ligaments and the remaining 17% in front of the ligaments. There was a high incidence of associated local injury, with 63% of patients having other scapular fractures, 58% having an acromioclavicular dislocation, and 21% having a clavicle fracture. Only 5% had an associated shoulder dislocation.

TABLE 10-8 EPIDEMIOLOGY OF GLENOID FRACTURES

	Fracture Type[a]				
	I	**II**	**III**	**IV**	**V**
Incidence (%)	85	3	1	6	5
Average age (y)	56.1	50.7	47	56	53.2
Associated injuries (%)	43.5	100	100	0	60

[a]For fracture types, see Figure 10-9.
Data from Ideberg R, Grevsten S, Larsson S. Epidemiology of scapular fractures: incidence and classification of 338 fractures. Acta Orthop Scand 1995;66:395–397.

Associated Injuries

There is a high incidence of other injuries in patients who present with scapula fractures (Tables 10-8 to 10-10). They are mostly in the thorax and shoulder and may be very severe. The literature indicates that the injury severity score (ISS) is higher in multiply injured patients with a scapular fracture than in those without. In addition to the injuries listed in Table 10-10, there is a relatively high incidence of head and abdominal trauma. There is also a high incidence

TABLE 10-9 EPIDEMIOLOGY OF ACROMION FRACTURES

	Fracture Type[a]			
	IA	**IB**	**II**	**III**
Incidence (%)	12	44	28	16
Average age (y)	22.7	39.5	35.8	40.2
Associated injuries (%)	0	63.6	100	100

[a]For fracture types, see Figure 10-11.
Data from Kuhn JE, Blasier RB, Carpenter JE. Fractures of the acromion process: a proposed classification system. J Orthop Trauma 1994;8:6–13.

of ipsilateral clavicle fracture, and the combination of clavicle and scapular damage should always point to the possibility of scapulothoracic dissociation (see Fig. 10-3). It has been estimated that about 66% of patients who present with a type I glenoid rim fracture have an associated shoulder dislocation.

DIAGNOSIS

Clinical History and Examination

- Patients with scapular fractures are often multiply injured.
- A complete history and physical examination according to ATLS principles is essential.
  - Damage to the thorax, lungs, brachial plexus, and great vessels should be particularly sought, and the presence of an ipsilateral clavicle fracture should be checked.
- There may be coexisting head, abdominal, spinal, and pelvic injuries, and these areas should be carefully examined.
- The scapular fracture may not be of pressing importance initially, but its presence should point to the possibility of the associated injuries listed in Table 10-10.
- Patients who have isolated scapular fractures present with a painful stiff shoulder.
- Careful examination of the neurological and vascular status of the ipsilateral arm is important.

Radiologic Examination

- Scapular fractures are notoriously difficult to visualize and are usually diagnosed initially from a chest X-ray or anteroposterior X-ray of the shoulder (Figs. 10-13 and 10-14), but axillary, lateral, or oblique views may show more detail and are particularly indicated if the shoulder is dislocated secondary to a glenoid rim fracture.
- The scapula is best visualized using CT scanning (Fig. 10-15), although they are sometimes difficult to interpret.
- The presence of other injuries means that CT or MRI scans of the head, spine, chest, abdomen, and pelvis may be required.

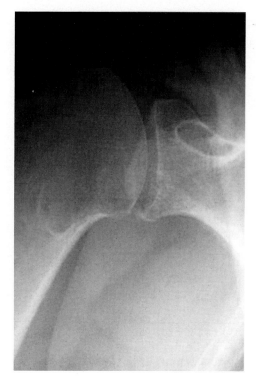

Figure 10-13   A type I glenoid rim fracture.

- Angiography may also be required if there is suspicion of damage to the great vessels.

TREATMENT

Fractures of the Scapular Body

- Most body fractures are treated nonoperatively.
- The fractures are often complex, but the fragments are held in position by the surrounding musculature.

TABLE 10-10 PREVALENCE OF OTHER INJURIES ASSOCIATED WITH SCAPULA FRACTURES

Injury	Incidence (%)	
	Range	Average
Rib fractures	48.1–53.5	37
Pneumothorax	10.2–62.5	26.9
Pulmonary contusion	15.2–58.9	27.7
Great vessel/myocardium	0–10.7	5.9
Brachial plexus	5.1–12.5	7.1
Clavicle fracture	25.6–39.2	30.4
Vertebral fracture	3.8–21.4	12
Pelvic fracture	7.7–32.9	19.6

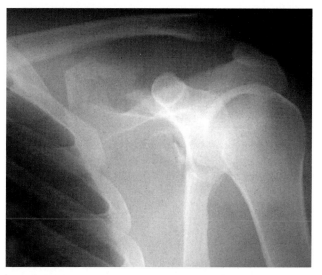

Figure 10-14   A type IV glenoid fracture emerging at the bottom of the glenoid.

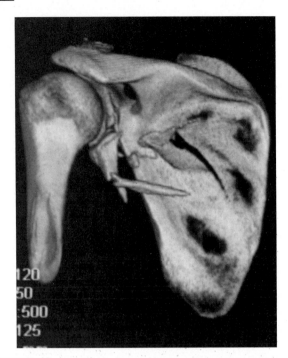

Figure 10-15   A CT scan of a scapula showing a comminuted type II fracture but also highlighting the damage to the scapular body.

The indication for surgery is if a spike of bone is displaced and may therefore enter the chest cavity or shoulder joint.
■ This can be treated by open reduction and internal fixation using a plate placed on the dorsolateral or dorsomedial surfaces of the scapula.
■ The requirement for surgery is rare.
■ Nonoperative management of all scapular fractures involves the use of a sling for 2 to 4 weeks followed by a course of physical therapy.

Neck Fractures

■ Displaced or angulated neck fractures should be treated operatively.
■ The exact amount of acceptable displacement or angulation of the neck is unknown, but it has been suggested that more than 1 cm of displacement or 40 degrees of angulation is an indication for surgical treatment.
■ The approach is posterior, with a plate being placed on the neck and dorsomedial surface of the scapula.
■ Remarkably little information is available about the success of treatment, but in one study 40% of nonoperatively treated patients had abduction weakness, 50% had subacromial pain, and 20% had a decreased range of motion.
  ■ This contrasts with no complications or pain in the operatively treated group, who had improved glenohumeral function.

Glenoid Fractures

■ About 66% of type I glenoid fractures are associated with shoulder instability.

■ Small peripheral glenoid rim fractures (see Fig. 10-13) may not be a problem, but it is recommended that shoulder stability be checked by arthroscopy or MRI imaging.
■ Larger fragments are associated with instability and should be fixed either arthroscopically or by open reduction and screw fixation using an anterior approach.
■ If there is evidence of residual glenohumeral instability, a type I fracture should be fixed regardless of its size.
■ Displaced type II–V fractures (Figs. 10-14 and 10-15) should be fixed internally.
  ■ The degree of acceptable displacement varies with the age and general health of the patient, but most surgeons would agree that a step-off of 5 mm requires surgery.
  ■ As with type I fractures, if there is evidence of instability associated with type II–V fractures, open reduction and internal fixation is required.
  ■ An anterior or posterior approach is required depending on the fracture pattern.

Spine Fractures

■ Spine fractures usually occur in association with body fractures.
■ Their treatment is nonoperative unless there is significant displacement, but this is extremely rare.

Acromion Fractures

■ Table 10-7 shows that surgeons rarely see displaced acromion fractures.
■ Type I fractures should be treated nonoperatively, but type II and III fractures are associated with significant local soft tissue damage, and internal fixation is recommended.
■ Intrafragmentary screw fixation or K-wires and tension banding can be used.
■ It is important to investigate the integrity of the rotator cuff in displaced fractures.
■ Acromial stress fractures have been reported, and these can be managed nonoperatively (see Chapter 6).

Coracoid Fractures

■ Most type I and II coracoid fractures are undisplaced.
■ Comparison of operative and nonoperative management has shown no differences in results between the two methods, and nonoperative management is recommended unless there is significant displacement.

COMPLICATIONS

■ The main complications of scapular fractures are shoulder stiffness, weakness, and pain.
■ The literature suggests about 64% of patients regain full movement, 76% have no pain, and 67% have normal power. The results are probably age dependent.
■ Nonunions are very rare but have been reported in fractures of the body, spine, coracoid, and acromion.
■ Treatment is by internal fixation if the nonunion is symptomatic.

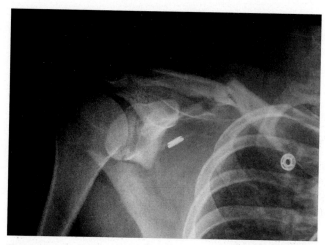

Figure 10-16 Floating shoulder with clavicle and scapular neck fractures.

FLOATING SHOULDER

The term *floating shoulder* is given to a combination of clavicle and scapular neck fractures (Fig. 10-16). Table 10-10 shows that about 30% of scapular fractures are associated with a clavicle fracture. The degree of instability depends on the extent of the associated soft tissue injury. Biomechanical analysis shows that the instability of a floating shoulder increases with damage to the acromioclavicular joint and the coracoacromial ligament. In the absence of these injuries, the floating shoulder is relatively stable.

It is the varying degree of stability that probably accounts for the argument between nonoperative and operative management. The rationale of operative management is that an unstable situation can be stabilized, allowing early movement and achieving better function. The literature does not support this philosophy, however, and the comparative results of operative and nonoperative management are given in Table 10-11. This indicates that the two methods of management give very similar results. There seems no doubt, however, that nonoperative management gives inferior results if the scapular neck fracture is displaced.

TREATMENT

- Treatment of undisplaced or minimally displaced floating shoulders can be nonoperative.

- If there is significant damage to the acromioclavicular joint or coracoacromial ligament, surgical stabilization of the clavicle and coracoacromial ligaments is advised.
- If the scapular neck is displaced, it should be reduced and plated through a posterior approach.

SCAPULOTHORACIC DISSOCIATION

EPIDEMIOLOGY AND ETIOLOGY

Scapulothoracic dissociation is the term applied to a closed forequarter amputation whereby the attachments of the shoulder girdle to the chest are disrupted (see Fig. 10-3). These injuries all follow high-energy trauma and are associated with considerable morbidity and mortality. Fewer than a hundred have been described in the literature. Initially all case reports involved arterial disruption and significant brachial plexus damage, but the condition can occasionally occur without these complications. The mortality rate is about 12%, and the incidence of brachial plexopathy averages 90%, with 80% of patients having severe vascular injury. Early amputation has been reported in about 22% of patients. The clavicle has been reported to be fractured in 58% of patients, with acromioclavicular disruption in about 22% of patients and sternoclavicular disruption in about 20% of patients. The increasing severity of injury is reflected in the scapulothoracic dissociation classification system of Zelle et al. (2004) (Table 10-12).

DIAGNOSIS

- The diagnosis is usually made by inference given the degree of injury, the swelling around the shoulder, and the presence of vascular and neurological abnormalities.
- Radiographs show lateral displacement of the scapula together with a clavicle fracture or dislocation of the sternoclavicular or acromioclavicular joint (see Fig. 10-3).

TABLE 10-11 RESULTS OF NONOPERATIVE AND OPERATIVE TREATMENT OF FLOATING SHOULDERS

Result	Nonoperative (%)		Operative (%)	
	Range	Average	Range	Average
Excellent/good	50–95	91.4	93.3–100	96.3
Pain free	50–84.6	59	42.8–75	61.5
Full range of motion	69.2–90	81.8	58.3–93.3	75

TABLE 10-12 CLASSIFICATION OF SCAPULOTHORACIC DISSOCIATION

Type	Description
1	Musculoskeletal injury alone
2A	Musculoskeletal injury with vascular disruption
2B	Musculoskeletal injury with incomplete neurological impairment of the upper extremity
3	Musculoskeletal injury with incomplete neurological impairment of the upper extremity and vascular injury
4	Musculoskeletal injury with complete brachial plexus avulsion

From Zelle BA, Pape HC, Gerich TG, et al. Functional outcome following scapulothoracic dissociation. J Bone Joint Surg (Am) 2004;86:2–8.

TREATMENT

- Most of the treatment of scapulothoracic dissociation relates to the management of the associated soft tissue injury.
- Vascular reconstruction, brachial plexus repair, soft tissue debridement, and amputation are the main operative procedures, but stabilization of the shoulder girdle is important, and clavicular plating and reconstruction of the sternoclavicular and acromioclavicular joints should be undertaken as required.
- Predictably the results are poor, with only 20% of patients achieving good results.

SHOULDER GIRDLE DISLOCATIONS

Shoulder girdle dislocations can occur at the sternoclavicular joint, acromioclavicular joint, and glenohumeral joint. Sternoclavicular dislocations are rare, but dislocations of the lateral two joints are relatively common.

Sternoclavicular Dislocation

EPIDEMIOLOGY AND ETIOLOGY

The strong ligaments that stabilize the sternoclavicular joint (see Fig. 10-1) prevent dislocation unless a significant force is applied. Dislocation may follow a direct force applied to the sternoclavicular joint or may occur if the shoulder is compressed and rolled forward. Most sternoclavicular dislocations occur in motor vehicle accidents or sporting injuries. The incidence has been reported to be 3% of all shoulder girdle injuries, and most authorities accept that the condition is more common than posterior glenohumeral dislocation.

CLASSIFICATION

Sternoclavicular dislocations are either anterior or posterior, with a 20:1 ratio in favor of anterior dislocation.

DIAGNOSIS

Clinical History and Examination

- Patients with anterior dislocation present with a prominent swelling at the sternoclavicular joint, and the medial end of the clavicle can be palpated.
- Posterior dislocations are more difficult to diagnose clinically, but sternoclavicular pain may be associated with flattening of the sternoclavicular joint.
- Because of the proximity of the great vessels, trachea, and esophagus, the patient may present with venous congestion, respiratory problems, choking, or dysphagia.
- It can be surprisingly difficult to distinguish between anterior and posterior sternoclavicular dislocations, and imaging may be required.

Radiologic Examination

- A routine chest X-ray or anteroposterior view of the sternoclavicular area may indicate a difference between the two sternoclavicular joints suggestive of a dislocation, but these radiographs are rarely diagnostic (Fig. 10-17).
- CT scanning should be used to diagnose the condition.
  - Both sternoclavicular joints should be scanned to permit comparison between the two sides (Fig. 10-18).
- If vascular damage is suspected in a posterior sternoclavicular dislocation, arteriography or MRI scanning may be required.

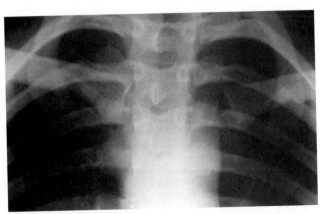

Figure 10-17   A-P radiograph showing a right-sided sternoclavicular dislocation.

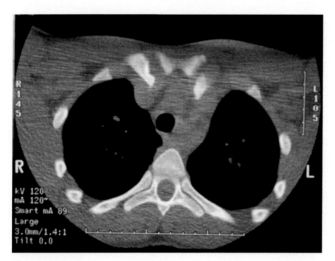

Figure 10-18   A CT scan showing a left-sided posterior sternoclavicular dislocation.

TREATMENT

- There is considerable debate about the role of nonoperative and operative management in anterior dislocation, but there are no good comparative data.
- Nonoperative management consists of relocation under anaesthesia, but the joint is inherently unstable.
- K-wiring has been used, but wire migration and persistent subluxation occur.
- Little morbidity seems to be associated with anterior dislocation, and it is suggested closed reduction be attempted if the patient presents acutely, but that the dislocation is accepted if this fails.
- Posterior dislocation should be treated by closed reduction.
    - A sterile towel clip can be used to pull the medial end of the clavicle upward and laterally.
- If closed reduction is impossible, open reduction can be undertaken.
- Following reduction, both anterior and posterior dislocations can be treated by the application of a sling for 2 to 3 weeks followed by a course of physical therapy.
- A figure-eight bandage can also be used, but little evidence indicates that this provides better results than a simple sling.

Acromioclavicular Dislocation

EPIDEMIOLOGY AND ETIOLOGY

Acromioclavicular injuries are common. Most are caused by a direct fall on the shoulder with the arm abducted. The causes the acromion to be driven downward and medially. Associated fractures of the clavicle and the coracoid process have been reported, and very rarely there may be a combined disruption to both the acromioclavicular and sternoclavicular joint.

CLASSIFICATION

The classification of acromioclavicular injury is shown in Table 10-13. It was originally described by Tossy in 1963 and modified by Rockwood in 1984. Types I–V are progressively more severe manifestations of the same injury caused by increasing soft tissue damage. The result is increasingly more displacement of the distal clavicle. Type VI dislocations are extremely rare and caused by high-energy injuries.

DIAGNOSIS

- In type I–V injuries, the distal clavicle is displaced upward (Fig. 10-19) and posteriorly, with a degree of posterior displacement depending on the extent of trapezius damage.
- Diagnosis depends on recognizing the degree of displacement.
    - Usually an anteroposterior radiograph or, preferably, one with a 10- to 15-degree cephalic tilt, will diagnose the dislocation and any associated fractures.
- Types I, II, IV–VI are usually straightforward to diagnose, and the difficulty lies in determining if the coracoclavicular ligaments are ruptured in type III lesions (see Fig. 10-19).
    - This may be detected by a stress radiograph with the patient holding a weight or by an ultrasound or MRI imaging.
- In type I lesions, the radiograph is normal, and a diagnosis is made from the history and by the presence of discomfort on palpation of the joint.

TABLE 10-13 CLASSIFICATION OF ACROMIOCLAVICULAR DISLOCATIONS

Type	Description
I	Sprain of acromioclavicular ligament
II	Acromioclavicular joint disrupted
III	Coracoclavicular ligaments disrupted. Possible deltoid or trapezius damage
IV	Clavicle displaced posteriorly into or through trapezius
V	Complete disruption of deltoid and trapezius insertion onto clavicle
VI	Inferior dislocation below acromion or coracoid

From Rockwood CA, Williams GR, Young CD. Injuries to the acromioclavicular joint. In: Rockwood CA, Green DP, eds. Fractures in adults, 2nd ed. Philadelphia: JB Lippincott, 1984.

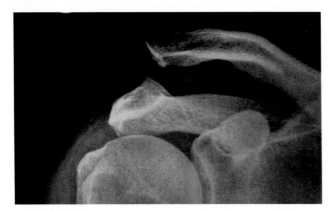

Figure 10-19 An A-P radiograph showing a type III acromioclavicular dislocation.

- In type II lesions, the distal clavicle is slightly elevated.
- In type III lesions, the joint is completely displaced.
- In type IV lesions, the joint may appear to be congruous because the distal clavicle has moved posteriorly rather than upward.
  - If this occurs, a lateral radiograph or CAT scan may confirm the diagnosis.

TREATMENT

- The requirement for operative treatment depends on the degree of displacement of the distal clavicle.
- There is universal agreement that type I and II lesions should be treated nonoperatively.
- A sling should be used for 10 to 14 days, followed by gradual mobilization with a physical therapy program.
- Type IV, V, and VI lesions all need to be treated surgically by open reduction, fixation with a coracoclavicular screw, reconstruction of the coracoclavicular ligament with a prosthetic ligament, and muscle repair.
- The debate concerns the management of type III lesions.
  - A number of different surgical techniques have been proposed, including the use of acromioclavicular K-wires with or without coracoclavicular ligament repair, coracoacromial ligament transfer, coracoclavicular reconstruction with a screw, and/or prosthetic ligament reconstruction and the use of a hook plate.
  - The use of K-wires is associated with poor fixation and pin migration, and acromioclavicular ligament transfer provides inadequate fixation in the long term.
  - In recent years the debate has therefore been among nonoperative management, coracoclavicular reconstruction, and the use of a hook plate.
  - Table 10-14 shows the incidence of excellent or good results for these treatment methods.
  - As with distal clavicle fractures, the use of a hook plate is less successful than coracoclavicular reconstruction with a screw and prosthetic ligament reconstruction.
  - The literature clearly shows, however, that the results of nonoperative management are as good as the results of surgical repair.

TABLE 10-14 EXCELLENT AND GOOD RESULTS FROM DIFFERENT TYPES OF TREATMENT OF TYPE III ACROMIOCLAVICULAR DISLOCATIONS

Treatment	Range (%)	Average (%)
Nonoperative	90.5–100	93.6
Coracoclavicular reconstruction	85.2–100	93.3
Hook plate	70–94.7	87

- Prospective comparative studies have confirmed this and have shown that shoulder function is gained more quickly with nonoperative treatment.
  - In recent years some surgeons have suggested that operative fixation should be confined to high-performance athletes, but given the results shown in Table 10-14 and the fact that residual deformity does not correlate with outcome, this view is illogical.

Suggested Treatment

- All type I, II, and III acromioclavicular dislocations should be treated nonoperatively.
- Types IV, V, and VI are treated by open reduction and coracoclavicular reconstruction using a coracoclavicular screw and a prosthetic ligament.

Sternoclavicular and Acromioclavicular Dislocations

A few cases of combined sternoclavicular and acromioclavicular dislocations have been reported. These are usually an anterior dislocation of the sternoclavicular joint and a posterior dislocation of the acromioclavicular joint. Most of the reported cases were treated nonoperatively, although in recent years acromioclavicular reconstruction has been undertaken more frequently.

Glenohumeral Dislocation

Glenohumeral dislocation is relatively common and particularly seen in young sportsmen in whom the redislocation rate is high. In recent years there has been a growing interest in the incidence and complications of glenohumeral dislocation in older patients, with the realization that the condition is associated with a higher incidence of rotator cuff tears. There has also been interest in the role of primary glenohumeral stabilization to prevent redislocation in younger patients.

EPIDEMIOLOGY

The incidence of shoulder dislocation in the overall population is between 1% and 2%. This is related to a number of factors, however, and particularly to gender and activity. The incidence in men is three times that of women, and in

TABLE 10-15 CLASSIFICATION OF GLENOHUMERAL DISLOCATION

Location	Position of Humeral Head
Anterior (96%–98%)	
Subcoracoid	Below coracoid process
Subglenoid	Below and anterior to glenoid
Subclavicular	Medial to coracoid process
Intrathoracic	Between ribs and thoracic cavity
Retroperitoneal	Behind kidney
Posterior (2%–4%)	
Subacromial	Below acromion
Subglenoid	Below and posterior to glenoid
Subspinous	Medial to acromion and inferior to spine
Inferior (luxatio erecta)	Below glenoid
Superior	Above level of acromion

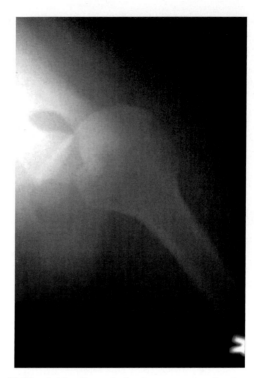

Figure 10-21   Axial radiograph showing a posterior glenohumeral dislocation. Note the impaction fracture.

sports such as ice hockey the incidence has been reported to be as high as 8%. The incidence of primary dislocation does not relate to age, although the incidence of redislocation clearly does.

CLASSIFICATION

Glenohumeral dislocation is best classified by the direction of dislocation (Table 10-15). Between 96% and 98% of all dislocations are anterior (Fig. 10-20), with the overwhelming majority subcoracoid in location. The other anterior dislocations listed in Table 10-15 are rare and associated with considerable force. Posterior dislocation (Fig. 10-21) accounts for 2% to 4%, with most being subacromial in location. Inferior and superior dislocations are very rare. In inferior dislocations, the head is displaced inferiorly and buttonholes the inferior shoulder capsule, causing the arm to be in full abduction. This condition is shown is known as luxatio erecta. In superior dislocation, there is significant damage to the acromion, coracoid, or proximal humerus as well as local muscular and ligamentous damage.

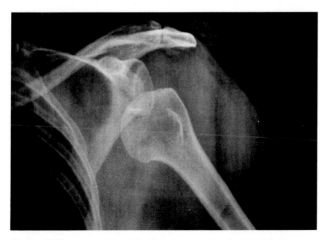

Figure 10-20   A-P radiograph of an anterior glenohumeral dislocation.

Associated Injuries

Most shoulder dislocations are isolated low-energy injuries. To permit the joint to dislocate, however, there has to be significant local soft tissue, or occasionally bony, damage. Tears of the glenoid labrum and capsule are common and frequently occur in the anteroinferior part of the glenoid. The Bankhart lesion involves avulsion of the labrum and capsule from the anterior scapula. At worst it may include a glenoid rim fracture (Ideberg type I). In posterior dislocations, there is rupture of the posterior capsule and teres minor. About 66% of patients have a posterior Bankhart lesion. In older patients the rotator cuff may be damaged in 60% to 90% of patients. Impaction fractures of the humeral head, the Hills-Sachs lesion, have been reported to occur in 47% to 82% of patients, the incidence rising in recurrent dislocation.

DIAGNOSIS

Clinical History and Examination

■ The patient usually presents with the history of a fall, usually with the arm in abduction, extension, and external rotation.
■ There may be a history of previous shoulder dislocation or of joint laxity.
■ Posterior dislocation may follow epileptic fits, electric shocks, or a fall on the flexed-adducted arm. In anyone who presents with restricted shoulder mobility, the possibility of a shoulder dislocation should always be considered.

- In patients with anterior dislocation, the humeral head may be palpable in the subcoracoid position.
  - There is usually a hollow posteriorly, and internal rotation and abduction are particularly restricted.
- In posterior dislocation, the arm is held in adduction, and internal rotation and external rotation is impossible.
  - There is flattening of the shoulder anteriorly with a prominence posteriorly.
  - Vascular and neural damage can occur and should always be looked for.

Radiologic Examination

- Most anterior dislocations are diagnosed on anteroposterior and lateral radiographs, although an axial or axillary view may be required.
- In posterior dislocations, the anteroposterior X-ray may look remarkably normal, but the normal overlap of the humeral head within the glenoid may be absent.
- An axial radiograph will confirm the diagnosis (see Fig. 10-21).
- Arthroscopy, ultrasound, and MRI scans may be used to investigate the integrity of the rotator cuff. MRI scans are particularly useful in diagnosing capsular and labral damage.
- MRI and CT scans are useful in diagnosing coexisting fractures.
- Doppler studies and angiography are indicated in the rare patient who presents with damage to the axillary artery.

TREATMENT

Nonoperative Treatment

- The initial treatment is nonoperative, with reduction of the shoulder joint. A number of techniques have been used (Table 10-16).

TABLE 10-16 METHODS FOR RELOCATING SHOULDER DISLOCATIONS

Method	Technique
Hippocratic method	Surgeon places foot on chest wall below shoulder. Applies traction to abducted arm
Stimson technique (posterior dislocation)	Patient prone on table with arm over side. 5- to 10-lb in hand
Milch technique	Arm abducted and externally rotated. Surgeon pushes humeral head into glenoid
Kocher technique	Arm externally rotated and adducted Gradual internal rotation

BOX 10-4 INDICATIONS FOR GLENOHUMERAL STABILIZATION

Soft tissue interposition
Glenoid rim fracture
Displaced greater tuberosity fracture
Rotator cuff tear
Young athlete (<20 years)

- The traditional method of management following reduction was to immobilize the shoulder in a sling for 4 to 6 weeks, but little evidence indicates that this reduces the redislocation rate, and mobilization can actually be started after about a week.

Surgical Treatment

- There are a number of indications for surgical treatment (Box 10-4).
- If there is soft tissue interposition from the long head of biceps, rotator cuff, or capsule, open reduction through an anterior approach is required.
- An associated glenoid rim fracture may make the shoulder joint unstable, and if this is the case the fracture should be fixed arthroscopically or through an anterior approach.
- Most greater tuberosity fractures associated with anterior shoulder dislocation will reduce to within 5 mm after relocation of the joint.
- If this does not occur, it is likely there is a significant rotator cuff tear and greater tuberosity fixation, and cuff repair should be undertaken.
- Occasionally the greater tuberosity fragment will be subacromial in location (see Fig. 11-5 in Chapter 11), and failure to reduce and fix the fragment will give rise to significant shoulder disability.
- The incidence of rotator cuff tears in patients over 40 years of age means that rotator cuff repair is often required.
- If there is clinical evidence of a rotator cuff tear 1 to 2 weeks after relocation, ultrasound or MRI imaging should be used to investigate the integrity of the cuff, which should be repaired if torn.
- The high incidence of recurrent dislocation in young patients has suggested to many surgeons that primary stabilization should be undertaken, and the evolution of arthroscopic shoulder surgery has provided surgeons with a minimally invasive surgical technique.
  - There is still debate about the usefulness of primary shoulder reconstruction after dislocation, but a number of studies comparing redislocation rates in young athletes after nonoperative and arthroscopic stabilization have been performed.
  - The average dislocation rate after nonoperative management in these studies in 88%, compared with 9% for the arthroscopically stabilized shoulder.
  - Further work is required, but there seems to be a role for primary arthroscopic stabilization in young athletes.

TABLE 10-17 INCIDENCE OF GLENOHUMERAL REDISLOCATION IN DIFFERENT AGE GROUPS

Age (y)	Incidence (%)
Overall	23–26
<20	34–64
20–29	28–37
30–40	9–12
>40	5–6

COMPLICATIONS

Redislocation

■ Recent literature indicates a significant incidence of redislocation, which is age related (Table 10-17).

■ The incidence of redislocation is about eight times higher if there is a glenoid rim or greater tuberosity fracture.

■ In patients 23 to 40 years of age, a moderate Hills-Sachs impaction fracture is associated with an increased rate of redislocation.

  ■ It has been shown that about 3% of patients sustain a redislocation within 1 week of the first dislocation.

  ■ Very early dislocation is higher in patients who have a high-energy injury, a neurological deficit, a rotator cuff tear, or when there is a coexisting fracture.

Nerve Injury

■ Nerve damage is surprisingly common after anterior shoulder dislocation and has been recorded as occurring in 21% of patients when assessed clinically and in 45% of patients when electrophysiological testing is used.

■ Axillary nerve and brachial plexus lesions are most commonly seen, but EMG studies of the peripheral nerves have shown that a solitary nerve lesion is present in about 50% of cases with mixed nerve lesions present in the other 50%.

TABLE 10-18 INCIDENCE OF PERIPHERAL NERVE LESIONS ASSOCIATED WITH SHOULDER DISLOCATION

Peripheral Nerve	Incidence (%)
Axillary	42
Suprascapular	14
Musculocutaneous	12
Ulnar	8
Radial	7
Median	4

■ The distribution of peripheral nerve lesions is shown in Table 10-18.

■ Analysis of brachial plexus lesions indicates that the posterior cord is the most commonly injured.

Vascular Damage

■ Vascular damage associated with shoulder dislocation is very rare, but when it occurs it usually involves the axillary artery, although damage to the subclavian artery has been documented.

■ The literature indicates that vascular damage is more common in the elderly, with 86% of patients with axillary artery injuries more than 50 years of age.

■ Patients normally present with absent pulses in the arm but may present with an axillary mass.

■ Vascular reconstruction is usually required.

SUGGESTED READING

Craig EV. Fractures of the clavicle. In: Rockwood CA, Matsen FA, eds. The shoulder. Philadelphia: WB Saunders, 1990.

Fann CY, Chiu FY, Chuang TY, et al. Transacromial Knowles pins in the treatment of Neer type 2 distal clavicle fractures. A prospective evaluation of 32 cases. J Trauma 2004;56:1102–1105.

Flinkkila T, Ristiniemi J, Hyvonen P, et al. Surgical treatment of unstable fractures of the distal clavicle: a comparative study of Kirschner wire and clavicular hook plate fixation. Acta Orthop Scand 2002;73:50–53.

Goss TP. Scapular fractures and dislocations: diagnosis and treatment. J Am Acad Orthop Surg 1995;3:22–33.

Hill JM, McGuire MH, Crosby LA. Closed treatment of displaced middle-third fractures of the clavicle gives poor results. J Bone Joint Surg (Br) 1997;79:537–539.

Ideberg R, Grevsten S, Larsson S. Epidemiology of scapular fractures: incidence and classification of 338 fractures. Acta Orthop Scand 1995;66:395–397.

Jubel A, Andermahr J, Schiffer G, et al. Elastic stable intramedullary nailing of midclavicular fractures with a titanium nail. Clin Orthop 2003;408:279–285.

Kitsis CK, Marino AJ, Krikler SJ, et al. Late complications following clavicular fractures and their operative management. Injury 2003;34:69–74.

Kuhn JE, Blasier RB, Carpenter JE. Fractures of the acromion process: a proposed classification system. J Orthop Trauma 1994; 8:6–13.

Marti RK, Nolte PA, Kerhoffs GM, et al. Operative treatment of mid-shaft clavicular nonunion. Int Orthop 2003;27:131–135.

McKee MD, Wild LM, Schemitsch EH. Midshaft malunions of the clavicle. J Bone Joint Surg (Am) 2003;85:790–797.

Neer CS. Nonunion of the clavicle. JAMA 1960;172:1006–1011.

Neer CS. Fractures of the distal third of the clavicle. Clin Orthop 1968;58:43–50.

Nordqvist A, Petersson CJ, Redlund-Johnell I. Mid-clavicle fractures in adults: end result after conservative management. J Orthop Trauma 1998;12:572–576.

Ogawa K, Yoshida A, Takahashi M, et al. Fractures of the coracoid process. J Bone Joint Surg (Br) 1995;77:425–428.

Robinson CM. Fractures of the clavicle in the adult. Epidemiology and classification. J Bone Joint Surg (Br) 1998;80:476–484.

Robinson CM, Court-Brown CM, McQueen MM, et al. Estimating the risk of nonunion following nonoperative treatment of a clavicular fracture. J Bone Joint Surg (Am) 2004;86:1359–1365.

Rockwood CA, Williams GR, Young CD. Injuries to the acromioclavicular joint. In: Rockwood CA, Green DP, eds. Fractures in adults, 2nd ed. Philadelphia: JB Lippincott, 1984.

Ring D, Jupiter JB. Injuries to the shoulder girdle. In: Browner BD, Jupiter JB, Levine AM, et al., eds. Skeletal trauma, 3rd ed. Philadelphia: WB Saunders, 2003.

Schandelmaier P, Blauth M, Schneider C, et al. Fractures of the glenoid treated by operation. A 5- to 23-year follow-up of 22 cases. J Bone Joint Surg (Br) 2002;84:173–177.

Te Slaa RL, Wijffels MP, Brand R, et al. The prognosis following acute primary glenohumeral dislocation. J Bone Joint Surg (Br) 2004;86:58–64.

Tossy JD, Mead NC, Sigmond HM. Acromioclavicular separations: useful and practical classification for treatment. Clin Orthop 1963;28:111–119.

Van Noort A, te Slaa RL, Marti RK, et al. The floating shoulder. A multicentre study. J Bone Joint Surg (Br) 2001;83:795–798.

Veysi VT, Mittal R, Agarwal S, et al. Multiple trauma and scapula fractures: so what? J Trauma 2003;55:1145–1147.

Webber MC, Haines JF. The treatment of lateral clavicle fractures. Injury 2000;31:175–179.

Wirth MA, Rockwood CA. Subluxations and dislocations about the glenohumeral joint. In: Bucholz RW, Heckman JD, eds. Rockwood and Green's fractures in adults, 5th ed. Philadelphia: Lippincott Williams & Wilkins, 2001.

Zelle BA, Pape HC, Gerich TG, et al. Functional outcome following scapulothoracic dissociation. J Bone Joint Surg (Am) 2004; 86:2–8.

PROXIMAL HUMERAL FRACTURES

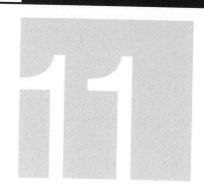

Much of the literature concerning the treatment of proximal humeral fractures has documented the results of various treatment methods, including wiring, plating, intramedullary nailing, and hemiarthroplasty, with surgeons usually claiming good results. Very few comparative studies of different treatment methods have been undertaken, however, and thus the indications for treatment of different fractures remain confused. In recent years there has been a realization that the majority of proximal humeral fractures occur in elderly patients and that nonoperative management may give equivalent or better results than surgery in this group of patients. But the indications for nonoperative and operative treatment for many proximal humeral fractures remain to be defined. A number of controversies about the treatment of proximal humeral fractures are listed in Box 11-1.

SURGICAL ANATOMY

The basic osteology of the proximal humerus is well known and illustrated in Figure 11-1. The anatomical neck lies behind the articular surface, and the surgical neck connects the humerus to the shaft. The lesser and greater tuberosities lie between the surgical and anatomical neck. It is the relative displacement of the anatomical and surgical necks

and the two tuberosities that defines the different types of proximal humeral fracture.

The rotator cuff muscles insert into the proximal humerus behind the insertion of the joint capsule. The teres minor inserts onto the back of the greater tuberosity and for about 1 cm down the proximal humeral shaft. Infraspinatus runs above teres minor and inserts onto the greater tuberosity behind supraspinatus, which runs under the acromion and inserts into the tip of the greater tuberosity. Subscapularis runs anteriorly from the scapula and inserts into the lesser tuberosity with a few fibers inserting onto the proximal humeral shaft.

The rotator cuff and proximal humerus are most easily exposed by dissecting through the outer layer of muscles. These are deltoid and pectoralis major. The deltoid arises from the lateral clavicle, acromion, and spine of the scapula

BOX 11-1 CONTROVERSIES IN THE MANAGEMENT OF PROXIMAL HUMERAL FRACTURES

Is the Neer or OTA (AO) classification better? Are either predictive of outcome?
Should fractures in the elderly be treated surgically?
What is the best treatment for two-part fractures?
Should hemiarthroplasty be used for all three- and four-part fractures?
How useful is percutaneous screw fixation of three- and four-part fractures?
Is there a difference between valgus impacted and head rotation fractures?

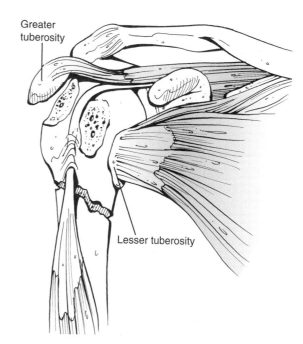

Figure 11-1   The anatomy of the proximal humerus showing the head and greater and lesser tuberosities.

and inserts into the deltoid tuberosity on the humeral diaphysis. Pectoralis major arises from the chest wall and the clavicle and inserts into the anterior aspect of the proximal humeral diaphysis. The cephalic vein lies between the muscles and serves as a marker for the deltopectoral intermuscular space, which has to be opened to allow access to the anterior shoulder. The short head of biceps and coracobrachialis lie between the deltoid and pectoralis major and the anterior rotator cuff. They originate from the coracoid process. The musculocutaneous nerve pierces coracobrachialis about 4 cm below the coracoid and is at risk in anterior shoulder surgery. The axillary nerve arises behind the proximal humerus and can also be damaged by a proximal humeral fracture or surgery. The main arterial supply to the area is the axillary artery, which gives rise to the anterior and posterior circumflex humeral arteries that anastomose around the surgical neck of the humerus and supply ascending branches to the humeral head. Damage to the vascular supply by fracture may cause avascular necrosis.

CLASSIFICATION

The original classification was put forward by Codman, who recognized that proximal humeral fractures result in fractures of the anatomical neck, surgical neck, and both tuberosities. This classification was extended by Neer (1960), who defined 15 different fractures based on the fracture morphology and degree of displacement. He defined a displaced fragment as one with more than 1 cm displacement or more than 45 degrees of angulation. Using these criteria, he defined proximal humeral fractures as minimally displaced, displaced two-part anatomical neck, surgical neck, and greater and lesser tuberosity fractures. He also defined three- and four-part displaced fractures as those that had displacement of either one or both the tuberosities together with a surgical neck fracture. In addition, he recognized two-, three- and four-part fracture dislocations and head-splitting fractures. The main advantage of Neer's classification was the recognition that displacement is important.

TABLE 11-1 DISTRIBUTION OF PROXIMAL HUMERAL FRACTURES ACCORDING TO THE NEER CLASSIFICATION

Neer Type	Distribution (%)
Minimally displaced	49
Two-part anatomical neck	0.3
Two-part surgical neck	28
Two-part greater tuberosity	4
Two-part lesser tuberosity	0
Three-part fracture	9.3
Four-part fracture	2
Two-part fracture dislocation	5.2
Three-part fracture dislocation	0.2
Four-part fracture dislocation	1.1
Head-splitting fracture	0.7

From Court-Brown CM, Garg A, McQueen MM. The epidemiology of proximal humeral fractures. Acta Orthop Scand 2001;72:365–371.

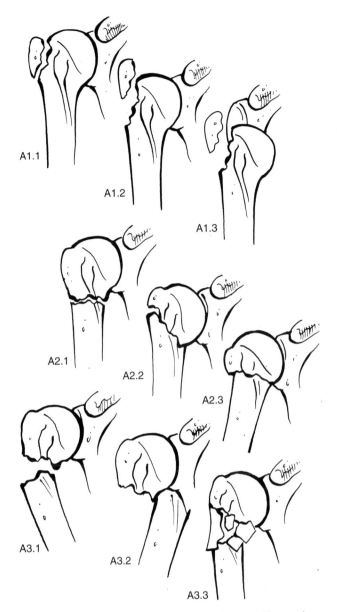

Figure 11-2 The OTA (AO) classification of proximal humeral fractures.

The OTA (AO) classification has 27 subtypes and therefore better defines the different fractures (Fig. 11-2). Type A fractures are unifocal fractures, with A1 fractures involving the greater tuberosity. A2 and A3 fracture are surgical neck fractures with A2 impacted and A3 nonimpacted. In A1 fractures, the suffixes 0.1 to 0.3 refer to the displacement of the greater tuberosity or glenohumeral dislocation. In A2 and A3 fractures, the suffixes 0.1 to 0.3 refer to different fracture types as shown in Figure 11-2. Type B fractures are bifocal with B1 fractures showing metaphyseal impaction. B2 fractures are nonimpacted, and B3 fractures are associated with glenohumeral dislocation. The suffix 0.1 to 0.3 refers to the different fracture patterns that are shown in Figure 11-2. Type C fractures are fractures of the anatomical neck, with C1 fractures showing slight displacement and C2 fractures showing marked displacement. C3 fractures are either associated with a dislocation or/and head-splitting fractures.

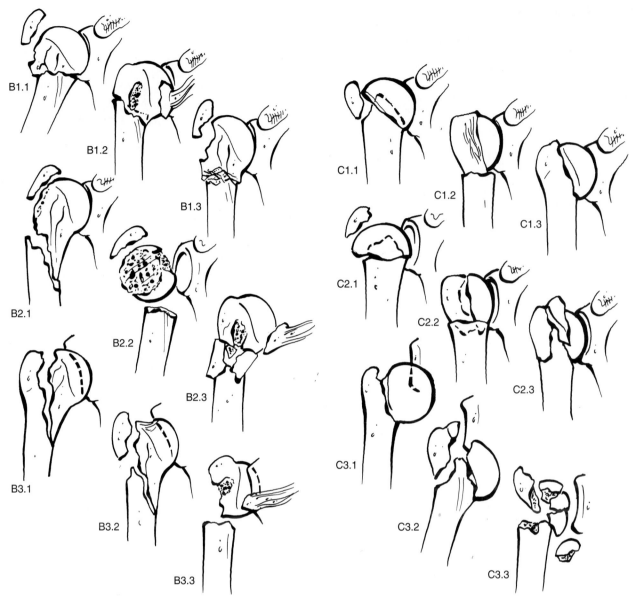

Figure 11-2 *(continued)*

Again the suffix 0.1–0.3 denotes different fracture configurations. The OTA (AO) classification is more comprehensive but does not take fracture displacement into account. It is therefore best to combine the OTA (AO) classification with Neer's displacement criteria, which is done in this chapter.

EPIDEMIOLOGY

The basic epidemiology of proximal humeral fractures is shown in Table 11-2. It is a fracture of the fit elderly, with analysis showing that about 90% of patients live at home at the time of fracture. Very few proximal humeral fractures are open, and in about 90% of patients there is no other musculoskeletal injury. About two thirds of proximal humeral fractures are type A unifocal fractures, with only 6% a type C fracture. The most common fracture type is the B1.1 bifocal impacted valgus fracture, involving both the surgical neck and the greater tuberosity. Altogether about 21% of proximal humeral fractures are impacted valgus fractures (A2.3, B1.1, C1.1, and C2.1). Table 11-1 shows the distribution of fractures if Neer's criteria are used.

DIAGNOSIS

History and Physical Examination

- As shown in Table 11-2, patients who present with proximal humeral fractures tend to be elderly.
- They present with a painful shoulder and a very restricted range of motion.

TABLE 11-2 EPIDEMIOLOGY OF PROXIMAL HUMERAL FRACTURES

Proportion of all fractures	5.7%
Average age	64.5 y
Men/women	30%/70%
Incidence	31.6/10^5/y
Distribution	Type F
Open fractures	0%
Most common causes	
Fall	76.2%
Motor vehicle accident	5.7%
Fall involving stairs	5.4%
OTA (AO) classification[a]	
Type A	67%
Type B	27%
Type C	6%
Most common subgroups[a]	
B1.1	15%
A3.2	13%
A2.2	13%
A1.2	10%

[a]OTA (AO) types and subgroups taken from Court-Brown CM, Garg A, McQueen MM. The epidemiology of proximal humeral fractures. Acta Orthop Scand 2001;72:365–371.

■ Nerve damage is not uncommon, and therefore a neurological examination of the arm should be undertaken.

■ In view of the age of the patients, a thorough social history is important because the fracture may well prevent an independent existence, at least on a temporary basis.

■ If the fracture has occurred in a high-energy injury, an examination according to ATLS principles is mandatory.

Radiologic Examination

■ Adequate information to diagnose and classify the fracture should be obtained from anteroposterior and axial radiographs (Fig. 11-3).

■ An axillary view can also be useful. CT scans can show the extent of the fracture but are rarely required.

■ MRI scans may help delineate the extent of associated soft tissue damage in fracture dislocations.

TREATMENT

Minimally Displaced Fractures

■ About 56% of type A, 41% of type B, and 15% of type C fractures are minimally displaced (Fig. 11-4).

■ There is universal acceptance these fractures should be managed nonoperatively, and the results of nonoperative management are generally good (Table 11-3).

■ Most patients are pain free and have a good range of motion after treatment.

■ Analysis shows that the results are age dependent, with most patients under 50 achieving normal shoulder function.

■ Poor results tend to occur in older patients who have coexisting medical comorbidities.

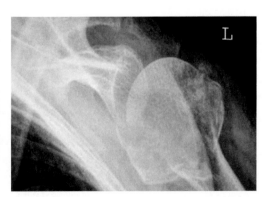

Figure 11-3 A-P and axial radiographs showing a proximal humeral fracture.

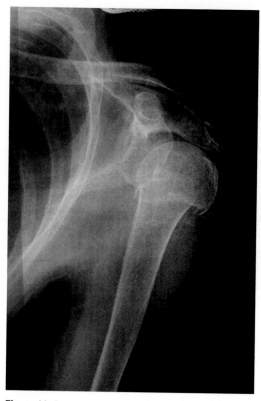
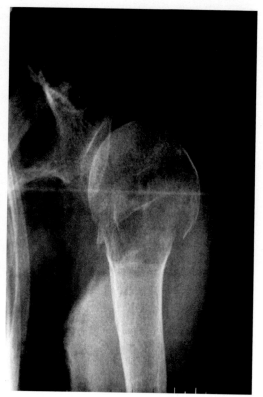

Figure 11-4   A-P and axial radiographs of a minimally displaced proximal humeral fracture. The A-P shows a valgus position of the head, but it is less than 45 degrees.

Displaced Fractures

Two-Part Fractures

Greater Tuberosity Fractures

■ Greater tuberosity fractures account for about 19% of proximal humeral fractures (Fig. 11-5).

■ About 4% are undisplaced (A1.1), 5% are associated with glenohumeral dislocation (A1.3), and the remaining 10% are displaced (A1.2).

■ These fractures occur in younger patients with an average age of about 55 years.

■ All greater tuberosity fractures should be regarded as possible rotator cuff tears.

■ The true incidence of rotator cuff tears associated with greater tuberosity fractures is unknown, but it seems likely they are more common in older patients, high-energy injuries, and where there is significant tuberosity displacement.

■ It has become accepted that displacement of more than 5 mm is an indication for surgical reconstruction of the greater tuberosity.

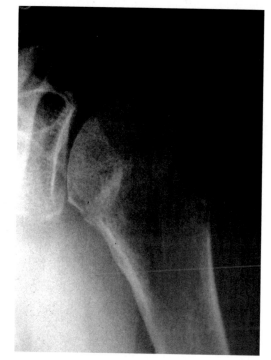

Figure 11-5   A greater tuberosity (A1.2) fracture showing significant displacement.

TABLE 11-3 RESULTS OF THE NONOPERATIVE TREATMENT OF MINIMALLY DISPLACED PROXIMAL HUMERAL FRACTURES

Result	Range (%)	Average (%)
Excellent/good	77–93.7	85.9
Average range of movement[a]	82.5–88	86.2
No pain	56.7–72	68.1

[a]The average range of motion is expressed as a percentage of the normal shoulder.

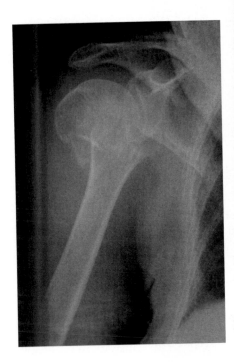
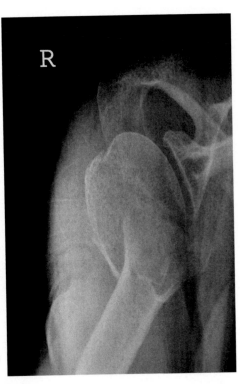

Figure 11-6 A-P and axial radiographs of a two-part (A3.2) surgical neck fracture. Note the posterior angulation on the axial view. This is common in this fracture.

- All greater tuberosity fractures should have an ultrasound examination or an MRI scan to check the integrity of the rotator cuff.
- If the tuberosity is displaced by more than 5 mm or imaging shows a cuff tear, operative treatment is indicated.
- Surgery can be through an anterior approach or a lateral deltoid splitting approach.
- The tuberosity can be fixed by an intrafragmentary screw if the bone fragment is large enough or with interosseous sutures or a suture anchor if screw fixation is impossible.
- Rotator cuff tears must be repaired.

Surgical Neck Fractures

- About 47% of proximal humeral fractures are in the surgical neck, although Table 11-1 shows that only 28% are significantly displaced.
- The majority of surgical neck fractures are translated fractures (A3.2) or impacted varus fractures (A2.2).
- Translated surgical neck fractures (Fig. 11-6) have received considerable attention in the literature.

- Suggested methods of treatment include nonoperative management, percutaneous K-wires, antegrade and retrograde intramedullary nailing, and plating.

Nonoperative Treatment

- Table 11-4 shows that nonoperative management is associated with better results than percutaneous K-wire fixation or plating, despite the much higher average age of the patients in published series.
- As with all treatment methods, the results of nonoperative management are age dependent, but they also relate to the degree of initial displacement. In a large study of nonoperative managed patients, it was shown those patients aged 50 to 59 years recovered 92% of shoulder function, whereas patients over 80 years recovered only 72%. Operative treatment did not improve the results, however.
- Tables 11-4 and 11-5 suggest that nonoperative management remains the treatment of choice for older patients with displaced two-part surgical neck fractures.
- The treatment involves using a sling for 2 weeks and then instituting a physical therapy program.

TABLE 11-4 RESULTS OF THE TREATMENT OF TWO-PART SURGICAL NECK FRACTURES

	Nonoperative		K-wires		Plate	
	Range	Average	Range	Average	Range	Average
Age (y)	66–77	72	43–61	56.5	46–62	56
Result/complication (%)						
Excellent/good	65–81.8	69.1	38.1–85.7	50	40–100	67
Fixation failure	—	—	14.3–42.8	35.7	0–54.5	31.8
Infection	—	—	0	0	0–50	4.5
Pin infection	—	—	0–23.8	17.9	—	—

TABLE 11-5 RESULTS OF ANTEGRADE AND RETROGRADE NAILING IN TWO-PART SURGICAL NECK FRACTURES

	Antegrade		Retrograde	
	Range	Average	Range	Average
Age (y)	48–71	63.1	29.2–69.5	60.1
Result/complication (%)				
Excellent/good	69.6–85.7	78.2	53.3–100	82.1
Fixation failure	0–15	7.7	2.9–23.5	12.7
Infection	0	0	0	0
Elbow dysfunction	—	—	0–36.8	25.7

Surgical Treatment

Percutaneous K-Wire Fixation
- This technique is widely talked about, but there is little evidence to justify its use.
- K-wires are inserted using either an antegrade or retrograde technique under fluoroscopic control after fracture reduction.
- The technique is much more difficult than it appears, and the difficulty of transfixing the fracture combined with pin loosening in osteopenic bone leads to high pin failure and infection rate (Table 11-4).
- The literature clearly indicates that the results are age dependent, with a study reporting 100% excellent results in patients under 50 compared with 13% excellent results in patients over 50 years of age. Because displaced two-part fractures are rare in patients under age 50, the technique has little place. Although it is very useful in displaced proximal humeral physeal fractures in adolescents (Fig. 11-7), it should not be used in the over-50 age group.

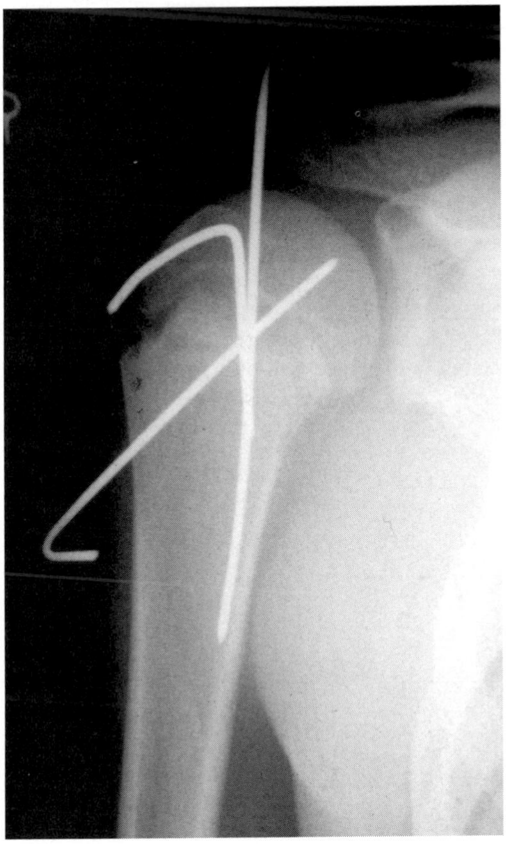

Plating
- Many surgeons have utilized T- or L-shaped neutralization plates or blade plates to treat displaced two-part surgical neck fractures (Fig. 11-8).
- As with percutaneous K-wire fixation, the results for those under 50 are much better than in older patients. A study comparing plate use in both age groups showed 75% excellent results in the under-50 group compared with 7% in patients over age 50. This accounts for the high incidence of fixation failure seen in Table 11-4. The technique can give good results in young patients but rarely in the elderly. It is likely the new generation of locking plates will improve these results.

Figure 11-7   K-wire fixation of a proximal humeral physeal fracture.

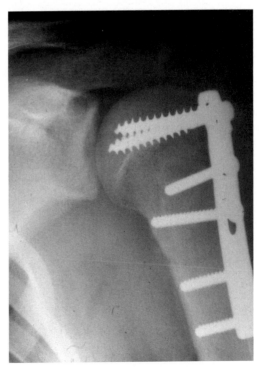

Figure 11-8   T-plate fixation of a proximal humeral fracture.

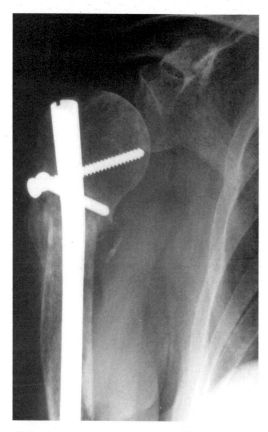

Figure 11-9   Antegrade nailing of a proximal humeral fracture.

Antegrade Intramedullary Nailing

■ The results of both antegrade (Fig. 11-9) and retrograde nailing of two-part surgical neck fractures are shown in Table 11-5.

■ The average age of the series dealing with this technique lies between those with K-wires and plating and nonoperative management, but it is clear the results are better than those associated with K-wires and plating.

■ The problem associated with antegrade nailing is rotator cuff damage.

■ Antegrade nailing is usually undertaken through a deltoid splitting approach under fluoroscopic control.

■ A statically locked short intramedullary nail is usually used.

■ As with all methods of treatment, better results are gained in younger patients, but unlike K-wiring and plating, the difference between the results in the young and older groups is less marked.

Retrograde Intramedullary Nailing

■ The results of retrograde nailing using two or more flexible intramedullary pins are similar to those of antegrade nailing and indeed to those of nonoperative management in patients of a similar age.

■ Retrograde nailing is undertaken using multiple thin nails inserted from above the olecranon fossa.

■ The obvious drawback is that the nails tend to back out, causing loss of elbow extension, usually of less than 20 degrees. This typically resolves after nail removal.

■ This technique is less popular than the other techniques listed in Tables 11-4 and 11-5 but does give good results.

Two-Part Varus Impacted Fractures

■ These are extremely common (Fig. 11-10), accounting for 13% of all proximal humeral fractures, and it is surprising only one study of their treatment has been done.

■ In a series of 133 consecutive fractures, the average age was 68 years, and 89% of patients were over 50 years of age.

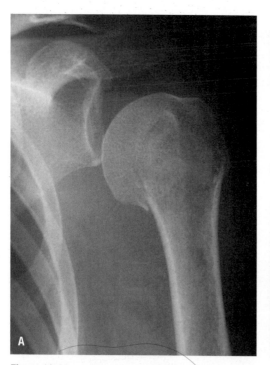
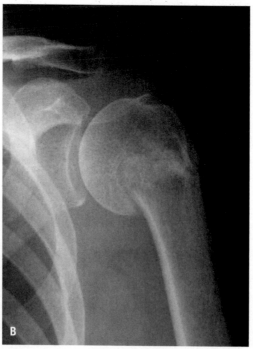

Figure 11-10   (A) Impacted varus (A2.2) proximal humeral fracture. (B) The same fracture after 3 months. This is the only fracture configuration to worsen with time.

- Nonoperative management was used, and 78% of patients had excellent or good results.
- There is understandable concern that increasing varus angulation causes increased impingement between the greater tuberosity and the acromion and therefore increased pain and decreased function.
- Analysis shows, however, that although the outcome of A2.2 fractures is age dependent, it is independent of the degree of varus of the humeral head.
- Nonoperative management is therefore indicated in these fractures.

Lesser Tuberosity Fractures

- These are extremely rare and treated in the same way as greater tuberosity fractures.
- If displaced, they should be internally fixed and if undisplaced can be treated nonoperatively. As with greater tuberosity fractures, imaging of the rotator cuff is indicated with repair undertaken as required.

Three- and Four-Part Fractures

- These fractures are associated with damage to the vasculature of the humeral head, and the incidence of avascular necrosis (Fig. 11-11) is therefore higher than in two-part fractures.
- Table 11-1 shows they are relatively uncommon.
- The literature dealing with their management is confusing. Different studies appear to show very different results. Three variables must be taken into consideration, however.
  - First is that the average age of the patient is very different, and the prognosis is unquestionably better

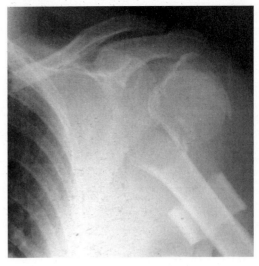

Figure 11-12 A three-part (B2.2) proximal humeral fracture.

for younger patients regardless of the method of management.
- Second, it can be difficult to diagnose three-part (Fig. 11-12) and four-part (Fig. 11-13) fractures from standard radiographs, and several papers have included a number of less severe injuries.
- Third, the prognosis for three- and four-part impacted valgus fractures is better for three- and four-part fractures with head rotation as originally described by Neer. The incidence of avascular necrosis is less, and reconstructive surgery has a higher success rate. Thus the results of studies of three- and four-part fractures depend on the ratio of valgus impacted to head rotation fractures.

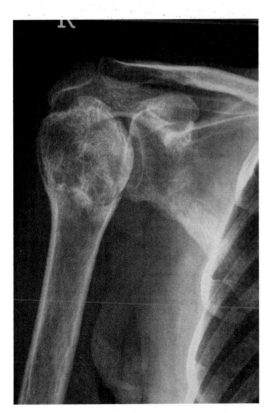

Figure 11-11 Avascular necrosis of the humeral head following a fracture.

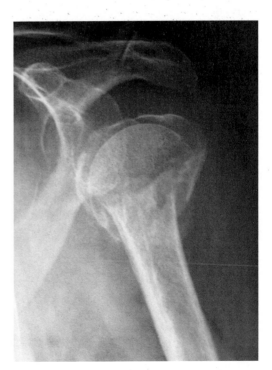

Figure 11-13 A four-part (C2.3) proximal humeral fracture.

TABLE 11-6 RESULTS OF THE TREATMENT OF THREE-PART PROXIMAL HUMERAL FRACTURES

	Nonoperative		Plate		Percutaneous screw		Screw/Cerclage	
	Range	Average	Range	Average	Range	Average	Range	Average
Age (y)	70–77	72.7	62–72	66.6	48.1–54	51.6	48–64	51.4
Result/complication (%)								
Excellent/good	47.1–77.8	63	42.9–70.6	63.1	83.3–88.9	86.7	90.0–100	92.9
Avascular necrosis	0–11.1	1.8	0–28.6	2.7	0	0	0–4.5	3.6
Infection	—	—	0–14.3	2.0	0	0	0	0
Fixation failure	—	—	0–7.3	2.0	0	0	0	0

Treatment

NonoperativeTreatment

■ Tables 11-6 and 11-7 show the results of nonoperative treatment in the management of three- and four-part fractures.

■ As with two-part fractures (Table 11-4), the patients tend to be older, and a poorer prognosis can therefore be expected.

■ The results for three-part fractures are at least equivalent to those of plating and are only slightly worse than those of two-part fractures.

■ The results of the use of nonoperative management in four-part fractures are poor, however.

Surgical Treatment

Plating

■ The results of plating of three- and four-part fractures are poor.

■ Table 11-6 shows that the technique is no better than nonoperative management in three-part fractures.

■ In four-part fractures, it is better than nonoperative management but worse than percutaneous screw fixation or the use of sutures or cerclage wires (Table 11-7).

■ There is no evidence that the technique should be used, although, as with two-part fractures, the new locking compression plates may improve results.

Percutaneous Screw Fixation

■ This technique is designed for valgus impacted fractures (Fig. 11-14).

■ Under fluoroscopic control, minimal dissection techniques are used to reduce the fragments into an ana-tomical position, and percutaneous screws are used to fix the fracture.

■ The data in Tables 11-6 and 11-7 show better results in both three- and four-part fractures, although the average age of the patients in these series is much younger. There is no good information about the use of this technique in older patients.

Suture-Cerclage Wire

■ It is possible to reduce and hold the tuberosities with nonabsorbable sutures or use a cerclage wire or tension band to hold the reduced tuberosities to the humeral shafts.

■ The soft tissue dissection is less than with plating, but again Tables 11-6 and 11-7 show that although good results can be obtained, it is younger patients who have been treated.

K-Wires and Tension Banding

■ This technique is rarely used.

■ Good results have been reported, but they have not been duplicated by many surgeons.

■ The technique cannot be recommended in three- and four-part fractures.

Intramedullary Nailing

■ Good results have been published, but there are very few good studies, and up to 71% fixation failure has been reported.

■ Both antegrade and retrograde nailing provide good results in two-part fractures, but these techniques are not appropriate for more complex injuries.

TABLE 11-7 RESULTS OF THE TREATMENT OF FOUR-PART PROXIMAL HUMERAL FRACTURES

	Nonoperative		Plate		Percutaneous screw		Screw/Cerclage	
	Range	Average	Range	Average	Range	Average	Range	Average
Age (y)	70–77	72.7	62–72	66.4	49.5–54	51.6	48–55	51.5
Result/complication (%)								
Excellent/good	11.1–60	28.6	0–85.7	48.1	73.2–75	74.3	72.7–81.8	77.3
Avascular necrosis	0–20	7.1	10–75	22.2	11.1–26.3	18.9	9.1–18.1	13.6
Infection	—	—	0–14.3	1.2	0	0	0	0
Fixation failure	—	—	0–10	4.3	0	0	0	0

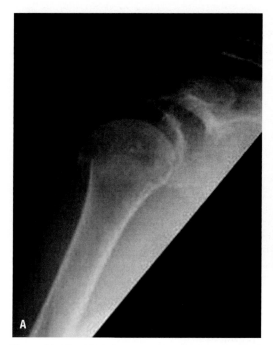 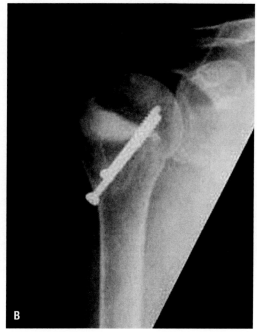

Figure 11-14   (A) A three-part (C2.1) valgus impacted proximal humeral fracture. (B) This has been treated with percutaneous screw fixation and calcium phosphate cement.

Hemiarthroplasty
- The results of the use of hemiarthroplasty prostheses (Fig. 11-15) to treat three- and four-part fractures are given in Table 11-8.
- A number of different implants are used, but the literature suggests little difference between them.
- They are inserted through an anterior deltopectoral approach with the tuberosities reconstructed after the prosthesis has been inserted.

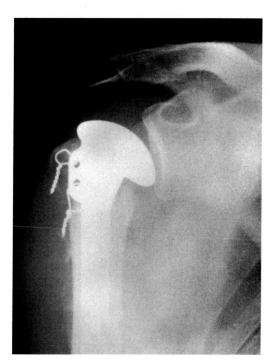

Figure 11-15   A Neer hemiarthroplasty prosthesis.

- Table 11-8 shows these prostheses are usually used in older patients and only about 50% of patients will get excellent or good results.
  - As with other techniques, this is age dependent.
  - Over 85% of patients have little or no pain and regain reasonable movement.
  - Patient satisfaction is high, and the operation is better than nonoperative management in the fit elderly.
- There has only been one prospective study comparing hemiarthroplasty with nonoperative management in elderly patients.
  - This showed that function was relatively poor in both groups, but the patients who had arthroplasties had better pain relief.
- There has been no prospective study comparing hemiarthroplasty with operative reconstruction.
- Recent analyses of hemiarthroplasty have shown the survival of these prostheses is excellent, with 96.9% survival at 1 year and 93.9% at 10 years.

TABLE 11-8 RESULTS OF THE USE OF HEMIARTHROPLASTY

	Range	Average
Age (y)	62–82	67.8
Result		
Excellent/good (%)	40–90.9	52.6
No/slight pain (%)	74.1–100	87.6
Forward elevation (degrees)	55–128	104.6
External rotation (degrees)	12–43	27.9
Internal rotation	T12–L4	L2

BOX 11-2 FACTORS PROVED TO AFFECT FUNCTION AFTER HEMIARTHROPLASTY

Age
Neurological deficit
Timing of surgery
Displacement of prosthesis
Displacement of tuberosities
Union of tuberosities
Alcohol consumption
Tobacco usage
Experience of surgeon

- A number of factors have been shown to correlate with improved shoulder function after hemiarthroplasty (Box 11-2).
- Age is certainly a significant predictor of outcome, but the skill with which the prosthesis is inserted and the tuberosities reconstructed is also important.
- Poor results can be expected if the tuberosities do not unite.
- A recent study has shown that experienced surgeons gain better results.
- Timing of surgery is also important, with the best results obtained if the operation is undertaken within a week of fracture.
- Results worsen progressively with increasing delay.

Fracture Dislocations and Head-splitting Fractures

- Three- and four-part fracture dislocations and head-splitting fractures are very rare (Table 11-1), altogether accounting for 2% of proximal humeral fractures.
- The prognosis is worse than for three- and four-part fractures, with very high rates of avascular necrosis and shoulder dysfunction often recorded.
- Hemiarthroplasty provides the best treatment method.

Valgus Impacted Fractures

- These fractures (Figures 11-4, 11-13, and 11-14) have assumed greater importance in the past 20 years.

- They represent about 21% of proximal humeral fractures. About 48% are minimally displaced, 31% are two-part, 18% are three-part, and 3% are four-part fractures.
- The average age of patients with a valgus impacted fracture is 72 years.
- The incidence of avascular necrosis is less than in fractures associated with rotation of the head.
- Minimally displaced and two-part valgus impacted fractures are usually treated nonoperatively, with 90% and 72% excellent and good results obtained, respectively.
- Nonoperative treatment of three-part surgical neck and greater tuberosity fractures results in about 63% excellent and good results.
- Four-part impacted valgus fractures are best treated by percutaneous screw fixation, with good results obtained (Table 11-7).
- Operative treatment of three-part valgus impaction fractures is indicated if there is excessive valgus.
  - These fractures have been treated successfully with reduction, the insertion of calcium phosphate cement to fill the void in the humeral head, and either screw fixation or plate fixation (see Fig. 11-14).
  - Unfortunately there is, as yet, no definition as to what constitutes extreme valgus of the humeral head, but consideration should be given to operative treatment of three-part impacted valgus fractures that show significant valgus of the head, particularly if they occur in younger patients.

Suggested Treatment

The suggested treatment of proximal humeral fractures is given in Table 11-9.

COMPLICATIONS

Nonunion

- The implication in some texts is that proximal humeral nonunion (Fig. 11-16) is common, but this is not the case.

TABLE 11-9 SUGGESTED TREATMENT FOR DIFFERENT PROXIMAL HUMERAL FRACTURES

Type	Criteria	Suggested Treatment
Minimally displaced		Nonoperative
Two-part surgical neck	Patient age <65 y	Antegrade or retrograde nailing
	Patient age >65 y	Nonoperative
Two-part greater tuberosity	Displacement <5 mm	Nonoperative
	Displacement >5 mm	Screw or suture fixation
Three-part and four-part impacted valgus	Patient age <65 y	Percutaneous screw fixation
	Patient age >65 y	Nonoperative
Three-part head rotation		Percutaneous screw fixation
Four-part head rotation		Hemiarthroplasty
Two-part fracture dislocation		Reduce and as for fracture
Three- and four-part fracture dislocation		Hemiarthroplasty
Head-splitting fracture		Hemiarthroplasty

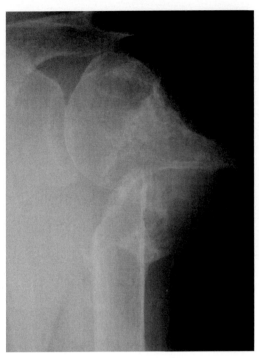

Figure 11-16   A proximal humeral nonunion.

- In a study of 1,027 consecutive proximal humeral fractures, only 11 (1.1%) occurred.
- Five (45.4%) were OTA (AO) type A3 fractures, and three (27.3%) were B2 fractures.
- Overall, 7.7% of proximal humeral fractures associated with metaphyseal comminution developed nonunion.
- Nonunion can be extremely disabling. The humeral head becomes stuck and movement is at the site of the nonunion.
- Treatment depends on the age and degree of infirmity of the patient. Symptomatic nonunion is best treated by internal fixation and bone grafting in younger patients and by hemiarthroplasty in older patients in whom pain relief is the most important outcome.
- Good results have been reported with locked antegrade nails and bone grafting.
- The results of hemiarthroplasty are also encouraging, but function is not generally as good as for primary hemiarthroplasty.

Malunion

- Malunion is relatively common after proximal humeral fractures but rarely requires surgery.
- In younger patients, however, repositioning of displaced tuberosities may improve shoulder function, and a proximal humeral osteotomy and refixation can be carried out.
- More commonly, hemiarthroplasty is the treatment of choice for symptomatic proximal humeral malunion.

Avascular Necrosis

- Tables 11-6 and 11-7 give the incidence of avascular necrosis in three- and four-part fractures.

TABLE 11-10 INCIDENCE OF NERVE DAMAGE IN PROXIMAL HUMERAL FRACTURES

	Incidence (%)	
Nerve	Minimally displaced	Displaced
Suprascapular	40	64
Axillary	51	72
Radial	25	46
Musculocutaneous	23	42
Median	13	24
Ulnar	5	5

Data from Visser CP, Croene LN, Brand R, et al. Nerve lesions in proximal humeral fractures. J Elbow Shoulder Surg 2001;10:421–427.

- If symptomatic this should be treated by hemiarthroplasty.

Heterotopic Ossification

- Heterotopic ossification has been reported to occur in up to 56% of hemiarthroplasty procedures. In 50% to 65% of cases, it is minor.
- When it is more severe and symptomatic, excision can be carried out, with indomethacin or radiation therapy used to minimize the risk of recurrence.

Axillary Artery Damage

- This is extremely rare and has been reported in less than 20 cases.
- It occurs in high-energy injuries, usually in younger patients.
- The head of the humerus is forced into the axilla, damaging the artery.
- Vascular reconstruction is usually required.

Neurological Damage

- Neurological damage is surprisingly common after proximal humeral fractures. A list of the nerves associated with proximal humeral fractures is given in Table 11-10.
- In brachial plexus injuries, the posterior cord is usually involved.
- There is significant nerve damage even in minimally displaced fractures, although its incidence is higher in displaced fractures. (The results in Table 11-10 were gained using EMG studies, and if clinical examination is used the incidence will be less.)
- Treatment is expectant and recovery usually complete.

SUGGESTED READING

Boileau P, Walch G, Krishnan SG. Tuberosity osteosynthesis and hemi-arthroplasty for four part fractures of the proximal humerus. Tech Shoulder Elbow Surg 2000;1:96–109.

Court-Brown CM, Garg A, McQueen MM. The epidemiology of proximal humeral fractures. Acta Orthop Scand 2001;72:365–371.

Court-Brown CM, Garg A, McQueen MM. The translated two-part fracture of the proximal humerus. Epidemiology and outcome in the older patient. J Bone Joint Surg (Br) 2001;83:799–804.

Esser RD. Treatment of three- and four-part fractures of the proximal humerus with a modified cloverleaf plate. J Orthop Trauma 1994;8:15–22.

Habernek H, Schneider R, Popp R, et al. Spiral bundle nailing for subcapital humeral fractures: preliminary report of the method of Henning. J Trauma 1999;46:400–406.

Jakob RP, Miniaci A, Anson PS, et al. Four-part valgus impacted fractures of the proximal humerus. J Bone Joint Surg (Br) 1991;73:295–298.

Koval KJ, Gallagher MA, Marsicano JG, et al. Functional outcome after minimally displaced fractures of the proximal humerus. J Bone Joint Surg (Am) 1997;79:203–207.

Lin J, Hou SM, Hang YS. Locked nailing for displaced surgical neck fractures of the humerus. J Trauma 1998;45:1051–1057.

Müller ME, Nazarian S, Koch P, et al. The comprehensive classification of fractures of long bones. Berlin: Springer-Verlag, 1990.

Neer CS. Displaced proximal humeral fractures. I. Classification and evaluation. J Bone Joint Surg (Am) 1970;52:1077–1089.

Norris TR, Green A. Proximal humeral fractures and glenohumeral dislocations. In: Browner BD, Jupiter JB, Levine AM, et al., eds. Skeletal trauma, 3rd ed. Philadelphia: WB Saunders, 2003.

Park MC, Murthi AM, Roth NS, et al. Two-part and three-part fractures of the proximal humerus treated with suture fixation. J Orthop Trauma 2003;17:319–325.

Resch H, Povacz P, Frolich R, et al. Percutaneous fixation of three- and four-part fractures of the proximal humerus. J Bone Joint Surg (Br) 1997;79:295–300.

Robinson CM, Page RS. Severely impacted valgus proximal humeral fractures. Results of operative treatment. J Bone Joint Surg (Am) 2003;85:1647–1655.

Robinson CM, Page RS, Hill RM, et al. Primary hemi-arthroplasty for treatment of proximal humeral fractures. J Bone Joint Surg (Am) 2003;85:1215–1223.

Stableforth PG. Four-part fractures of the neck of the humerus. J Bone Joint Surg (Br) 1984;66:104–108.

Visser CP, Croene LN, Brand R, et al. Nerve lesions in proximal humeral fractures. J Elbow Shoulder Surg 2001;10:421–427.

Zyto K, Ahrengart L, Sperber A, et al. Treatment of displaced proximal humeral fractures in elderly patients. J Bone Joint Surg (Br) 1997;79:412–417.

HUMERAL DIAPHYSEAL FRACTURES

Fractures of the humeral diaphysis differ from other long-bone fractures in that nonoperative management remains the standard treatment method for most fractures. Plating, intramedullary nailing, and external fixation are used, but they are mainly restricted to specific indications such as open fractures, pathological fractures, floating elbows, and multiply injured patients. Radial nerve palsy can be associated with both the fracture and the treatment method, and there is still debate about how both primary and secondary radial nerve lesions should be treated. A number of current controversies regarding the treatment of humeral diaphyseal fractures are listed in Box 12-1.

SURGICAL ANATOMY

There are two compartments in the arm, the anterior and posterior (Fig. 12-1). These contain a number of muscles that insert into and originate from the humerus. The posterior aspect of the humerus mainly gives rise to the lateral and medial heads of the triceps. The brachialis muscle arises from the anterior aspect of the bone, with brachioradialis and extensor carpi radialis longus arising from the lateral aspect of the distal half of the humerus. The rotator cuff muscles insert into the proximal humerus with pectoralis major, latissimus dorsi, and teres major inserting anteriorly into the proximal third of the bone. The deltoid

inserts laterally, approximately halfway down the bone with coracobrachialis inserting medially at the same level.

The main vascular supply is the brachial artery, which arises from the axillary artery at the lower border of teres major. Proximally it lies medial to the humerus, but it passes in front of the bone as it nears the elbow. The median nerve arises from the medial and lateral cords of the brachial plexus and runs with the brachial artery through the arm (Fig. 12-1). The ulnar nerve arises from the medial cord of the brachial plexus and runs with the brachial artery in the proximal half of the arm before entering the posterior compartment where it descends on the medial head of the triceps. The musculocutaneous nerve arises from the lateral cord of the brachial plexus, pierces coracobrachialis, and descends between biceps and brachialis, ending as the lateral cutaneous nerve of the forearm. The radial nerve arises from the posterior cord of the brachial plexus and passes behind the humerus in a shallow groove in the mid-diaphysis. It enters the anterior compartment through the lateral intermuscular septum and descends between brachialis and brachioradialis. It is at risk of injury in the mid-diaphysis and distally.

BOX 12-1   CURRENT CONTROVERSIES IN HUMERAL DIAPHYSEAL FRACTURES

Is functional bracing the best treatment method?
What are the indications for humeral plating?
Antegrade or retrograde nailing?
Are retrograde flexible nails useful?
What is the incidence of primary and secondary nerve palsy?
Should the radial nerve be explored?
How should humeral nonunions be treated?

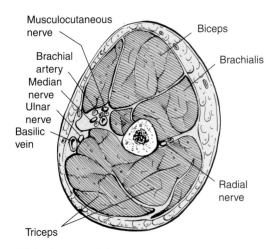

Figure 12-1   Anatomy of the upper arm.

CLASSIFICATION

The OTA (AO) classification is used for humeral diaphyseal fractures (Fig. 12-2). Type A fractures are simple unifocal fractures, with A1 fractures being spiral, A2 being oblique, and A3 being transverse. The suffix 0.1–0.3 indicates the location of the fracture with 0.1 proximal, 0.2 referring to fractures in the middle third, and 0.3 to fractures in the distal third. Type B fractures are wedge fractures with B1 a spiral wedge, B2 a bending wedge, and B3 a fragmented wedge. The suffix 0.1–0.3 means the same as in type A fractures. Type C fractures are complex with C1 fractures spiral, C2 segmental, and C3 comminuted. The suffix 0.1–0.3 refers to the number of intermediate fragments or segments in C1 and C2 fractures. In C3 fractures it refers to the extent of the comminution, with C3.1 fractures having two or three intermediate fragments, C3.2 fractures having limited comminution, and C3.3 fractures having extensive comminution.

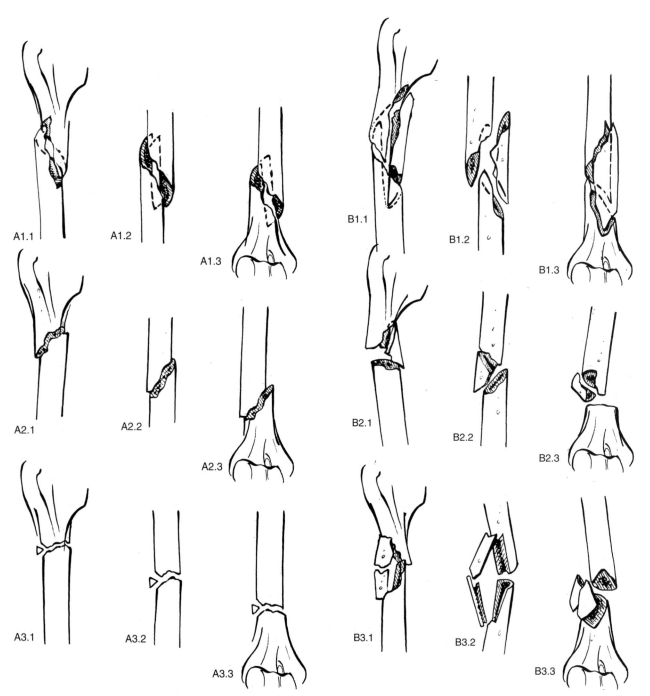

Figure 12-2   The OTA (AO) classification of humeral diaphyseal fractures.

EPIDEMIOLOGY

The epidemiology of humeral diaphyseal fractures is shown in Table 12-1. More women are affected, and there is a type H distribution (see Chapter 1). About 66% are at least 60 years of age. Open fractures are unusual, although they are more commonly seen in level 1 trauma centers. Most

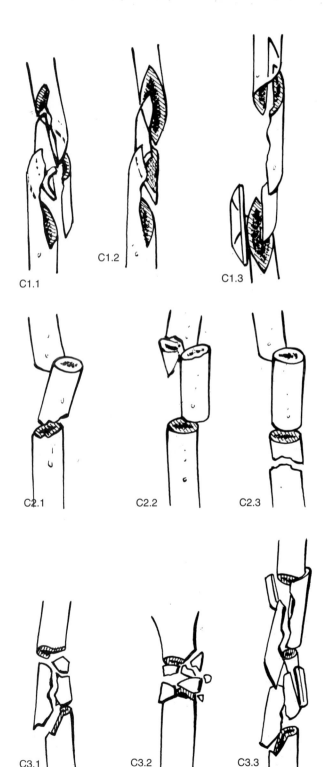

C1.1   C1.2   C1.3

C2.1   C2.2   C2.3

C3.1   C3.2   C3.3

Figure 12-2 *(continued)*

TABLE 12-1 EPIDEMIOLOGY OF HUMERAL DIAPHYSEAL FRACTURES

Proportion of all fractures	1.2%
Average age	54.8 y
Men/women	42%/58%
Incidence	$12.9/10^5$/y
Distribution	Type H
Open fractures	4.4%
Most common causes	
Fall	56.5%
Motor vehicle accident	11.6%
Fall height	7.2%
Pathological	4.4%
OTA (AO) classification	
Type A	62.3%
Type B	27.9%
Type C	8.8%
Most common subgroups	
A1.1	17.6%
A1.2	17.6%
B1.1	11.8%
A3.2	10.3%

fractures are type A unifocal fractures with type C fractures uncommon. Table 12-2 shows an analysis of the different causes of injury. Most humeral diaphyseal fractures follow a simple fall and occur in older patients. Motor vehicle accidents account for about 12% of fractures and have the highest incidence of type C fractures. About 5% of humeral fractures are pathological, with virtually all type A fractures. It is well recorded that some distal spiral humeral diaphyseal fractures occur as a result of sudden muscle action. They are associated with throwing grenades, javelins, or baseballs! They also occur in arm wrestling.

Associated Injuries

Young patients presenting with humeral diaphyseal fractures after high-energy injuries are frequently multiply injured. Analysis of the patients detailed in Tables 12-1 and 12-2 shows that about 5% of patients with humeral diaphyseal fractures present with spinal fractures or complex foot fractures and about 4% present with pelvic or proximal tibial fractures. Older patients tend to present with other fractures in the ipsilateral arm, usually distal radial fractures (5%).

TABLE 12-2 EPIDEMIOLOGY OF DIFFERENT CAUSES OF HUMERAL FRACTURE

Cause	Age (y)	OTA (AO) Type (%)		
		A	B	C
Fall	64.2	66.6	28.2	5.1
Motor vehicle accident	22.5	42.9	28.6	28.6
Fall (height)	34.0	60.0	20.0	20.0
Pathological	72.0	100.0	—	—

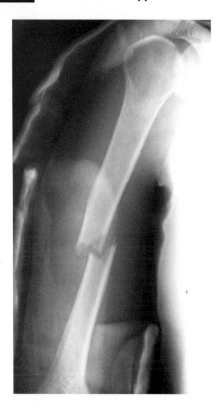
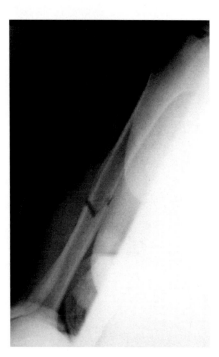

Figure 12-3 A-P and lateral radiographs of an A3.2 humeral diaphyseal fracture.

DIAGNOSIS

History and Physical Examination

- Most patients who present with humeral diaphyseal fractures are older and have isolated injuries.
- They present with a painful deformed arm that may be associated with a radial nerve palsy.
- In view of the frequency of radial nerve involvement and the fact that a palsy may develop secondarily after treatment, it is important to undertake a neurological examination of the arm and document the findings.
- In multiply injured patients, a thorough examination according to ATLS principles is mandatory.

Radiologic Examination

- Standard anteroposterior and lateral radiographs (Fig. 12-3) are usually sufficient to diagnose a humeral diaphyseal fracture.
- Further imaging is rarely required.
- Arterial involvement is rare but may occur, requiring Doppler and angiographic studies.

TREATMENT

Nonsurgical Treatment

- The standard treatment for humeral diaphyseal fractures remains nonoperative.
- In 1977 Sarmiento and his colleagues suggested the use of a plastic functional brace that could be removed and

reapplied to replace the earlier plaster U-slab (Fig. 12-4). Analysis shows that functional bracing gives better overall results than a U-slab, particularly with respect to elbow mobility.
- The results of fracture bracing are shown in Table 12-3. This shows a high percentage of excellent and good results with a relatively low incidence of nonunion, refracture, and secondary nerve palsy.
- The technique is associated with some impairment of shoulder and elbow function, however. The most common shoulder movements affected are external rotation, which is impaired in 30% of patients, and flexion (15%), although about 10% of patients also have impaired abduction. Elbow flexion and extension are both impaired in about 8% of patients.
- The results in Table 12-3 are good and suggest that functional bracing should remain the treatment of choice for most humeral fractures, but note that a number of papers dealing with this method of management have documented the results of selected patients whose fractures tend to be less severe.
- Distal diaphyseal fractures (Fig. 12-5) are difficult to control in a cast or brace. Plating is often used.
- In nonoperative management, it is suggested a hanging cast be used for 1 to 2 weeks, following which a functional brace is applied. Physical therapy can be started soon after the application of the brace.

Surgical Treatment

Plating

- Humeral diaphyseal plating is undertaken through either an anterolateral approach or a posterior approach.

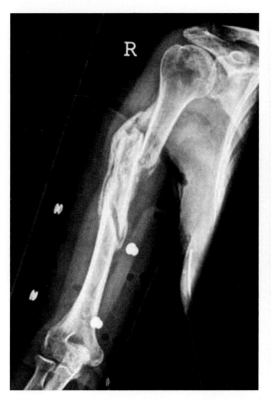
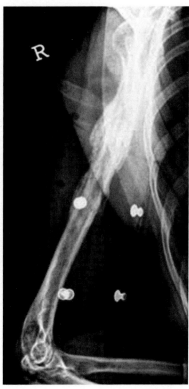

Figure 12-4 A-P and lateral radiographs of a humeral diaphyseal fracture treated with a functional brace. Note the malunion, but good function was achieved.

- The former is more useful for proximal and middle third fractures and the latter for distal third fractures or if the surgeon wishes to visualize the radial nerve.
- A 4.5 mm DCP or LC-DCP is usually used (Fig. 12-5), although locking plates are increasingly employed in older patients.
- Primary plating theoretically facilitates early joint movement, and in multiply injured patients humeral fixation aids patient mobility.
- The theoretical disadvantages are the likely higher incidence of infection and iatrogenic radial nerve damage than with bracing. Table 12-3 shows that this is in fact the case, although the incidence of both is relatively low.
- Shoulder and elbow mobility is improved after plating, and the incidence of nonunion is the same as in nonoperative treatment (Table 12-3).
- There is a low incidence of fixation failure.
- The studies included in Table 12-3 not infrequently used primary bone grafting in type B and C fractures, and evidence indicates that if primary bone grafting is not used with plate fixation, the incidence of nonunion is about 16%.

TABLE 12-3 RESULTS OF FUNCTIONAL BRACING AND PLATING

	Functional Bracing		Plating	
	Range	Average	Range	Average
Age (y)	25–57	38	31.5–51.1	39.9
Result/complication (%)				
Excellent/good	86.4–94	89.9	87.2–94.1	89.5
Normal/good shoulder function	85.1–94.2	89.2	94.1–100	98.5
Normal/good elbow function	92–97	93.1	91.3–100	96.7
Nonunion	2.6–13.4	4.2	1.9–8.5	4.2
Infection	0	0	0–6.5	3.4
Radial nerve damage	0–4.5	1.7	0–5.1	2.2
Refracture	0–3	0.7	0	0
Iatrogenic fracture	0	0	0–4.3	0.2
Fixation failure	0	0	0–4.9	2.1

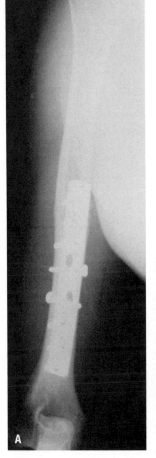
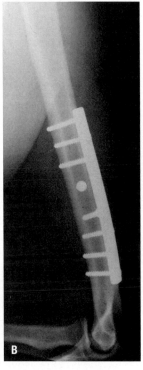
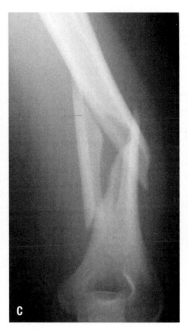
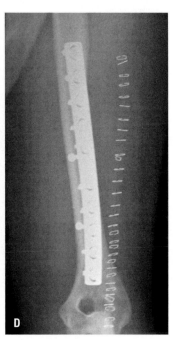

Figure 12-5 (**A,B**) A-P and lateral radiographs of a humeral diaphyseal fracture treated with an interfragmentary screw and a dynamic compression plate. (**C,D**) Pre- and post-operative radiographs of a typical distal humeral (B1.3) fracture that requires plating.

■ The average age of the series using plating as primary treatment is relatively low, and many of the patients were multiply injured. In older patients the incidence of fixation failure is higher, but the new locking plates may well extend the role of humeral plating.

Intramedullary Nailing

■ There are three main techniques for nailing humeral diaphyseal fractures.

■ The original technique involved the use of multiple flexible wires or nails passed in a retrograde fashion from a point just above the olecranon fossa.

■ In recent years interest has been expressed in the use of interlocking nails inserted in either an antegrade or retrograde manner.

Flexible Retrograde Nailing

■ Flexible nails or wires can either be inserted centrally above the olecranon fossa or through bilateral epicondylar portals.

  ■ The latter tends to be associated with poor results, and a central entry portal should be used.

■ The nails are inserted under fluoroscopic control, and if thin wires are used, up to 12 may be needed to stabilize the fracture.

■ The results of retrograde nailing using flexible nails are shown in Table 12-4. The overall results are similar to nonoperative management and plating, but there is a higher incidence of elbow dysfunction because of the requirement of a distal entry point and problems with nail migration, which is seen in about 5% of patients.

■ Distal heterotopic bone formation also occurs in about 4% of patients.

■ Overall results are good, although it should be remembered that the pins are unlocked and supplementary bracing is often required as is later pin removal.

Antegrade Interlocking Nailing

■ Antegrade nails are inserted through the head of the humerus and can be locked proximally and distally (Fig. 12-6).

■ Ideally, the nails should be inserted outside the rotator cuff, but most humeral nails are not flexible, and although such an entry point is desirable, it is rarely possible. Shoulder pain and disability is the main complication of the technique.

■ Table 12-4 shows that the results of locked antegrade nailing are worse than those of the other treatment methods, mainly because of shoulder dysfunction.

TABLE 12-4 RESULTS OF RETROGRADE PINNING AND NAILING AND ANTEGRADE NAILING

	Retrograde Flexible Pinning		Retrograde Locked Nailing		Antegrade Locked Nailing	
	Range	Average	Range	Average	Range	Average
Age (y)	24.6–40	34.1	39.2–54.2	51.7	32–64.6	49.8
Result/complication (%)						
Excellent/good	86.9–93.1	90.4	84.6–91.2	88.8	29.4–92.1	77.8
Normal/good shoulder function	90.5–100	95.8	88.9–100	92.6	29.4–92.1	77
Normal/good elbow function	66.6–100	89.1	55.6–88.2	82.4	93.3–100	97.2
Nonunion	0–10.7	6.2	0–8	4.5	0–23.3	11.6
Infection	0–3.6	1.7	0	0	0–6.7	1.8
Radial nerve damage	0	0	0–4.3	3.2	1–12-5	3.4
Iatrogenic fracture	0	0	5.9–13.3	7.1	0–31.2	5.1

■ There is also a higher incidence of nonunion, probably secondary to fracture distraction during nailing and iatrogenic extension of the fracture.

■ In addition to increased fracture comminution, closed nailing has also been reported associated with fractures at the tip of the nail, and fractures can propagate through to the elbow joint.

■ Care must be taken when inserting proximal and distal cross screws not to damage local vessels or nerves.

■ Table 12-4 shows that antegrade nailing is associated with a slightly higher incidence of secondary radial nerve palsy, and obviously if the radial nerve is caught in a fracture site it is at risk of being damaged by the reamers or nail.

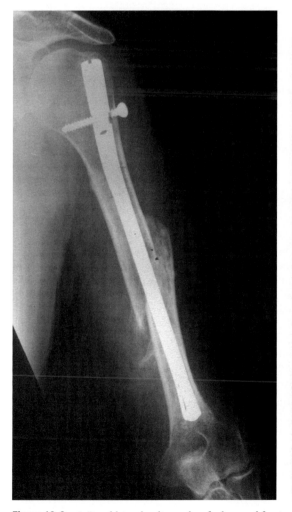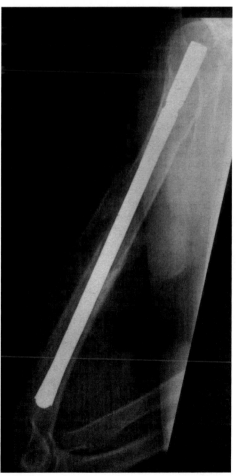

Figure 12-6 A-P and lateral radiographs of a humeral fracture treated with an antegrade intramedullary nail.

- Rotator cuff damage
- Adhesive capsulitis
- Impingement syndrome
- Proximal nail prominence
- Articular cartilage damage
- Prominent proximal cross screw

- Closed nailing should never be used if there is a nerve palsy present.
- Shoulder pain has a number of causes (Box 12-2).
  - The most common cause is rotator cuff damage.
  - The average age of the patients in Table 12-4 that were treated by antegrade nailing is 50 years; thus rotator cuff problems can be expected.
  - In young patients the cuff can be repaired, but in older patients repair is more difficult.
  - The nail must be buried in the bone because if it is left prominent, shoulder function is usually poor.
- The results in Table 12-4 relate to closed antegrade nailing. If open nailing is undertaken, the incidence of nonunion is much higher.

Retrograde Locked Nailing

- Locked nails can be inserted into the humeral intramedullary canal through an entry porthole just above the olecranon fossa (Fig. 12-7).
- This minimizes the shoulder problems associated with antegrade nailing but leads to increased elbow dysfunction.
- The results of retrograde locked nailing are shown in Table 12-4. Overall the results are better than those of antegrade nailing but not as good as those of plating (Table 12-3).
- Table 12-4 shows a higher incidence of iatrogenic fracture, mainly because of the stresses placed on the distal humeral cortex just above the nail entry point.
  - This may fracture as the nail is inserted, particularly if the humeral diaphyseal fracture is distal in location.
- As with antegrade nailing, closed retrograde nailing is associated with a slightly high incidence of radial nerve damage than nonoperative management, plating, or flexible nailing.

External Fixation

- External fixation is rarely used for the treatment of humeral diaphyseal fractures.
- Muscle penetration is inevitable and leads to joint stiffness.
- The technique is used in open fractures and particularly favored in missile or gunshot injuries where up to 78% excellent and good results have been reported.
- In severe injuries, a transarticular frame across the elbow may be necessary, but as with other long-bone injuries, ideally a unilateral periarticular joint-sparing frame should be used where possible (see Chapter 35).

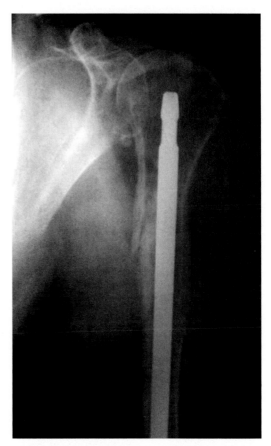

Figure 12-7 The use of a retrograde intramedullary nail to treat a humeral nonunion. The nonunion occurred in a patient treated with radiotherapy for breast carcinoma 21 years earlier.

- The general principles of open fracture management detailed in Chapter 4 should be followed.

Indications for Operative Treatment

Tables 12-3 and 12-4 show that nonoperative treatment with a functional brace provides good results in the majority of humeral diaphyseal fractures. Given the shoulder dysfunction and relatively high rate of nonunion associated with antegrade nailing, and the elbow dysfunction and incidence of iatrogenic fracture associated with retrograde nailing, it is suggested these techniques are not used routinely and that plating is the method of choice when internal fixation is required. Suggested indications for operative treatment are given in Box 12-3.

BOX 12-3 INDICATIONS FOR OPERATIVE TREATMENT

- Open fractures
- Irreducible fractures
- Multiply injured patients
- Failure of nonoperative treatment
- Floating elbow
- Pathological fractures

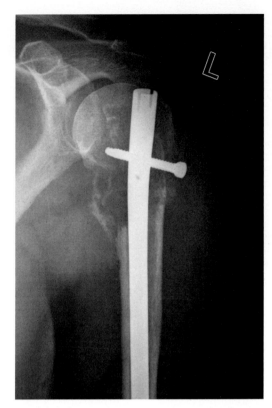

Figure 12-8 A pathological fracture of the proximal humeral diaphysis treated with a locked intramedullary nail.

Pathological Fractures

■ About 5% of humeral fractures are pathological (Fig. 12-8).

■ Closed nailing provides a good method of managing these fractures, and satisfactory pain relief and reasonable shoulder mobility can be expected.

TABLE 12-5 COMPLICATIONS AND RESULTS OF TREATMENT OF FLOATING ELBOWS

Result/Complication	Range	Average
Excellent/good (%)	44.4–71.4	56.2
Vascular injury (%)	5.6–28.6	15.7
Nerve injury (%)	28.6–63.2	51
Infection (%)	14.3–15.8	15.1
Nonunion (%)	0–42.1	23.5
Elbow arc (degree)	94–113	102

■ Most metastatic deposits are proximal and better stabilized by antegrade locked nailing.

Floating Elbow

■ The term *floating elbow* refers to the presence of ipsilateral humeral and forearm fractures (Fig. 12-9).

■ These usually occur in multiply injured patients, and the literature suggests about 60% of patients have an open humerus or forearm fracture, and about 60% have other musculoskeletal injuries.

■ About 16% have vascular damage requiring reconstruction, and about 50% have nerve damage (Table 12-5).

■ The nerve damage may involve the brachial plexus or any of the peripheral nerves, with the radial nerve most commonly affected.

■ Treatment is by fixation of both the humerus and forearm fracture.

■ Even with good treatment, however, only 45% of patients get excellent or good results, with the main problem elbow dysfunction.

■ A recent study has also shown that grip strength averages 35% when compared with the normal side.

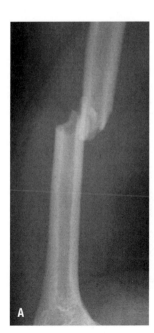

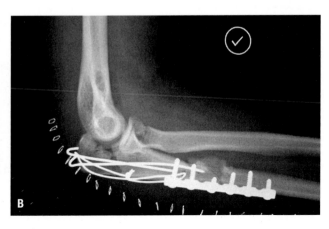

Figure 12-9 (A) A floating elbow. (B) The humerus was plated, and the ulna fixation is shown here. Note the considerable articular damage in this high-energy injury.

TABLE 12-6 SUGGESTED TREATMENT FOR HUMERAL DIAPHYSEAL FRACTURES

Injury	Treatment
Closed fractures	Functional bracing
	Consider plating in distal fractures
Open fractures	Plating
Floating elbows	Plating
Multiply injured	Plating
Failed nonoperative treatment	Plating
Pathological fracture	Intramedullary locked nailing
Nonunion	Plating and bone grafting
	(Locked plating in osteoporotic nonunions)

BOX 12-4 CAUSES OF PRIMARY AND SECONDARY RADIAL NERVE PALSY

Primary
Neuropraxia: closed and open fractures
Axonotmesis: closed and open fractures
Neurotmesis: usually open fractures

Secondary
Holstein-Lewis lesion
Mid-diaphyseal fracture entrapment
Iatrogenic neuropraxia
Trapped under plate
Reaming or nailing damage
Distal cross screw damage
Perineural fibrosis
Callus formation
Lateral intramuscular septum

■ Analysis of an article dealing with floating elbows indicates it is mainly the extent and severity of the nerve damage that dictates the overall prognosis.

Suggested Treatment

Suggested treatment of humeral diaphyseal fractures and nonunions is given in Table 12-6.

COMPLICATIONS

Nerve Damage

■ The brachial plexus and all of the peripheral nerves of the arm can be damaged in humeral diaphyseal fractures, but the radial nerve is particularly susceptible to injury.
■ The incidence of radial nerve damage varies with the type of injury.
   ■ In low-energy injuries usually treated by bracing, the incidence is reported as 7% to 11%.
   ■ In higher energy injuries in multiply injured patients, the published incidence is 15% to 34%, and in a series dealing exclusively with open humeral fractures, the incidence was 55%.
■ There is universal agreement that most radial nerve palsies are neuropraxias and 90% of palsies will resolve within 4 months. Thus routine exploration of radial nerve in closed fractures is not indicated.
■ Primary exploration of the nerve is only indicated in open fractures, often caused by gunshot or missiles, where the nerve may be lacerated and repair may be attempted.
■ The treatment of secondary radial nerve palsy is different.
■ The causes of both primary and secondary radial nerve damage are listed in Box 12-4.
   ■ The nerve may be trapped in the fracture. This commonly occurs in low spiral fractures below where the nerve penetrates the lateral intermuscular septum.
   ■ It may be caught in the fracture after reduction. This is called the Holstein-Lewis lesion (Fig. 12-10).
   ■ The nerve may also be trapped in the mid-diaphysis, although this is uncommon.

■ There are also reports of entrapment in callus and at the lateral intermuscular septum.
■ The most common cause of secondary radial nerve palsy is an iatrogenic neuropraxia during internal fixation.
■ These palsies will recover, but the nerve may be trapped under a plate or injured by passing a reamer or a nail down the intramedullary canal.
■ Distal cross screws may also damage the radial nerve distally.
■ Secondary nerve palsy following closed reduction of a fracture should be explored to ensure the nerve is free.

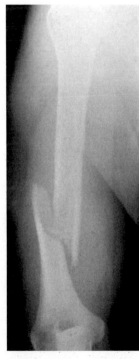

Figure 12-10   A-P radiograph of a spiral (A1.3) fracture in which the radial nerve may become trapped—the Holstein-Lewis lesion.

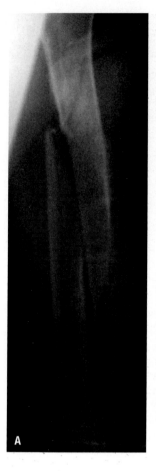

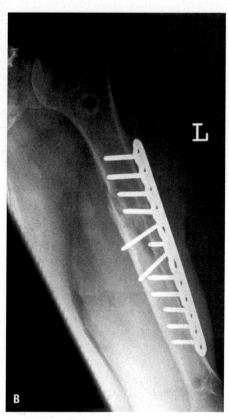

Figure 12-11   A-P radiographs of a humeral nonunion (**A**) successfully treated with a locking compression plate and bone graft (**B**).

- If the radial nerve lesion occurs after plating and the surgeon is certain the nerve is undamaged, a positive outcome is anticipated.
- If the nerve has not been well visualized during the plating procedure, however, the assumption must be made it has been damaged, and exploration is required.
- Similarly, if a radial nerve lesion occurs after closed nailing, exploration must be undertaken.
- Palsies secondary to callus, peroneal fibrosis, or entrapment by the lateral intermuscular septum occur later and are treated operatively.
- There are case reports of both ulnar and median nerve palsies following humeral diaphyseal fractures.
  - These can be treated in the same way as radial nerve injuries with exploration undertaken in open injuries and in closed injuries if there is no return of function after 3 months.
  - Nerve conduction studies can be used.

Nonunion

- Tables 12-3 and 12-4 show that the incidence of nonunion has been reported to be as high as 23%, although an overall average value of about 6% to 8% is probably accurate.
- The incidence of nonunion depends on the age of the patient, the degree of soft tissue damage, and the method of fixation.

- About 90% of humeral nonunions are atrophic and 10% are hypertrophic, suggesting an avascular cause for most nonunions.
- Treatment is usually by plating (Fig. 12-11) or intramedullary nailing, although the Ilizarov external fixator has been used.
- Bone grafting is usually used, although a number of surgeons have investigated the use of exchange intramedullary nailing without open bone grafting.
- The results of plating, intramedullary nailing with and without supplementary bone graft, and Ilizarov external fixation are shown in Table 12-7.
  - The best results are obtained from plating and bone grafting.
  - Similar union rates can be expected from nailing and grafting and from the use of an Ilizarov fixator, but, as with primary nailing (Table 12-4), exchange nailing is associated with shoulder dysfunction.
  - There are fewer excellent and good results associated with the Ilizarov device because of shoulder dysfunction, nerve damage from the fine wires, and refracture.
  - The results of plating in Table 12-7 come from studies using conventional plating techniques.
  - Early results with locking plates (Fig. 12-11) in osteoporotic humeral nonunions are good, with one study reporting 100% union and 91.7% excellent and good results in 24 patients with an average age of 72 years.

TABLE 12-7 RESULTS OF THE TREATMENT OF HUMERAL NONUNIONS WITH PLATES, INTRAMEDULLARY NAILING WITH AND WITHOUT BONE GRAFT, AND ILIZAROV EXTERNAL FIXATION

Result/Complication	Plates (%)		Intramedullary Nail (no Graft) (%)		Intramedullary Nail (Graft) (%)		Ilizarov (%)	
	Range	Average	Range	Average	Range	Average	Range	Average
Union	90.1–100	95.6	28.5–46.1	44	66.6–100	95.7	93.3–93.7	93.4
Excellent/good	76.5–90.1	86.8	15.3–28.6	20	66.6–91.3	87.2	62.5–83.3	76.1
Normal/good shoulder function	73.3–96.1	87.5	38.5–42.8	40	66.6–91.3	78.7	62.5–83.3	76.1
Infection	0–6.7	0.9	0	0	0–4.3	2.1	0–6.6	4.3
Nerve lesion	0–5.9	3.6	0	0	0–4.3	2.1	10–18.7	13
Refracture	—	—	—	—	—	—	6.2–13.3	10.9

- Table 12-7 shows that exchange humeral nailing without grafting is ineffective.
  - This is very different from the femur and tibia, and surgeons have attributed the lower success rate to fracture distraction.
  - It is more likely associated with humeral avascularity, and this is borne out by the high incidence of atrophic, rather than hypertrophic, nonunions.
- The treatment of infected humeral nonunion is difficult.
- The incidence of deep infection is low, with 6.7% the highest incidence recorded. Most infections are appropriately treated, and therefore infected nonunions are rare.
- An analysis of 15 patients showed that the use of functional bracing was uniformly unsuccessful in gaining union.
- This contrasted with a 70% union rate in nonunions treated by resection, operative fixation, and bone grafting.
- The treatment of osteomyelitis is discussed in Chapter 40.

Malunion

- Symptomatic malunions of the humerus are unusual.
- Up to 30% angular deformity of the humerus is acceptable both cosmetically and functionally.
- The most common deformity associated with functional bracing is varus, which rarely exceeds 10 degrees.
- If symptomatic malunion occurs, osteotomy, plating, and bone grafting is the best treatment method.

SUGGESTED READING

Bell MJ, Beauchamp CG, Kellam JK, et al. The results of plating humeral shaft fractures in patients with multiple injuries. J Bone Joint Surg (Br) 1985;67:293–296.

Chapman JR, Henley MB, Agel J, et al. Randomized prospective study of humeral shaft fracture fixation: intramedullary nails versus plates. J Orthop Trauma 2000;14:162–166.

Farragos AF, Schemitsch EH, McKee MD. Complications of intramedullary nailing for fractures of the humeral shaft: A review. J Orthop Trauma 1999;13:258–267.

Holstein A, Lewis GB. Fractures of the humerus with radial nerve paralysis. J Bone Joint Surg (Am) 1963;45:1382–1388.

Keller A. The management of gunshot fractures of the humerus. Injury 1995;26:93–95.

McKee MD, Miranda MA, Riemer BL, et al. Management of humeral nonunion after failure of locking intramedullary nails. J Orthop Trauma 1996;10:492–499.

Menon DK, Dougall TW, Pool RD, et al. Augmentative Ilizarov external fixation after failure of diaphyseal union with intramedullary nailing. J Orthop Trauma 2002;16:491–497.

Ring D, Jupiter JB, Quintero J et al. Atrophic ununited diaphyseal fractures of the humerus with a defect. Treatment by wave-plate osteosynthesis. J Bone Joint Surg (Am) 2000;82:867–871.

Ring D, Kloen P, Kadzielski J, et al. Locking compression plates for osteoporotic nonunions of the diaphyseal humerus. Clin Orthop 2004;425:50–54.

Rodriguez-Merchan EC. Compression plating versus hackethal nailing in closed humeral shaft fractures failing nonoperative reduction. J Orthop Trauma 1995;9:194–197.

Rommens PM, Verbruggen J, Broos PL. Retrograde locked nailing of humeral shaft fractures. J Bone Joint Surg (Br) 1995;77B: 84–89.

Sarmiento A, Kinman PB, Calvin EG, et al. Functional bracing of fractures of the shaft of the humerus. J Bone Joint Surg (Am) 1977;59(Suppl):596–601.

Sarmiento A, Zargorski JB, Zych GA, et al. Functional bracing for fractures of the humeral diaphysis. J Bone Joint Surg (Am) 2000;82:478–486.

Solomon HB, Zadnik M, Eglseder WA. A review of outcomes in 18 patients with floating elbow. J Orthop Trauma 2003;17: 563–570.

DISTAL HUMERAL FRACTURES

The recent literature concerning distal humeral fractures has dealt mainly with the treatment and complications of intra-articular fractures and largely ignored the problems associated with extra-articular fractures. There is an increased awareness of the importance of partial articular distal humeral fractures, although few studies have been undertaken. A few advances in the treatment of distal humeral fractures have been made in the last 20 years, but a number of current controversies, listed in Box 13-1, remain.

SURGICAL ANATOMY

The lower part of the humerus is divided into medial and lateral columns. It is flattened anteroposteriorly and essentially triangular in shape (Fig. 13-1). Medial and lateral epicondyles are situated on both sides of the distal humerus. Between them are the trochlea and capitellum. The trochlea is spool shaped and bounded by medial and lateral ridges. It articulates with the olecranon. The capitellum is spherical and articulates with the head of the radius. Posteriorly, there is a large fossa, the olecranon fossa, which accepts the tip of the olecranon on full extension. Anteriorly, there are two small fossae above the trochlea and capitellum to permit full flexion. The capsule surrounds the trochlea, capitellum, and all three fossae.

BOX 13-1 CURRENT CONTROVERSIES IN DISTAL HUMERAL FRACTURES

How common are extra-articular distal humeral fractures?
What is the prognosis for transcondylar fractures?
What is the optimal treatment of capitellar fractures?
Olecranon osteotomy or triceps split for intra-articular fracture?
How successful is the treatment of intra-articular fractures?
Internal fixation or primary arthroplasty in the elderly?
How should nonunions be treated?

The muscles of the common flexor origin, pronator teres, flexor carpi radialis, flexor digitorum superficialis, palmaris longus, and flexor carpi ulnaris arise from the outer surface of the medial epicondyle. The muscles of the common extensor origin, extensor carpi radialis longus, extensor digitorum, extensor digiti minimi, and extensor carpi ulnaris arise from the lateral epicondyle. The lateral epicondyle also gives rise to anconeus and the superficial portion of supinator muscle.

The brachial artery runs anteriorly across the elbow under the bicipital aponeurosis to divide into the ulnar and radial arteries at the level of the neck of the radius. The median nerve runs with the brachial artery. The ulnar nerve passes behind the medial epicondyle and enters the forearm by passing between the two heads of flexor carpi ulnaris. The radial nerve lies laterally on the capsule of the elbow joint and on supinator muscle. All three nerves are at risk of damage in distal humeral fractures, but the location of the ulnar nerve places it at greatest risk.

CLASSIFICATION

There are many distal humeral classifications. Most have dealt with intra-articular fractures, but a number have included both extra-articular, condylar, and capitellar fractures. The OTA (AO) classification has incorporated previous classifications and is shown in Figure 13-2. Type A fractures are extra-articular with A1 fractures involving the epicondyles. A2 fractures are simple extra-articular fractures, and A3 fractures are multifragmentary extra-articular fractures. In A1 fractures, the suffix 0.1–0.3 refers to the involved epicondyle and whether or not the medial epicondyle is incarcerated in the joint. In the A2 fractures, 0.1–0.3 refers to the direction of the fracture, with the transcondylar fracture being A2.3. In A3 fractures, 0.1–0.3 refers to the degree of comminution.

Type B fractures are partial articular fractures with B1 fractures involving the lateral condyle, B2 fractures the medial condyle, and B3 fractures the capitellum and trochlea. In B1 and B2 fractures, 0.1–0.3 refers to the extent of the injury (see Fig. 13-2), and in B3 fractures 0.1–0.3 refers to

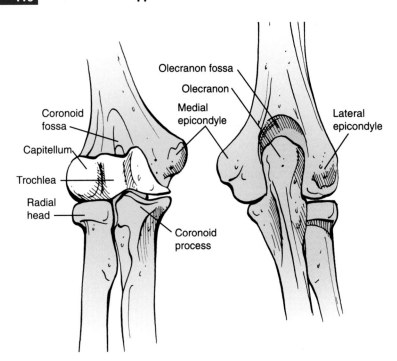

Figure 13-1   The anatomy of the distal humerus.

whether the capitellum, trochlea, or both areas are involved. All B3 fractures are shear fractures.

Type C fractures are complete articular fractures. C1 fractures have a simple articular and metaphyseal morphology, C2 fractures have a comminuted metaphysis, and C3 fractures have both articular and metaphyseal comminution. In C1 fractures, 0.1–0.2 refer to the displacement of the articular fragments, with 0.3 used for T-shaped epiphyseal fractures. In C2 and C3 fractures, 0.1–0.3 refers to increasing comminution.

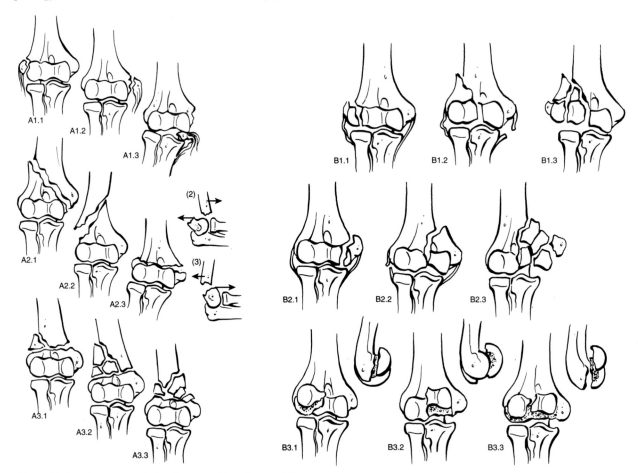

Figure 13-2   The OTA (AO) classification of distal humeral fractures.

EPIDEMIOLOGY

The epidemiology of distal humeral fractures is shown in Table 13-1. They are relatively rare injuries and have a type E (see Chapter 1) distribution with a fairly even age distribution in men and a unimodal peak in elderly women. Like distal femoral fractures, they are often thought of as high-energy intra-articular fractures in young patients, but the majority of fractures are in fact osteopenic. Table 13-1 shows that type A extra-articular fractures are as common as type C intra-articular fractures. The most common three subgroups are extra- or partial articular, with the most common intra-articular fracture the C1.2 displaced simple fracture.

An analysis of the main causes of distal humeral fractures is shown in Table 13-2. This shows that the overwhelming majority of fractures are isolated fractures in older patients. The fact that falls are associated with the highest incidence of type C fractures confirms the association with osteopenia. Sports injuries are relatively common, with many fractures extra-articular.

Associated Injuries

Most distal humeral fractures are isolated injuries. Because the majority of fractures occur in older women, the associated musculoskeletal injuries tend to occur in the ipsilateral arm. Analysis shows that about 13% present with

TABLE 13-1 EPIDEMIOLOGY OF DISTAL HUMERAL FRACTURES

Proportion of all fractures	0.5%
Average age	56.4 y
Men/women	29%/71%
Incidence	$5.8/10^5/y$
Distribution	Type E
Open	7.2%
Most common causes	
Fall	68.4%
Motor vehicle accident	13.1%
Sport	12.9%
Fall height	9.7%
OTA (AO) classification	
Type A	38.7%
Type B	24.1%
Type C	37.2%
Most common subgroups	
A1.2	10.3%
A2.3	9.4%
B3.1	7.2%
C1.2	7.2%

Data on causes and fracture types taken from Robinson CM, Hill RMF, Jacobs N, et al. Adult distal humeral metaphyseal fractures: Epidemiology and results of treatment. J Orthop Trauma 2003;17:38–47.

ipsilateral proximal forearm fractures, and about 6% have either proximal femoral or distal radial fractures. In young patients presenting with high-energy injuries, there may be other musculoskeletal injuries.

DIAGNOSIS

History Physical and Examination

- Most patients present with isolated fractures following a low-energy injury. They have a painful deformed elbow.
- Unlike supracondylar fractures in children, vascular injuries in adults are exceptionally rare, but a thorough neurological examination of the affected arm is essential because primary nerve lesions occur in about 4% of patients with distal humeral fractures.
- Because postoperative secondary nerve lesions also occur, any preoperative nerve palsy should be carefully recorded. In multiply injured patients, a complete examination according to ATLS principles is mandatory.

TABLE 13-2 MAIN CAUSES OF DISTAL HUMERAL FRACTURES

Cause	Age (y)	OTA (AO) Type (%)		
		A	B	C
Fall	57	33.3	25.1	41.6
Motor vehicle accident	33.2	33.3	30.9	35.7
Sport	22.9	65.8	14.6	19.5

Data from Robinson CM, Hill RMF, Jacobs N, et al. Adult distal humeral metaphyseal fractures: Epidemiology and results of treatment. J Orthop Trauma 2003;17:38–47.

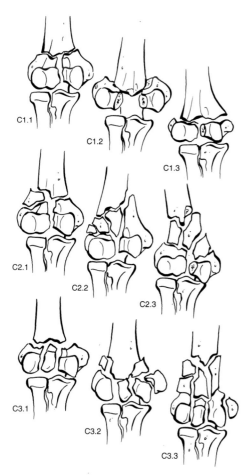

C1.1 C1.2 C1.3 C2.1 C2.2 C2.3 C3.1 C3.2 C3.3

Figure 13-2 *(continued)*

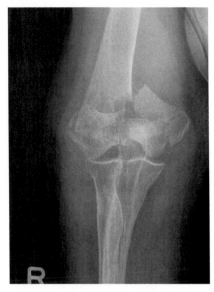

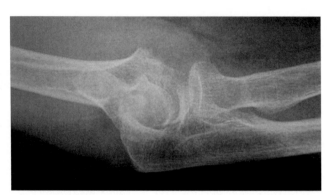

Figure 13-3 A-P and lateral radiographs of a C2.1 distal humeral fracture.

Radiologic Examination

- Standard anteroposterior and lateral radiographs are usually adequate to diagnose distal humeral fractures (Fig. 13-3).
- CT scans may help identify the extent of intramedullary or metaphyseal comminution but may not provide much intraoperative assistance.
- CT scans are very helpful, however, in B3 fractures, in which radiographs may not fully delineate the degree of comminution or show whether a capitellar fracture extends over the lateral ridge of the trochlea.
- The signs of a capitellar fracture on standard anteroposterior and lateral radiographs may be quite subtle (Fig. 13-4), revealing only a slight foreshortening of the capitellum on the anteroposterior radiograph or a double arc sign on the lateral radiograph.

TREATMENT

Type A Fractures

- Given their frequency, there is very little information in the literature about the treatment of extra-articular distal humeral fractures (Fig. 13-5) in adults.
- A1 fractures tend to occur in young adults, and A2 and A3 fractures in older patients.
- Nonoperative management should be reserved for undisplaced fractures and for elderly infirm patients in whom surgical intervention is contraindicated.

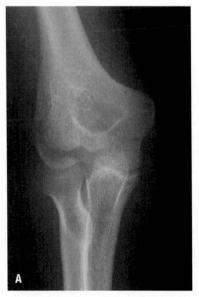

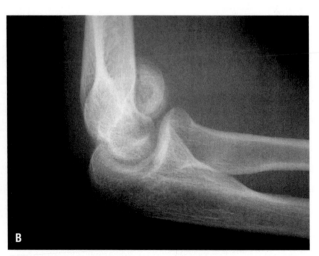

Figure 13-4 (A,B) A-P and lateral radiographs of a B3.1 capitellar fracture. (C,D) Treated with a headless Acutrak screw through a lateral approach.

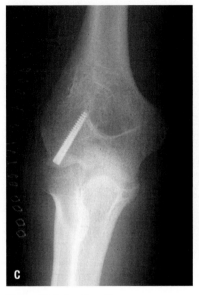

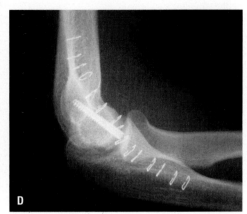

Figure 13-4 *(continued)*

- Most displaced fractures should be treated operatively using two plates (Fig. 13-5).
- A1 fractures are best treated with intrafragmentary screws (see Fig. 34-18 in Chapter 34), and A2 and A3 fractures with medial and lateral plates (Fig. 13-5).
- Low A3.2 transcondylar fractures in the elderly are probably best treated by primary arthroplasty (Fig. 13-6).
- What little information there is indicates a 4% nonunion rate in operatively managed type A fractures compared with 14% in nonoperatively managed fractures.
- The greatest difference is seen in A2 fractures, where the relative nonunion rates are 2.3% and 20%, respectively.

Type B Fractures

- The treatment of displaced medial or lateral condylar fractures is by intrafragmentary screws (see Fig. 34-18 in Chapter 34), supplemented, if required, by an antiglide plate placed on the ipsilateral supracondylar ridge.
  - This is particularly useful in B1.2, B1.3, B2.2, and B2.3 fractures.
- The treatment of B3 fractures is very different.
- About 80% of B3 fractures are B3.1 capitellar fractures. These are best treated by the use of intrafragmentary headless screws (see Fig. 13-4), which can be placed from

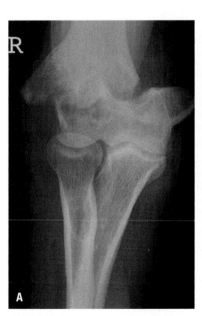

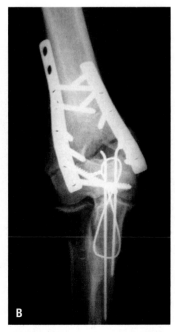

Figure 13-5 (A) An extra-articular A2.2 distal humeral fracture treated with two plates. (B) An olecranon osteotomy was used.

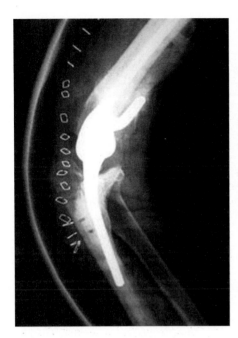

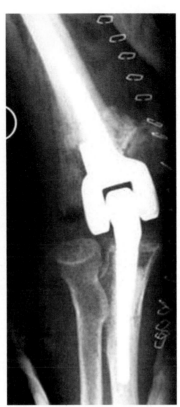

Figure 13-6 The use of a Coonrad-Morrey semiconstrained elbow prosthesis in the treatment of a distal humeral fracture in an elderly patient.

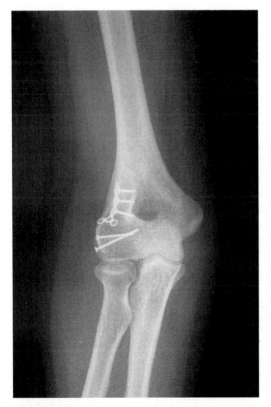

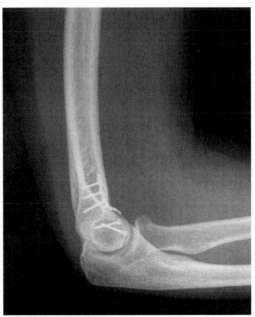

Figure 13-7 A-P and lateral radiographs of a B3.1 fracture treated with a mini fragment screw and antiglide plate.

TABLE 13-3 RESULTS OF INTERFRAGMENTARY SCREW FIXATION OF CAPITELLAR FRACTURES

Result/Complication	Range (%)	Average (%)
Excellent/good	75–100	91.7
No pain	66.6–100	83.3
Nonunion	0	0
Avascular necrosis	0–20	4.2

TABLE 13-4 RESULTS OF BICOLUMN PLATING OF TYPE C DISTAL HUMERAL FRACTURES

	Range	Average
Age (y)	36.2–57	49.6
Result/complication (%)		
Excellent/good	53.2–76.5	65.7
Nonunion	0–7.8	5
Infection	0–13	5.7
Fixation failure	2.6–7.9	4
Nerve damage	0–16.9	9.1
Heterotopic ossification	0–49.1	12.8

posterior to anterior using a posterior approach or, more easily, from anterior to posterior using a lateral approach.

■ An alternative is to use an intrafragmentary screw passed from anterior to posterior supplemented by a mini fragment antiglide plate, which is placed just over the upper edge of the capitellar fragment (Fig. 13-7). This does not impede flexion.

■ In comminuted capitellar fractures, multiple screws may be required.

■ Avascular necrosis occurs if the capitellar fragment is not reduced or if the capitellar fragment is made up of only the articular surface.

■ Closed reduction can be used, but the results are less good, and a comparison of screw fixation with K-wire fixation undoubtedly favors screw fixation.

■ Fractures of the trochlea are treated in the same way as fractures of the capitellum, but a medial approach is required.

■ The results of internal fixation of capitellar fractures are shown in Table 13-3.

■ The series that Table 13-4 comprises are very small, but the results are good.

Type C Fractures

■ In the early 1980s, there was a change from nonoperative treatment and treatment using screw fixation to rigid internal fixation using two plates (Fig. 13-8).

■ Since then, the surgical technique has remained essentially unchanged.

■ A posterior approach is used, and either an olecranon osteotomy or a triceps-splitting approach can be employed. The literature suggests no significant difference in results between the two approaches, and because the

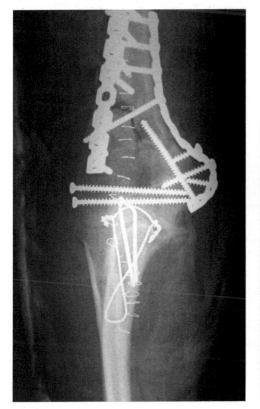

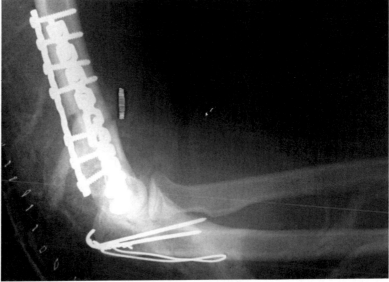

Figure 13-8   The use of two reconstruction plates to treat a type C distal humeral fracture.

TABLE 13-5 RESULTS OF INTERNAL FIXATION AND ARTHROPLASTY IN TYPE C FRACTURES IN THE ELDERLY

	Internal Fixation		Arthroplasty	
	Range	Average	Range	Average
Age (y)	73.6–80	78.7	72–84.6	74.4
Result/complication (%)				
Excellent/good	66.6–84.6	80.4	90–95.2	93.2
Nonunion	3.4–8.3	7.5	—	—
Infection	0–8.3	2	0	0
Fixation failure	8.2–25	11.5	0–5	1.7
Heterotopic ossification	8.3	8.3	0–10	3.3

use of an olecranon osteotomy results in better visualization, it is preferred.
- A transverse or chevron type of intra-articular osteotomy can be used, or an extra-articular osteotomy may be undertaken.
  - The former gives better visualization, and the literature does not indicate that either the transverse or chevron osteotomy is superior. Either can therefore be used.
- Care must be taken to protect the ulnar nerve as the triceps is mobilized.
- Two plates should be used, ideally placed at right angles to each other.
- The lateral plate is placed posteriorly, and the medial plate is placed on the medial aspect of the medial supracondylar ridge.
- Usually reconstruction or one-third tubular plates are used, although location-specific distal humeral plates are available.
- The results of this type of management are shown in Table 13-4.
  - Despite low rates of nonunion, infection, and fixation failure, the incidence of excellent and good results averages about 65%.
- This is because patients are usually left with a degree of impaired elbow mobility.
  - Worse results can be expected in older patients, C3 fractures, polytrauma patients, patients with other injuries in the same arm, or if the surgery is delayed.
  - A recent analysis has indicated that in severe fractures the average block to extension is about 25 degrees, with an overall flexion/extension arc of about 105 degrees obtained after treatment.
  - Elbow rotation is about 75% of normal.
  - About 4% of olecranon osteotomies remain ununited and may require secondary surgery.
  - Olecranon osteotomies are usually closed with K-wires and a tension band (see Chapter 34), and a secondary operation to remove the wires is often required.

Fractures in the Elderly

- An alternative surgical technique in elderly patients is the use of a primary semiconstrained elbow arthroplasty (see Fig. 13-6).

- If elbow arthroplasty is being considered, the patient should be warned that heavy lifting must be avoided postoperatively.
- The results of both internal fixation and elbow arthroplasty in type C distal humeral fractures in elderly patients are given in Table 13-5.
  - The percentage of excellent and good results is higher than in Table 13-4, but the patient numbers are much smaller.
- Both methods of management give reasonable results, but predictably there is a relatively high failure of fixation, more heterotopic ossification, and a greater incidence of nonunion in the internally fixed patient.
- The results of arthroplasty are clearly very good and, as with other fractures in the elderly, it is likely elbow arthroplasty will become more widely used to treat type C and A2.3 fractures in the elderly.

Suggested Treatment

Table 13-6 gives a summary of the treatment of the different types of distal humeral fractures.

TABLE 13-6 SUGGESTED TREATMENT OF DISTAL HUMERAL FRACTURES

Fracture Location	Treatment
Type A	
Epicondyle	Intrafragmentary screws
Metaphyseal	Bicolumn plates
Transcondylar (elderly)	Arthroplasty
Type B	
Lateral/medial condyles	Screw ± antiglide plate
Capitellum/trochlea	Interfragmentary screws
Type C	
Young patient	Bicolumn plates
Elderly patient	Arthroplasty
(C2 or C3 fracture)	

TABLE 13-7 RESULTS OF INTERNAL FIXATION AND ARTHROPLASTY IN TREATMENT OF DISTAL HUMERAL NONUNION

Result/Complication	Internal Fixation (%)		Arthroplasty (%)	
	Range	Average	Range	Average
Excellent/good	35–73.3	51.4	57.1–86.1	78
Nonunion	1.9–20	6.9	—	—
Infection	0–3.8	2.3	5.2–7.1	6
Nerve damage	5–13.3	9.2	5.2–7.1	6

COMPLICATIONS

Nonunion

- Tables 13-4 and 13-5 give the incidence of nonunion after plate fixation of distal humeral fractures. This is less than the incidence of nonunion after transcondylar fractures in older patients (see Fig. 13-5), and it is interesting that the literature dealing with the treatment of distal humeral nonunion includes many A2 fractures.
- The treatment of distal humeral nonunion is essentially the same as the primary treatment of distal humeral fractures, where the choice is among stabilization, bone grafting, and arthrolysis or prosthetic replacement. The results of both procedures are shown in Table 13-7.
- Stabilization and bone grafting results in a 93% union rate, but the overall results of prosthetic replacement are clearly better, and arthroplasty should be used for older patients, with stabilization and bone grafting reserved for younger patients.

Malunion

- Symptomatic malunion in older patients is treated by prosthetic replacement of the elbow joint.
- In younger patients, however, an intra-articular osteotomy, stabilization, and bone grafting is the treatment of choice.
- This is a difficult procedure, but in expert hands about 75% excellent or good results can be expected, and the largest series has shown an increase in the flexion/extension arc from 43 degrees before surgery to 96 degrees after surgery.

Nerve Damage

- Primary nerve damage occurs in about 4% of patients with distal humeral fractures if assessed by clinical examination. About 66% of cases involve the ulnar nerve, 25% the median nerve, and 7% the radial nerve. Most are neuropraxias and can be expected to resolve.
- The incidence of secondary nerve lesions is shown in Table 13-4. These virtually always involve the ulnar nerve, and again they are normally neuropraxias.

- Ulnar nerve transposition is recommended if the nerve is seen to be in direct contact with the plate during surgery.
- Postoperative ulnar neuropraxia can be treated expectantly, but persistent symptoms should be investigated with nerve conduction studies, and a decompression or transposition may be required.

SUGGESTED READING

Frankle MA, Hersocovici D, DiPasquale TG, et al. A comparison of open reduction and internal fixation and primary total elbow arthroplasty in the treatment of intra-articular distal humerus fractures in women older than age 65. J Orthop Trauma 2003;17: 473–480.

Helfet DL, Kloen P, Anand N, et al. Open reduction and internal fixation of delayed unions and nonunions of fractures of the distal part of the humerus. J Bone Joint Surg (Am) 2003;85: 33–40.

Holdsworth BJ, Mossad MM. Fractures of the adult distal humerus. Elbow function after internal fixation. J Bone Joint Surg (Br) 1990;72:362–365.

John H, Rosso R, Neff U, et al. Operative treatment of distal humeral fractures in the elderly. J Bone Joint Surg (Br) 1994;76: 793–796.

Jupiter JB, Neff U, Holzach P, et al. Intercondylar fracture of the humerus. J Bone Joint Surg (Am) 1985;67:226–239.

Kamineni S, Morrey BF. Distal humeral fractures treated with non-custom total elbow replacement. J Bone Joint Surg (Am) 2004; 86:940–947.

McKee MD, Jupiter JB. Fractures of the distal humerus. In: Browner BD, Jupiter JB, Levine AM, et al., eds. Skeletal trauma, 3rd ed. Philadelphia: Saunders, 2003.

McKee MD, Jupiter JB, Bamberger HB. Coronal shear fractures of the distal end of the humerus. J Bone Joint Surg (Am) 1996;78: 49–54.

McKee MD, Wilson TL, Winston L, et al. Functional outcomes after surgical treatment of intraarticular distal humeral fractures through a posterior approach. J Bone Joint Surg (Am) 2000;82: 1701–1707.

Müller ME, Nazarian S, Koch P, et al. The comprehensive classification of fractures of long bones. Berlin: Springer-Verlag, 1990.

Ring D, Jupiter JB, Gulotta L. Articular fractures of the distal part of the humerus. J Bone Joint Surg (Am) 2003;85:232–238.

Robinson CM, Hill RMF, Jacobs N, et al. Adult distal humeral metaphyseal fractures: epidemiology and results of treatment. J Orthop Trauma 2003;17:38–47.

Ruedi TP, Murphy WM, ed. AO principles of fracture management. Stuttgart: AO Publishing-Thieme, 2000.

14

PROXIMAL FOREARM FRACTURES AND ELBOW DISLOCATIONS

The management of fractures and dislocations of the proximal forearm and elbow can be very challenging. Radial head fractures have always been problematic, and until the use of radial head spacers became popular in the 1970s, dislocations associated with severe radial head fractures were very difficult to treat. There is still considerable debate about the merits of internally fixing radial head fractures and whether excision arthroplasty of the radial head produces good results. In recent years the importance of coronoid fractures has been recognized, as have the associations among elbow dislocation, radial head fracture, and coronoid fracture—the so-called terrible triad of elbow injuries. Elbow dislocations without an associated fracture are relatively common, but there is still debate about whether soft tissue repair improves the overall prognosis. Box 14-1 contains a number of current controversies related to fractures of the proximal forearm and dislocation of the elbow.

SURGICAL ANATOMY

The elbow joint consists of the distal humerus, described in Chapter 13, the head of the radius, and the proximal ulna (Fig. 14-1). The key components of the proximal ulna are the olecranon fossa and the coronoid process. The elbow is essentially a hinge joint and therefore has strong medial and lateral collateral ligaments. The tissues of the anterior and posterior capsule are weak and contain many oblique fibers, which permit the elbow's extensive range of movement. The annular ligament encircles the head of the radius and is attached to the proximal ulna, anterior and posterior to the radial notch, thus securing the proximal radioulnar joint. The lateral collateral ligament arises from the lateral humeral epicondyle and is attached to the lateral and posterior parts of the annular ligament. The medial collateral ligament runs from the medial humeral epicondyle to an area between the coronoid process and the olecranon.

A number of muscles arise from and insert into the proximal forearm. Supinator muscle arises from a depression below the radial notch of the ulnar. It attaches around the proximal radius. The biceps attaches to the radial tuberosity just below the radial neck, and the brachialis attaches to the proximal ulnar just below the coronoid process. The triceps attaches to the olecranon. The anconeus muscle attaches to the lateral border of the olecranon.

The brachial artery enters the cubital fossa on the brachialis muscle and divides into the radial and ulnar arteries. The median nerve enters the cubital fossa with the brachial artery, gives off some branches to the muscles on the medial side of the cubital fossa, and leaves the fossa between the two heads of pronator teres. The ulnar nerve passes behind the medial epicondyle of the humerus and enters the forearm between the heads of flexor carpi ulnaris. The radial nerve divides into its deep and superficial branches at the level of the lateral epicondyle of the humerus. Both branches continue into the forearm. The deep branch enters supinator muscle, and a superficial branch runs into the forearm under cover of the brachioradialis muscle.

CLASSIFICATION

There are separate classifications for radial head and neck fractures, coronoid fractures, and olecranon fractures, but the OTA (AO) classification has combined them (Fig. 14-2).

BOX 14-1 CURRENT CONTROVERSIES CONCERNING PROXIMAL FOREARM FRACTURES

Mason II fractures: Do they require internal fixation?
Mason III fractures: nonoperative management, reconstruction, or excision?
Is radial head replacement better than excision arthroplasty?
Olecranon fractures: tension band wiring or plating?
What is the significance of a coronoid fracture?
Is there a spectrum of elbow dislocations?
How should elbow dislocations be treated?
Radioulnar dissociation: treatment and prognosis

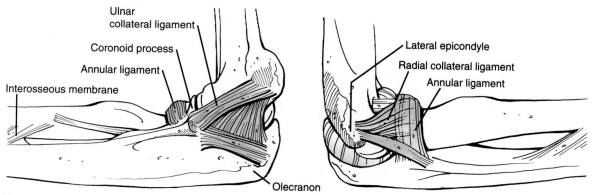

Figure 14-1 The anatomy of the proximal forearm.

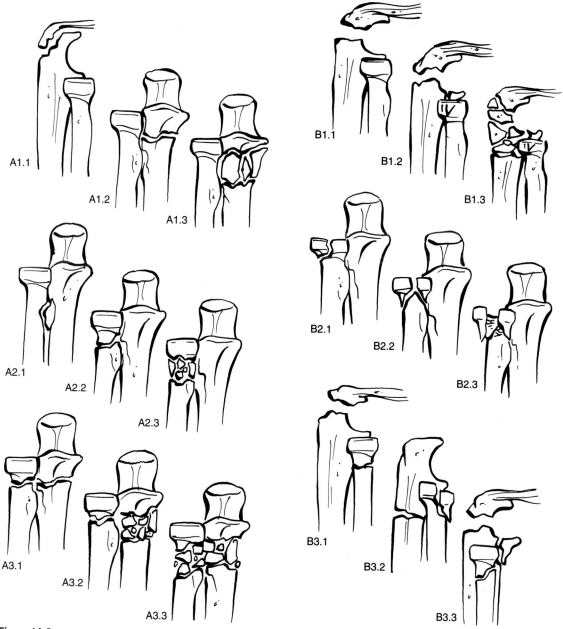

Figure 14-2 The OTA (AO) classification of proximal forearm fractures.

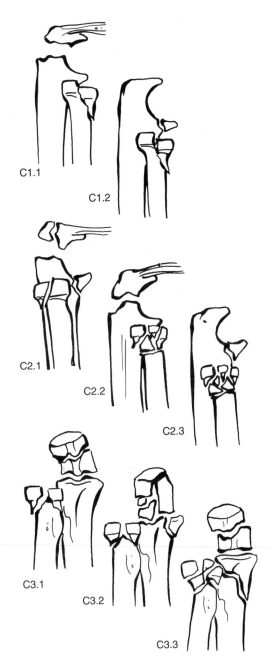

Figure 14-2 *(continued)*

TABLE 14-1 OVERALL EPIDEMIOLOGY OF PROXIMAL FOREARM FRACTURES

Proportion of all fractures	5.0%
Average age	45.7 y
Incidence	$55.5/10^5/y$
Distribution	Type D
Men/women	46%/54%
Open fractures	1.3%
Most common causes	
Fall	59.6%
Motor vehicle accident	13.1%
Sport	10.1%
Fall height	9.1%
OTA (AO) classification	
Type A	20.9%
Type B	77.4%
Type C	1.7%
Most common subgroups	
B2.1	49.8%
A2.2	18.8%
B1.1	18.5%
B2.3	3.7%

Type A fractures are extra-articular with A1 fractures involving the ulna, A2 the radius, and A3 both the radius and ulna. In type A fractures, the suffix 0.1–0.3 refers to the location of the fracture or degree of fragmentation. Type B fractures are partial articular fractures, with B1 fractures involving the ulna, B2 the radius, and B3 both bones. As in type A fractures, the suffix 0.1–0.3 refers to the location of the fracture and the degree of fragmentation.

Type C fractures are complete articular fractures affecting both bones. C1 fractures are simple fractures of both bones. The C2 group contains simple fractures of one bone and multifragmentary fractures of the other. The C3 group contains multifragmentary fractures of both bones. Again, the suffix 0.1–0.3 refers to the location and degree of fragmentation of the fractures. There is no C1.3 fracture. The main drawback of the OTA (AO) classification is that it does not deal with elbow fracture dislocations.

EPIDEMIOLOGY

Table 14-1 gives the basic epidemiology of proximal forearm fracture. Overall they have a type D distribution (see Chapter 1) affecting young men and women and older women. Table 14-2 shows that the age and sex distribution

TABLE 14-2 BASIC EPIDEMIOLOGY OF THE DIFFERENT PROXIMAL FOREARM FRACTURES

Fracture Location	Prevalence (%)	Average Age (y)	Men/Women (%)	Distribution
Olecranon	19.9	58.2	47/53	F
Radial head	56.4	39.1	46/52	H
Radial neck	19.9	43.6	44/56	A
Proximal radius and ulna	3.7	61.2	36/64	F

TABLE 14-3 CAUSES OF PROXIMAL FOREARM FRACTURES

Cause	Age (y)	OTA (AO) Type (%)		
		A	B	C
Fall	53.9	22.0	75.1	2.8
Motor vehicle accident	30.4	23.1	76.9	—
Sport	26.5	16.6	83.3	—
Fall (height)	41.9	18.5	81.5	—

differs between the different proximal forearm fractures, however. Overall there is an approximately equal gender ratio, and open fractures are rare. The overwhelming majority of proximal forearm fractures are OTA (AO) type B, with about half of all proximal forearm fractures being isolated simple radial head fractures. Radial neck fractures and olecranon fractures each comprise about 20% of proximal forearm fractures. The main subgroups associated with significant soft tissue damage and elbow dislocation (A1.3, B1.3, B2.3, B3.3, and C2.3) account for about 6% of proximal forearm fractures. Table 14-3 shows the epidemiology of proximal forearm fractures with reference to the cause of injury. The osteopenic nature of these fractures is highlighted by the absence of type C fractures in higher energy injuries.

Associated Injuries

Most proximal forearm fractures are isolated injuries, and if other musculoskeletal injuries occur, they tend to be in the ipsilateral arm. Analysis suggests that about 2.7% of proximal forearm fractures are associated with proximal humeral fractures, 1.7% with distal radial fractures, and 1.3% with distal humeral fractures. There is also evidence that about 4.8% of proximal forearm fractures are associated with elbow dislocation.

DIAGNOSIS

History and Physical Examination

- The majority of proximal forearm fractures and dislocations follow low-energy injuries and are not associated with other musculoskeletal injuries or injuries to other body systems.
- If they occur in a polytrauma patient, a thorough examination according to ATLS principles is essential.
- The usual presentation is with a painful elbow following a fall, motor vehicle accident, or sports injury.
- Neurological damage is very rare, but occasionally an ulnar neurapraxia will occur.
- If there is an associated dislocation, careful examination of the vascular and neurological status of the arm should be undertaken and the results recorded.

Radiologic Examination

- It is unusual to require views other than a standard anteroposterior and lateral radiograph to diagnose proximal forearm fractures.
- The fat-pad sign may be useful. It is caused by elevation of the anterior and posterior fat pads from the distal humerus and appears as areas of translucency on the lateral radiograph with the elbow flexed to 90 degrees.
  - The fat-pad sign has been demonstrated to be useful in children in diagnosing proximal forearm fractures, but in adults the sensitivity for radial head/neck fractures is 85.4% and the specificity only 50%. The sign is probably more useful when absent.
- MRI scanning has been shown to be useful in demonstrating interosseous membrane damage, but it is not used routinely.

RADIAL HEAD FRACTURES

Radial head fractures (B2 fractures) account for 56% of all proximal forearm fractures (Table 14-2). The OTA (AO) classification is shown in Figure 14-2, but many surgeons use the Mason (1954) classification shown in Figure 14-3. Mason type I fractures are undisplaced, type II fractures are displaced marginal fractures, and type III fractures are comminuted. The classification was later modified by Johnson (1962), who added type IV fractures associated with dislocation. Mason I and II fractures comprise the OTA (AO) B2.1 subgroup (50%), with Mason III fractures making up the B2.2 and B2.3 subgroups (6%).

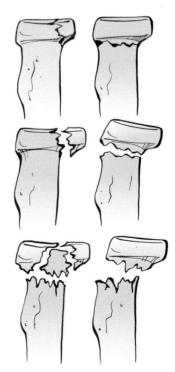

Figure 14-3 The Mason (1954) classification of proximal radial fractures.

TREATMENT

Mason I Fractures

- There is universal agreement that Mason I (Fig. 14-4) undisplaced radial head fractures should be treated nonoperatively.
- In recent years there have been few studies of this fracture, but the results from the literature are given in Table 14-4.
- This shows that good results are not universal. Some of the early articles indicated that if the undisplaced fractures involve only one third of the radial head, about 90% excellent or good results could be expected. Because more of the head was involved, the results tended to worsen.
- Nonoperative management involves the use of a sling followed by early mobilization as the pain settles.
- Use of a full arm cast with the elbow flexed results in impaired extension compared with the use of a sling.

- Better results are obtained with early movement.
- Physical therapy may be required.
- Aspiration of the elbow joint facilitates early movement, but by 3 months the beneficial effects of aspiration have disappeared.

Mason II Fractures

- There has been considerable debate about whether Mason II fractures (Fig. 14-4) should be treated nonoperatively or by internal fixation usually using headless screws (see Chapter 34) (Fig. 14-5).
- The overall results of nonoperative and operative management are shown in Tables 14-4 and 14-5. Operative management appears to be associated with better results, although not with a better rotation arc. This reinforces the results of a prospective randomized study that showed better results with operative management.
- It would seem likely that the results of nonoperative treatment might correlate with the degree of depression

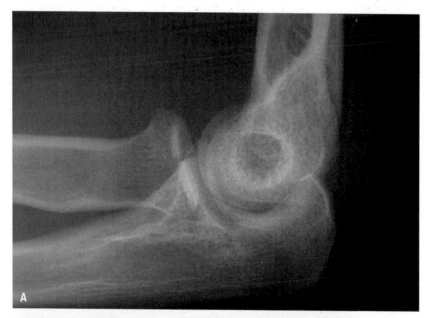

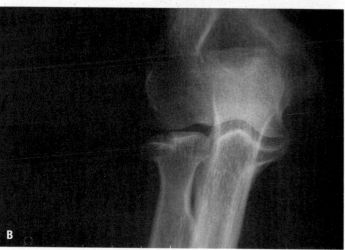

Figure 14-4 A-P radiographs showing Mason I (**A**), Mason II (**B**), and Mason III (**C**) fractures.

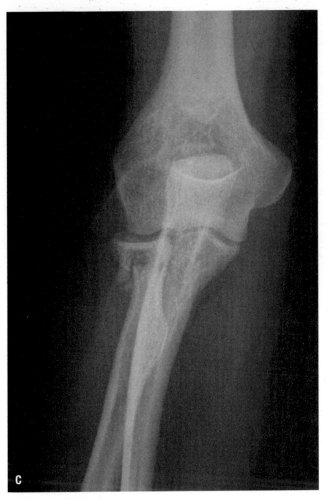

Figure 14-4 *(continued)*

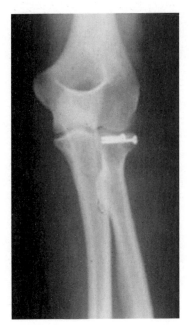

Figure 14-5 An A-P radiograph of a Mason II fracture fixed with two screws.

of the radial head fragment, but this does not appear to be the case. There are no studies specifically comparing operative and nonoperative fracture in minimally displaced Mason II fractures.

Mason III Fractures

■ Tables 14-4 and 14-5 show that the results of the operative treatment of Mason III fractures are worse than those of Mason II fractures, although the rotational arc seems to be less affected than the flexion arc.

■ Nonoperative management appears to be associated with better results, and a recent study of 100 Mason II and III fractures treated nonoperatively showed 84% excellent and good results with no nonunions, avascular necrosis, proximal radioulnar synostosis, or heterotopic ossification.

■ The alternative methods of Mason type III fractures are radial head excision or proximal radial replacement.

Radial Head Excision

■ Radial head excision (Fig. 14-6) may be undertaken primarily for unreconstructable Mason III radial head fractures or secondarily because of late pain and disability after both operative and nonoperative treatment.

■ The operation is straightforward, but care must be taken not to damage the posterior interosseous nerve lying within supinator muscle.

■ The results of both early and late excision of the radial head are shown in Table 14-6.

■ It seems apparent that the results of early radial head excision are similar to those of nonoperative management and better than those of surgical reconstruction.

TABLE 14-4 RESULTS OF NONOPERATIVE MANAGEMENT OF RADIAL HEAD FRACTURES

| | Mason Type | | | | | |
| | I | | II | | III | |
Result	Range	Average	Range	Average	Range	Average
Excellent/good (%)	68.2–100	87.3	43.7–100	75.6	50–93.7	80.4
Flexion arc (degrees)	—	—	121–134	130	—	—
Rotation arc (degrees)	—	—	167–170	169	—	—

TABLE 14-5 RESULTS OF OPERATIVE MANAGEMENT IN MASON II AND III FRACTURES

| | Mason Type | | | |
| | II | | III | |
Result	Range	Average	Range	Average
Excellent/good (%)	16.6–100	90.2	33.3–100	70
Flexion arc (degrees)	119–149	133	111–135	120
Rotation arc (degrees)	117–176	155	127–176	153

TABLE 14-6 RESULTS OF EARLY AND LATE RADIAL HEAD EXCISION

| | Early | | |
Result/Complication	Range	Average	Late
Excellent/good (%)	37.5–95.2	78.6	76.2
Flexion (degree)	117–135	128	117
Rotation arc (degree)	153–169	160	130
Radial shortening (%)	8.3–93.3	52.9	—
Wrist pain (%)	11.1–26.7	18.6	Uncommon
Osteoarthritic elbow (%)	57.7–100	63.1	77
Grip strength (%)	83–100	92	80
Cubitus valgus (%)	30–100	52.9	—

Late results taken from Broberg MA, Morrey BF. Results of delayed excision of the radial head after fracture. J Bone Joint Surg (Am) 1986;68:669–674.

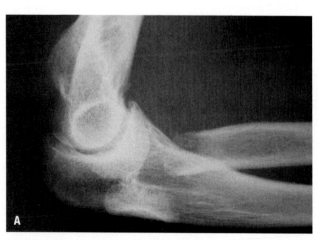
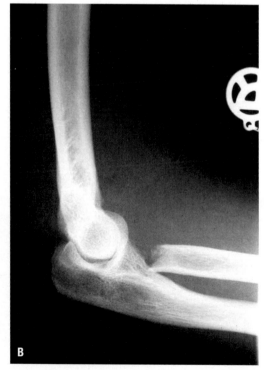

Figure 14-6   A type III radial neck fracture (**A**) treated by radial head excision (**B**).

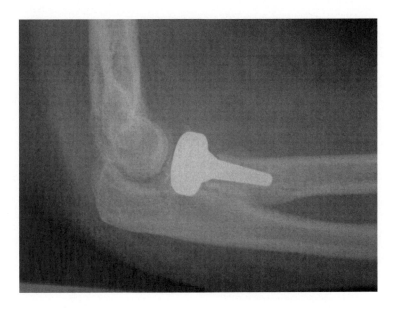

Figure 14-7 A radial head prosthesis.

Table 14-6, however, shows two problems associated with radial head excision, both related to increased mediolateral instability of the elbow.

■ The loss of the radial head increases the degree of cubitus valgus in about 50% of patients by about 8 degrees on average. This may increase tension on the ulnar nerve.

■ In adults the radius will shorten in about 50% of cases. If the shortening is less than 3 mm, the symptoms are usually minor, but almost 20% of patients present with wrist pain following radial head excision.

■ Late radial head excision gives results not dissimilar to early excision, although the flexion arc is poorer and the incidence of wrist pain is less.

■ This suggests that late radial head excision is a reasonable alternative if nonoperative management of type III radial head fractures is unsuccessful.

Radial Head Replacement
■ Early radial head replacements were made of acrylic or silastic and often failed after a relatively short time.

Modern prostheses are metal and may act as an uncemented spacer or a cemented prosthesis (Fig. 14-7).

■ Radial head replacements can be inserted early or late, with late insertion usually undertaken for late pain and elbow dysfunction.

■ The results of both early and late radial head replacement are given in Table 14-7. This shows that the results are not dissimilar from radial head excision, although radial shortening, and presumably wrist pain, is less.

■ The type III fractures in Table 14-7 tended to be worse than those analyzed in Tables 14-4, 14-5, and 14-6 in that there were more associated bone and soft tissue injuries.

■ Radial head replacement is a reasonable option, however, for severe type III fractures and will probably prove better than both operative reconstruction and radial head excision.

■ Late replacement predictably gives poorer results than early replacement, but the papers dealing with its use emphasize that it improves the patient's preoperative symptoms.

TABLE 14-7 RESULTS OF EARLY AND LATE RADIAL HEAD REPLACEMENT

Result	Type III Early Range	Type III Early Average	Type III Late Range	Type III Late Average	Type IV Early Range	Type IV Early Average	Type IV Late Range	Type IV Late Average
Excellent/good (%)	75–100	85	75	75	75–100	85	66	66
Flexion arc (degrees)	119–136	130	115–137	128	103–138	120	94–97	95
Rotation arc (degrees)	144–170	154	130–149	141	139–170	143	107–142	119
Grip strength (%)	90	90	92.5	92.5	87–98	88.5	83.3	83.3
Radial shortening (mm)	0.7	0.7	2.4	2.4	0	0	3	3

- It is therefore useful if patients present with pain and elbow dysfunction after radial head excision.

Type IV Fractures

- Type IV radial head fractures are associated with elbow dislocation (see Fig. 14-17).
- The results of radial head replacement in these fractures are shown in Table 14-7.
- The goal is elbow stabilization and good late function, and Table 14-7 shows this is achieved by early radial head replacement.
- The results of early head replacement of type IV fractures are slightly worse overall than those of type III fractures, but this is understandable given the increased soft tissue injury associated with type IV fracture-dislocations.
- The articles included in Table 14-7 tended to include all types of fracture-dislocation associated with a radial head fracture as a type IV lesion. Thus Table 14-7 covers a spectrum of different pathologies. Elbow fracture dislocations are discussed later in this chapter.

COMPLICATIONS

- The main complications of radial head fracture are elbow pain and restriction of function.
- These have usually been treated by radial head excision but increasingly are being treated by radial head replacement.
- The results of both procedures are given in Tables 14-6 and 14-7. Nonunion of radial head fractures is very rare and treated by radial head excision or replacement.
- There is a very low incidence of associated ulnar or posterior interosseous neuropraxia.
- Radial head excision is associated with wrist pain and dysfunction, valgus instability, and loss of grip strength.
  - These are often improved by radial head replacement.
- Osteoarthritis and heterotopic ossification both occur after radial head excision, but both tend to be fairly minor and rarely require treatment.

RADIAL NECK FRACTURES

Isolated radial neck fractures (A2.2 and A2.3) account for about 20% of proximal forearm fractures. The epidemiology of radial neck fractures is shown in Table 14-2. They have a type A distribution (see Chapter 1) and an approximately equal sex distribution. There are very few papers dealing with radial neck fractures in adults, and the literature dealing with radial head fractures tends to combine radial neck and head fractures with the assumption that the Mason classification should be used to determine management of radial neck fractures as well (see Fig. 14-3). Mason type I radial neck fractures are undisplaced, type II are displaced but reconstructable, and type III are unreconstructable.

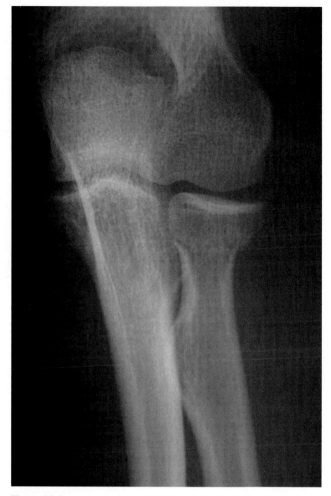

Figure 14-8 A lateral radiograph of a Mason I radial neck fracture.

TREATMENT

- Most radial neck fractures are undisplaced Mason I fractures and treated nonoperatively (Fig. 14-8).
- Unfortunately there are no criteria to decide what degree of radial neck displacement requires intervention in Mason II or III fractures.
- It has been suggested that an examination under anaesthesia should be undertaken, and if there is a block to rotation, reduction and internal fixation should be carried out.
  - There are no trials of this method of management, but empirically it is reasonable and many surgeons use it.
- Internal fixation is best undertaken with a 2-mm blade plate or T-plate (Fig. 14-9).
- A lateral approach is used and the annular ligament divided.
- Care must be taken not to damage the posterior interosseous nerve lying within supinator muscle.
- Other suggested methods of management include closed reduction with a periosteal elevator followed by the use of a cast, the use of percutaneous K-wires, or the insertion of retrograde flexible nails.
- Plate fixation is the method of choice, however.

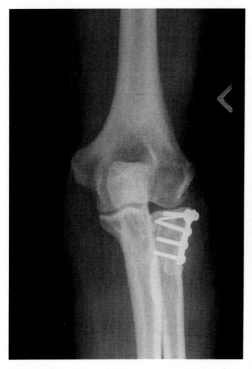
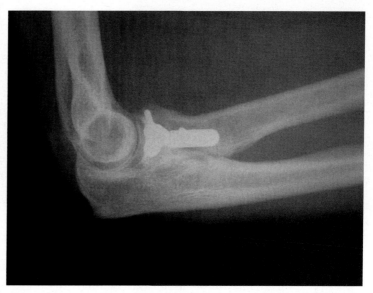

Figure 14-9 A Mason II fracture treated with a mini T-plate.

COMPLICATIONS

- The same complications occur in radial neck fractures as in radial head fractures, namely pain and elbow dysfunction.
- These can be treated by radial head excision or replacement.
- There is a higher incidence of radial neck nonunion with up to 5% reported, although the true incidence is unknown.
- Treatment is usually by radial head excision or replacement.

OLECRANON FRACTURES

Isolated olecranon fractures account for about 20% of proximal forearm fractures with the majority simple fractures. The basic epidemiology of olecranon fractures is given in Table 14-2, which shows they have a type F osteoporotic fracture distribution (see Chapter 1). There are a number of classifications of olecranon fractures, and that of Schatzker is shown in Figure 14-10. It illustrates the

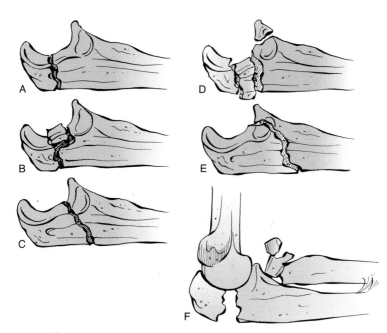

Figure 14-10 The Schatzker (1987) classification of proximal ulnar fractures.

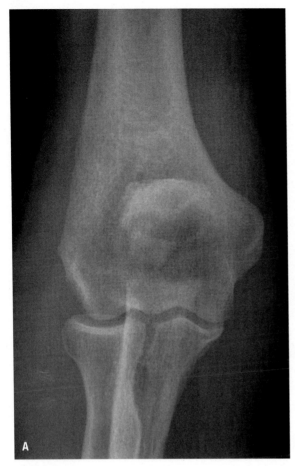
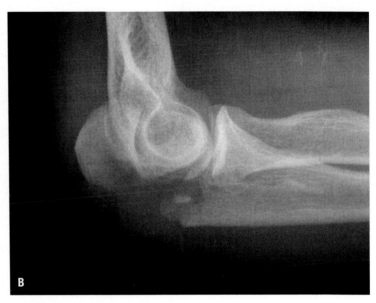

Figure 14-11   A Schatzker-type A olecranon fracture (**A,B**) treated with tension band wiring (**C,D**).

major differences between the different olecranon fracture types. Type A fractures are transverse, type B are transverse-impacted, type C are oblique, type D are comminuted, type E are oblique-distal, and the type F fracture is really a trans-olecranon elbow dislocation often associated with a Mason III radial head fracture. Some surgeons have included these as Mason IV fractures (Table 14-7), although strictly they represent a different type of injury.

TREATMENT

Olecranon Excision

■ Excision of the olecranon fragment with suturing of the triceps to the distal ulnar was popular in elderly patients until relatively recently.

■ Even in older patients, however, olecranon excision is associated with some loss of extension power, although elbow motion is usually preserved.

■ The literature indicates that an excision of more than 70% of the olecranon may be associated with ulnar subluxation.

■ Biomechanical testing has shown that open reduction and internal fixation restores the normal biomechanics of the elbow joint, whereas olecranon excision results in abnormally elevated joint stresses.

■ The widespread use of the technique can not be recommended because of the loss of triceps strength, a particular problem in elderly patients who rely on their arms to raise themselves from a sitting position.

Internal Fixation

■ A number of different internal fixation methods have been devised to treat olecranon fractures. The more common methods are intramedullary screw fixation, the use of a figure-eight wire either by itself or supplemented by flexible nails, the AO technique of K-wires supplemented by a figure-eight tension band (tension band wiring), or plating.

■ Many biomechanical studies have investigated the different methods of applying both smooth and threaded wires and tension banding to the olecranon, but no clinical evidence indicates that the exact position of the K-wires or the type of tension banding is crucial.

■ If a wiring system is used, two K-wires should be passed over the fracture and a figure-eight loop tightened between the ulnar and the proximal ends of the wires (Fig. 14-11).

■ Olecranon plating should be distinguished from the use of a plate to treat a proximal ulna fracture associated with an elbow dislocation.

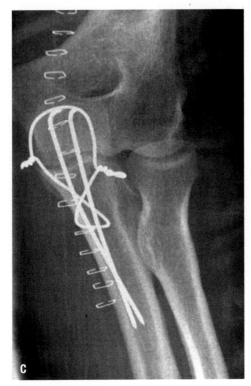

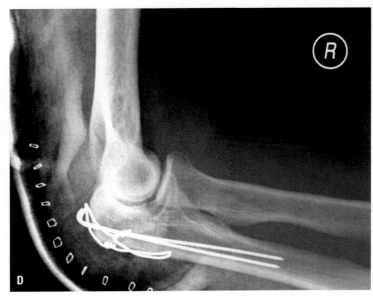

Figure 14-11 *(continued)*

- These can often be treated with a conventional plate, but olecranon plating requires the use of a plate placed posteriorly over the proximal ulnar and curved around the olecranon (Fig. 14-12).
- A one-third tubular or reconstruction plate is usually used, although location-specific prebent olecranon plates are available.
- Both tension band wiring and proximal plating are popular, and the results of both techniques are shown in Table 14-8.
- It is important to remember that the articles dealing with plating tend to consider more difficult fractures including Mason IV and Schatzker-type F fractures. Thus the results for plating are clearly better than those of tension band wiring.

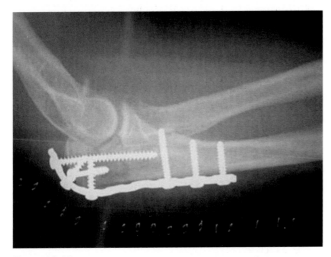

Figure 14-12 An olecranon fracture treated by plate fixation.

- The nonunion rate is less, and there are fewer problems with symptomatic hardware requiring removal. Forearm rotation appears less after plating, but this may relate to the severity of the fractures that are often treated by this technique.
- The only prospective study comparing plating and tension band wiring has shown that plating gives better results.

COMPLICATIONS

- The main complications of tension band wiring and plating are shown in Table 14-8.
- The principal problem is that of prominent hardware if tension band wiring is used.
  - This is usually solved by removal of the implants, which has been reported to be required in up to 80% of patients.
  - Nonunions are unusual but easily treated by refixation and bone grafting.

CORONOID FRACTURES

Isolated fractures of the coronoid are very rare, and it is likely all coronoid fractures represent elbow dislocation or, at the very least, a severe soft tissue injury to the joint. The classification (Regan and Morrey, 1989) is straightforward and shown in Figure 14-13.

TABLE 14-8 RESULTS OF OLECRANON TENSION BAND WIRING AND PLATING

Result/Complication	Tension band wiring		Plating	
	Range	Average	Range	Average
Excellent/good (%)	47.3–87.8	72.9	64.7–92	81.8
Nonunion (%)	2.4–10.5	3.9	0	0
Infection (%)	2.1–10.5	3.2	0–15.4	3.3
Flexion arc (degree)	120–125	121	110–128	122
Rotation arc (degree)	173–175	173	112–175	149
Ulnar nerve lesion (%)	1–5.2	1.7	0–4	2.1
Symptomatic hardware (%)	7.3–42.1	18.3	0–8	5

TREATMENT

- Treatment depends on the size of the coronoid fragment and the extent of any associated musculoskeletal injury.
- Type I lesions are treated nonoperatively, but an examination of the elbow is required, and MRI scanning may be used to investigate the extent of any associated soft tissue injuries.
- Types II and III lesions usually present as part of the terrible triad of elbow dislocation, radial head fracture, and coronoid fracture.
- It is important to restore elbow stability by radial head reconstruction or replacement and by coronoid fixation.
- This is best done by an intrafragmentary screw placed from the posterior surface of the ulnar, although the proximal ulnar may have to be reconstructed first to allow the screw to be placed.
- Alternatively, a wire loop can be used to maintain the position of the smaller coronoid fragment.

ELBOW DISLOCATION

Elbow dislocation accounts for about 20% of all dislocations. The most common mechanism is a fall on an outstretched hand with the elbow extended and the arm abducted, although elbow dislocations may also follow sports injuries and motor vehicle accidents. The classification is defined by the direction taken by the radius and ulnar (Fig. 14-14). About 80% to 90% of dislocations are posterior or posterolateral. Usually the forearm bones remain together, but very rarely they diverge (see Fig. 14-14).

All elbow dislocations are associated with significant soft tissue damage. In posterior or posterolateral dislocations there is medial collateral ligament damage with injury to the anterior capsule and brachialis muscle. These dislocations are usually relatively straightforward to treat, but the difficulty of treatment correlates with the increasing musculoskeletal damage. Elbow dislocations can be separated into four types depending on the degree of musculoskeletal damage (Box 14-2).

DIAGNOSIS

History and Physical Examination

- Most elbow dislocations are isolated injuries (Fig. 14-15) with the patient presenting with a deformed painful elbow following a fall or sports injury.
- If the dislocation has occurred in a motor vehicle accident, a complete examination according to ATLS principles is required.

BOX 14-2 THE FOUR STAGES OF ELBOW DISLOCATION

1. Soft tissue damage only
2. Type I with a coronoid process fracture
3. Lateral column fracture
   a. Radial head or neck
   b. Capitellum
   c. Lateral humeral condyle
4. Proximal ulnar fracture
   a. Intact radial head—Monteggia variant
   b. Fractured radial head

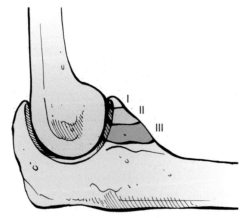

Figure 14-13 The Regan and Morrey (1989) classification of coronoid process fractures.

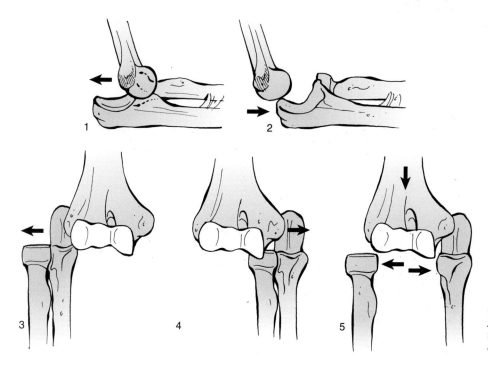

Figure 14-14 The classification of elbow dislocation by McKee and Jupiter (2003). 1 is posterior, 2 is anterior, 3 is lateral, 4 is medial, and 5 is divergent.

- Brachial artery damage is very rare, but a vascular examination should be undertaken.
- The neurological status of the arm should also be checked and recorded.

Radiologic Examination

- Standard anteroposterior and lateral radiographs are adequate to diagnose a dislocation.
- MRI scans are not required in acute situations but might be used to investigate recurrent elbow instability.

TREATMENT

Type I Dislocations

- Elbow dislocations associated with soft tissue injury (see Fig. 14-15) are treated by reduction under regional or general anaesthesia.
- The stability of the joint can then be assessed.
- There is no evidence, however, that the surgical repair of damaged soft tissues is worthwhile. A randomized prospective study of repair versus nonoperative

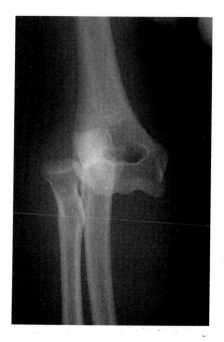

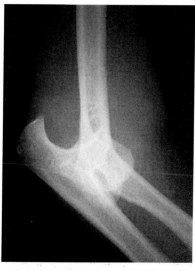

Figure 14-15 A-P and lateral radiographs showing a type I elbow dislocation with soft tissue damage only (see Box 14-2).

management showed no difference in elbow mobility, weakness, or discomfort, and operative repair of the soft tissues following elbow dislocation is unnecessary.

■ Nonoperative management consists of 7 to 10 days immobilization in a well-padded splint with the elbow at 90 degrees, followed by a program of physical therapy.

■ It is essential that check radiographs be obtained 3 to 5 days after reduction to ensure the reduced position is maintained.

■ In unstable dislocations it may be impossible to maintain reduction, and soft tissue reconstruction is advised. An external fixator may be used to stabilize the joint.

■ In stable dislocations the average loss of extension is about 10 degrees, with about 15% of patients complaining of weakness and 30% of pain on effort.

  ■ The severity of the symptoms depends on the extent of the soft tissue injury.

  ■ In patients in whom an external fixator is required to stabilize the joint, a flexion arc of about 100 degrees can be expected.

  ■ Open reduction of the elbow joint is indicated only if closed reduction fails.

  ■ In some dislocations, damage to the ulnar component of the lateral collateral ligament causes late posterolateral rotatory instability of the elbow.

  ■ If this occurs, ligamentous repair is required.

Type II Dislocations

■ If an elbow dislocation is associated with a coronoid process fracture (Fig. 14-16), the stability of the joint must be assessed after reduction.

■ If a type I coronoid fracture exists, the joint will probably be stable, and the same treatment method used for type I dislocations can be employed.

■ If the joint is unstable on examination, however, the coronoid fracture must be reduced and fixed, with an intrafragmentary screw or wire loop.

Type III Dislocations

■ The next stage of complexity is if the lateral column of the elbow is fractured.

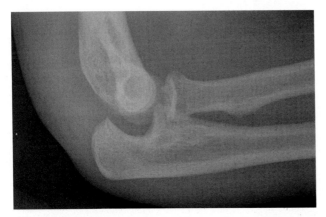

Figure 14-16   A lateral radiograph showing a coronoid fracture in a type II elbow dislocation (see Box 14-2).

■ This usually takes the form of a proximal radial fracture (Fig. 14-17) and is defined as a Mason type IV radial head fracture.

■ The treatment is radial head replacement and the results are given in Table 14-7.

■ If the lateral humeral condyle or capitellum is fractured, they must be fixed internally using the techniques described in Chapter 13.

Type IV Dislocations

■ The most difficult elbow dislocation to treat is if the proximal ulna is fractured.

■ This is rarely an olecranon fracture but usually involves the ulna proximal to the olecranon (Fig. 14-18), and there may be severe comminution extending over the proximal third of the ulna.

■ If the radial head is intact, it represents a variant of the Monteggia fracture dislocation.

  ■ Under these circumstances the ulnar is plated and stability restored.

  ■ If the coronoid is fractured, it must be reduced and fixed, and if the radial head is fractured, it must be reconstructed or replaced.

  ■ The literature indicates that if this policy is followed, about 88% of patients have excellent or good results with a flexion arc averaging about 115 degrees and a rotation arc of about 170 degrees.

COMPLICATIONS

■ The main complications of elbow dislocation are discomfort and restriction of elbow function whose severity is related to the degree of musculoskeletal damage.

■ Post-traumatic proximal radioulnar synostosis has been described and again relates to the extent of the musculoskeletal injury.

  ■ The condition is unusual and treated by surgical resection.

■ Post-traumatic ulnar and posterior interosseous neuropathies have been described.

  ■ These are usually neuropraxias and can be expected to resolve.

■ Continuing ulnar nerve symptoms may be treated by anterior transposition.

RADIOULNAR DISSOCIATION

Radioulnar dissociation was described by Essex-Lopresti in 1951 and often called the Essex-Lopresti lesion. It refers to the problems associated with concurrent damage to the proximal radius and the distal radioulnar joint. There is debate about whether there is physical damage to the interosseous membrane between the radius and ulnar, as has been shown in cadaver studies, or whether the condition is caused by an instability of the interosseous membrane secondary to the obliquity of its

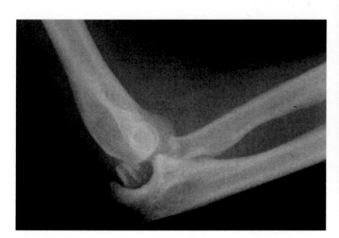

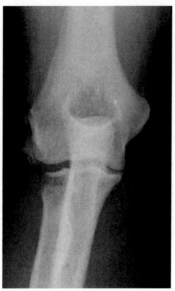

Figure 14-17 A-P and lateral radiographs of a type III dislocation showing a lateral column fracture (see Box 14-2).

fibers, which permits shortening or rotation of the radius. It seems most likely it is the latter because radial head excision without distal radioulnar joint damage may result in proximal radial migration, relative ulnar lengthening, and wrist pain (Table 14-6). It is possible, however, that a high-energy injury may cause direct damage to the interosseous membrane.

■ The problem with combined proximal and distal damage is that the distal injury is often missed.

■ If both lesions are detected and treated early, the literature suggests the outcome for the elbow is good, with 80% excellent and good results, but it is less good for the wrist, with only 40% excellent or good results.

■ Where the diagnosis is made late, only 27% of patients get excellent or good results in the elbow and 20% in the wrist.

■ It is very important to examine the wrist carefully in any patient who presents with a proximal radial injury.

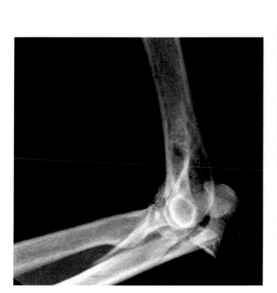

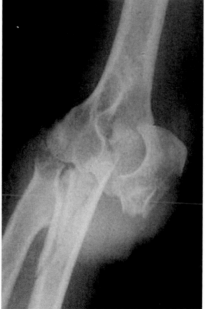

Figure 14-18 A-P and lateral radiographs of a type IV dislocation with an ulnar fracture (see Box 14-2).

TABLE 14-9 SUGGESTED TREATMENT FOR PROXIMAL FOREARM FRACTURES AND DISLOCATIONS

Injury	Treatment
Radial head	
Mason type	
I	Nonoperative
II	Internal fixation
III	Nonoperative. Late excision or replacement if symptomatic
IV	Internal fixation or replacement
Radial neck	
Undisplaced	Nonoperative
Displaced	Internal fixation
Olecranon	Plating
	Tension band wiring if fragment too small
Dislocation type	
I	Closed reduction
II	Coronoid fixation if elbow unstable
III	Radial head reconstruction or replacement
	Internal fixation distal humerus
IV	Proximal ulnar plating
	Radial head reconstruction or replacement

Suggested Treatment

The suggested management of proximal forearm fractures and dislocations is shown in Table 14-9.

SUGGESTED READING

Bakalim G. Fractures of the radial head and their treatment. Acta Orthop Scand 1970;42:320–331.

Beingessner DM, Dunning CE, Gordon KD, et al. The effect of radial head excision and arthroplasty on elbow kinematics and stability. J Bone Joint Surg (Am) 2004;86:1730–1739.

Broberg MA, Morrey BF. Results of delayed excision of the radial head after fracture. J Bone Joint Surg (Am) 1986;68:669–674.

Broberg MA, Morrey BF. Results of treatment of fracture-dislocations of the elbow. Clin Orthop 1987;216:109–119.

Edwards G, Jupiter JB. The Essex-Lopresti lesion revisited. Clin Orthop 1988;234:61–69.

Janssen RPA, Vegter J. Resection of the radial head after Mason type-III fractures of the elbow. Follow up at 16 to 30 years. J Bone Joint Surg (Br) 1998;80:231–233.

Johnston GW. A follow up of one hundred cases of fracture of head of the radius with a review of the literature. Ulster Med J 1962;31:51–56.

Josefsson PO, Gentz CF, Johnell O, et al. Surgical versus nonsurgical treatment of ligamentous injuries following dislocation of the elbow joint. J Bone Joint Surg (Am) 1987;69:605–608.

Mason ML. Some observations on fractures of the head of the radius with a review of one hundred cases. Br J Surg 1954;42:123–132.

McKee MD, Jupiter JB. Trauma to the adult elbow. In: Browner BD, Jupiter JB, Levine AM, et al., eds. Skeletal trauma, 3rd ed. Philadelphia: Saunders, 2003.

Müller ME, Nazarian S, Koch P, et al. The comprehensive classification of fractures of long bones. Berlin: Springer-Verlag, 1990.

O'Driscoll SW, Jupiter JB, King GJW, et al. The unstable elbow. J Bone Joint Surg (Am) 2000;82:724–738.

Regan W, Morrey B. Fractures of the coronoid process of the ulna. J Bone Joint Surg (Am) 1989;71:1348–1354.

Ring D, Jupiter JB. Fracture-dislocation of the elbow. J Bone Joint Surg (Am) 1998;80:566–580.

Ruedi TP, Murphy WM, eds. AO principles of fracture management. Stuttgart: AO Publishing-Thieme, 2000.

Schatzker J. Olecranon fractures. In: Schatzker J, Tile M, eds. The rational basis of operative fracture care. New York: Springer-Verlag, 1987.

FRACTURES OF THE FOREARM DIAPHYSIS

There has been little disagreement about the optimal method of managing fractures of the radial and ulnar diaphyses since the 1970s when plating was popularized. Prior to that, surgeons had used both nonoperative management and intramedullary nailing using flexible pins or nails, but the literature of the time is clear that rigid internal fixation with plates was associated with a lower rate of nonunion and improved function. This was particularly true of Galeazzi fractures, which involve dislocation of the distal radioulnar joint. Surgeons reported 0% to 8% excellent or good results with nonoperative management and about the same following K-wire fixation.

Surgeons have continued to plate forearm fractures and have used different types of plate. There has been particular interest in the management of open forearm fractures and fractures associated with proximal or distal dislocations. A number of the current controversies concerning the treatment of forearm diaphyseal fractures are listed in Box 15-1.

SURGICAL ANATOMY

The forearm bones are the radius and ulna. There are proximal and distal radioulnar joints that are dislocated following forearm fractures. The radius rotates around the ulnar, the degree of rotation influenced by the integrity of the distal and proximal radioulnar joints and the bow of

the radius. There are two compartments in the forearm through which run the muscles that control the wrist and hand (Fig. 15-1). In the flexor compartment, the muscles are arranged in superficial and deep groups. The superficial group consists of pronator teres, flexor carpi radialis, palmaris longus, flexor carpi ulnaris, and flexor digitorum superficialis. These mainly arise from the medial epicondyle of the humerus. Pronator teres inserts into the lateral aspect of the radius and palmaris longus into the palmar aponeurosis of the hand, but the rest form tendons that pass under the flexor retinaculum into the hand.

The deep muscles arise from the radius and ulna and the adjacent interosseous membranes. They are flexor digitorum profundus, flexor pollicis longus, and pronator quadratus. Pronator quadratus arises from the distal ulna and inserts into the distal radius. The remaining muscles form tendons that pass under the flexor retinaculum into the hand.

The ulnar nerve enters the forearm between the two heads of flexor carpi ulnaris and lies between the flexor carpi ulnaris and flexor digitorum profundus. Near the

BOX 15-1 CURRENT CONTROVERSIES IN THE TREATMENT OF FOREARM FRACTURES

Are DCP or LC-DCP plates better in forearm fractures?
Is routine bone grafting required?
How should open forearm fractures be treated?
Is forearm nailing useful?
Should forearm plates be removed?
How common are Monteggia and Galeazzi fracture dislocations?
Does the distal radioulnar joint need K-wire fixation in Galeazzi fracture dislocations?
How common is forearm compartment syndrome?

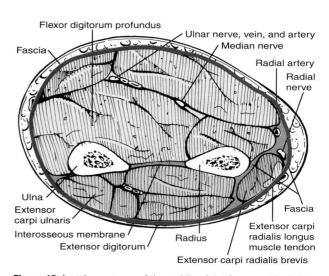

Figure 15-1 The anatomy of the middle of the forearm. The bold lines mark the myofascial compartments.

pisiform bone it pierces the deep fascia and leaves the forearm by passing in front of the flexor retinaculum to form superficial and deep branches. The median nerve enters the forearm between the two heads of pronator teres and gives off the anterior interosseous nerve at that point. The median nerve runs under flexor digitorum superficialis and leaves the forearm through the carpal tunnel. The anterior interosseous nerve descends over the front of the interosseous membrane, passing between flexor digitorum profundus and flexor pollicis longus, and runs onto the front of the wrist joint.

The extensor compartment also contains superficial and deep layers of muscle. The superficial muscles are brachioradialis, extensor carpi radialis longus and brevis, extensor digitorum, extensor digiti minimi, extensor carpi ulnaris, and anconeus. Anconeus arises from the lateral humeral epicondyle and inserts into the lateral ball of the olecranon, but the other muscles arise from the common extensor origin and the lateral supracondylar ridge of the humerus. Brachioradialis inserts into the lateral aspect of the distal radius, but the other muscles give rise to tendons that enter the hand.

The deep muscles are supinator, abductor pollicis longus, extensor pollicis brevis, and longus and extensor indicis. These muscles arise from the posterior aspect of the radius and ulnar and the interosseous membrane. Supinator inserts into the proximal ulna, but the others end as tendons that pass into the hand.

The deep branch of the radial nerve penetrates supinator muscle to enter the posterior compartment as the posterior interosseous nerve. It descends under extensor digitorum and extensor pollicis longus to the dorsum of the wrist joint. The superficial branch of the radial nerve lies under brachioradialis until about 5 cm above the wrist where it pierces the deep fascia.

The vascular supply of the forearm is from the radial and ulnar arteries, which arise from the brachial artery at the level of the radial neck. The ulnar artery lies between the superficial and deep flexor muscles on flexor digitorum profunda. Near the wrist it becomes superficial between the tendons of flexor carpi ulnaris and flexor digitorum superficialis and pierces the deep fascia proximal to the flexor retinaculum. The radial artery descends in the lateral part of the front of the limb to the distal radius where it turns around the lateral border of the wrist.

CLASSIFICATION

The best classification of forearm diaphyseal fractures is the OTA (AO) classification, shown in Figure 15-2. Type A fractures contain the unifocal simple fractures with A1 ulnar fractures, A2 radial fractures, and A3 fractures in both bones. In the A1 and A2 groups, the suffix 0.1–0.3 refers to the position of the fracture and the presence of a proximal or distal dislocation. A1.1 and A2.1 fractures are oblique, A1.2 and A2.2 fractures are transverse, A1.3 refers to a proximal Monteggia dislocation, and A2.3 refers to a distal Galeazzi fracture dislocation. In A3 fractures, 0.1–0.3 refers to the position of the radial fracture with 0.1 proximal, 0.2 in the middle third, and 0.3 distal.

The classification of type B fractures is very similar, although the actual fracture is an intact or fragmented wedge. In B1 and B2 fractures, 0.1 signifies an intact wedge, 0.2 a fragmented wedge, and 0.3 a fracture dislocation, with B1.3 fractures having a proximal Monteggia fracture dislocation and B2.3 fractures having a distal Galeazzi fracture dislocation. B3 fractures involve both bones, with B3.1 fractures having an ulnar wedge and simple radial fracture, B3.2 having a radial wedge and simple ulnar fracture, and B3.3 having wedge fractures of both bones. Type C fractures are bifocal or complex fractures. C1 fractures contain segmental or comminuted ulnar fractures, C2 contain the equivalent fractures of the radius, and C3 contain segmental or comminuted fractures involving both bones.

EPIDEMIOLOGY

Table 15-1 shows the overall epidemiology of forearm diaphyseal fractures. Overall they have a type D pattern (see Chapter 1), but Table 15-2 shows that the different forearm diaphyseal fractures have different age and sex distributions, with fractures of both bones occurring mainly in young men. About 10% of diaphyseal fractures are open and most have an OTA (AO) type A or B pattern. About 54% of fractures are isolated ulna fractures, and the rest are equally distributed between isolated radial fractures and fractures of both bones. Both Galeazzi and Monteggia fracture dislocations are relatively common.

Table 15-3 shows the epidemiology of the different causes of forearm diaphyseal fractures. The most common causes are sports injuries or a direct blow to the forearm. Both of these tend to occur in young men, whereas falls from a standing height tend to cause fractures in older women. Type

TABLE 15-1 OVERALL EPIDEMIOLOGY OF FRACTURES OF THE RADIAL AND ULNAR DIAPHYSES

Proportion of all fractures	1.2%
Average age	34.6 y
Men/women	64%/36%
Distribution	Type D
Incidence	$13.8/10^5/y$
Open fracture	9.5%
Most common causes	
Sport	25.7%
Assault/blow	20.3%
Fall	17.6%
Motor vehicle accident	14.9%
OTA (AO) classification	
Type A	76.7%
Type B	16.4%
Type C	6.8%
Most common subgroups	
A1.2	24.3%
A1.1	17.6%
A3.2	9.5%
A2.2	9.5%

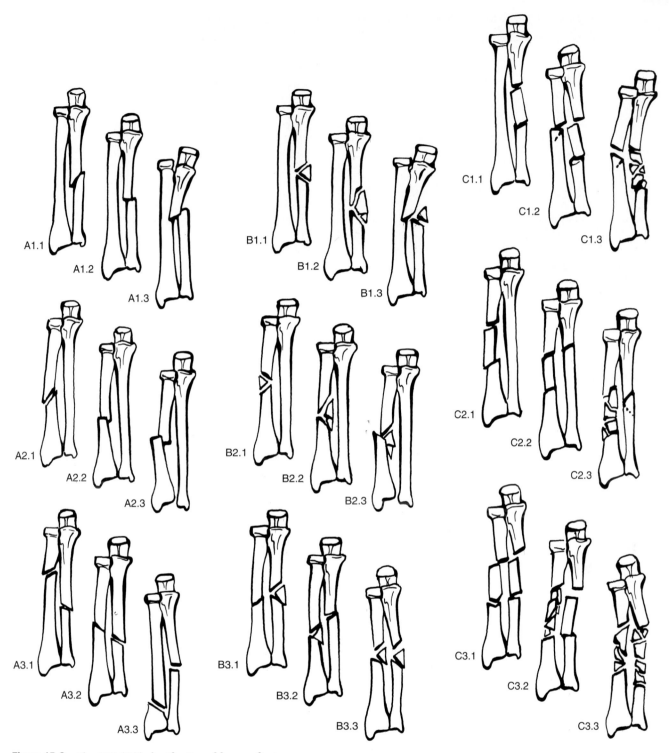

Figure 15-2   The OTA (AO) classification of forearm fractures.

TABLE 15-2 BASIC EPIDEMIOLOGY OF THE DIFFERENT FOREARM DIAPHYSEAL FRACTURES

Fracture Location	Prevalence (%)	Average Age (y)	Men/Women (%)	Dislocation	Distribution
Ulna	54.1	38.2	55/45	Monteggia 12.5%	A
Radius	23.0	35.9	76/24	Galeazzi 23.5%	H
Radius and ulna	22.9	25.8	67/33	—	B

TABLE 15-3 CAUSES OF FOREARM DIAPHYSEAL FRACTURES

Cause	Average Age (y)	OTA (AO) Type (%)		
		A	B	C
Sport	20.2	78.9	10.5	10.5
Assault/blow	38.5	60.0	40.0	—
Fall	45.0	76.9	23.1	—
Motor vehicle accident	41.1	72.7	18.2	9.1

C fractures tend to follow sports injuries, motor vehicle accidents, and falls from a height.

Associated Injuries

Most radius and ulna fractures are isolated, although Table 15-2 shows that associated Monteggia and Galeazzi dislocations are not unusual. Other injuries tend to be in the ipsilateral arm, with the most common metacarpal fractures, which occur in about 7% of cases.

DIAGNOSIS

History and Physical Examination

■ Most fractures of the radius and ulnar are isolated fractures occurring during a sporting activity or from a direct blow or fall.
■ Vascular complications are very rare, but there may be damage to the posterior interosseous, ulnar, or median nerves, and a careful neurological examination of the arm is essential.
■ Compartment syndrome may also occur, and surgeons should be particularly aware of this problem in high-energy or gunshot injuries in young men.
■ If the forearm fractures result from motor vehicle accidents, there may be other significant injuries, and a thorough examination according to the ATS principles is essential.
■ Surgeons should be aware that the patient may have a floating elbow with ipsilateral fractures of the humerus and forearm (see Chapter 12).
■ Vascular and neurological damage is more common after these injuries.

Radiologic Examination

■ Fractures of the radial and ulnar diaphyses are diagnosed with standard anteroposterior and lateral radiographs (Fig. 15-3).

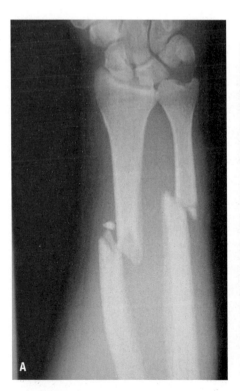
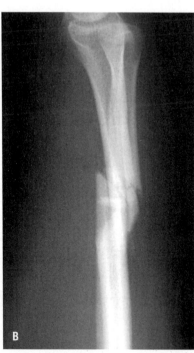

Figure 15-3   A-P and lateral radiographs of an A3.2 fracture of the radius and ulna (**A,B**) treated by plating (**C,D**).

■ Further imaging is rarely required, but it is important to include the elbow and wrist in the radiographic series because there may be dislocation of the radiocapitellar joint, a Monteggia fracture dislocation (Fig. 15-4), or a Galeazzi fracture dislocation (Fig. 15-5).

TREATMENT

Radius and Ulna Fractures

■ There is virtually unanimous agreement among orthopaedic surgeons that plating is the best way of treating diaphyseal forearm fractures, regardless of whether the fracture only involves the radius or ulna or both bones.

■ Nonoperative management is reserved for undisplaced fractures and still used for isolated ulnar fractures associated with minimal displacement.

■ There is no place for nonoperative management in other forearm fractures because nonunion, malunion, and forearm dysfunction are common.

■ Most surgeons use separate radial and ulnar incisions and 3.5-mm dynamic compression plates (DCP) to treat both radius and ulna.

■ Standard OTA (AO) fixation techniques (see Chapter 32) are used.

■ In recent years a number of surgeons have used LC-DCP plates because of the problems associated with periosteal damage if conventional plating techniques are used.

■ It is very difficult to separate the results of plating of both forearm bones from those of the treatment of isolated radius and ulna fractures in the literature.

TABLE 15-4 RESULTS OF PLATING RADIAL AND ULNAR DIAPHYSEAL FRACTURES

Result/Complication[a]	Range (%)	Average (%)
Excellent/good	69.1–100	84.9
Open	18.5–38	23.6
Nonunion	0–7.4	3.7
Infection	0–7.4	2.5
Fixation failure	0–7.1	2.5
Radioulnar synostosis	0–5.4	0.9
Nerve damage	0–21.4	4.1

[a]The results include isolated and both bone fractures.

The results of mixed series of radial and ulnar diaphyseal fractures treated by plating are shown in Table 15-4.

■ This indicates that the overall results are good. In closed fractures, over 90% of the patients show excellent or good results.

■ The incidence of nonunion is low.

■ Many of the early series used routine bone grafting, but later studies have shown this is only necessary in the rare fractures associated with bone loss.

■ In other fractures, the results of primary fixation with or without bone grafting are equivalent.

■ The incidence of fixation failure and radioulnar synostosis is low.

■ Table 15-4 contains results of the use of both 3.5-mm DCPs and LC-DCPs, but a prospective randomized

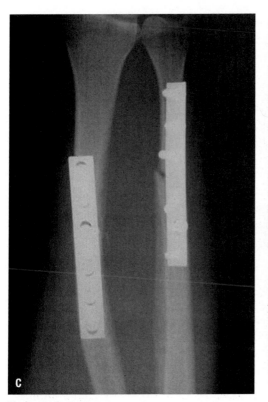

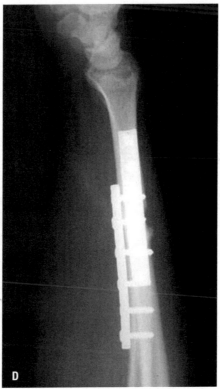

Figure 15-3 *(continued)*

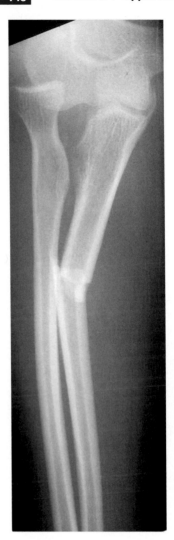

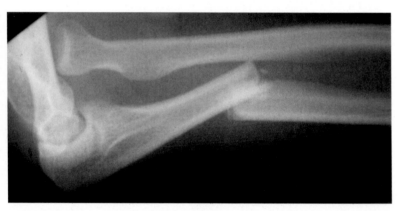

Figure 15-4   A-P and lateral radiographs of a Bado type I Monteggia fracture dislocation.

study has shown no difference in the results for the use of both plates, and it would appear that the benefits of LC-DCP plates are theoretical.

■ There are few studies of isolated radius or ulna fractures not associated with a proximal or distal dislocation. Plating of these fractures is associated with good results, with virtually 100% of isolated radial fractures and about 85% of isolated ulnar fractures having excellent or good results.

  ■ The difference is probably because most isolated radial fractures occur in young patients following low-energy trauma.

■ There is little information about forearm function after fixation of both bones of the forearm, but a study from Schemitsch and Richards (1992) does provide useful information.

■ The effect of plating fractures of the radius and ulnar on forearm function is shown in Table 15-5.

  ■ Elbow rotation, the arc of wrist movement, and grip strength are particularly affected.

■ The use of plates to treat open fractures of the forearm has been studied, and the overall results are shown in Table 15-6.

■ These results are very similar to those of closed fractures (Table 15-5), although Gustilo I and II fractures are associated with about 90% excellent and good results compared with about 70% excellent or good results for Gustilo type III fractures.

TABLE 15-5 FUNCTIONAL RESULTS OF PLATING RADIAL AND ULNAR DIAPHYSEAL FRACTURES

Result	Average Value	Average Decrease[a]
Wrist arc (degrees)	123	12
Elbow arc (degrees)	136	5
Rotation arc (degrees)	137	30
Grip strength (%)	76	24

[a]The average decrease represents the loss of movement or strength compared with the normal forearm.
Data from Schemitsch EH, Richards RR. The effect of malunion on functional outcome after plate fixation of both bones of the forearm in adults. J Bone Joint Surg (Am) 1992;74:1068–1078.

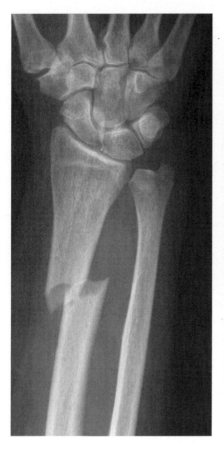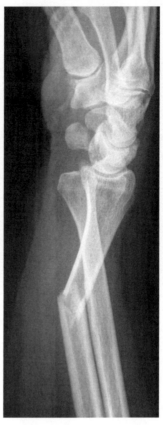

Figure 15-5 A Galeazzi (A2.3) fracture dislocation.

- The results for Gustilo type IIIb and IIIc fractures are uniformly poor, but this relates to the considerable soft tissue injury associated with the fracture.
- Grip strength after open fracture is about 10% less than following closed fracture, although the forearm rotation arc is equivalent.

External Fixation

- External fixation has been used to treat forearm fractures, but there are few results, and the problems of malunion and joint stiffness associated with external fixation suggest it should not be used routinely.
- It has been used successfully for the primary management of wartime injuries, and it seems likely that temporary skeletal stabilization in the seriously injured patient will be the main indication for its use.

Intramedullary Nailing

- Unlocked intramedullary nails or pins were popular until compression plating was introduced.
  - Results were poor in complex fractures.
- Locked ulnar nailing has been used (Fig. 15-6) and 90% excellent and good results claimed, although there are no functional results and the technique can not be recommended for routine use at this time.
- It is a useful technique, however, in the management of pathological fractures in patients with a poor prognosis.

Isolated Ulnar Fractures

- Isolated ulnar fractures have been treated by a variety of different methods including above-elbow casts, below-elbow casts, functional braces, compression plating, and locked intramedullary nailing.
- Biomechanical data have shown that where the ulnar displacement is less than 50% of the bone diameter (Fig. 15-7), the interosseous membrane is intact and the fracture is stable in rotation.
  - Thus nonoperative management may be expected to give good results in these fractures.
- The results of the management of isolated ulnar fractures are shown in Table 15-7.
  - This shows no advantage in using a cast instead of a functional brace, which can be removed at 2 to 3 weeks.
- Locked nailing gives poor results compared with plating and cast management.

TABLE 15-6 RESULTS OF PLATING OPEN FOREARM FRACTURES

Result/Complication	Range (%)	Average (%)
Excellent/good	83.3–85.1	84.2
Nonunion	5.9–8.9	8.3
Infection	4.3–5.9	4.7

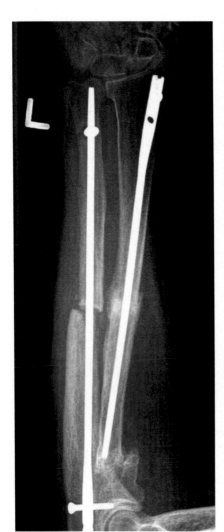
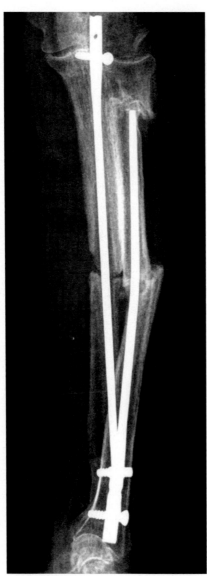

Figure 15-6 AP and lateral radiographs of locking nails used to treat radial and ulna nonunions in a young woman with osteogenesis imperfecta.

TABLE 15-7 RESULTS OF DIFFERENT TREATMENT METHODS IN THE MANAGEMENT OF ISOLATED ULNA FRACTURES

Treatment	Union (wk)	Result		
		Excellent/Good (%)	Nonunion (%)	Complications (%)
Above-elbow cast	8.6	88	2	2
Below-elbow cast	9.1	90	4	4
Functional brace	9.7	96	2	2
Plate	12.1	84	2	8
Locked nail	10.4	72	0	?

Data from Mackay D, Wood L, Rangan A. The treatment of isolated ulnar fractures in adults: a systematic review. Injury 2000;31:565–570.

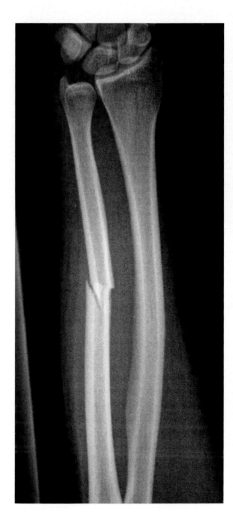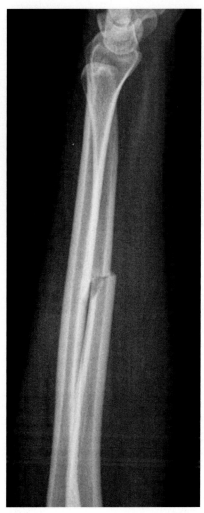

Figure 15-7 A-P and lateral radiographs of a minimally displaced (A1.1) isolated ulna fracture.

■ For ulnar fractures with up to 50% translation, a functional brace should be used. For fractures associated with greater displacement compression, plating is the method of choice.

Isolated Radial Fractures

■ The literature contains little information about these fractures, except that the outcome of compression plating is uniformly excellent and good.
■ Functional bracing is advised for undisplaced fractures, and plating is suggested for displaced fractures.

Monteggia Fracture Dislocation

The Monteggia fracture dislocation (see Fig. 15-4) involves a fracture of the ulna associated with the dislocation of the radial head. Table 15-2 shows they are relatively common. Monteggia fracture dislocations were classified into four types by Bado (1962). The classification depends on the direction of the radial head (Fig. 15-8). In type I lesions, the head is anterior to the distal humerus. In type II lesions, it is posterior, and in type III lesions, it is lateral. In type IV fracture dislocations, a dislocation of the radial head is associated with a fracture of both the radius and ulna. Most authorities indicate that about 60% of Monteggia fracture dislocations are type I, 15% are type II, 10% are type III, and 10% are type IV. Type III lesions occur virtually only in children.

■ Treatment of Monteggia fracture dislocation is plate fixation of the ulna and accurate reduction of the radial head.
  ■ The literature suggests this management method is associated with about 80% excellent or good results, with an average flexion arc of 112 degrees and a rotation arc of 128 degrees.
  ■ The incidence of radioulnar synostosis is about 6%.
■ There is a relatively high incidence of nerve palsies in Monteggia fracture dislocations, which commonly affect the radial nerve but may affect the ulna and median nerves.
■ The literature suggests the overall incidence of nerve injury is about 4%. Most are neuropraxias that improve without treatment.

Galeazzi Fracture Dislocation

■ The Galeazzi fracture dislocation (see Fig. 15-5) involves a fracture of the radius with an associated dislocation of the distal radioulnar joint.

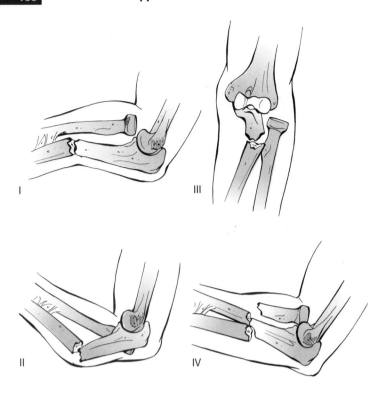

Figure 15-8 The Bado (1967) classification of Monteggia fracture dislocations.

■ This is associated with significant damage to the interosseous membrane and triangular fibrocartilage of the wrist, rendering the distal ulnar very unstable.

■ Nonoperative management is associated with very poor results mainly because of distal ulnar instability, and the correct treatment is plate fixation of the radius and accurate reduction of the distal ulnar using a K-wire to maintain the reduced position if the distal radioulnar joint remains unstable after plating.

■ A recent analysis of Galeazzi fracture dislocations showed that about 55% of radial fractures in Galeazzi lesions are within 7.5 cm of the radiocarpal joint. About 65% of these lesions were associated with an unstable distal radioulnar joint after plating of the radius. The remaining 45% of radial fractures were more than 7.5 cm from the radiocarpal joint, and only 6% of these lesions were associated with persistent distal radioulnar joint instability after radial plating.

■ Thus the more distal the radial fracture, the greater the likelihood of distal radioulnar joint instability and the requirement for ancillary K-wire fixation of the joint after radial plating.

■ If this management method is used, 95% excellent or good results can be expected.

Bipolar Fracture Dislocation

■ The combination of a Monteggia and Galeazzi fracture dislocation has been termed *bipolar fracture dislocation.*

■ It is extremely rare.

■ It is always caused by high-energy injury and should be treated by plating of the radius and ulnar fractures and stabilization of the proximal and distal radioulnar joints using K-wire fixation of the distal radioulnar joint if required.

■ One series of 10 patients has been published, which documented 80% excellent or good results with an average elbow flexion/extension arc of 124 degrees, a rotation arc of 113 degrees, and a wrist flexion/extension arc of 134 degrees. There was one case of radioulnar synostosis.

Floating Elbow

Floating elbow is discussed in Chapter 12.

Suggested Treatment

The suggested treatment of treatment of diaphyseal fractures of the forearm is given in Table 15-8.

COMPLICATIONS

A number of complications are related to fractures of the forearm and their treatment.

Plate Removal

■ Of the number of complications associated with plate removal, the best known is refracture.

■ The literature gives a range of values of refracture between 2.9% and 30.4%, with an average of 6.1%.

■ Refracture usually occurs within 9 months of plate removal and often within a few weeks, although it may occur after many years (see Fig. 6-2).

TABLE 15-8 SUGGESTED TREATMENT OF FOREARM DIAPHYSEAL FRACTURES

Injury	Treatment
Radius and ulna	
Undisplaced	Forearm cast
Displaced	DCP or LC-DCP plating
	Bone graft if bone defect present
Isolated ulna	
<50% translation	Functional brace
>50% translation	Plating
Isolated radius	
Undisplaced	Functional brace
Displaced	Plating
Monteggia fracture dislocation	Ulnar plating. Closed reduction of radial head
Galeazzi fracture dislocation	Radial plating.
	K-wiring of distal radioulnar joint if unstable

- Different plate types are associated with different refracture rates (Table 15-9).
- Obviously the more rigid the plate, the higher the refracture rate.
- A 4.5-mm DCP should not be used to plate the radius and ulna, and few surgeons use one-third tubular plates because they are too flimsy.
- About 5% of patients who have a DCP or LC-DCP will refracture.
  - To minimize the risk, the plate should not be removed for about a year after fracture, and the patient should be advised to refrain from energetic activities for about 3 months after plate removal.
- Neurological damage is the most severe complication of plate removal.
  - The literature shows that about 30% of patients have increased sensory loss after plate removal.
- Forearm plates should be retained unless there is a good reason to remove them.

Malunion

- Gross malunion is unusual with plate fixation, but it is relatively easy to alter the bow of the radius by applying a plate.
- Schemitsch and Richards (1992) have shown that a good or excellent arc of rotation results from accurate reconstruction of the radial bow.

TABLE 15-9 REFRACTURE RATE FOR DIFFERENT TYPES OF PLATES USED FOR FOREARM FIXATION

Plate	Refracture Rate (%)
3.5-mm one-third tubular plate	0
3.5-mm DCP	5.6
3.5-mm LC-DCP	4.3
4.5-mm DCP	21.0

- They showed that when the location of the maximum bow of the radius was within 5% of that of the normal arm, optimal function could be expected.
- Care must therefore be taken to reduce the forearm fracture accurately.

Compartment Syndrome

- About 8% of compartment syndromes presenting to a trauma unit occur in the forearm.
- They usually occur in young men and follow a high-energy injury.
- Analysis of the incidence of compartment syndrome in a series of forearm fractures shows an incidence of 0% to 10%, with a probable average incidence of about 4% for forearm fractures secondary to nongunshot injuries and 10% for fractures caused by low-velocity gunshot wounds.
- As with all compartment syndromes, early diagnosis and fasciotomy is important, and good results will follow appropriate treatment.
- Compartment monitoring is recommended.

Nonunion

- Nonunion is rare after plate fixation of the forearm (Table 15-4).
- It should be treated by bone grafting and refixation if fixation failure has occurred.

Nerve Damage

- Nerve damage is relatively common in high-energy injuries and can occur with any forearm fracture (see Table 15-4).
- All the nerves in the forearm can be affected.
- If they are transected, nerve repair should be undertaken, but later tendon transfer is often required.
- Neuropraxia should be treated nonoperatively, and about 90% can be expected to resolve.

Proximal Radioulnar Synostosis

- Crossed union between the radius and ulna is relatively unusual (Table 15-4) but has been estimated at 6% following Monteggia fracture dislocation.
- Good results have been reported following excision of the synostosis with adjuvant postexcision radiation therapy.
- Using this protocol there is about a 6% incidence of recurrence.

SUGGESTED READING

Bado JL. The Monteggia lesion. Clin Orthop 1967;50:71–86.

Chapman MW, Gordon JE, Zissimos AG. Compression plate fixation of acute fractures of the diaphysis of the radius and ulna. J Bone Joint Surg (Am) 1989;71:159–169.

Gustilo RB, Anderson JT. Prevention of infection in the treatment of 1,025 open fractures of long bones: retrospective and prospective analysis. J Bone Joint Surg (Am) 1976;58:453–458.

Jupiter JB, Kellam JF. Diaphyseal fractures of the forearm. In: Browner BD, Jupiter JF, Levine AM, et al., eds. Skeletal trauma, 3rd ed. Philadelphia: WB Saunders, 2003.

Jupiter JB, Leibovic SJ, Ribbans W, et al. The posterior Monteggia lesion. J Orthop Trauma 1991;5:395–402.

Lenihan MR, Brien WW, Gellman H, et al. Fractures of the forearm resulting from low-velocity gunshot wounds. J Orthop Trauma 1992;6:32–35.

Leung F, Chow SP. A prospective, randomized trial comparing the limited contact compression plate with the point contact fixator for forearm fractures. J Bone Joint Surg (Am) 2003;85:2343–2348.

Mackay D, Wood L, Rangan A. The treatment of isolated ulnar fractures in adults: a systematic review. Injury 2000;31:565–570.

McQueen MM, Gaston P, Court-Brown CM. Acute compartment syndrome. Who is at risk? J Bone Joint Surg (Br) 2000;82:200–203.

Moed BR, Kellam JF, Foster JR, et al. Immediate internal fixation of open fractures of the diaphysis of the forearm. J Bone Joint Surg (Am) 1986;681008–1017.

Müller ME, Nazarian S, Koch P, et al. The comprehensive classification of fractures of long bones. Berlin: Springer-Verlag, 1990.

Ring D, Jupiter JB, Simpson NS. Monteggia fractures in adults. J Bone Joint Surg (Am) 1998;80:1733–1744.

Rosson JW, Shearer JR. Refracture after removal of plated from the forearm: an avoidable complication. J Bone Joint Surg (Br) 1991;73:415–417.

Ruedi TP, Murphy WM, eds. AO principles of fracture management. Stuttgart: AO Publishing-Thieme, 2000.

Sarmiento A, Latta LL, Zych G, et al. Isolated ulnar shaft fractures treated with functional braces. J Orthop Trauma 1999;12:420–423.

Schemitsch EH, Richards RR. The effect of malunion on functional outcome after plate fixation of both bones of the forearm in adults. J Bone Joint Surg (Am) 1992;74:1068–1078.

Solomon HB, Zadnik M, Eglseder WA. A review of outcomes in 18 patients with floating elbow. J Orthop Trauma 2003;17:563–570.

FRACTURES OF THE DISTAL RADIUS AND ULNA

Fracture of the distal radius is defined as occurring between the flare of the metaphysis of the radius and the radiocarpal joint, thus involving the distal 3 to 4 cm of the radius. It is one of the most common fractures, but controversy remains centered around the appropriate management and likely functional outcome of these injuries. The principal current controversies about distal radial fractures and their management are listed in Box 16-1.

SURGICAL ANATOMY

The distal radius and ulna are one half of the wrist joint, which exists to subserve hand function. The wrist itself includes both the radiocarpal and distal radioulnar joints.

The articular surface of the radius is triangular with the apex of the triangle at the radial styloid. The base of the triangle is the sigmoid notch, which is the ulnar surface of the radius and articulates with the ulnar head to form the distal radioulnar joint (DRUJ). The articular surface is divided into two concave facets for articulation with the scaphoid and the lunate.

The dorsal surface of the radius is convex and irregular. Lister's tubercle acts as a fulcrum for the tendon of extensor pollicis longus (EPL), which lies in a groove on the ulnar side of the tubercle. The extensor tendons lie in six dorsal compartments, a knowledge of which is essential for

safe surgical approaches to the dorsum of the distal radius (Fig. 16-1).

The volar side of the distal radius is flat and makes a smooth curve concave from proximal to distal. The radiocarpal ligaments are attached to the volar surface distally, and proximally the bone is covered by the transverse fibers of the muscle belly of pronator quadratus, which is attached to the radial side of the bone.

The distal radioulnar joint is formed by the sigmoid notch of the radius and the ulnar head. Rotation of the radius around the ulna occurs at this joint along with some translation of the ulna, which causes dorsal prominence of the ulna in pronation and anterior displacement of the ulna in supination.

Much of the stability of the distal radioulnar joint is conferred by the triangular fibrocartilage. This arises from a wide base on the ulnar side of the lunate facet and attaches by a narrow point to the base of the ulnar styloid, and it is situated between the triquetrum and the ulnar head. Its surfaces are covered with hyaline cartilage. Other stabilizers of the distal radioulnar joint are the tendons of extensor carpi ulnaris and flexor carpi ulnaris, pronator quadratus, and the interosseous membrane of the forearm.

BOX 16-1 CURRENT CONTROVERSIES IN THE MANAGEMENT OF DISTAL RADIAL FRACTURES

Which distal radial fractures require surgical treatment?
Does anatomy relate to function? What is an acceptable position?
Which fractures require surgical treatment?
How should metaphyseal instability be treated?
How should intra-articular fractures be treated?
If external fixation is used, which is the best type?
If a cast is used, how long should it be kept on?
Should the ulnar styloid be fixed?
How useful are locked plates?

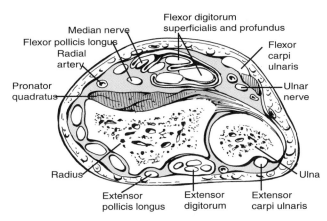

Figure 16-1 A cross section of the distal radius showing the six extensor compartments. Note the smooth surface on the volar side compared to the irregular dorsal surface.

CLASSIFICATION

The classification most commonly used is the OTA (AO) classification of the distal radius. This is a morphological classification, which does not take displacement into account. It is not a predictive classification system.

The OTA (AO) type A fracture is extra-articular, the type B is partial articular (i.e., involving only part of the articular surface), and the type C is a complete articular fracture with the articular surface completely detached from the diaphysis. Differentiation between groups (A1, A2, A3, etc.) depends on anatomy, complexity, and com-

minution (Fig. 16-2). Thus the A1 fracture is a fracture of the ulna, the A2 fracture is an extra-articular fracture without metaphyseal comminution, and the A3 fracture is extra-articular with metaphyseal comminution. The B1 fracture is a styloid fracture, the B2 is a dorsal partial articular fracture, and the B3 is a volar partial articular fracture. The C1 fracture is a complete articular fracture with a simple articular component and no comminution. The C2 fracture is a simple articular fracture with metaphyseal comminution; the C3 fracture has a complex articular pattern with increasing metaphyseal comminution.

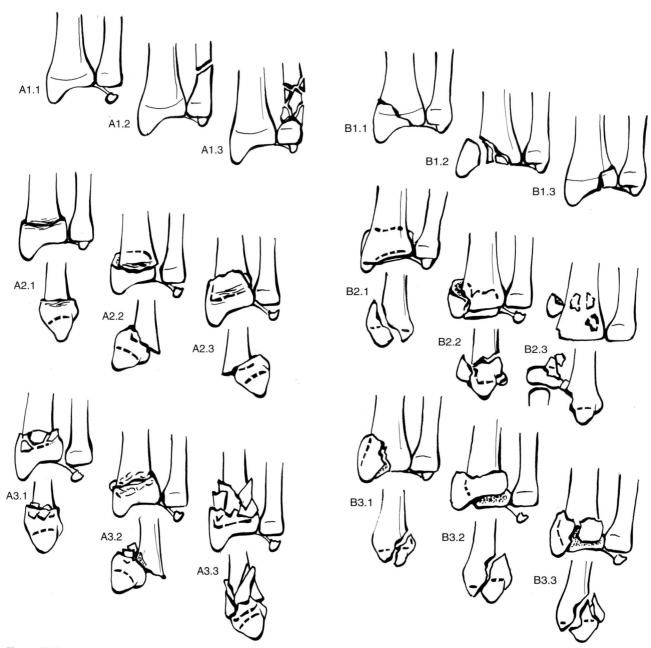

Figure 16-2   OTA (AO) classification of fractures of the distal radius and ulna.

Fractures of the distal ulna in association with fractures of the distal radius are classified according to a Q modifier in the OTA (AO) classification. Q1 is a fracture of the base of the ulnar styloid; Q2 is a simple fracture of the ulnar neck; Q3, a comminuted fracture of the ulnar neck; Q4, a fracture of the ulnar head; Q5, a fracture of the ulnar head and neck; Q6, a diaphyseal fracture of the ulna.

The Frykman classification system is also used by some clinicians. This is based on whether or not the fracture is articular (including both radiocarpal and distal radioulnar joints) and the presence or absence of an ulnar fracture (Table 16-1).

TABLE 16-1 FRYKMAN CLASSIFICATION OF DISTAL RADIUS FRACTURES

	Frykman Class	
Fracture Location	Without Ulnar Fracture	With Ulnar Fracture
Extra-articular	1	2
Intra-articular radiocarpal	3	4
Intra-articular DRUJ	5	6
Intra-articular radiocarpal and DRUJ	7	8

EPIDEMIOLOGY

The basic epidemiology of distal radial fractures is shown in Table 16-2. This shows they are predominantly an injury of the middle-aged to elderly woman. They are therefore associated with postmenopausal osteopenia or osteoporosis, and like other osteoporotic fractures they are increasing in incidence. Thus prevention of these injuries should concentrate on both detecting and treating osteoporosis and on strategies to reduce the risk of falling in older individuals. Fracture of the distal radius occurs in the fit patient; in 80% of all fractures, the patient is independent for all the activities of daily living prior to the injury.

The majority of distal radial fractures occur in low-energy injury. Because of the osteopenic nature of the bone, approximately two thirds of the fractures have metaphyseal comminution implying metaphyseal instability. Half of the total are OTA (AO) type A3.2 or C2.1, which are extra-articular or minimal articular fractures with metaphyseal comminution. It is generally agreed that the incidence of distal radial fractures increases in the winter months attributable to icy conditions.

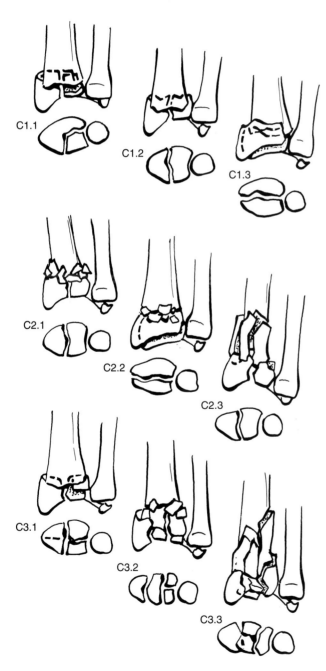

Figure 16-2 *(continued)*

TABLE 16-2 EPIDEMIOLOGY OF DISTAL RADIAL FRACTURES

Proportion of all fractures	17.5%
Average age	55.5 y
Men/women	31%/69%
Distribution	Type A
Incidence	$195.2/10^5/y$
Open fractures	0.7%
Most common causes	
Fall	76.2%
Sport	12.5%
Height	5.4%
OTA (AO) classification	
Type A	47.8%
Type B	10.2%
Type C	41.9%
Most common subgroups	
A3.2	25.8%
C2.1	22.9%
A2.1	15.3%
C1.2	7.1%

TABLE 16-3 AVERAGE AGES AND OTA (AO) TYPES OF THE DIFFERENT CAUSES OF INJURY IN DISTAL RADIUS FRACTURES

Cause	Average Age (y)	OTA (AO) Type (%)		
		A	B	C
Fall	64	48.8	9.0	42.2
Sports	32	45.5	19.4	35.1
Fall from height	47	26.5	11.9	61.6

There is a smaller number of older men sustaining these fractures. As medicine becomes more successful in prolonging life, there is an increasing incidence of osteopenic elderly men with distal radial fractures compared with 50 years ago. Younger individuals, especially men, are more likely to sustain higher energy injury with severe intra-articular fractures, although these are a small proportion of the overall numbers. The average ages of the patients sustaining the different types of injury are shown in Table 16-3.

Associated fractures are unusual and occur in less than 1% of cases. The most common are the contralateral distal radius, proximal femur, and proximal humerus. In high-energy injury, it is important to exclude carpal injury.

The ages and AO type according to the mechanism of injury are shown in Table 16-3. Not surprisingly there are more intra-articular injuries in younger patients with the higher energy types of injury.

FRACTURES OF THE DISTAL RADIUS

DIAGNOSIS

Radiologic Examination

■ The distal end of the normal radius slopes in a volar and ulnar direction.
■ The average volar angle ranges from 7 to 12 degrees in the sagittal plane.
■ Deformity in this plane is calculated from a lateral radiograph by measuring the angle between a line perpendicular to the long axis of the radius and a line joining the volar and dorsal margins of the articular surface (Fig. 16-3).
■ When the articular surface is tilted dorsally, this angle is termed the *dorsal angle*.
■ When the articular surface is tilted in a volar direction, this is termed *volar angulation* and generally measured as a negative value.
■ The length of the radius can be expressed in two ways: measurement of the height of the tip of the radial styloid

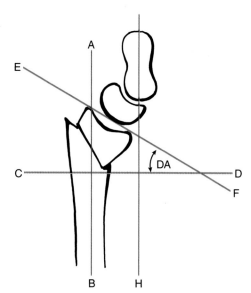

Figure 16-3   The dorsal angle is measured on the lateral view by finding the angle between a line perpendicular to the long axis of the radius and a line joining the dorsal and volar extremities of the radiocarpal joint. Carpal alignment is assessed by the point of intersection of the line parallel to the long axis of the radius and a line parallel to the long axis of the capitate. If these intersect outwith the carpus, the carpus is malaligned.

compared to the distal articular surface of the ulnar head or measurement of the ulnar variance, which is the vertical distance between a line parallel to the ulnar side of the radial articular surface and a line parallel to the articular surface of the distal ulna (Fig. 16-4).
■ Radiographs of the uninjured wrist are ideally required to determine normal ulnar variance in an individual, although in most cases the medial corner of the radius and the ulnar head are level.

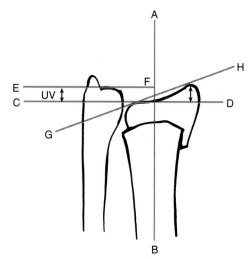

Figure 16-4   Measurement of radial shortening is either by comparison of the relative heights of the radial styloid and the ulnar head or of the relative heights of the ulnar corner of the radius and the ulnar head.

BOX 16-2 RADIOLOGIC MEASUREMENTS PREDICTING POOR FUNCTIONAL OUTCOME

- Positive ulnar variance >3 mm
- Carpal malalignment
- Dorsal angle >10 degrees
- Articular step-off or gap >2 mm

BOX 16-3 FACTORS INCREASING METAPHYSEAL INSTABILITY IN FRACTURES OF THE DISTAL RADIUS

Patient characteristics
Increasing age
Loss of independence

Fracture characteristics
Metaphyseal comminution
Positive ulnar variance on initial radiographs
Initial dorsal angulation

- In fractures of the distal radius, the radius is commonly shorter than the ulna (positive ulnar variance).
- Carpal alignment depends on the preservation of normal distal radial anatomy.
- When distal radial alignment is correct, the capitate sits directly above the long axis of the radius on a lateral radiograph.
- Carpal alignment is measured by calculating the point of intersection of a line drawn along the long axis of the radius and a line drawn along the long axis of the capitate on the lateral radiograph.
- If the point of intersection is within the confines of the carpus, the carpus is aligned; if outside the carpus, the carpus is malaligned (see Fig. 16-3).

The Relation of Anatomy to Function

- It is now generally agreed that either extra- or intra-articular deformity of the distal radius after a fracture is likely to cause a functional deficit, usually either pain (either radiocarpal or arising from the DRUJ), reduction in the range of motion (especially rotation of the forearm), or weakened grip strength.
- The radiological factors implicated in a poor functional outcome are listed in Box 16-2.
  - The strongest associations with poor function are with carpal malalignment and positive ulnar variance.
- Carpal malalignment is an indirect method of measuring dorsal tilt.
- The accurate measurement of dorsal tilt depends on a true lateral radiograph, which can be difficult to obtain; carpal malalignment does not depend on the positioning of the wrist.
- Both dorsal tilt and ulnar variance will cause malalignment of the distal radioulnar joint.
- An articular step-off or gap of more than 2 mm is generally considered to cause increasing evidence of radiographic degenerative changes.
- An acceptable radiological position can be defined as a dorsal angle less than 10 degrees or volar angle greater than –15 degrees, no carpal malalignment, positive ulnar variance of less than 3 mm, and an articular step or gap of less than 2 mm.

Instability of the Distal Radius

- Instability of the distal radius is considered to occur when the reduced position cannot be maintained in a forearm cast and is usually applied to metaphyseal alignment (Fig. 16-5).

- Various predictive factors for malalignment have been described and are listed in Box 16-3.

History and Physical Examination

- The history is most commonly one of a fall from standing height onto the outstretched hand, although a smaller number of cases may have a higher energy injury.
- Pain is usually localized around the wrist itself.
- The patient may also complain of swelling and deformity if the fracture is displaced.
- A neurological history should be taken at an early stage to exclude neurological injury such as a carpal tunnel syndrome complicating the fracture.
- Severe pain with or without neurological symptoms may indicate the presence of an acute compartment syndrome, which, although rare, can occur, especially in a high-energy injury.
- In the displaced fracture, deformity is usually obvious: the dinner fork or silver fork deformity in dorsally displaced fractures and a similar although more proximal deformity in palmar displaced fractures.
- In undisplaced fractures, the key to the diagnosis is the finding of local tenderness over the distal radius.

TREATMENT

EXTRA-ARTICULAR AND MINIMAL ARTICULAR FRACTURES

Undisplaced Fractures

- There is no disagreement that the undisplaced or minimally displaced fracture of the distal radius should be managed nonoperatively in a forearm cast (see Figure 31-7 in Chapter 31) or splint (see Figure 31-15 in Chapter 31).
- Excellent functional results are obtained in over 90%, provided the fracture does not displace.
- The minimally displaced fracture should be followed radiologically at 1 week to 10 days after injury to ensure maintenance of position because up to 10% can displace within the cast.

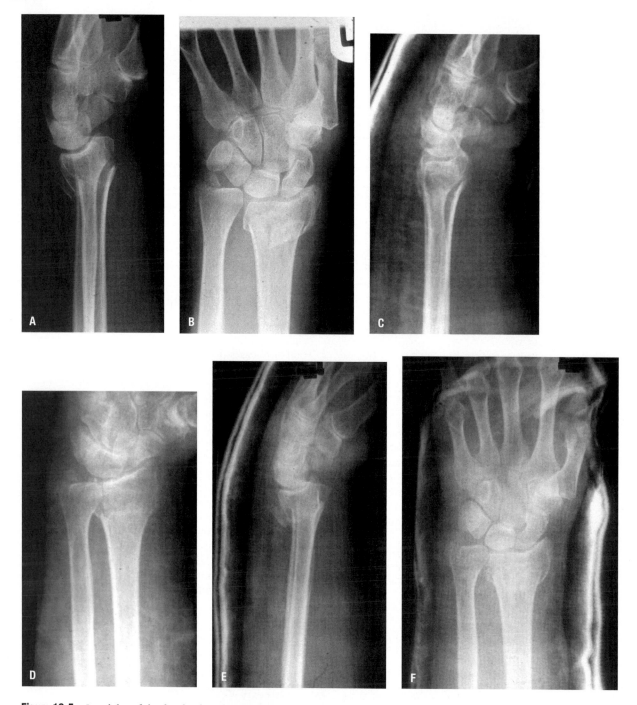

Figure 16-5   Instability of the distal radius. (**A,B**) The initial films show a displaced fracture of the distal radius with dorsal angulation, radial shortening and carpal malalignment. (**C,D**) After reduction there is good restoration of the length and dorsal angle; the carpus is well aligned. (**E,F**) One week later the fracture has redisplaced.

■ The only remaining debate in the undisplaced fracture of the distal radius is the length of time immobilization is required, if at all.

■ Early mobilization of the wrist allows more rapid functional recovery and earlier resolution of swelling, with no increase in pain and no loss of anatomical position.

■ The undisplaced or stable minimally displaced fracture should be mobilized as soon as comfort allows, usually at around 3 weeks.

Dorsal Displacement

Nonsurgical Treatment

■ The majority of displaced fractures of the distal radius are treated nonoperatively in the first instance unless there is articular displacement or predictable severe metaphyseal instability.

■ Reduction is performed under a regional block or general anaesthetic.

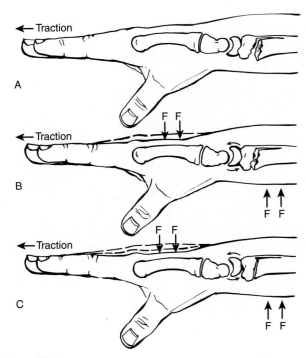

Figure 16-6   Agee's maneuver places a volar translation force on the distal radial fragment, which allows the lunate to tilt the distal fragment in a volar direction.

- It can be attempted using a hematoma block (injection of local anaesthetic into the fracture hematoma) but is less successful both radiologically and in terms of pain relief than regional or general anaesthetic.
- Reduction can be achieved either manually or using finger traps.
- Traction is first applied to regain length, followed by some flexion and ulnar deviation.
  - If this does not restore the volar tilt, Agee's maneuver of palmar translation of the hand relative to the forearm may be successful in achieving volar tilt (Fig. 16-6).

- The reduced fracture should then be immobilized in a forearm cast (see Fig. 31-7 in Chapter 31).
  - This should either be a dorsal slab or a split full cast.
- There is no anatomical advantage but possible functional disadvantage in the use of a full long arm cast, which can result in permanent loss of rotation.
- Early hand movement should be encouraged with elevation to reduce postinjury swelling.
- The cast or slab can be completed when swelling diminishes.
- All displaced fractures requiring reduction should be reviewed radiologically and clinically within 10 days of injury to identify metaphyseal instability.
- Further treatment is then instituted if indicated.
- If the fracture is stable, the cast should be retained for 3 to 6 weeks.
- There is no advantage in retaining the cast for longer, but there is some evidence that a shorter period in a cast (3 weeks) leads to a more rapid recovery.
- Physical therapy should be prescribed after cast removal for patients with pain, restricted forearm rotation, and poor function because these are predictors of a poorer outcome.
- Reported results of nonoperative treatment of displaced fractures of the distal radius are detailed in Table 16-4.
- These results do not separate stable and unstable displaced fractures, which explains the high malunion rate and the relatively low rate of excellent and good functional results compared to the surgical methods of treatment.
- The complication rate of nonoperative treatment is similar to many surgical methods.
- In the elderly patient with low demands on wrist function, displacement leading to malunion should be accepted.
  - Little benefit has been shown from primary manipulation in these patients because the fracture is almost inevitably unstable.
  - Reduction should not be attempted in the frail elderly, but a forearm cast (see Figure 31-7 in Chapter 31) should be used for pain relief.

TABLE 16-4 RESULTS OF THREE OF THE TECHNIQUES OF MANAGEMENT OF DISTAL RADIUS FRACTURES

Result	Cast[a] (%)		Bone Substitutes[a] (%)		Volar Plate[b] (Volar Displaced Fractures) (%)	
	Range	Average	Range	Average	Range	Average
Excellent/good	32–94	68	45–82	64	82–84	83
Malunion	15–88	48	18–29	22	11–28	16
Complications	6–45	23	15–46	26	33–41	36

[a]Cast and bone substitute management figures relate to the treatment of both stable and unstable fractures.
[b]Volar plating in this context is in fractures with volar displacement.

BOX 16-4 INDICATIONS FOR SURGERY IN DORSALLY DISPLACED EXTRA-ARTICULAR OR MINIMAL ARTICULAR FRACTURES

- ■ Redisplacement in cast
- ■ Predicted instability
- ■ Open fractures[a]
- ■ Acute carpal tunnel syndrome[a]
- ■ Irreducibility[a]

[a]Uncommon indications.

Surgical Treatment

- ■ Instability of a dorsally displaced fracture of the distal radius in a fit patient is the most common indication for surgical treatment.
  - ▨ This may be predicted instability or redisplacement in a cast (see Fig. 16-5).
- ■ Other less common causes are listed in Box 16-4.

External Fixation

- ■ There are three main types of external fixation (see Chapter 35) employed in the treatment of distal radial fractures: bridging (Fig. 16-7), augmented bridging (Fig. 16-8), and nonbridging external fixation (Fig. 16-9).
- ■ Table 16-5 summarizes the published results of external fixation of the distal radius. Such a distillate of published results should be interpreted with care.
- ■ Nonbridging external fixation has the lowest malunion rate and the highest proportion of excellent to good functional results of the three techniques.

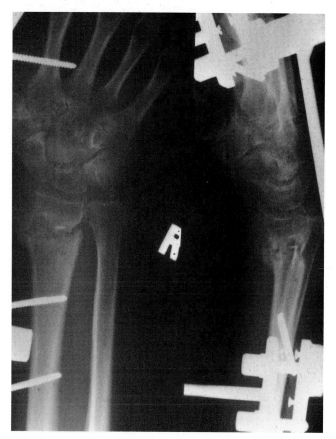

Figure 16-7   Bridging external fixation with pins in the second metacarpal and pins in the radius proximal to the fracture site. The fixator is therefore bridging the radiocarpal, midcarpal, and carpometacarpal joints and applying an indirect reduction force to the distal radius.

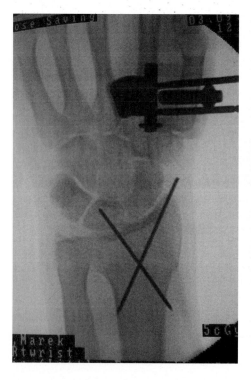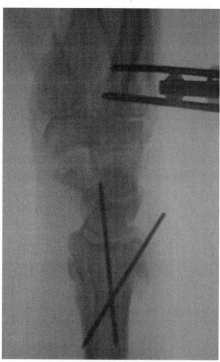

Figure 16-8   Augmentation of a bridging external fixator, usually with K-wires, helps maintain the reduction.

Chapter 16 / Fractures of the Distal Radius and Ulna

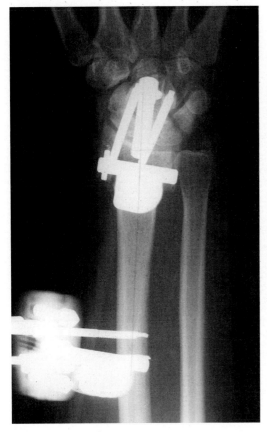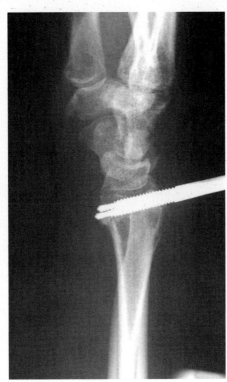

Figure 16-9 Nonbridging external fixation with pins in the distal radial fragment, allowing direct control of the reduction and its maintenance.

- The outcome of bridging external fixation is improved by augmentation with internal fixation, usually percutaneous wires.
- Complication rates with external fixation are comparable to or slightly higher than other techniques, although a number of these are superficial pin track infections that do not alter the final outcome.
- They are more common after nonbridging external fixation, presumably because of active wrist movement.
- Any technique of managing the unstable distal radial fracture will likely have some cases of malunion.
- Both nonbridging and augmented bridging external fixation are relatively new techniques, and there is a paucity of information as yet published.

- Although nonbridging external fixation is likely to reduce the rate of dorsal malunion significantly, it risks volar malunion in the presence of volar comminution if the fracture is overreduced.
- Complex regional pain syndrome type 1 (CRPS1) is most prevalent with bridging external fixation without augmentation and least prevalent in nonbridging external fixation. This may be because the latter does not risk distracting the radiocarpal and intercarpal joint.

Percutaneous Wiring
- Although a popular technique, percutaneous wiring of the distal radius (Fig. 16-10; see also Fig. 34-1 in Chapter 34)

TABLE 16-5 RESULTS OF THE THREE DIFFERENT TYPES OF EXTERNAL FIXATION FOR DORSALLY DISPLACED UNSTABLE FRACTURES OF THE DISTAL RADIUS

Result	Bridging (%)		Augmented Bridging (%)		Nonbridging (%)	
	Range	Average	Range	Average	Range	Average
Excellent/good	57–94	80	65–96	84	79–97	91
Malunion	6–47	24	0–10	5	0	0
Complications	12–53	33	16–24	20	19–47	33

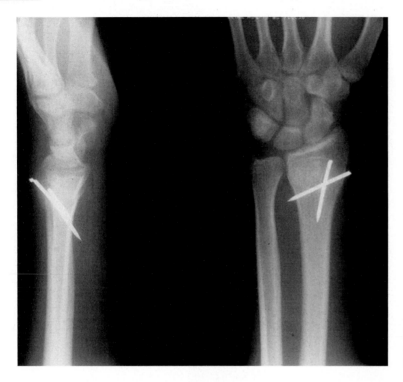

Figure 16-10   Kapandji or intrafocal wiring of the distal radius where wires are introduced percutaneously into the fracture site and used to assist the reduction.

has never been demonstrated to be effective, especially in older more osteopenic patients.

- Table 16-6 shows that the malunion rate for percutaneous wiring appears to be less than that for cast management, although it remains unacceptably high.
- Studies on percutaneous wiring, however, do not always select only unstable fractures for inclusion, and randomized studies show no benefit with percutaneous wiring compared to cast management.
- It is agreed that the radiological results after percutaneous wiring worsen with age when instability is most likely. This is reflected in the functional outcome.
- Complication rates are similar to those of other methods of treatment.

Plating

- Dorsal plating (Fig. 16-11) is the most invasive method of treating the unstable dorsally displaced fracture of the distal radius.
- Malunion remains a problem, but, like nonbridging external fixation, it is most likely to be volar in cases with volar comminution.

- Functional outcome is comparable to external fixation as is the complication rate (see Table 16-6).
  - Analyzing the specific complications, however, reveals that tendon rupture or irritation rates are very high, resulting in a significant rate of secondary surgery for plate removal.
  - Tendon rupture, unlike some other complications, is likely to compromise the final functional outcome.
- A recent development in the management of dorsally displaced fractures of the distal radius is locked volar plating (Fig. 16-12) (see Chapter 32). Very few studies have as yet been published, but the results look promising (see Table 16-6). As experience accumulates, it is likely that pitfalls of this technique will become obvious.

Bone Substitutes

- Calcium phosphate bone cements have recently become available and are used as a paste that is injected into the defect in the metaphysis to support the distal radius fracture while healing (see Fig. 16-13).
- The results of the published literature are summarized in Table 16-4.

TABLE 16-6 RESULTS OF INTERNAL FIXATION TECHNIQUES FOR DORSALLY DISPLACED UNSTABLE FRACTURES OF THE DISTAL RADIUS

Result	Percutaneous Wiring (%)		Dorsal Plating (%)		Locked Plating (%)	
	Range	Average	Range	Average	Range	Average
Excellent/good	38–94	79	67–100	85	92–100	96
Malunion	9–38	17	0–33	15	0–6	3
Complications	13–33	21	7–50	27	3–32	12

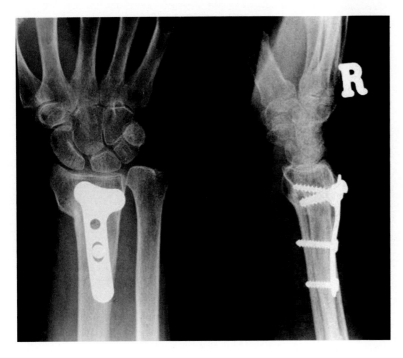

Figure 16-11 Dorsal plating of the distal radius. The end of the plate is rather prominent, suggesting the possibility of tendon rupture. This patient ruptured the extensor pollicis longus tendon 10 weeks after plating.

- There remains a significant rate of malunion when these substitutes are used in isolation and supported with a plaster cast.
- It is generally recommended that bone substitute should be used as an adjunct to other forms of fixation.
- They can also be used to support the reduction of an articular fracture in association with internal fixation.
- Complication rates of bone substitutes are similar to other methods of treatment.

- One complication specific to bone mineral substitute is extrusion of cement into either the soft tissues or the radiocarpal or distal radioulnar joints.
- Neither seems to cause significant problems, although there may be a risk of tendon rupture from dorsal extrusion.

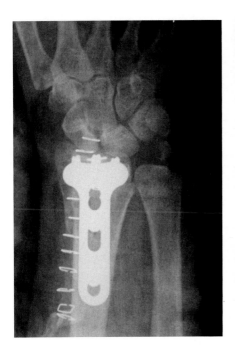

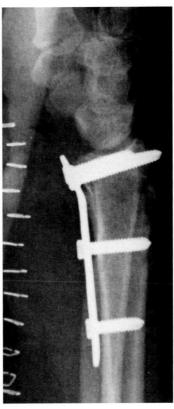

Figure 16-12 A locking plate applied to the volar surface of the distal radius used to treat an unstable dorsally displaced fracture of the distal radius.

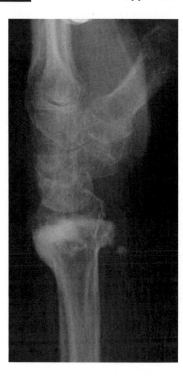

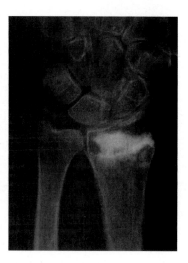

Figure 16-13   Calcium phosphate cement used to support the reduction of an unstable distal radius fracture.

Volar Displacement

- There is little disagreement that distal radius fractures with volar displacement should be treated with a plate contoured to the volar surface of the distal radius and then supported by a forearm cast for a few weeks.
- These fractures may be partial articular fractures or extra-articular with volar comminution.
- Severe complete articular fractures of the distal radius with volar displacement are considered in the section on intra-articular fractures.

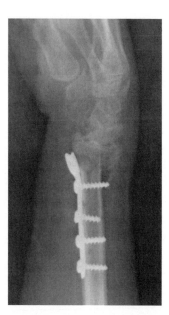

Figure 16-14   This volar plate has been used to maintain the reduction of a volar displaced fracture. Because of inadequate contouring of the plate in the presence of dorsal comminution, a dorsal malunion has resulted.

- Patient satisfaction after volar plating for volar displaced fracture is relatively high (see Table 16-4).
- Complications remain common as in other treatment methods.
- The most common treatment-related problem is malunion. It is iatrogenic and results from poor contouring of the plate, which can push the distal radius into dorsal malunion if there is dorsal comminution (Fig. 16-14).

INTRA-ARTICULAR FRACTURES OF THE DISTAL RADIUS

- Fractures of the distal radius with intra-articular displacement often require a combination of treatment methods, including open reduction and internal fixation, external fixation, and percutaneous internal fixation (Fig. 16-15).
- Internal fixation may be with wires, screws, or plates.
- Location-specific plates supporting individual fragments are available and can be used with small incisions to avoid a large approach with soft tissue stripping.
- Adjunctive techniques include the use of bone graft or bone substitutes to support the articular reduction and the use of arthroscopy to improve the articular reduction.
  - Although both these techniques may be helpful, their superiority to techniques without their use has yet to be proven.
  - Accompanying arthroscopy is a high prevalence of diagnosed associated carpal injuries averaging 70%. The diagnosis of carpal injury does not seem to affect the functional results, however, and the clinical importance of these findings has yet to be established.
- The results of these techniques are summarized in Table 16-7.
- Excellent and good functional results are reported as highest with external fixation and indirect reduction and

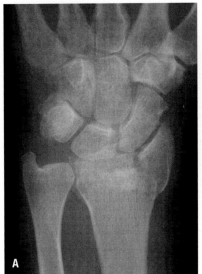
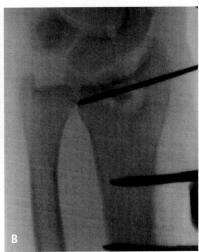
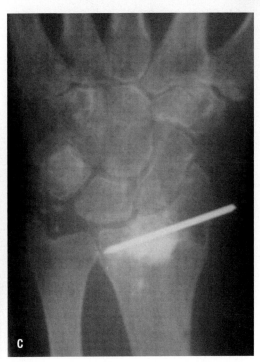

Figure 16-15 (A) A displaced intra-articular fracture of the distal radius with a depressed die-punch fragment. (B) The die-punch fragment has been reduced by percutaneous methods and fixed with a K-wire. (C) The reduction has been supported with a calcium phosphate bone cement. Bone graft can also be used.

lowest with a combination of open reduction, internal fixation, and external fixation, with slightly better joint alignment achieved with the former technique.

■ These results were supported by a recent report of a randomized study of external fixation and indirect reduction versus open reduction and internal fixation.

RADIOCARPAL FRACTURE-DISLOCATION

■ Radiocarpal fracture-dislocation is rare and can be either volar or dorsal in direction.
■ It is differentiated from the partial articular fracture with severe displacement by loss of contact between the proximal carpal row and the articular surface of the distal radius (Fig. 16-16).
■ Most occur as a result of high-energy injury and may be associated with other injury either locally or distant.
■ Closed reduction is usually possible but may need to be supplemented with external fixation, ligamentous repair, or internal fixation of an associated radial-styloid fracture.

Suggested Treatment

■ The recommended treatment for distal radial fractures is presented in Table 16-8.

TABLE 16-7 RESULTS OF THE DIFFERENT TYPES OF MANAGEMENT OF DISPLACED INTRA-ARTICULAR FRACTURES OF THE DISTAL RADIUS

Result	ORIF (%)		Combined ORIF/External Fixation (%)		External Fixation/Percutaneous Reduction and Fixation (%)	
	Range	Average	Range	Average	Range	Average
Excellent/good	56–94	80	59–86	73	70–92	85
Malunion						
Joint	3–24	16	29	29	2–10	7
Metaphyseal	0–24	9	23	23	2–24	14
Complications	10–50	30	0–29	17	14–20	15

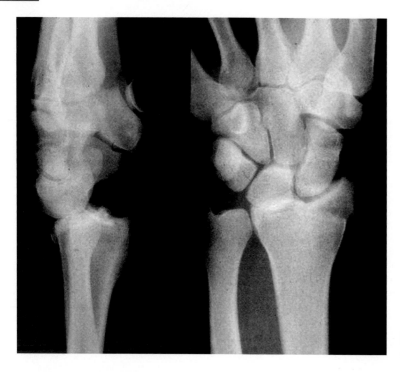

Figure 16-16 A radiocarpal fracture dislocation with displacement of a radial styloid fracture.

COMPLICATIONS

■ Fracture-related and treatment-related complications are shown in Table 16-9.

Malunion

■ Malunion is the most common treatment-related complication of distal radius fracture.
■ It is usually considered as occurring with more than 10 degrees of dorsal angulation, more than 15 degrees of volar angulation or in the presence of secondary carpal malalignment.

■ Symptomatic malunion should be treated by distal radial osteotomy, which is usually successful in relieving symptoms and improving function.

Nerve Compression or Injury

■ This complication is a regular occurrence after distal radial fracture.
■ The most common nerve affected is the median nerve, although occasionally compression of the ulnar or radial nerves is found.
■ Symptoms of median nerve compression that are deteriorating indicate a need for immediate carpal tunnel decompression.

TABLE 16-8 RECOMMENDED TREATMENT FOR DISTAL RADIAL FRACTURES

Injury	Treatment
Undisplaced	Forearm cast
Dorsal displacement (extra-articular or minimal articular displacement)	
Stable after reduction	Closed reduction and forearm cast
Unstable after reduction	
Distal fragment >1 cm	Nonbridging external fixator or locking volar plate
Distal fragment <1 cm	Augmented bridging external fixation
Volar displacement	Volar plate
	Locking plate if osteopenic
Intra-articular	
Partial articular	Percutaneous reduction and internal fixation
	ORIF if irreducible percutaneously
Complete articular	Bridging external fixation
	Percutaneous reduction and fixation. ORIF if irreducible percutaneously.
Frail elderly	Forearm cast

TABLE 16-9 COMPLICATION RATES OF FRACTURES OF THE DISTAL RADIUS

Complication	Range (%)	Average (%)
All	6–53	25
Malunion	0–79	22
Osteoarthrosis (articular fractures)	0–82	49
Infection		
Minor	0–46	11
Major	0–8	1
Nerve compression/injury	0–28	7
Tendon rupture	0–40	6
CRPS type 11	0–49	5
Nonunion	Rare (<1)	<1

■ No advantage has been demonstrated in prophylactic carpal tunnel decompression in asymptomatic patients.
■ Radial nerve damage can be caused by the incision for proximal pin placement in external fixation or by compression from plaster casts.
■ Injury to the radial nerve can lead to a painful neuroma.

Complex Regional Pain Syndrome Type 1

■ CRPS type 1, or reflex sympathetic dystrophy, occurs in varying amounts after distal radius fracture.
■ It may be associated with carpal tunnel syndrome or with distraction of the radiocarpal joint with the use of bridging external fixation.
■ Early diagnosis and treatment is essential (see Chapter 41), but this complication usually leads to a poor functional outcome.

Tendon Rupture

■ The extensor pollicis longus tendon is the most common tendon to rupture after distal radius fracture.
■ This can occur either spontaneously or after surgical intervention, most commonly dorsal plating, and is characterized by lack of interphalangeal joint extension of the thumb or an inability to elevate the thumb with the palm of the hand flat on the table.
■ In spontaneous cases, the tendon usually ruptures some time after the fracture, with a median time of 6 weeks, although the range of rupture time has been reported between 2 weeks and 1 year.
■ It is thought that the rupture occurs because of tendon entrapment between the extensor retinaculum and callus on the distal radius.
■ This can cause either an attrition rupture or poor vascularization and obstruction of the flow of synovial fluid, causing degenerative necrosis of the tendon.
■ Either of these could be the cause of higher rates of rupture after dorsal plating.
■ It is recommended that after dorsal plating the extensor retinaculum be placed under the tendons to avoid attrition from the plate.

■ The prevalence of EPL rupture is seen in Table 16-9. If dorsal plating were excluded, the actual prevalence is probably lower and has been reported as low as 0.3%.
■ Treatment of EPL rupture is by tendon transfer, usually with extensor indicis proprius.
■ If this is either unsuitable or unavailable, extensor communis to the little finger, extensor carpi radialis longus, or a free tendon graft may be used.
■ Extensor indicis proprius transfer has excellent results in 80% to 90% of cases, although a possible disadvantage is weakness of independent extension of the index finger.
■ Other tendon ruptures have been described after fracture of the distal radius including flexor tendon ruptures after volar plating and rupture of all the extensor tendons.

Posttraumatic Osteoarthrosis

■ Osteoarthrosis following distal radial fracture is unusual in extra-articular or undisplaced articular fractures, but its prevalence is high after displaced intra-articular fractures.
■ Most reports, however, are of radiological osteoarthrosis, which is frequently asymptomatic.
■ Treatment of disabling symptomatic osteoarthrosis is by radiocarpal arthrodesis.

Other

■ Infection is relatively common after surgical treatment of distal radius fractures, but the majority are superficial pin track infections with external fixation.
  ■ Major infections are unusual (see Table 16-9).
■ Distal radioulnar joint pain is relatively common after distal radial fracture but usually resolves spontaneously in the absence of malunion or rotational contracture.
  ■ Perseverance of disabling distal radioulnar joint pain is an indication for a reconstructive procedure.
■ Nonunion after distal radius fracture is rare but when present can be treated with internal fixation and bone grafting. Arthrodesis occasionally is required.

FRACTURES OF THE DISTAL ULNA

■ Most fractures of the distal ulna are associated with distal radius fractures and usually well aligned and stable after reduction and stabilization of the distal radius.
■ Residual malalignment or instability after distal radial reduction may compromise DRUJ function, however, and are an indication for fixation with small plates if possible.
■ Unstable fractures of the ulna have also been implicated in the rare development of distal radial nonunion.
■ Ulnar head fractures are uncommon but usually require fixation with screws or wires to restore DRUJ alignment and function.
■ Ulnar diaphyseal fractures should be managed as outlined in Chapter 15.

BOX 16-5 INJURIES OCCURRING WITH DRUJ DISLOCATION

Without fracture (simple)
TFCC injury
Volar radioulnar ligament/capsule
Dorsal radioulnar ligament/capsule

With fracture (complex)
Galeazzi
Distal radius
Ulnar styloid
Essex Lopresti

BOX 16-6 STABILIZERS OF THE DRUJ

- TFCC
- Dorsal radiocarpal ligaments
- Volar radiocarpal ligaments
- Extensor carpi ulnaris
- Flexor carpi ulnaris
- Interosseous membrane

joint (Box 16-6), the principal of which is the triangular fibrocartilage complex (TFCC).

Diagnosis

History and Physical Examination
- The diagnosis of an isolated distal radioulnar joint dislocation is made clinically and radiographically.
- On clinical examination there is swelling around the distal radioulnar joint.
- If the swelling does not obscure the ulnar head, it can be seen to be prominent in dorsal dislocation.
- In volar dislocation, the wrist appears narrow with a depression in place of the normal prominence of the ulnar head.
- Rotation of the forearm is always reduced with a block to supination in a dorsal dislocation and to pronation in a volar dislocation.

Radiologic Examination
- The radiographic diagnosis is made with a true lateral X-ray of the wrist when the diagnosis should be obvious (Fig. 16-17).
- On the anteroposterior view, there is usually overlap of the radius and ulna, with volar dislocation and widening of the joint with dorsal dislocation.

INJURIES TO THE DISTAL RADIOULNAR JOINT

DISTAL RADIOULNAR JOINT DISLOCATION

- DRUJ dislocation may occur in isolation (simple) or associated with a fracture (complex) (Box 16-5).
- Those in association with Galeazzi fractures and Essex Lopresti lesions are discussed in Chapter 15.
- Isolated DRUJ dislocation is uncommon.
- Dorsal dislocation is probably the more common and occurs with hyperpronation of the forearm.
- Volar dislocation occurs with hypersupination.
- Dislocation in either direction results in damage to some or all of the stabilizers of the distal radioulnar

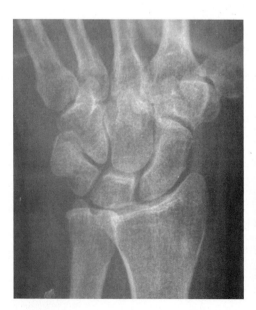
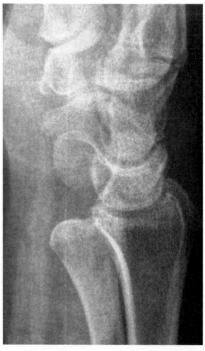

Figure 16-17 A volar dislocation of the DRUJ.

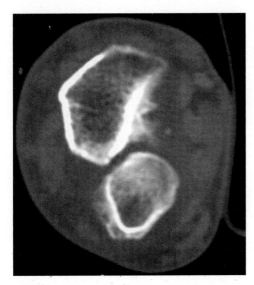

Figure 16-18 A CT scan of the patient in Figure 16-17. Lines drawn through the dorsal ulnar and radial borders and through the volar ulnar and radial borders should contain the ulna if the joint is aligned.

- A single axial CT scan may be used where there remains doubt about the diagnosis.
- Lines drawn through the dorsal ulnar and radial borders and through the volar ulnar and radial borders should contain the ulna (Fig. 16-18).

Treatment

- Isolated DRUJ dislocations are usually easily reduced by rotation of the forearm while applying pressure to the ulnar head.
- Excessive force must be avoided as occasional cases are irreducibly closed because of interposition of one or more of the extensor tendons.
- In these cases open reduction should be performed.
- For dorsal dislocation, the forearm should be supinated and for volar, pronated.
- An above-elbow cast is then applied in supination for dorsal dislocation or pronation for volar dislocation and should be retained for 6 weeks.
- If the dislocation has required open reduction or is unstable after closed reduction, the ulna should be transfixed to the radius in the reduced position with K-wires or screws.
- These should be removed at 6 weeks and active movement encouraged.

INJURIES TO THE TRIANGULAR FIBROCARTILAGE COMPLEX

- The triangular fibrocartilage complex (TFCC) is one of the main stabilizers of the DRUJ, and so damage to its structural integrity can produce symptoms of DRUJ pain with or without instability.
- These injuries can occur in isolation or in association with fracture of the ulnar styloid.
- If there is doubt about the diagnosis arthrography, MRI scanning or arthroscopy may be helpful.

BOX 16-7 CAUSES OF DRUJ PAIN

- Malunion of the distal radius
    - Radial shortening leading to ulnar carpal impingement
    - Dorsal tilt leading to malalignment of the DRUJ
    - Incongruence of the sigmoid notch
    - Distal radioulnar joint instability
- Ulnar styloid nonunion
- Posttraumatic osteoarthritis
- TFCC tears
- Extensor carpi ulnaris tenosynovitis

- For isolated tears of the TFCC, several methods of treatment have been suggested.
- Proponents of nonoperative treatment have shown that the natural history of the acute TFCC tear without DRUJ instability is good. Positive results have also been obtained from open or arthroscopic debridement or repair with or without ulnar shortening in the presence of volar plus deformity.
- Where the TFCC disruption is associated with instability of the DRUJ, operative repair (either arthroscopic or open) is indicated.
- When instability is associated with a fracture of the base of the ulnar styloid, the TFCC is likely to remain attached to the ulnar styloid fragment.
- Operative stabilization of the fracture, usually with K-wires, tension banding, or intraosseous suturing, is then required.
- If the DRUJ remains unstable, transfixion of the ulna to the radius is necessary.

DISTAL RADIOULNAR JOINT PAIN

- DRUJ pain is recognized commonly after distal radial fracture and occasionally following injury without fracture.
- Possible causes are listed in Box 16-7.
- Treatment may be nonoperative with immobilization and intra-articular injections of anti-inflammatory agents.
- Surgical treatment is either directed at a specific identified problem or is by radial osteotomy to realign the distal radioulnar joint in cases of malunion.

SUGGESTED READING

Fernandez DL, Jupiter JB. Fractures of the distal radius. A practical approach to management. New York: Springer-Verlag, 1996.

McQueen MM. Redisplaced fractures of the distal radius. A randomised prospective study of bridging versus non-bridging external fixation. J Bone Joint Surg (Br) 1998;80;665–669.

McQueen MM, Hajducka C, Court-Brown CM. Unstable fractures of the distal radius. A randomised prospective study of four treatment methods. J Bone Joint Surg (Br) 1996;78:404–409.

Ring D, Jupiter JB. Percutaneous and limited open fixation of fractures of the distal radius. Clin Orthop 2000;375:105–115.

Ruch DS, Weiland AJ, Wolfe SW, et al. Current concepts in the treatment of distal radial fractures. Instr Course Lect 2004; 53: 389–401.

HAND FRACTURES AND DISLOCATIONS

17.1 Carpal Injuries

17.2 Metacarpal Injuries

17.3 Phalangeal Injuries

17.4 Finger Dislocations

Hand fractures are very common, although comparatively few studies of their treatment have been done. The exception is the scaphoid fracture, which has been the subject of considerable interest because of its frequency and the comparatively high rate of nonunion associated with traditional nonoperative treatment. Metacarpal and phalangeal fractures are routinely seen in outpatient fracture clinics, but surgeons frequently find them difficult to treat. The recent introduction of mini fragment plates and headless screws has expanded the scope of surgical treatment, but traumatic hand surgery is difficult, and the literature remains unclear about indications and results of surgical management. More sophisticated imaging techniques have improved our understanding of carpal instability, but many surgeons still find the concepts of carpal instability confusing, which leads to difficulties in treatment. Some of the current controversies related to fractures of the hand are listed in Box 17-1.

ANATOMY

Carpus

The carpus is a complex arrangement of bones, joints, and ligaments. There are two carpal rows: the proximal containing the lunate, triquetrum and pisiform, and the distal row comprising the hamate, capitate, trapezoid, and trapezium (Fig. 17-1). The scaphoid acts as a link between the two rows and is oriented at approximately 45 degrees to each.

The *scaphoid* has been described as a small tubular bone that has been twisted into an S shape. It lies within the radiocarpal joint with over three quarters of its surface covered by articular cartilage. It is concave on its

ulnar side where it articulates with the capitate. It articulates with the lunate medially and the radius laterally and distally with the trapezium and trapezoid. The middle third of the scaphoid narrows to form a waist. The distal third expands to form the tubercle of the scaphoid on its volar surface.

The blood supply of the scaphoid enters through soft tissue attachments. Approximately 80% of the scaphoid is supplied by vessels that enter along the spiral groove or ridge in the middle third of the scaphoid. The distal 20% is supplied by vessels entering the tubercle and distal pole. Thus the blood supply of the proximal pole is retrograde and may be endangered by a fracture.

The *lunate*, or semilunar bone, as its name suggests, is half-moon shaped. It carries a proximal facet for the radius, which extends further on the dorsal than on the palmar surface. On each side are facets for the adjoining scaphoid

---

BOX 17-1 CURRENT CONTROVERSIES IN HAND FRACTURES

- Which type of cast should be used for scaphoid fractures?
- How reliable are clinical signs in diagnosing scaphoid fractures?
- Which scaphoid fractures should be fixed primarily?
- What is the best technique?
- How should scapholunate dissociation be treated?
- What angulation is acceptable in metacarpal neck fractures?
- Which metacarpal fractures need surgical treatment?
- How should phalangeal fractures be treated?
- How should fracture-dislocations of the proximal interphalangeal joint be treated?

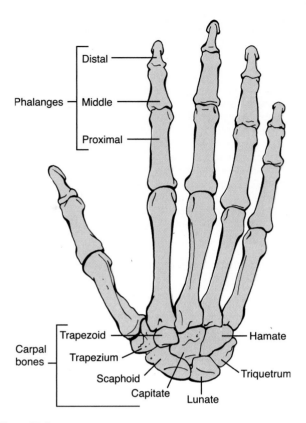

Figure 17-1 The osteology of the hand.

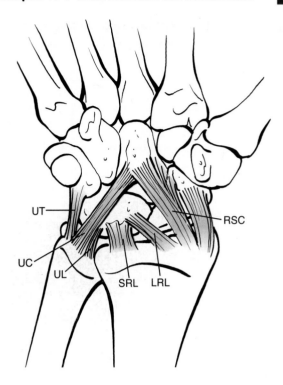

Figure 17-2 The palmar extrinsic ligaments. UT, ulnotriquetral ligament. UC, Ulnocapitate ligament. UL, Ulnolunate ligament. SRL, Short radiolunate ligament. LRL, Long radiolunate ligament. RSC, Radioscaphocapitate ligament.

and triquetrum, which are continuous distally with the articular facet for the capitate.

The *triquetrum* articulates with the lunate laterally and the hamate distally through concavities on each surface. There is also an articular facet on the palmar side for the pisiform.

The *trapezium* articulates with the adjacent *trapezoid,* and together they cover the distal articular surface of the scaphoid. There is a distal saddle-shaped facet for the separate synovial joint with the thumb metacarpal. The trapezoid articulates with the second metacarpal with a small contribution to this joint from the trapezium.

The *capitate* is the largest carpal bone. It has a convex proximal articular surface that fits the concavity of the lunate and a distal articulation with the base of the third metacarpal and a small proportion of the fourth metacarpal.

The *hamate* articulates proximally with the triquetrum and distally with the bases of the fourth and fifth metacarpals. On its palmar surface it has a hooklike flange that overhangs the carpus and to which the flexor retinaculum is attached.

The stability of the scaphoid and carpus depends on a complex combination of extrinsic and intrinsic ligaments. The most important palmar extrinsic ligaments are illustrated in Figure 17-2. The ulnocarpal and radiocarpal ligaments form the arcuate ligament complex, proximal to the apex of which is a relatively weak area of the capsule termed the space of Poirier. It is through this

area that the midcarpal joint dislocates in a perilunate dislocation.

When seen through an open approach to the volar aspect of the wrist, the palmar extrinsic ligaments appear to be a single sheet of capsule, but they can be individually identified arthroscopically. The ligaments and their functions are described in Table 17-1.

The role of the dorsal ligaments has been increasingly appreciated in recent years. The interosseous ligaments play a key part in carpal stability: disruption of the scapholunate ligament causes scapholunate dissociation and abnormal carpal motion, and disruption of the lunatotriquetral ligament contributes to a volar intercalated segment instability (VISI). Interosseous ligaments are also present in the distal carpal row, and along with the congruous articular surfaces they form a single functioning unit.

Metacarpals

The metacarpals have expanded bases (see Fig. 17-1) by which they articulate with the distal carpal row and with each other, excepting the thumb metacarpal, which has a saddle-shaped facet for the trapezium. The heads have rounded articular facets that extend further on the flexor than the extensor surfaces. The second to fifth metacarpals together form a concavity for the palm and are joined by the deep transverse ligament of the palm. The first metacarpal shaft is at right angles to the plane of the other four with its flexor surface facing across the palm.

TABLE 17-1 CARPAL LIGAMENTS AND THEIR FUNCTIONS

	Ligament	Function
Palmar radiocarpal	Radioscaphocapitate (RSC)	Fulcrum for scaphoid flexion
	Radiolunate (long LRL, short SRL)	Acts as "labrum" on distal radius
		Supports proximal pole of scaphoid
		Prevents ulnar translation of carpus
	Radioscapholunate (RSL)	Conduit for vessels and nerves
		Developmental remnant
Palmar ulnocarpal	Ulnolunate (UL)	Stabilization of ulnocarpal and DRUJ
	Ulnotriquetral (UT)	Stabilization of ulnocarpal and DRUJ
	Ulnocapitate (UC)	Stabilization of ulnocarpal and DRUJ
Palmar midcarpal	Scaphotrapeziotrapezoid	Stabilizers of scaphoid, triquetrum,
	Scaphocapitate (SC)	and midcarpal joint
	Triquetrocapitate (TC)	
	Triquetrohamate (TH)	
Dorsal	Dorsal radiocarpal (DRC)	Controls ulnar translation, stabilizes lunate
	Dorsal intercarpal (DIC) (triquetrum to scaphoid waist)	Stabilizes scaphoid
	Dorsal scaphotriquetral (DST)	Supports capitate head
Interosseous (intrinsic)	Scapholunate (SL)	Dorsal limits scapholunate translation
	Lunatotriquetral (LT)	Palmar limits scaphoid rotation
		Dorsal limits LT rotation
		Palmar limits LT translation

The metacarpophalangeal joints are stabilized by collateral ligaments that run from the sides of the metacarpal heads to the sides of the bases of the proximal phalanges and by the volar plates, which are thick plates of fibrocartilage that prevent hyperextension.

Phalanges

There are two phalanges in the thumb and three in each of the other digits. Each of the five proximal phalanges has a concave facet on its base with which it articulates with the convex metacarpal head. The proximal and distal interphalangeal joints are very similar, with the base of the middle and distal phalanges split into two concavities with a central ridge dividing them. These articulate with the trochlear-shaped ends of the proximal and middle phalanges, which extend onto the flexor but not the extensor surfaces. The interphalangeal joints are stabilized by collateral ligaments palmar or volar plates similar to those in the metacarpophalangeal joints. The distal phalanges expand distally to form the ungual tuberosities.

TABLE 17-2 TENDON ATTACHMENTS IN THE HAND

Tendon	Attachment
Flexor carpi radialis	Second and third metacarpal bases
Flexor carpi ulnaris	Pisiform, pisohamate, and pisometacarpal ligaments
Flexor digitorum profundus	Base distal phalanges
Flexor digitorum superficialis	Base middle phalanges
Flexor pollicis longus	Base terminal phalanx of thumb
Extensor carpi ulnaris	Base fifth metacarpal
Extensor carpi radialis brevis	Base middle metacarpal
Extensor carpi radialis longus	Base index metacarpal
Extensor digitorum	Central slip base of middle phalanx, lateral slip base of distal phalanx
Interossei, lumbricals, extensor indicis, extensor digiti minim	Extensor expansion
Abductor pollicis longus	Base thumb metacarpal
Extensor pollicis brevis	Base proximal phalanx thumb
Extensor pollicis longus	Base terminal phalanx thumb

TABLE 17-3 INTRINSIC MUSCLES IN THE HAND

Muscle Group	Muscles	Origin	Attachment
Thenar	Abductor pollicis brevis	Flexor retinaculum	Base proximal phalanx
	Opponens pollicis	Flexor retinaculum	Radial border thumb metacarpal
	Flexor pollicis brevis	Flexor retinaculum	Base proximal phalanx
Adductor pollicis	Adductor pollicis	Shaft middle metacarpal, bases second and third metacarpals, capitate	Base proximal phalanx of thumb
Hypothenar	Flexor digiti minimi	Flexor retinaculum, hook of hamate	Base proximal phalanx
	Opponens digiti minimi	Flexor retinaculum, hook of hamate	Shaft fifth metacarpal
	Abductor digiti minimi	Flexor retinaculum, pisiform	Base proximal phalanx
Interossei	Palmar	Flexor surface of own metacarpal	Extensor expansion
	Dorsal	Flexor/dorsal surface of adjacent metacarpals	Extensor expansion
Lumbricals	Lumbricals	Profundus tendons	Extensor expansion

Muscles and Tendons

The tendons in the hand are those of the forearm muscles. Their attachments are listed in Table 17-2. All the muscles in the hand are intrinsic to the hand. Their origins and attachments are listed in Table 17-3.

Nerves

The *median nerve* enters the hand through the carpal tunnel deep to the flexor retinaculum. Just proximal to this it gives off a palmar branch, which supplies the skin over the thenar eminence. It then divides into three branches. The medial branch divides into two common digital nerves and supplies the adjacent sides of the ring and middle fingers, the adjacent sides of the index and middle fingers, and the second lumbrical muscle. The lateral branch supplies the digital nerves to the radial surface of the index finger, the whole of the thumb, and a branch to the first lumbrical. The motor branch is given off just distal to the flexor retinaculum and supplies the thenar muscles.

The *ulnar nerve* enters the hand superficial to the flexor retinaculum. Just proximal to this it gives off a dorsal branch, which supplies sensation to the ulnar side of the dorsum of the hand. At the radial border of the pisiform, it divides into superficial and deep branches. The superficial branch becomes the digital nerves to the ulnar one and a half fingers. The deep branch passes between the origins of flexor and abductor digiti minimi where it enters Guyon's canal lying on the hook of the hamate and passing between the base of the fifth metacarpal and the origin of opponens digiti minimi. It then supplies branches from a deep palmar arch to the hypothenar muscles, the two ulnar lumbricals, the interossei, and adductor pollicis.

The *radial nerve* has no motor function in the hand. Its terminal branch emerges from deep to the brachioradialis tendon a few centimeters proximal to the radial styloid and then splits into several branches that cross the roof of the anatomical snuffbox and supply the sensation to the dorsum of the hand on its radial side.

EPIDEMIOLOGY

Hand fractures are relatively common. Their epidemiology, described in Table 17-4, shows they make up about 24% of all fractures. They are more common in men, and metacarpal and phalangeal fractures are more common than carpal fractures.

TABLE 17-4 EPIDEMIOLOGY OF HAND FRACTURES

Proportion of all fractures	24%
Average age	32.8 y
Men/women	77%/23%
Incidence	$267/10^5/y$
Fracture types	
Carpus	11.1%
Metacarpus	48.7%
Phalanges	40.1%

17.1 CARPAL INJURIES

The prevalence of the different carpal fractures is shown in Table 17.1-1. This shows that over 80% of carpal fractures involve the scaphoid, with the triquetrum the next most affected bone. Fractures of the lunate, hamate, trapezium, capitate, and pisiform comprise less than 9% of carpal fractures.

Most carpal fractures are isolated injuries, although damage to the intercarpal ligaments may occur. About 11% of patients have other musculoskeletal injuries, most of which are in the ipsilateral arm. The majority are fractures of the distal radius or proximal forearm.

SCAPHOID FRACTURES

EPIDEMIOLOGY

The epidemiology of scaphoid fractures is shown in Table 17.1-2. They have a type B (see Chapter 1) distribution tending to occur most frequently in young men. They usually occur following simple falls or sports injuries.

CLASSIFICATION

Scaphoid fractures are generally described depending on their position in the scaphoid (tubercle, distal, waist, proximal pole) and by the presence or absence of displacement or comminution.

Herbert's classification system is the only systematic classification system in common use (Table 17.1-3). There are four types with types A and B pertaining to acute fractures (Fig. 17.1-1).

This classification is based on stability but makes little allowance for comminution, which has a significant effect on the stability of the fracture. Displacement should also be considered, although this may be difficult to assess on plain radiographs.

DIAGNOSIS

History and Physical Examination

- The history of a scaphoid fracture is usually pain on the radial side of the wrist or at the base of the thumb after a fall, often during a sporting activity.
- The typical patient is a young man.
- The diagnosis of scaphoid fracture can be difficult even in experienced hands because of the failure of X-rays to demonstrate all fractures.
- Accurate clinical examination remains an important adjunct in order to identify those patients with possible occult fractures.
- Swelling and tenderness in the anatomical snuffbox should be sought, with the cardinal sign considered anatomical snuffbox tenderness.
  - Although highly sensitive, this sign has low specificity (i.e., a large number of false positives).
- This also applies to tenderness over the scaphoid tubercle and pain on longitudinal compression of the thumb.
- The scaphoid shift test is described in the section in this chapter on carpal instability.
- Although described for the diagnosis of carpal ligamentous injuries, it can be used for the diagnosis of occult scaphoid fractures.
- It can be seen from Table 17.1-4 that no single clinical sign has high sensitivity and specificity.
- When anatomical snuffbox tenderness, tubercle tenderness, and pain on longitudinal compression are all present on initial examination, however, the sensitivity is 100% and the specificity rises to 74%, with a positive predictive value of 58% and a negative predictive value of 100%.

Radiologic Examination

- Because of the low specificity of clinical signs, accurate radiologic diagnosis is essential to reduce either misdiagnosis or overdiagnosis and unnecessary treatment.

TABLE 17.1-1 PREVALENCE OF FRACTURES IN THE DIFFERENT CARPAL BONES

Carpal Bone	%
Scaphoid	82.4
Triquetrum	8.8
Lunate	3.1
Hamate	2.5
Trapezium	1.9
Capitate	0.6
Pisiform	0.6

TABLE 17.1-2 EPIDEMIOLOGY OF SCAPHOID FRACTURES

Proportion of all fractures	2.2%
Proportion of hand injuries	9.2%
Average age	30.1 y
Men/women	72%/28%
Incidence	24.5/10^5/y
Distribution	Type B
Open fractures	0%
Most common causes	
Fall	38.9%
Sport	25.2%
Assault	11.4%

TABLE 17.1-3 CLASSIFICATION OF SCAPHOID FRACTURES

Type	Description
A	Stable acute fractures
	■ Fracture appears incomplete (only one cortex involved)
	■ Union usually rapid
	■ Minimal treatment
A1	Tubercle fracture
A2	Incomplete fracture through the waist of the scaphoid
B	Unstable acute fractures
	■ Likely to displace in plaster
	■ Delayed union common
	■ Internal fixation
B1	Distal oblique fracture
B2	Complete waist fracture
B3	Proximal pole fracture
B4	Transscaphoid perilunate dislocation
B5	Comminuted fracture
C	Delayed union
	■ Widening of fracture line
	■ Cysts adjacent to fracture
	■ Relative density of the proximal fragment
D	Established nonunion
D1	Fibrous nonunion
D2	Pseudarthrosis

■ There are usually four standard radiologic views (Fig. 17.1-2):
- ■ Posteroanterior view with the wrist in full ulnar deviation
- ■ Posteroanterior view with the wrist in full radial deviation
- ■ 45-degree oblique view
- ■ Lateral view with the wrist in the neutral position

■ Some authorities recommend the same views in the uninjured wrist, which allows detection of shortening in the scaphoid and radial deviation implying instability.

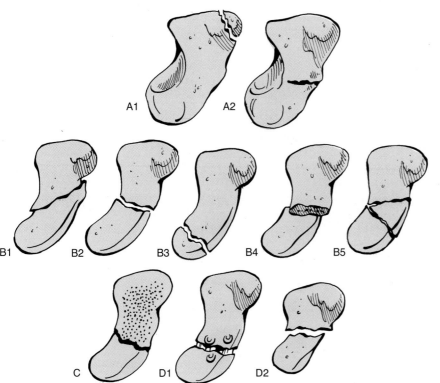

Figure 17.1-1 The Herbert classification of scaphoid fractures. See Table 17.1-3.

TABLE 17.1-4 RELIABILITY OF THE CLINICAL SIGNS OF SCAPHOID FRACTURE

Clinical sign	Sensitivity (%)	Positive predictive value (%)	Specificity (%)	Negative predictive value (%)
Anatomical snuffbox tenderness (ASB)	100	30	19	100
Scaphoid tubercle tenderness	100	34	30	100
Longitudinal compression	100	40	48	100
Reduced range of movement in thumb	66	41	66	85
Swelling in ASB	61	50	52	58
Pain in ASB on ulnar deviation/pronation	83	44	17	56
Pain in ASB on radial deviation/pronation	70	45	31	56
Pain on thumb/index pinch	48	44	31	41
Scaphoid shift test	66	49	31	69

- The 45-degree oblique view is used to increase the detection of a fracture.
- The lateral view is to assess the alignment of the carpus: The distal articular surface of the lunate should be roughly perpendicular to the long axis of the capitate and the radius.
- Dorsiflexion of the lunate implies severe carpal instability and a flexion deformity of the scaphoid (see Fig. 17.1-2), indicating a dorsal intercalated segment instability (DISI) pattern.
- The scaphoid is difficult to define on the lateral film, but when seen its long axis should be approximately 45 degrees to the long axis of the lunate.
  - Reduction of this angle also implies carpal instability.
- A further posteroanterior view of the wrist with the beam tilted by 20 degrees toward the elbow is useful to detect a scaphoid waist fracture (Fig. 17.1-3).
- Scaphoid fractures can be difficult to detect with plain films even when special projections are included.
  - This is demonstrated by the prevalence of false-negative examinations, which can be up to 14%.

- Thus repeated radiographs in patients with persisting symptoms and signs of scaphoid fracture are recommended at around 2 weeks after injury. This is usually sufficient to make a diagnosis.
- If uncertainty remains, consider further investigation, which may take the form of ultrasound, bone scan, MRI, or CT scanning.
  - Ultrasound has the benefit of being relatively inexpensive and noninvasive. Sensitivity rates vary from 50% to 78%, although specificity is usually around 90%. This may be related to the experience of the ultrasonographer.
  - Bone scans and MRI and CT scans have similar detection rates, although MRI scanning may have an advantage in detecting other occult carpal injuries.
  - Radiographs are an unreliable method of assessing the amount of displacement or union of a scaphoid fracture. The appearances of both are very dependent on the orientation of the X-ray.
  - Displacement is probably best assessed by CT scanning.

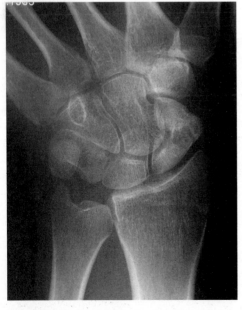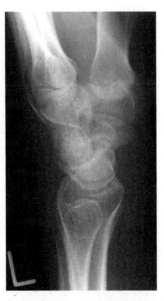

Figure 17.1-2   The standard radiologic views of the scaphoid. There is dorsiflexion of the lunate with a DISI deformity.

- Union is best assessed by monitoring the size of the gap at the fracture site by plain radiographs or MRI or CT scanning.
  - Although the presence of a gap, especially if it is increasing, is suggestive of nonunion, the possibility of a partial union should be considered.
- Avascular necrosis can occur in the proximal fragment of the scaphoid after fracture and is diagnosed from plain radiographs in the presence of the loss of normal trabeculation, cystic change, and deformity of the proximal fragment.
  - This should be distinguished from bone ischemia, which causes increased density of the proximal pole without collapse and implies the possibility of recovery by revascularization.

TREATMENT

Fractures of the Scaphoid Waist

- Fractures of the waist of the scaphoid are the most common scaphoid fractures and may be managed with or without surgery.

Nonsurgical Treatment

- Management in a plaster cast remains the mainstay of the treatment of acute scaphoid waist fractures.
- Debate centers around the type of cast used, with some authorities recommending long arm thumb spicas, some recommending short arm thumb spicas, and some recommending a short forearm cast not including the thumb.
  - There is little indication for long arm casts in scaphoid fractures.
  - One study did show an advantage in terms of healing times in long arm casts but was not blinded and no functional results were presented.
  - A further randomized study showed no benefit in including the thumb.

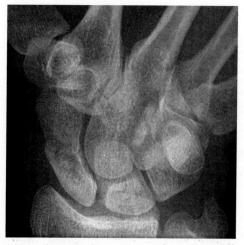

Figure 17.1-3 A 20-degree tilted anteroposterior view of the scaphoid.

- Wrist flexion and ulnar deviation have been advocated in order to close any gap in the scaphoid.
- Plaster treatment is usually required for 8 weeks but may be more prolonged with delayed union.
- The morbidity of plaster cast management is low, although functional results are poorly reported.
- Nonunion rates can be high, and improvements in treatment will come from addressing this problem.

Surgical Treatment

- Earlier attempts at operative stabilization of acute scaphoid fractures used open methods, but with the introduction of headless cannulated screws designed specifically for scaphoid fixation, closed fixation is becoming more popular.
  - This can be achieved either retrograde from the scaphoid tubercle (Fig. 17.1-4) or antegrade with an entry point in the distal pole.

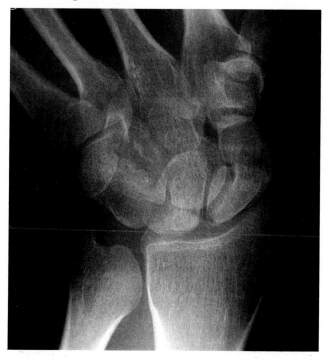

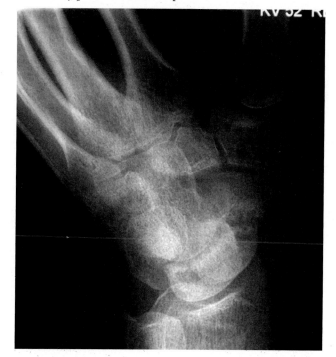

Figure 17.1-2 (continued)

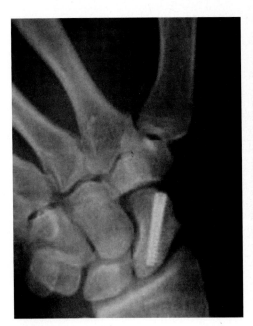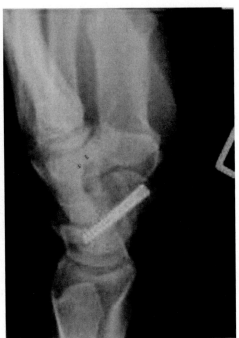

Figure 17.1-4 A scaphoid series showing the use of an Acutrak screw.

■ Careful intraoperative assessment of guide wire and screw positioning and screw length is essential with this technique to avoid unwanted screw protrusion.

■ There is also evidence that the more central the screw in the scaphoid, the higher the chance of successful union.

■ There have been a number of studies of undisplaced scaphoid fractures, indicating that operative stabilization, especially if closed, allows earlier return to work and sporting activities probably because this technique abolishes the need for prolonged cast immobilization.

■ Nonunion rates may be lower, but this has not yet been proven in undisplaced fractures.

■ It is accepted that unstable fractures with displacement or comminution require fixation.

■ The morbidity of early fixation of scaphoid waist fractures is low. Infection rates are extremely low.

■ Osteoarthrosis of the scaphotrapezial joint has been noted radiologically on longer follow-up, but this is generally asymptomatic.

■ The outcome of operative treatment of scaphoid waist fractures is shown in Table 17.1-5.

Fractures of the Scaphoid Proximal Pole

■ Fractures of the proximal pole of the scaphoid are a special situation because of the vascular supply of the scaphoid.

TABLE 17.1-5 RESULTS OF THE TREATMENT OF SCAPHOID WAIST AND PROXIMAL POLE FRACTURES

Result/Complication	Nonoperative		CRIF		ORIF	
	Range	Average	Range	Average	Range	Average
Waist fractures						
Good/excellent	92–97	95	87–92	90	91–100	95
Nonunion	5–15	8	0–8	4	0–11	3
Avascular necrosis	10–17	13	<1	<1	3–7	5
Proximal pole fractures[a]						
Good/excellent	N/A	N/A	N/A	N/A	75	75
Nonunion	18–67	40	N/A	N/A	0–8	4
Avascular necrosis	40	40	N/A	N/A	4–8	6

[a]Series based on small numbers.

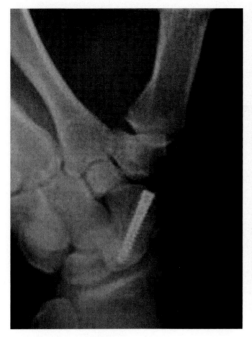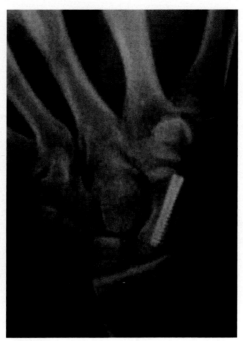

Figure 17.1-4 *(continued)*

- Fracture at this level often disturbs the blood supply of the proximal pole, making these fractures at high risk of nonunion and avascular necrosis (see Table 17.1-5).
- Because the proximal pole is small with few soft tissue attachments, these fractures are usually unstable.
    - For these reasons and because conservative management even when successful requires prolonged immobilization, most authorities recommend early internal fixation and bone grafting of proximal pole fractures.
- In most cases an antegrade screw is inserted from the proximal to the distal pole to ensure good fixation.
- The results of treatment of proximal pole fractures of the scaphoid where available from the literature are detailed in Table 17.1-5.

Fractures of the Scaphoid Distal Pole

- Tubercle fracture of the scaphoid is the most common to occur in the distal pole.
    - These are avulsion fractures and most easily seen on a semipronated view.
- Because of the excellent vascularity in this area, these usually heal with 3 to 4 weeks of immobilization in a cast.
- Rare cases of nonunion can be treated by excision.
- Body fractures in the distal third are rare but usually heal with 6 to 8 weeks of immobilization in a cast.

Suggested Treatment

- The management of scaphoid fractures is summarized in Table 17.1-6.

TABLE 17.1-6 SUGGESTED TREATMENT OF SCAPHOID AND CARPAL FRACTURES AND DISLOCATIONS

Injury Location	Treatment
Scaphoid	
Type A	Scaphoid or forearm cast for 6–8 wk
Type B	Primary percutaneous screw fixation
Proximal pole	Antegrade screw +/− bone graft
Other fractures	Retrograde screw
Type C	ORIF +/− bone graft
Type D	ORIF + bone graft
Other carpal fractures	
Undisplaced	Scaphoid or forearm cast for 3–4 wk
Displaced	Internal fixation
With intercarpal dislocation	Internal fixation and ligamentous repair
Carpal dislocations	
Perilunate	Ligamentous repair + intercarpal fixation
Scapholunate	
Stable	Forearm cast for 4–6 wk
Unstable	Ligamentous repair + intercarpal fixation
Lunatotriquetral	Forearm cast for 4–6 wk
Midcarpal instability	Forearm cast for 4–6 wk

Scaphoid Nonunion

■ The management of scaphoid nonunion is discussed in Chapter 39.

NONSCAPHOID CARPAL FRACTURES

EPIDEMIOLOGY

The epidemiology of the nonscaphoid carpal fractures is shown in Table 17.1-7. These fractures are unusual and shown a different epidemiological pattern from scaphoid fractures (see Table 17.1-2). They have a type A distribution (see Chapter 1) affecting younger men and older women. This is reflected in the higher average age. Most are caused by simple falls.

DIAGNOSIS AND TREATMENT

Triquetrum

■ Fractures of the triquetrum are the second most common carpal fracture after the scaphoid.
■ Isolated fractures of the triquetrum are usually seen as a flake fracture from the dorsal aspect of the triquetrum on a lateral radiograph (Fig. 17.1-5).
■ These fractures may be caused by impingement of the ulnar styloid on the triquetrum in forced dorsiflexion and ulnar deviation.
■ Closed treatment in a cast or splint for 2 to 3 weeks is required until acute symptoms settle.
■ Fracture of the triquetral body is much more serious, usually occurring in association with a perilunate dislocation.
■ In these circumstances internal fixation is usually indicated.

Lunate

■ Lunate fractures may involve the volar pole, body, or margins of the bone.
■ They are often high-energy injuries and require a high degree of suspicion because they may be associated with carpal dislocation or subluxation (Fig. 17.1-6).

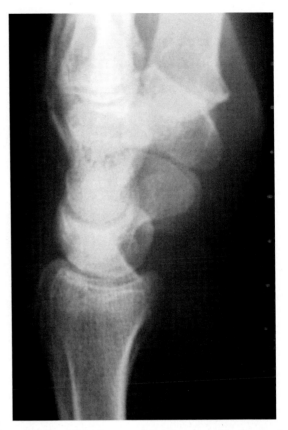

Figure 17.1-5   A flake fracture of the triquetrum. The fracture is seen on the dorsum of the bone.

■ Changes on plain radiographs may be subtle, and CT scanning is often required.
■ Displacement of the fracture or carpal disruption are indications for surgery.

TABLE 17.1-7 EPIDEMIOLOGY OF NONSCAPHOID CARPAL FRACTURES	
Proportion of all fractures	0.5%
Proportion of hand injuries	2.0%
Average age	46.7 y
Men/women	71%/29%
Incidence	5.2/10^5/y
Distribution	Type A
Open fractures	0%
Most common causes	
Fall	60.7%
Sport	21.4%

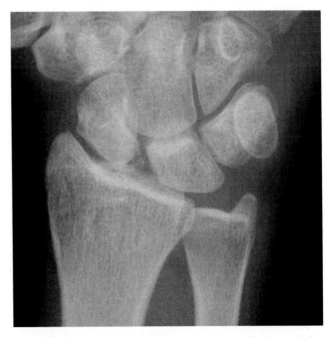

Figure 17.1-6   A marginal lunate fracture associated with scapholunate dissociation.

Hamate

- Fractures of the hook of the hamate are frequently missed.
- They should be suspected if there is tenderness in the ulnar side of the palm of the hand after injury.
- Ulnar nerve symptoms may be present from damage to the nerve, which is contained in Guyon's canal at this point.
- Radiographs are often inconclusive but should include a carpal tunnel view. CT scanning may be necessary to make the diagnosis.
- Treatment is generally by cast immobilization unless there is a large displaced fragment, which may require internal fixation.
- The most common complication is nonunion, which may be treated by excision.
- Fractures of the body of the hamate are very rare and may be associated with fracture dislocation of the fourth and fifth carpometacarpal joints.
- Internal fixation is only required for significant displacement.

Trapezium

- The more common fracture of the trapezium is a body fracture, which is seen either as a vertical line (Fig. 17.1-7) or as a comminuted area.
  - The cause is usually an axial load on the thumb.
- Trapezial fractures may be associated with dislocation of the carpometacarpal joint of the thumb.

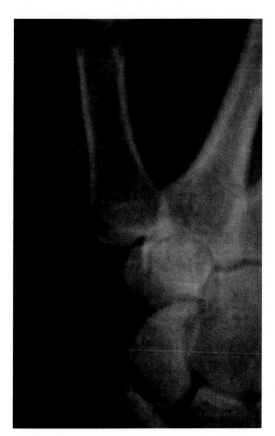

Figure 17.1-7   A vertical fracture of the body of the trapezium.

- Internal fixation is required for displacement.
- Trapezial ridge fractures are similar to hamate hook fractures and may occur with avulsion of the attachment on the flexor retinaculum.
  - They are usually treated nonoperatively but may require excision for nonunion.

Capitate

- Fracture of the capitate may be isolated or in association with a more complex injury to the carpus.
  - One such is the naviculocapitate syndrome when the capitate head may be rotated through 180 degrees.
- If a capitate fracture is suspected, CT scanning may be required to make a definitive diagnosis.
- Cast treatment is adequate for undisplaced fractures.
- Internal fixation with wires, headless screws, or plates is required in cases of displacement.
- Complications include nonunion, avascular necrosis of the capitate head, and posttraumatic arthritis.

Pisiform

- Pisiform fracture is suggested by a history of a direct blow to the ulnar side of the hand and local pain and tenderness.
  - Ulnar nerve symptoms may be present.
- Carpal tunnel views or CT scanning may be required in addition to the normal carpal series of radiographs to make the diagnosis.
- Nonoperative management is recommended unless symptomatic nonunion ensues when excision is usually effective.

Trapezoid

- The trapezoid acts as a keystone of the carpal arch and is held by tight ligamentous connections.
  - Fracture is therefore very rare.
- CT scanning will usually detect the injury.
- Cast management is normally required for 3 to 4 weeks except in the extremely rare cases of displacement when surgery is necessary.

Suggested Treatment

- The management of other carpal fractures is summarized in Table 17.1-6.

ACUTE CARPAL LIGAMENT INJURY

CLASSIFICATION

There are a number of ways of classifying acute carpal ligament injury. Three of those are shown in Table 17.1-8. Instability may also be adaptive secondary to malalignment outside the

TABLE 17.1-8 CLASSIFICATIONS OF CARPAL INSTABILITY

Classification	Types	Description
Linscheid	Dorsal intercalated segment instability (DISI)	Lunate extended (>15 degrees capitolunate, >60 degrees scapholunate)
		Dorsal subluxation of capitate
	Volar intercalated segment instability (VISI)	Lunate flexed (>30 capitolunate, < 30 degrees scapholunate
Taleisnik	Static	Standard X-rays show malalignment of carpus
	Dynamic	Abnormal alignment only when carpus is stressed
Dissociative/nondissociative	Dissociative	Disruption of normal kinematics within a carpal row
	Nondissociative	Disruption between carpal rows

carpus such as in distal radius malunion. There may also be complex combinations of different types of instability.

Mayfield described four stages of ligament disruption in progressive perilunate instability (Table 17.1-9). Fractures associated with perilunate dislocation may result in transscaphoid, transcapitate, or transtriquetral perilunate dislocation. These are described as greater arc injuries, in contrast to lesser arc injuries, which only involve ligamentous structures (Fig. 17.1-8).

DIAGNOSIS

History and Physical Examination

■ In most cases a history of trauma is obtained and may range from low- to high-energy fracture.
■ In acute high-energy injury, there is usually clear evidence of clinical abnormality: deformity, gross swelling, and bruising.
■ A careful neurological examination is necessary because carpal tunnel syndrome is a common complication of carpal injury.
■ In less severe injury there may be symptoms of pain on movement or a popping feeling in the wrist.
■ Palpation to elicit tenderness may be helpful in localizing the pathology.

TABLE 17.1-9 MAYFIELD'S STAGES OF PERILUNATE INSTABILITY

Stage	Malalignment
I	Scaphoid rotation
	Scapholunate dissociation
II	Dislocation of the capitate
	Capitolunate dissociation
III	Lunatotriquetral dissociation
IV	Complete lunate dislocation

■ There are a number of specific tests for ligamentous disruption in the carpus (Table 17.1-10).
　■ All of these tests must be interpreted with care because there are a number of false-positive and false-negative results.
■ The opposite wrist must also be tested because there is a range of ligamentous laxity in normal individuals.

Radiologic Examination

■ Radiographic examination should consist of a minimum of three views: posteroanterior, lateral, and a 45-degree pronated oblique view.

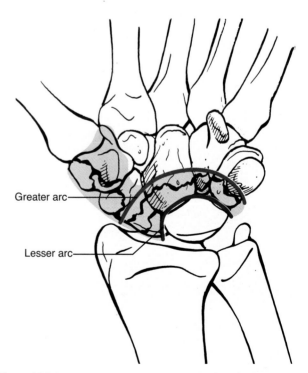

Greater arc
Lesser arc

Figure 17.1-8   Greater and lesser arc injuries. Greater arc injuries include bony disruption. Lesser arc injuries are ligamentous.

TABLE 17.1-10 TESTS FOR LIGAMENTOUS DISRUPTION IN THE CARPUS

Test	Description	Positive Finding	Diagnosis
Scaphoid shift test	Pressure is placed on the scaphoid tubercle while the wrist is brought from radial to ulnar deviation	"Clunk" as the scaphoid subluxes dorsally out of the scaphoid fossa.	Scapholunate disruption
Midcarpal shuck test	Pressure is placed on the dorsum of the capitate as the wrist is moved from radial to ulnar deviation	"Clunk" as the lunate reduces from the palmar flexed position.	Midcarpal instability
Lunatotriquetral ballottement	Lunate is fixed with thumb and index finger of one hand while the triquetrum is displaced palmarly and dorsally with the thumb of the other hand	Pain	Lunatotriquetral instability or arthritis

- The PA view should be inspected for an increased scapholunate gap suggesting scapholunate dissociation (Fig. 17.1-9).
  - Gilula's lines (Fig. 17.1-10) should be three smooth arcs; a break in any of these indicate likely carpal malalignment.

- If the lunate shape is triangular rather than quadrilateral, there may be perilunate instability.
- If the scaphoid is foreshortened with a signet ring appearance of a bicortical density, there may be scapholunate dissociation or a VISI deformity.

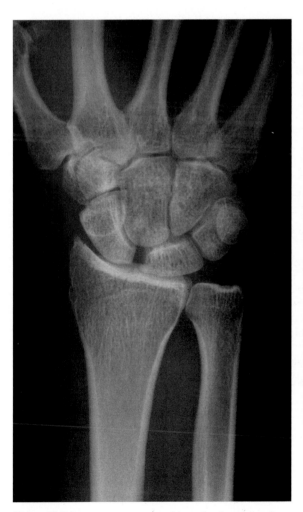
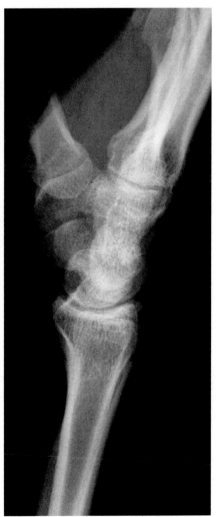

Figure 17.1-9   Anteroposterior and lateral radiographs of a scapholunate dissociation showing the characteristic gap between the scaphoid and lunate.

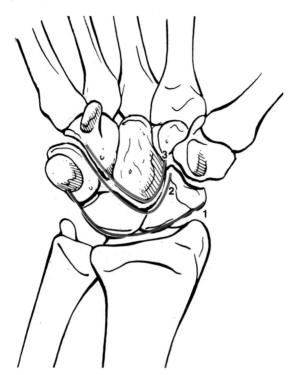

Figure 17.1-10   Gilula's lines. (1) A line around the proximal aspect of the proximal carpal row. (2) A line around the distal aspect of the proximal carpal row. (3) A line around the proximal aspect of the distal carpal row. Each line should have a smooth curve.

- The carpal height should be measured: The height from the radius to the base of the third metacarpal should be approximately half that of the third metacarpal height.
- On the lateral view, scapholunate and capitolunate angles should be inspected for possible DISI or VISI deformities (see Table 17.1-8).
- There are a number of specific instability views. The two in most common use are the clenched fist view (Fig. 17.1-11), which may demonstrate scapholunate widening in scapholunate dissociation, and a traction view to accentuate any abnormality.
- Posteroanterior and lateral views in radial and ulnar deviation may also be helpful.
- There is no consensus about the best method of diagnosing carpal ligament injuries, although a number of other investigations may be helpful (Table 17.1-11).
- With gross malalignment, standard views are sufficient.

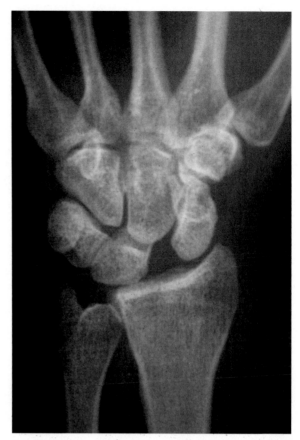

Figure 17.1-11   The clenched fist view demonstrating increased scapholunate widening.

- A combination of studies may be required in cases of more subtle injury.

DISLOCATIONS OF THE CARPUS

TREATMENT

Scapholunate Dissociation

- Treatment of scapholunate dissociation depends on whether the injury is acute or chronic, stable or unstable.
- Stable injuries with no evidence of carpal malalignment imply the ligament is intact, although it may be attenuated.

TABLE 17.1-11 RADIOLOGIC DIAGNOSIS OF CARPAL LIGAMENT INJURY

Diagnostic Modality	Positive Finding	Advantage/Disadvantage
Cineradiography	Dyssynchronous movement	False-negative rate
Arthrography	Abnormal communication between joints	Low correlation between symptoms and abnormality
CT	Presence of occult fractures	Poor for ligamentous injury
MRI	Demonstration of ligament or bone injury	Dependent on equipment and skill of radiologist
Ultrasound scan	Absence of specific ligament	Dependent on equipment and skill of radiologist
Arthroscopy	Visualization of hemorrhage, increased intercarpal gap	Dependent on skill of surgeon
		May detect clinically silent lesions
		Invasive, requires anesthetic

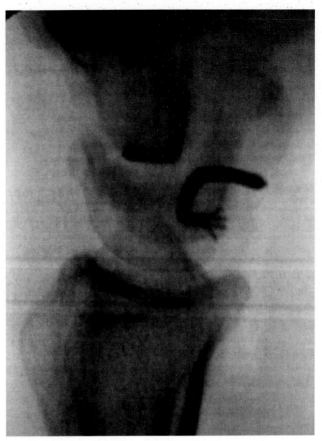

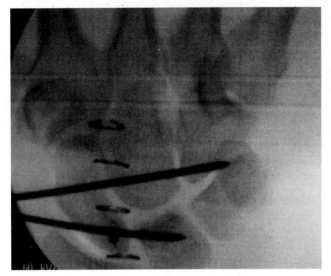

Figure 17.1-12 Anteroposterior and lateral radiographs showing reduction and K-wire fixation of a scapholunate dissociation.

- They may be treated with a short arm cast for a few weeks.
- The diagnosis must be firmly established because a missed unstable acute injury will become chronic with fewer treatment options available and a likely poorer outcome.
- In acute unstable injuries, primary repair is recommended preferably with suture anchors.
  - The repair should be supported by K-wire fixation maintaining the reduced position of the scaphoid (Fig. 17.1-12).
- Dorsal capsulodesis techniques can be used to reinforce the ligamentous repair.
  - This involves advancement of the dorsal wrist capsule to the distal pole of the scaphoid to restrict palmar flexion and dorsal shift of the scaphoid permanently.
- In chronic injuries, tendon weave techniques or localized carpal fusion may be necessary.
- Total wrist fusion is a salvage technique.

Perilunate Dislocation

- This usually, although not exclusively, occurs due to high-energy injury.
- All the ligaments attaching the lunate to the carpus are disrupted.
- The carpus lies dorsal to the lunate; the lunate may either lie in its normal position (dorsal perilunate dislocation) or is dislocated in a volar direction (lunate dislocation).
- These are unstable injuries and require surgery to ensure a good outcome.
- If closed reduction and casting alone is used, there is a high proportion (around 60%) of cases that lose the initial reduction, and clinical results rarely achieve excellence.
- If it is anticipated that surgery will be delayed, a closed reduction should be performed.
- Closed reduction is performed in dorsal perilunate dislocations by extending the wrist with some traction and applying pressure dorsally to the capitate.
- If there is a lunate dislocation, reduction should be attempted by first flexing the wrist to relax the palmar ligaments. Palmar pressure is then applied over the lunate to return it to its fossa on the radius. The wrist is then flexed to reduce the capitate.
  - If this maneuver is not successful, open reduction is indicated.
- Surgical treatment aims to restore and maintain normal carpal alignment and repair disrupted ligaments.
- Both volar (carpal tunnel) and dorsal approaches to the carpus may be necessary.
  - Kirschner wires may be used as "joy sticks" to correct rotation of the scaphoid or lunate.
- Additional K-wires or screws are required to stabilize the reduction (see Fig. 17.1-12), usually from scaphoid to lunate and triquetrum or capitate to lunate.

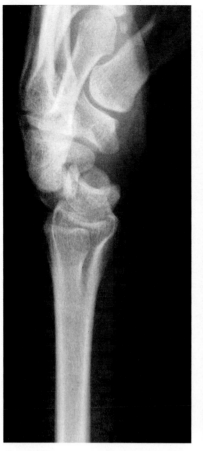
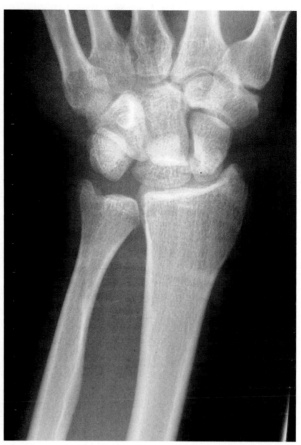

Figure 17.1-13   A transscaphoid perilunate dislocation.

■ Ligamentous repair should use suture anchors where possible.

■ Fluoroscopy should be used to confirm correct carpal reduction.

■ Should there be an associated scaphoid fracture (transscaphoid perilunate dislocation) (Fig. 17.1-13), this should be treated by internal fixation.

  ■ A volar approach with bone grafting may be required because the scaphoid is frequently comminuted.

■ Associated radial or ulnar styloid fractures if sufficiently large should also be stabilized by internal fixation because they carry important ligamentous attachments.

■ In cases with median nerve symptoms that have not resolved after closed reduction, carpal tunnel decompression is indicated.

Lunatotriquetral Dissociation

■ These are rarely recognized injuries and lead to ulnar-sided wrist pain after often minor injury.

■ The diagnosis is made by the history, the finding of point tenderness over the lunatotriquetral joint, and a positive lunatotriquetral ballottement test (see Table 17.1-10).

■ Occasionally Gilula's proximal row line (see Fig. 17.1-10) will be disrupted.

■ Treatment is usually nonoperative with pinning, ligament debridement, or localized fusion reserved for chronic symptoms.

Midcarpal Instability

■ In this condition there is a sudden extension of the proximal row of the carpus with ulnar deviation and sudden flexion with radial deviation.

■ Patients will complain of a painful clunk with ulnar deviation and pronation.

■ Treatment is usually nonoperative.

■ Soft tissue reconstruction or localized intercarpal arthrodesis can be used in refractory cases.

Suggested Treatment

■ The management of carpal dislocation is summarized in Table 17.1-6.

RESULTS AND COMPLICATIONS

The outcome of carpal dislocations and fracture dislocations is poorly documented, probably because of the rarity of these injuries. Patients should be warned that the likely outcome of successful treatment is some residual pain with restriction of the wrist flexion/extension arc and approximately 20% weakness of grip. Unsuccessful treatments may lead to posttraumatic arthritis. Other complications include nonunion or avascular necrosis with related fractures.

17.2 METACARPAL INJURIES

EPIDEMIOLOGY

Metacarpal fractures are the most common fracture affecting the hand. Their epidemiology is shown in Table 17.2-1. They have a type B (see Chapter 1) distribution predominantly occurring in young men. Open fractures are uncommon, and most fractures follow a direct blow or assault or a simple fall. About 60% of metacarpal fractures occur in the little finger.

Table 17.2-2 shows the distribution of the different types of metacarpal fractures. Basal fractures are most commonly seen in the thumb with extra-articular epibasal fractures and Bennett fracture dislocations the most common. In the other fingers, basal metacarpal fractures occur with approximately equal frequency comprising 14% to 18% of metacarpal fractures. Diaphyseal fractures are most common in the ring and middle finger metacarpals and least common in the thumb. Predictably, neck fractures of the little finger metacarpal are more common than the neck fractures of the other metacarpals. Metacarpal head fractures are most commonly seen in the index finger.

Associated Injuries

Metacarpal fractures are usually isolated injuries. About 19% of patients have other fractures, but 80% of these are in an adjacent metacarpal.

CLASSIFICATION

The classification of metacarpal fractures differentiates between the head and the neck, the diaphysis, and the base of the metacarpal. Fractures of the neck are extra-articular and vary in complexity from a simple fracture to a comminuted fracture. Fractures of the head are by definition intra-articular and separated by the plane of the fracture.

Fractures of the shaft of the metacarpal are similar to those of any long bone. They may be spiral, transverse, or oblique, with or without varying degrees of comminution from a simple wedge to a comminuted fracture.

Fracture patterns at the bases of the metacarpals are illustrated in Figures 17.2-1 and 17.2-2 and are either intra- or extra-articular with varying degrees of complexity. In the thumb metacarpal, the type B fracture is also known as Bennett's fracture. This occurs when there is an avulsion of the main part of the metacarpal from the volar ulnar part of the metacarpal base. The main part of the metacarpal including the majority of the carpometacarpal joint subluxes radially and dorsally. The three-part fracture at the base of the thumb metacarpal is known as Rolando's fracture.

DIAGNOSIS

History and Physical Examination

- The history is usually of either a punch or a fall onto the clenched fist.
- Pain and swelling is evident around the affected area.
- Metacarpal shortening can be identified by loss of prominence of a metacarpal head with the metacarpophalangeal joints flexed; this may also be a sign of apex dorsal angulation when the metacarpal head "drops."
- In this case there may also be a prominence dorsally over the fracture site, although this may be obscured by swelling.
- Radial/ulnar deviation should be assessed with the fingers in extension.
- Overlap of the digits or malrotation of the plane of the nail when viewed end on is indicative of malrotation at the fracture site.
  - This is commonly missed because it may not be evident radiologically.

Radiologic Examination

- Anteroposterior, lateral, and oblique views with the hand pronated and supinated (Fig. 17.2-3) are required to identify the site and type of the fracture and the degree of displacement.
  - The anteroposterior view (Fig. 17.2-3A) allows assessment of shortening and radial and ulnar displacement.

TABLE 17.2-1 EPIDEMIOLOGY OF METACARPAL FRACTURES

Proportion of all fractures	11.7%
Proportion of hand injuries	48.7%
Average age	29.9 y
Men/women	85%/15%
Incidence	130.3/10⁵/y
Distribution	Type B
Open fractures	1%
Most common causes	
Blow/assault	47.2%
Fall	20.5%
Sport	15.4%
Metacarpal	
Thumb	10.0%
Index	7.9%
Middle	7.2%
Ring	14.8%
Little	60.2%

TABLE 17.2-2 DISTRIBUTION OF THE TYPES OF METACARPAL FRACTURES

Fracture	Common Name	Prevalence (%)				
		Little	Ring	Middle	Index	Thumb
Base						
Epibasal (A)		9.5	13.9	8.2	7.4	
Two-part (B)	Bennett	1.7	1.0	4.1	3.6	32.3
Three-part (C)	Epibasal	4.6	0	2.0	7.4	38.2
Comminuted (D)	Rolando	0.7	0	0	0	14.7
Shaft						
Spiral/oblique		9.2	23.7	46.9	18.5	2.9
Transverse		13.9	25.7	6.1	7.4	1.5
Wedge/comminuted		3.2	0	2.0	1.9	1.5
Neck		54.0	29.7	20.4	37.0	4.4
Head		3.2	5.9	10.2	16.7	4.4

- The lateral view is the only view in which dorsal or volar angulation can be assessed (Fig. 17.2-3B).
  - It must be remembered that there is a natural concavity of the metacarpal heads that can make the fifth metacarpal head appear prominent in the palm of the hand in the lateral view.
- Oblique views are necessary if there is doubt about the diagnosis.
  - Oblique views with the forearm supinated or pronated demonstrate the second and fifth carpometacarpal joints, respectively.
- The thumb metacarpal is well visualized with anteroposterior, lateral, and oblique views, although care should

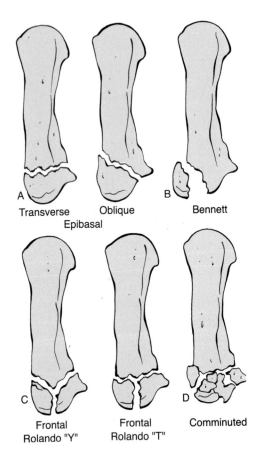

Figure 17.2-1 Classification of fractures of the base of the thumb metacarpal.

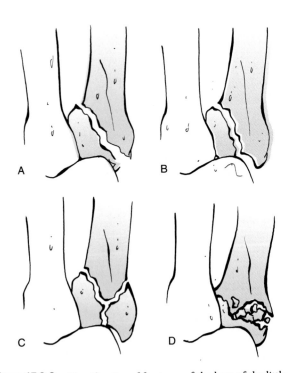

Figure 17.2-2 Classification of fractures of the base of the little finger metacarpal. (**A**) Epibasal. (**B**) Two part. (**C**) Three part. (**D**) Comminuted with impaction.

be taken to obtain a true lateral view with the hand pronated by 20 degrees.

■ A traction view can be helpful to assess the probability of closed reduction being successful.

TREATMENT

Metacarpal Head Fractures

■ Fractures of the metacarpal head may be difficult to visualize on standard radiographs, and CT scanning may be necessary to fully identify the fracture configuration.

■ These are usually intra-articular fractures to which the basic principles of stable fixation and early mobilization should be applied.

■ If undisplaced, metacarpal head fractures should be treated nonoperatively with early mobilization.

■ Displaced fractures should be treated with open reduction and internal fixation with screws for partial articular and with a small T-plate for complete articular fractures.

■ Complications include infection, particularly in human tooth injury, stiffness, and avascular necrosis.

Metacarpal Neck Fractures

■ If there is significant palmar displacement of the metacarpals, two problems may theoretically result.

■ The palmar displacement can cause an imbalance in the extrinsic tendons resulting in a claw deformity.

■ Prominence of the metacarpal head in the palm of the hand may cause discomfort gripping.

Nonsurgical Treatment

■ Undisplaced metacarpal neck fractures do not require any specific treatment.

■ A period of 2 weeks in neighbor strapping is usually sufficient, although some patients do not require any immobilization.

■ Finger motion should be encouraged.

■ There is considerable controversy about the degree of angulation that can be accepted after fracture of the metacarpal neck, although rotational deformity should always be reduced.

■ The published indications for reduction in metacarpal neck fractures are shown in Box 17.2-1.

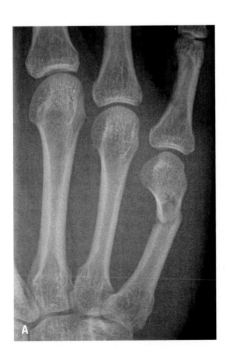
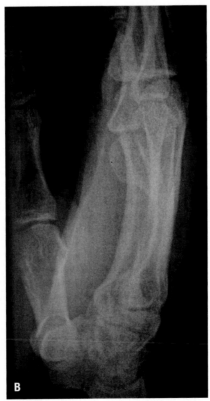
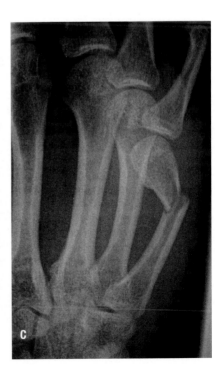

Figure 17.2-3   Anteroposterior (**A**), lateral (**B**), and oblique (**C**) views of a metacarpal fracture of the little finger.

BOX 17.2-1 INDICATIONS FOR REDUCTION IN METACARPAL NECK FRACTURES

- Angulation
    30–70 degrees for second and fifth metacarpals
    >15 degrees for middle metacarpals
- Malrotation
- Shortening >5 mm
- Finger clawing

BOX 17.2-2 INDICATIONS FOR REDUCTION OF METACARPAL SHAFT FRACTURES

- Angulation
    40–70 degrees angulation in fourth and fifth metacarpals
    >15-degree angulation in second and third metacarpals
- Malrotation
- Shortening >5–10 mm

- The majority of displaced metacarpal neck fractures are treated nonoperatively.
- If closed reduction is required, it can be achieved by flexing the metacarpophalangeal joints to 90 degrees and using the proximal phalanx to push the metacarpal head dorsally and to control rotation (Jahss's technique).
- If reduction is necessary, some form of external splintage is required.
    - This may be with an aluminium splint (see Fig. 31-25 in Chapter 31), a cast, or a functional brace.
- The fingers should be held in 80 to 90 degrees of metacarpophalangeal joint flexion with the proximal interphalangeal joint straight.
- Flexion of the proximal interphalangeal joint is contraindicated because it will cause disabling flexion contractures in the long term.
- The results of nonoperative management of metacarpal neck fractures are poorly reported, but good and excellent results are around 95%.
- There is general agreement that the main problem with nonoperative treatment is the persistent bony swelling associated with malunion.
- Patients should be warned that they may experience pain with vigorous use and cold intolerance within the first year after fracture, but that these will resolve.

Surgical Treatment
- The indications for surgery in metacarpal neck fractures are similar to those for reduction (see Box 17.2-1).
- In practice, the most common reason for surgery is either unacceptable angulation in an unstable fracture or malrotation, which can be difficult to control nonoperatively.
- Operative treatment is usually achieved using closed reduction techniques (see earlier) and percutaneous wiring.
- This may be with transverse wires securing the unstable metacarpal to an intact neighbor (Fig. 17.2-4) or by intramedullary pinning techniques (see Fig. 34-5 in Chapter 34).
    - If transverse wires are used, it is important to use two distal wires if there is sufficient space; otherwise postoperative malalignment may ensue.
- The hand may be mobilized immediately.
- Open reduction and internal fixation is rarely required, usually only where the fracture is irreducibly closed,

multiple complex fractures are present, or there is an open injury.
- The results of operative treatment of metacarpal neck fractures are not well documented, but closed reduction and percutaneous wiring can be expected to give a high proportion of good and excellent results.

Metacarpal Shaft Fractures

- There are many similarities between the treatment of metacarpal neck and shaft fractures.
- Undisplaced metacarpal shaft fractures do not require specific treatment, although neighbor strapping may be used for up to 2 weeks to alleviate local discomfort.
- Finger motion should be encouraged.
- As in the metacarpal neck, there is no absolute level of angulation above which agreement exists that reduction is required.
- It is generally agreed that less angulation is acceptable in the second and third metacarpals than in the fourth and fifth because the latter are more mobile.
- Less angulation is acceptable in the metacarpal shaft than in the neck.
- Shortening is well tolerated, but malrotation should not be accepted.
- Indications for reduction in metacarpal shaft fractures are shown in Box 17.2-2.

Nonsurgical Treatment
- The majority of isolated metacarpal shaft fractures are treated nonoperatively.
- Reduction can be achieved using the same technique as for reduction of metacarpal neck fractures.
    - Pressure applied over the apex of the displacement can also be helpful.
- The hand is then immobilized in an aluminium splint with the metacarpophalangeal joint at 80 to 90 degrees of flexion and the proximal interphalangeal joint straight.
- Plaster of Paris or a fracture brace may also be used.
- The results of nonoperative management of metacarpal shaft fractures are poorly reported but summarized in Table 17.2-3.
- Initial displacement if not reduced does not deteriorate with nonoperative management.

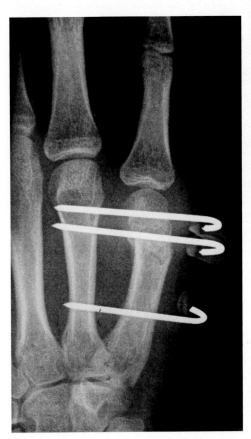
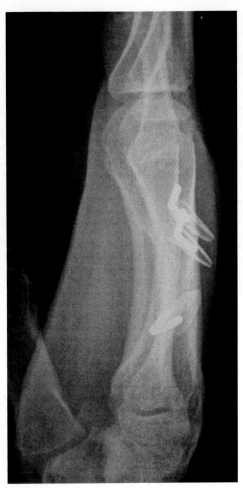

Figure 17.2-4 The use of transverse K-wires to treat a fifth metacarpal neck fracture.

■ No relationship between function and fracture angulation has as yet been demonstrated.

Surgical Treatment
■ The indications for operative treatment of metacarpal shaft fractures are detailed in Box 17.2-3.

■ These are variable and relative and depend on the functional demands of the patient.
■ Closed reduction and internal fixation techniques utilize either transverse (see Fig. 17.2-4) or intramedullary (see Fig. 34-5 in Chapter 34) K-wires using the same techniques as for neck fractures.

TABLE 17.2-3 RESULTS OF TREATMENT OF METACARPAL SHAFT FRACTURES

Result/Complication	Nonoperative (%)		Closed Reduction/ Internal Fixation (%)		Open Reduction/ Internal Fixation (%)	
	Range	Average	Range	Average	Range	Average
Good/excellent	98–100	99	100	100	70–79	75
Major complications	<1	<1	<1	<1	19–29	24
Nonunion	<1	<1	<1	<1	0–18	6
Hand stiffness	<1	<1	<1	<1	0–20	8
Hardware complications	N/A	N/A	6–16	7	8	8
Malunion/loss of reduction	11–18	15	Transverse: 0	0	<1	<1
				13		
			Medullary: 5–21			

H

BOX 17.2-3 INDICATIONS FOR OPERATIVE TREATMENT OF METACARPAL SHAFT FRACTURES

- Displacement
  - 40–70 degrees angulation in fourth and fifth metacarpals
  - >15-degree angulation in second and third metacarpals
- Rotational shortening >5–10 mm
- Irreducible fractures
- Multiple metacarpal fractures
- Open fracture with displacement
- Bone loss

- Open reduction and internal fixation is with plates (Fig. 17.2-5) or with interfragmentary screws in the spiral fracture.
- The results of operative treatment of metacarpal shaft fractures are shown in Table 17.2-3.
  - Comparing these results with the results of nonoperative treatment indicates that the latter is appropriate for the majority of fractures.
  - Major complications are unusual when metacarpal fractures are treated by nonoperative means or with closed reduction and fixation.
- Open reduction and internal fixation is a challenging technique and if not well performed may lead to a significant number of patients with nonunion or hand stiffness.

Multiple Metacarpal Fractures

- The presence of multiple fractures in the metacarpals implies increasing instability and soft tissue injury and constitutes a relative indication for surgical treatment.
- Whichever implant is used, it must confer sufficient stability to allow active hand mobilization and reduce the hand stiffness that is likely to accompany this severity of injury.
- Usually open reduction and internal fixation is required (Fig. 17.2-6).
- Transverse K-wire fixation may not be possible because it requires an intact metacarpal adjacent to the fracture.
- Intramedullary wiring does not confer sufficient rotational stability.
- Plating or intrafragmentary screws, depending on the configuration of the fracture, is usually necessary.
- In fractures that are severely comminuted, open, or with significant bone loss, the basic principles of wound debridement and skeletal stabilization should be used primarily.
  - This may require the use of external fixation either temporarily until there are suitable conditions for internal fixation or until fracture union.
- Adjunctive limited internal fixation may be required, especially with intra-articular injury.
- Bone grafting may be required to bridge an area of bone loss or severe comminution.

Fractures of the Metacarpal Bases

- Extra-articular fractures of the bases of the second to fifth metacarpals are usually undisplaced and can be successfully treated by nonoperative methods.
- If significantly displaced, they may require K-wire or plate fixation.
- Two-part intra-articular fracture of the base of the metacarpals especially the fourth and fifth, are likely to be associated with dislocation or subluxation of one or both carpometacarpal joints.
  - These may be difficult to visualize on standard A-P and lateral radiographs. Thirty-degree oblique radiographs in supination for the second carpometacarpal joint and in pronation for the fifth carpometacarpal joint are usually required.
- Fracture dislocation of the base of the fifth metacarpal is known as the reversed Bennett's fracture.
- These can usually be reduced closed by longitudinal traction followed by thumb pressure on the metacarpal base.
- Stabilization of either the fourth or fifth metacarpal base can be achieved by placing a K-wire across the

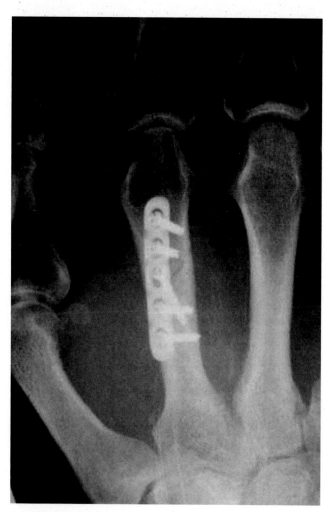

Figure 17.2-5   The use of a plate to treat a fracture of the index finger metacarpal.

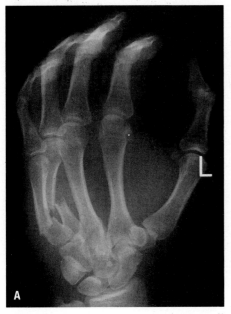
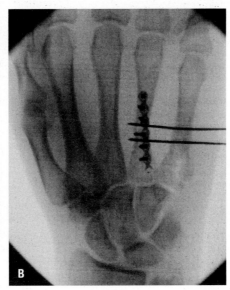

Figure 17.2-6   (A) Fractures of the fourth and fifth metacarpals. (B) Internal fixation using a combination of a plate and K-wires. Good stability was achieved.

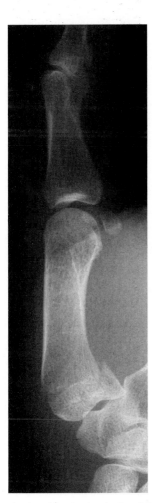

Figure 17.2-7   Undisplaced intra-articular basal fracture of thumb metacarpal. This was successfully treated in a cast.

carpometacarpal joint and into the adjacent intact metacarpal.

◼ Displaced three-part fractures may be difficult to reduce, especially if comminuted.

◼ Open reduction is indicated if closed reduction fails, especially in the second metacarpal where extensor carpi radialis brevis may be interposed in the fracture site.

◼ Where there is severe comminution, ligamentotaxis using external fixation combined with percutaneous K-wiring may be necessary.

◼ In severe cases, primary arthrodesis may be indicated, although this is most applicable to the second and third carpometacarpal joints, which normally have very little movement.

◼ Posttraumatic arthrosis is common radiologically and can cause pain on gripping and decreased grip power.

Fractures of the First Metacarpal Base

◼ Extra-articular fractures or undisplaced intra-articular fractures (see Fig. 17.2-7) of the thumb metacarpal are mostly treated successfully by closed reduction and a thumb spica cast.

◼ If closed reduction cannot be maintained in this manner, percutaneous wiring may be necessary.

◼ Open reduction and internal fixation is rarely required.

Bennett's Fracture

◼ Bennett's fracture can usually be reduced closed.

　◼ In this fracture the volar medial fragment of the metacarpal base is held in place by its ligamentous attachment (Fig. 17.2-8A).

- The metacarpal base dislocates dorsally and supinates because of the pull of abductor pollicis longus.
- Reduction requires traction on the thumb along with abduction, extension, and pronation of the metacarpal.

- Nonoperative management has been advocated after Bennett's fracture, but there is a significant risk of instability and malunion.
- Persistent subluxation of the carpometacarpal joint may lead to symptomatic arthritis. For these reasons stabilization is generally advised.

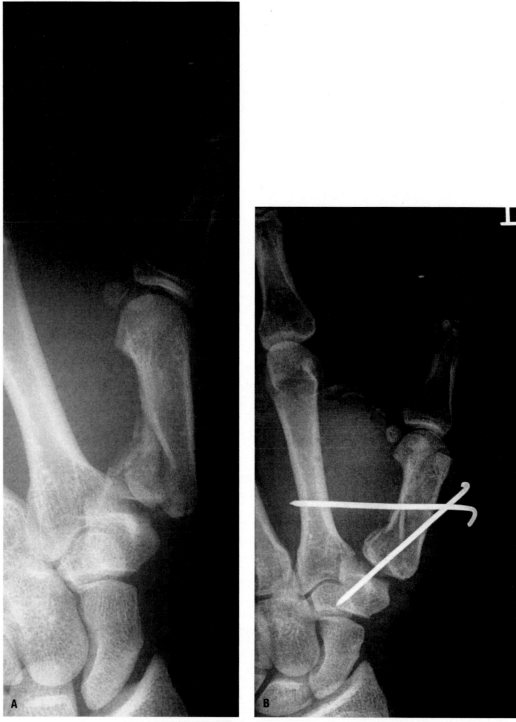

Figure 17.2-8 (**A**) A Bennett's fracture showing the volar medial fragment retained in the joint and dislocation of the remaining portion of the first metacarpal base. (**B**) K-wires used to treat the fracture.

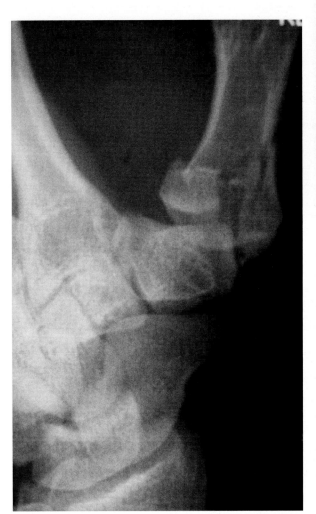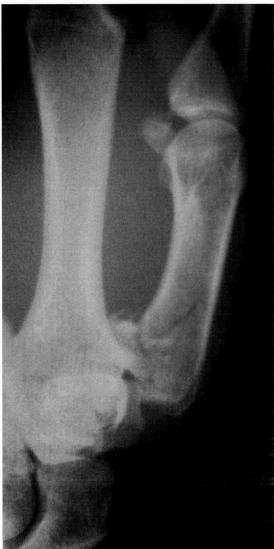

Figure 17.2-9   Anteroposterior and lateral radiographs of a Rolando fracture.

■ This can usually be obtained readily by insertion of two Kirschner wires, one across the carpometacarpal joint and one transmetacarpal between the first and second metacarpals (Fig. 17.2-8B).

■ It is not usually necessary to fix the volar medial fragment directly.

■ Open reduction and internal fixation should be reserved for fractures that cannot be adequately reduced closed (residual intra-articular displacement of >2 mm).

■ External fixation is occasionally employed in cases with severe soft tissue injury.

■ Although there is some controversy surrounding the outcome of Bennett's fracture, it is generally agreed that a better reduction of the joint will reduce the chances of the development of radiographic osteoarthrosis, although there seems to be little correlation between radiographic changes and symptoms.

　■ This correlation may depend more on the amount of articular impaction at the time of injury.

Rolando's Fracture

■ Rolando's fracture, or three-part fractures, of the first metacarpal base (Fig. 17.2-9) are more severe fractures and consequently have a poorer outcome.

■ If closed reduction is possible, closed K-wire fixation should be used to stabilize the fracture.

■ If a good reduction is unobtainable or uncontrollable by these means, open reduction and internal fixation may be required.

■ In severely comminuted fractures, external fixation may be indicated.

Suggested Treatment

■ The management of metacarpal fractures is summarized in Table 17.2-4.

TABLE 17.2-4 SUGGESTED TREATMENT OF METACARPAL FRACTURES

Fracture location	Treatment
Basal fractures (2–5)	
Undisplaced	Early mobilization
Displaced	Internal fixation. Percutaneous if possible
Basal fractures (thumb)	
Undisplaced	Cast immobilization: 3 wk
Displaced	Internal fixation. Percutaneous if possible
Shaft fractures	
Undisplaced	Mobilization; strapping if painful
Displaced (see Box 17.2-2)	Reduction and splinting for 4–6 wk
	Internal fixation if unsuccessful (K-wires)
Multiple fractures	Internal fixation (plates)
Neck fractures	
Undisplaced	Early mobilization
Displaced (see Box 17.2-1)	Percutaneous K-wires
Head fractures	
Undisplaced	Early mobilization
Displaced	ORIF

17.3 PHALANGEAL INJURIES

EPIDEMIOLOGY

Phalangeal fractures account for about 40% of hand fractures. They have a type B distribution (see Chapter 1). They commonly occur in sports injuries or, like metacarpal fractures, in blows or assaults. About 12.5% of phalangeal fractures are open, with 3% of proximal phalangeal, 5.7% of middle phalangeal, and 33.6% of distal phalangeal fractures open. Phalangeal fractures are most common in the little finger and least common in the index finger. A full breakdown of the different types of phalangeal fractures is shown in Table 17.3-1.

TABLE 17.3-1 EPIDEMIOLOGY OF PHALANGEAL FRACTURES

Proportion of all fractures	9.6%
Proportion of hand injuries	40.1%
Average age	36.2 y
Men/women	68%/32%
Incidence	$107.3/10^5$/y
Distribution	Type B
Open fractures	12.5%
Most common causes	
Sport	30.1%
Blow/assault	28.7%
Fall	20.0%
Phalanges	
Thumb	18.7%
Index	11.8%
Middle	17.4%
Ring	22.2%
Little	29.9%

Associated Injuries

As with metacarpal fractures, proximal phalangeal fractures are usually isolated injuries, although 17% have other fractures. However, 76% of these are also in the phalanges.

Table 17.3-2 shows that the highest incidences of proximal phalangeal fractures are seen in the thumb and little finger proximal phalanges with incidence decreasing toward the middle of the hand. Middle and distal phalangeal fractures tend to have a similar incidence in each finger, with the highest incidences seen in the middle finger. Epibasal proximal phalangeal fractures are relatively common in the little, ring, and index fingers and much less common in the index finger and thumb. In contrast, intra-articular basal fractures of the proximal phalanx are more common in the index finger and thumb. Epibasal fractures of the middle phalanx are uncommon in all fingers, and Table 17.3-2 shows that basal unicondylar fractures are most common in the middle phalanges of all fingers.

Diaphyseal fractures are most commonly seen in the proximal phalanges of the ring and index fingers and the distal phalanges of the middle finger and thumb. Neck fractures are most frequently seen in the distal phalanges.

PROXIMAL PHALANX

BASAL FRACTURES

Extra-Articular Fractures

◾ Extra-articular fractures of the base of the proximal phalanx can be difficult to assess radiologically.

TABLE 17.3-2 DISTRIBUTION OF THE DIFFERENT TYPES OF PHALANGEAL FRACTURES

	Prevalence (%)													
	Little			Ring			Middle			Index			Thumb	
Type	PP	MP	DP	PP	MP	DP	PP	MP	DP	PP	MP	DP	PP	DP
Overall	48.4	24.8	26.7	31.1	33.6	35.3	14.0	41.9	44.1	27.0	33.3	39.7	50.0	50.0
Base														
Epibasal	41.0	0	9.3	35.1	0	7.1	38.5	2.6	2.4	0	4.8	8.0	10.0	2.0
Unicondylar	7.7	62.5	53.5	10.8	70.0	33.3	23.1	74.4	19.5	17.6	76.2	28.0	52.0	28.0
Compression/ shear	11.6	17.5	4.7	8.1	7.5	2.4	7.7	5.1	0	17.6	4.8	0	10.0	0
Shaft														
Spiral/oblique	17.9	10.0	2.3	29.7	12.5	2.4	7.7	7.7	9.8	17.6	9.5	4.0	4.0	6.0
Transverse	3.8	2.5	9.3	0	2.5	9.5	0	5.1	4.9	11.8	0	0	4.0	18.0
Wedge/ comminuted	6.4	2.5	4.7	2.7	2.5	4.8	7.7	2.6	17.1	17.6	4.8	12.0	6.0	16.0
Neck	2.6	2.5	16.3	5.4	0	38.1	15.4	2.6	46.3	0	0	48.0	0	12.0
Head	9.0	2.5	0	8.1	5.0	2.4	0	0	0	17.6	0	0	14.0	18.0

■ They usually displace with apex volar angulation because of the pull of the central slip and lateral bands of the extensor tendon on the distal part of the phalanx, resulting in extension of the distal fragment while the intrinsic muscle attachments maintain the position of the proximal fragment (Fig. 17.3-1).

  ■ This displacement can be difficult to appreciate on a lateral X-ray because it is obscured by the proximal phalanges of the other digits.

■ Malunion with angulation of more than 25 degrees is recognized as resulting in limitation of movement at the proximal interphalangeal joint because of extensor tendon shortening.

■ Nonoperative treatment is usually successful, provided the metacarpophalangeal joint is placed in at least 70 degrees of flexion with the proximal interphalangeal joint straight.

■ The finger should be immobilized in this position in a splint or cast for 3 to 4 weeks.

■ Radiographic control during this time is necessary.

■ If the fracture should prove unstable, closed reduction and K-wiring should be used.

■ Open reduction and internal fixation is only indicated with severe soft tissue injury.

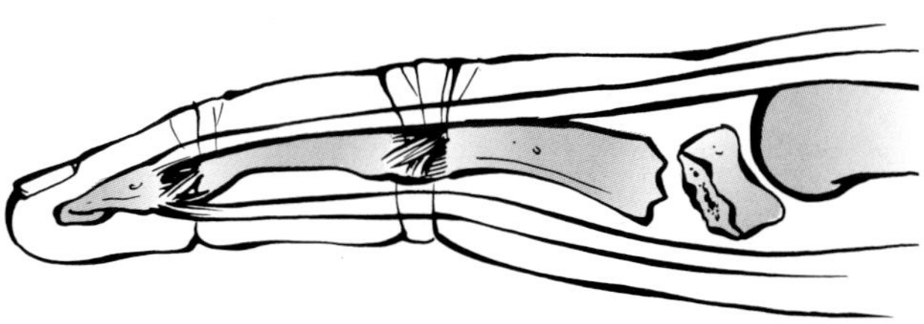

Intra-Articular Fractures

■ *Intra-articular* basal fractures of the proximal phalanx may be avulsion fractures, vertical shear fractures, or compression fractures (Fig. 17.3-2).

■ Avulsion fractures (Fig. 17.3-3A) are treated successfully with neighbor strapping to the finger adjacent to the injury, provided they are undisplaced or minimally displaced.

■ If significantly displaced, internal fixation is indicated to prevent chronic instability (Fig. 17.3-3B).

■ This can be achieved by tension band wiring techniques or screw fixation of larger fragments.

■ Neighbor strapping is recommended for 2 to 3 weeks postoperatively with active mobilization.

Figure 17.3-1 Displacement of an extra-articular basal fracture of the proximal phalanx.

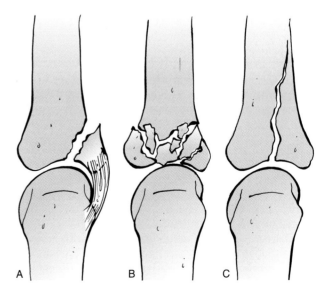

Figure 17.3-2 Types of intra-articular basal fractures of the proximal phalanx. (**A**) Collateral ligament avulsion. (**B**) Compression. (**C**) Shear.

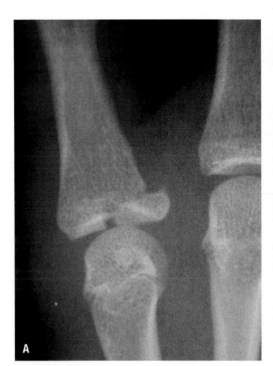 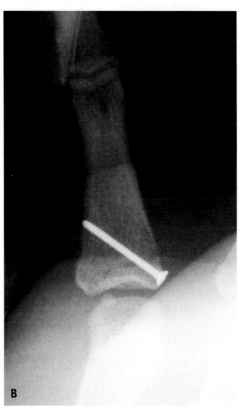

Figure 17.3-3   (A) An avulsion fracture of the base of the proximal phalanx. (B) This was fixed with an interfragmentary screw.

Vertical shear fractures if displaced require reduction and fixation. If closed reduction is possible, percutaneous fixation with K-wires should be used. If not, then open reduction and internal fixation with interfragmentary screw fixation is recommended (see Fig. 34-19 in Chapter 34).

Compression fractures of the base of the proximal phalanx are a more challenging situation. Closed reduction by ligamentotaxis may not be possible because all the fragments do not have soft tissue attachments. If there is significant (>1–2 mm) articular malalignment open reduction, elevation of the articular fragments, cancellous bone grafting, and internal fixation with K-wires, screw, or a mini T-plate may be required.

The limited reports of the outcome of these techniques for management of intra-articular basal fractures of the phalanges indicates that in approximately 75% of cases there is a good or excellent outcome.

SHAFT FRACTURES

Fractures of the shafts of the phalanges are usually classified by their morphology: transverse, spiral or oblique, wedge, or comminuted fractures.

Transverse fractures tend to angulate with a volar apex, although this can vary in the middle phalanx depending on the fracture's relationship to the attachment of the superficial finger flexor. Spiral fractures demonstrate rotational malalignment, whereas oblique fractures may rotate, angulate, or shorten. Comminuted fractures are most likely to shorten.

Treatment

Nonsurgical Treatment

- Undisplaced phalangeal shaft fractures are readily managed by neighbor strapping to an adjacent digit (see Fig. 31-21 in Chapter 31) for 2 to 3 weeks, during which time active mobilization is encouraged.
- The finger should be X-rayed approximately 1 week from injury to ensure the undisplaced position is maintained.
- Nonoperative management is also indicated for displaced fractures of the phalangeal shaft, which are stable after reduction.
- This may be by static or dynamic splintage, but whichever method is used the metacarpophalangeal joints must be held in at least 70 degrees of flexion.
- In static splints the proximal interphalangeal joint must be straight.
- Dynamic splinting, such as such as extension block casting, holds the metacarpophalangeal joints in 90 degrees of flexion but allows proximal interphalangeal joint flexion (see Fig. 31-23 in Chapter 31).
- With extension block casting, neighbor strapping may also be required to control rotation.
- X-rays approximately 1 week after splintage are required to confirm maintenance of the reduced position.

Surgical Treatment

- If a fracture is unstable after reduction, a number of techniques of internal fixation may be employed.
- General principles dictate that those methods with the least soft tissue dissection are preferable to avoid disturbance of the gliding structures in the finger.

TABLE 17.3-3 RESULTS OF TREATMENT OF PHALANGEAL SHAFT FRACTURES

	Incidence (%)			
	TAM >220 Degrees		Excellent/Good	
Treatment	Range	Average	Range	Average
Nonoperative	100	100	87–93	90
Closed K-wires	95	95	90–100	95
Tension band wiring	82–86	84	100	100[a]
Plating[b]	11–38	25	27–100	55

TAM, total active movement of the finger joints.
[a]Some authors consider TAM >50% to be a good result.
[b]Plating reports concentrate on more severe fractures.

- If closed reduction is possible, percutaneous Kirschner wires are usually recommended (see Fig. 34-8 in Chapter 34).
- If the fracture is transverse, intramedullary K-wires are required.
  - These may allow malrotation to occur, which should be prevented by additional external splinting.
- Transverse wires may be used for spiral or oblique fractures.
- In severely comminuted fractures, external splintage or K-wires may not be sufficient to control shortening.
  - In these rare cases, external fixation may be used.
- Open reduction and internal fixation is reserved for fractures that are irreducibly closed, either because of soft tissue interposition or because late diagnosis has allowed early healing.
- Interfragmentary screw fixation is preferred where the fracture morphology allows its use (see Fig. 34-19 in Chapter 34).
- Transverse or short oblique fractures can be treated with tension band wiring. Plating may be indicated for comminuted fractures to maintain length.

Results and Complications

- The results of the different methods of management can be seen in Table 17.3-3.
- It should be emphasized that some of these differences in outcome may be related to the severity of the initial fracture.
- The main complication of phalangeal shaft fractures is hand stiffness.
- Infection and nonunion are rare.

NECK FRACTURES

- These are uncommon injuries that are usually easily reduced but likely to be unstable. For that reason they usually require fixation with percutaneous intramedullary K-wires, introduced either through the metacarpophalangeal joint or the base of the proximal phalanx (see Fig. 34-8 in Chapter 34).

CONDYLAR FRACTURES

Condylar fractures of the middle or proximal phalanx are classified depending on whether they are unicondylar or bicondylar. Unicondylar fractures can be further subdivided depending on the amount of articular surface detached.

Unicondylar fractures result from a shearing force and if displaced will move laterally and may rotate because of the attachment of the collateral ligament (Fig. 17.3-4A).

Bicondylar fractures are usually caused by a compressive force, with the condyles separating and rotating, making closed reduction almost impossible.

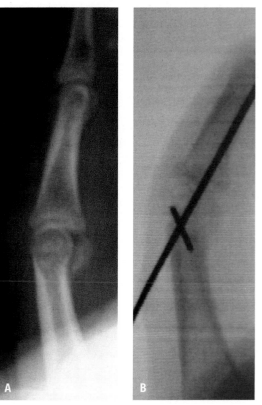

Figure 17.3-4 (**A**) An unicondylar phalangeal neck fracture. (**B**) Stabilized with K-wires.

Treatment

- Undisplaced unicondylar or bicondylar fractures may be treated by a splint or neighbor strapping.
- Displaced unicondylar fractures may be amenable to closed reduction and internal fixation with percutaneous wires (Fig. 17.3-4B).
  - This can be achieved by traction and varus or valgus pressure on the finger, depending on the size of the fracture.
  - The reduction can then be secured with percutaneous reduction forceps and percutaneous wires inserted.
- If there is irreducible rotation, open reduction and internal fixation with wires or screws may be required.
  - This is frequently challenging because the fragment may be small and difficult to control and secure.
- The same principles apply to bicondylar fractures, although these are more frequently irreducibly closed.
  - Mini plate fixation may be necessary in these cases.
- Mixed outcomes are reported for condylar fractures, with excellent and good results around 66%.
- Lack of extension is a common complication.
- Occasional cases of avascular necrosis of the condyle occur.

MIDDLE PHALANX

BASAL FRACTURES

Intra-articular fractures of the base of the middle phalanx may be separated into volar lip, dorsal lip, and "pilon"-type fractures. They may each be associated with subluxation or dislocation of the proximal interphalangeal joint.

Volar Lip Fractures

Volar lip fractures are the most common injury to the base of the middle phalanx and may be caused by hyperextension or axial compression. Hyperextension typically causes avulsion of the volar lip by the volar plate and usually involves less than 20% of the articular surface (Fig. 17.3-5). In this situation, comminution is rare. Axial compression is likely to result in more severe injury with articular comminution. Classification of these injuries depends on the size of the fracture and the amount of subluxation (Table 17.3-4). Thus a volar lip fracture of 25% of the joint surface with 30% of the joint uncovered would be a grade IIIb injury.

Undisplaced volar lip fractures may be treated by neighbor strapping, provided there is no joint subluxation. Results achieved with this form of treatment are over 90% excellent. Fair or poor results follow missed subluxation or are due to subsequent flexion contracture of the joint.

Fractures Associated with Subluxation or Dislocation

- Subluxation of the proximal interphalangeal joint may be subtle.
- A true lateral radiograph should show complete congruence of the joint with parallel joint lines.

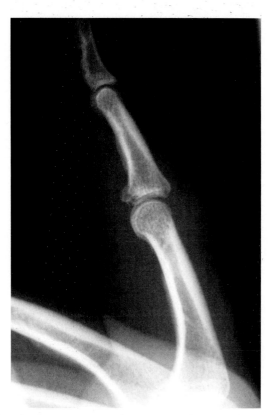

Figure 17.3-5   A volar lip fracture of the middle phalanx.

- Subluxation can be seen as divergence of the joint lines posteriorly, creating a V shape dorsally (Fig. 17.3-6).
- In fractures with an unstable joint, the dorsal subluxation usually occurs before full extension.
- Closed reduction is achieved with longitudinal traction and flexion of the joint.
- These injuries can then be managed by extension block splintage, provided the joint is stable when held in the flexed position (see Fig. 31-23 in Chapter 31).
- After reduction the joint should be slowly extended and the point of subluxation noted.
- A dorsal splint is applied with the wrist slightly extended, the MP joints in 70 degrees of flexion, and the PIP joint in slightly more flexion than the point of instability.

TABLE 17.3-4 SCHENCK'S CLASSIFICATION OF FRACTURES AND FRACTURE SUBLUXATION/DISLOCATION OF THE PROXIMAL INTERPHALANGEAL JOINT

Fracture Size	Grade	Extent of Dislocation/ Subluxation	Grade
<10%	I	<25%	A
11%–20%	II	25%–50%	B
21%–40%	III	>50%	C
>40%	IV	Total	D

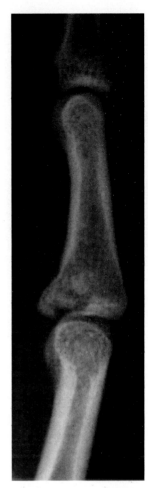

Figure 17.3-6 A fracture subluxation of the middle phalanx showing the characteristic dorsal V shape that indicates subluxation.

- The proximal phalanx is now taped to the splint, thus allowing active flexion of the proximal interphalangeal joint.
- The range of extension is gradually increased over a period of several weeks to full extension.
- Frequent review is required over the first few weeks to ensure that subluxation has not recurred.
- Extension block splinting can also be performed with a K-wire inserted percutaneously into the head of the proximal phalanx parallel to the shaft with the proximal interphalangeal joint in full flexion.
- The larger the fragment, the more likely the joint will be unstable.
  - With fragments greater than 50% of the joint surface, joint instability is almost inevitable because of disruption of the collateral ligament attachment.
- If more than 60 degrees of flexion is required to maintain stability or if the joint reduction is lost, extension block splinting is unlikely to be successful.
- With large noncomminuted fragments, open reduction and internal fixation may be possible.
- With comminution, ligamentotaxis using hinged external fixation or dynamic traction may be used, but the complication rates of these techniques are high and include loss of reduction, infection, joint contractures, pain, osteoarthritis, and loss of grip strength.

- In severe fractures it is more important to reduce the subluxation than to reconstruct the articular surface perfectly.

Dorsal Lip Fractures

- These are caused by an avulsion of a bony fragment by the central slip of the extensor mechanism and as such are incipient Boutonnière injuries.
- They should be treated by dynamic extension splinting for 6 weeks with active movement of the distal interphalangeal joints.

Pilon Fractures

- Pilon fractures are caused by axial loading and result in severe damage to the articular surface of the middle phalanx.
- Open reduction and internal fixation may be used but is technically complex with unpredictable outcomes.
- Traction with dynamic traction devices or hinged external fixation gives comparable outcomes with lower complication rates.
- Patients should be warned that the likely outcome is significant joint stiffness.
- Complications include loss of reduction and later osteoarthritis.

SHAFT, NECK, AND CONDYLAR FRACTURES

- These are treated in the same way as equivalent fractures of the proximal phalanx.

DISTAL PHALANX

- Fractures of the distal phalanx have been classified by Dobyns, taking into consideration both anatomic considerations and soft tissue injury (Table 17.3-5).

TABLE 17.3-5 DOBYNS' CLASSIFICATION OF DISTAL PHALANGEAL FRACTURES

Anatomic Site	Closed	Open
Tuft	Stable Heal in 6–8 wk	May be unstable Nail bed injury
Shaft	Usually undisplaced Heal in 8–12 wk	May be unstable Nail bed injury Nonunion possible
Base (physeal)	May be unstable May require reduction Healing: 6 wk	Nail root injury Usually displaced Open reduction usually required

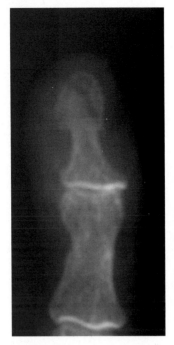
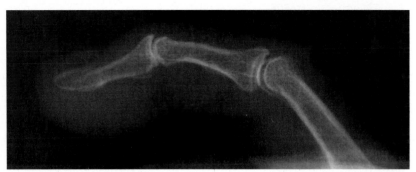

Figure 17.3-7   Anteroposterior and lateral radiographs of a tuft fracture.

TUFT FRACTURES

- Closed tuft fractures (Fig. 17.3-7) require little treatment, although a subungual hematoma may require evacuation for pain relief.
- Splintage is for comfort only, and active mobilization should start as soon as comfort allows.
- Open tuft fractures are mostly a soft tissue injury.
- A careful debridement and irrigation is required followed by soft tissue repair. This is usually sufficient to stabilize the tuft fracture.
- Shortening of the fingertip may be required if the soft tissues are not viable.
- Patients should be warned that the fingertip may remain tender for some months.
- Hypersensitivity can be a problem and require desensitization by a physical therapist.

SHAFT FRACTURES

- Closed shaft fractures of the distal phalanx are usually undisplaced or minimally displaced and stable.
  - They require minimal splintage for a short period only for discomfort.
- Open shaft fractures are usually associated with significant soft tissue injury.
  - Debridement, irrigation, and inspection of the nail bed are required.
  - Soft tissue interposition preventing fracture reduction may be found.
  - If unstable, the distal phalanx may require longitudinal K-wire fixation.

- The nail bed should be repaired and the nail replaced if possible because it will confer added stability to the fracture.
- Splinting is usually necessary for 2 to 3 weeks.

BASAL FRACTURES

- Basal fractures of the distal phalanx tend to be unstable.
- The extensor tendon remains attached to the proximal fragment; the flexor tendon flexes the distal fragment resulting in the typical apex dorsal angulation (Fig. 17.3-8).
- Closed fractures are usually easily reduced.
  - They should be splinted for 4 weeks with the distal interphalangeal joint maximally extended.
- Open fractures usually occur in association with severe soft tissue injury and are unstable.
  - After soft tissue debridement and fracture reduction, longitudinal K-wire support is usually required.
  - The distal interphalangeal joint should only be crossed if the proximal fragment is too small to allow adequate purchase of the K-wire.

MALLET INJURIES

- A mallet injury is damage to the extensor apparatus at the terminal phalanx, either in the substance of the tendon (tendinous mallet) or with an avulsion fracture (bony mallet).

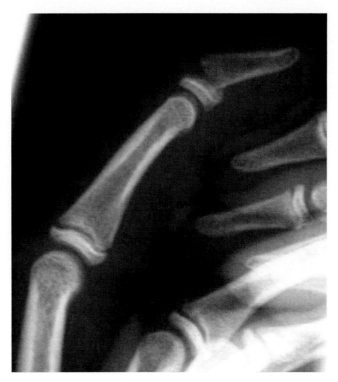

Figure 17.3-8   An extra-articular basal fracture of the distal phalanx.

- The clinical symptoms and signs are pain and swelling at the dorsum of the distal interphalangeal joint and an inability to extend the joint fully.
- Mallet injury often follows minor trauma when the dorsal interphalangeal joint is forcibly flexed against active extension.

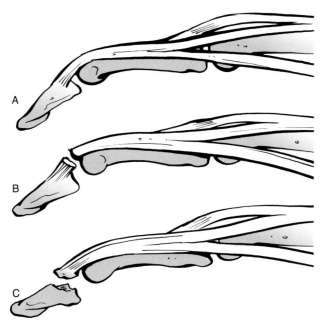

Figure 17.3-9   The Watson Jones classification of mallet injuries. (**A**) Stretching of the extensor mechanism. (**B**) Transection of the extensor mechanism. (**C**) A dorsal lip fracture.

TENDINOUS MALLET INJURY

- Tendinous mallet injuries may be classified into three types (Watson-Jones classification) (Fig. 17.3-9).
- Tendinous mallet injuries are almost exclusively managed nonoperatively.
  - The finger is placed in a splint with the distal interphalangeal joint extended (see Fig. 31-26 in Chapter 31).
    - This is retained for 6 to 8 weeks, after which night splinting is advised for 3 to 4 weeks.
- Results of splinting of the tendinous mallet injury are generally good, with around 85% good or excellent results.
- Complications are loss of extension and skin problems, although the latter are usually transient.
- Patient compliance may limit the adequacy of the result.

BONY MALLET INJURY

- Bony mallet injury may result from the same mechanism of injury as tendinous mallet fingers, from axial loading of the distal interphalangeal joint or from a sudden hyperextension injury.
- They usually involve more than one third of the articular surface.
- Like tendinous mallet finger, many bony mallet injuries can be successfully treated nonoperatively.
- Relative indications for surgery are given in Box 17.3-1.
- There are a number of surgical techniques, including extension block splinting, K-wire fixation, and tension band wiring.
- Surgery should be approached with caution because complication rates up to 53% have been reported, including skin problems, recurrent mallet deformity, permanent nail deformities, transient infection, and osteomyelitis.
  - Surgical treatment should therefore be reserved for refractory cases of bony mallet injury.

Suggested Treatment

- The management of phalangeal fractures is summarized in Table 17.3-6.

BOX 17.3-1 RELATIVE INDICATIONS FOR SURGERY OF BONY MALLET INJURIES

- Fractures involving more than 50% of the articular surface
- Fractures with volar subluxation of the distal phalanx
- Pilon-type fractures
- Displaced bony mallet of the thumb

TABLE 17.3-6 SUGGESTED TREATMENT OF PHALANGEAL FRACTURES

Fracture Location	Treatment
Proximal phalanx	
Basal fractures	
Extra-articular fractures	
Stable	Splinting for 3–4 wk
Unstable	K-wires
Intra-articular fractures	
Avulsion fractures	
Vertical shear fractures	
Compression fractures	
Undisplaced	Neighbor strapping for 3–4 wk
Displaced	Internal fixation. Percutaneous if possible
	+/− bone grafting in compression fractures
Shaft fractures	
Undisplaced	Neighbor strapping
Displaced	Reduction and splinting
	Internal fixation if unsuccessful
Neck fractures	
Usually unstable	K-wires
Condylar fractures	
Undisplaced	Splinting or strapping
Displaced	Internal fixation (open or closed)
Middle phalanx	
Basal fracture	
Intra-articular	
Volar lip fracture	
Undisplaced	Strapping
Subluxed/dislocated joint	Reduction and extension block splinting for 4 wk
Large intra-articular fragments	Internal fixation
Extensive comminution	External fixation or dynamic traction
Dorsal lip fracture	Dynamic extension splinting for 6 wk
Pilon fracture	External fixation or dynamic traction
Shaft, neck, and condylar fractures	As for proximal phalanx
Distal phalanx	
Basal fracture	
Closed	Splinting for 4 wk
Open	Debridement and K-wires
Shaft fracture	
Closed	Splinting for 2–3 wk
Open	Debridement and soft tissue repair
	K-wires if unstable
Tuft fracture	
Closed	Early mobilization
Open	Debridement and soft tissue repair
Mallet finger	
Soft tissue only	Mallet splinting for 6–8 wk
Dorsal fracture	Mallet splinting for 6–8 wk
	See text for surgical indications

17.4 FINGER DISLOCATIONS

CLASSIFICATION

Dislocations and ligament injuries in the hand are common, with the most common joint involved the proximal interphalangeal joint. They are classified as palmar, dorsal, or lateral dislocations depending on the position of the distal component. For example, a dorsal dislocation of the proximal interphalangeal joint occurs when the middle phalanx is displaced dorsally (Fig. 17.4-1).

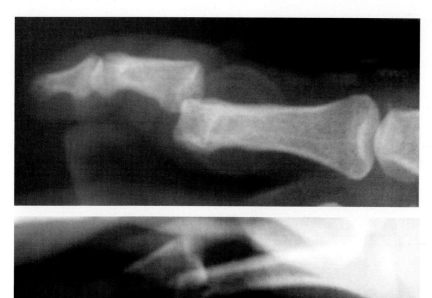

Figure 17.4-1 Anteroposterior and lateral radiographs of a dorsal PIP Joint dislocation.

DIAGNOSIS

- The dislocation is usually easily apparent on examination.
- X-rays must be obtained before reduction to determine the presence or absence of a fracture.
- After reduction the joint should be examined for stability both actively and passively.
- Collateral ligament integrity should be examined with varus and valgus stress and the palmar plate examined with dorsal to volar force.

TREATMENT

Proximal Interphalangeal Joint Dislocation

- Closed reduction is the recommended method of treatment for these injuries.
  - This is usually easily achieved by longitudinal traction and manipulation.
- Postreduction radiographs should be obtained to confirm a congruent reduction.
- If the joint is stable, neighbor strapping may be used for comfort for a short period, but active mobilization is encouraged early.
- If there is evidence of collateral ligament or volar plate injury, neighbor strapping or splintage in slight flexion is used for a maximum of 2 weeks.
- It is notable that stiffness is much more common than instability after these injuries.
- The patient should be warned that the joint may remain permanently thicker, and soreness with use may persist for up to 1 year.
- Occasionally dorsal dislocations are irreducible due to soft tissue interposition.

- This is an indication for open reduction.
- Volar dislocation is rare but may result in a Boutonnière deformity.
- Lack of active extension after reduction of a volar dislocation is an indication for surgical repair.

Distal Interphalangeal Joint Dislocation

- Dislocation of the distal interphalangeal joint is less common than that of the proximal interphalangeal joint.
  - They can usually be treated with closed reduction and splintage for a maximum of 10 days, followed by active mobilization.
- Palmar dislocation may result in a mallet injury, necessitating immobilization for 6 to 8 weeks.

Metacarpophalangeal Joint Dislocation

- Metacarpophalangeal joint dislocations are usually dorsal.
- They are less likely to be successfully reduced closed than interphalangeal joint dislocations because the palmar plate may become interposed between the joint surfaces, preventing reduction.
- Open reduction is then indicated through a dorsal approach, following which the joint is usually stable.
- The palmar plate should be protected by splintage to prevent hyperextension but allow active flexion for 3 to 4 weeks.

Carpometacarpal Joint of the Thumb

- This is a rare dislocation that occurs with supination of the metacarpal out of the joint. It should be reduced by pronation of the metacarpal.

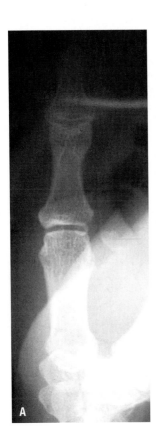 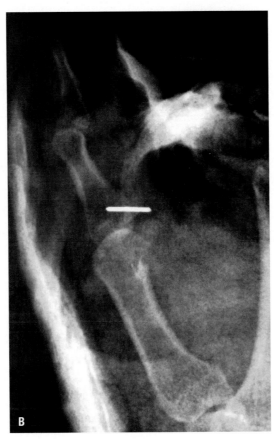

Figure 17.4-2 (A) An avulsion fracture of the ulnar collateral ligament insertion of the thumb. (B) Reconstructed with a K-wire.

■ These injuries are generally unstable and require Kirschner wire stabilization from the metacarpal into the trapezium and protection with a cast for 6 weeks.

Metacarpophalangeal Joint of the Thumb

■ Acute ligamentous injury to this joint is common and occurs with forced valgus and hyperextension.

■ It is associated with ski pole injury or artificial ski slopes when the thumb is caught in the diamond patterned matting as the skier falls.

■ The ulnar collateral ligament is most commonly injured.
  ■ Tenderness at the ulnar side of the joint should be sought, and joint stability must be assessed.

■ Complete disruption of the ulnar collateral ligament is likely if valgus stressing causes 30 degrees more instability than the opposite side.

■ Radiographic stress testing is unnecessary because this is a clinical diagnosis, but radiographs should be examined to document the possible presence of an avulsion fracture of the base of the proximal phalanx.

■ In collateral ligament injury with a stable joint, treatment is with a thumb spica cast for 3 to 4 weeks.

■ Patients should be warned of ongoing discomfort with use for several months.

■ With complete disruption of the ulnar collateral ligament, surgical exploration is recommended to exclude and repair a Stener lesion.

■ This occurs when the collateral ligament is displaced proximally and the adductor aponeurosis is interposed between the torn ligament and its attachment to the proximal phalanx.
  ■ An exception to this is when there is a relatively undisplaced avulsion fracture, in which case there cannot be a Stener lesion.

■ Alternatively, wide displacement of the avulsion fracture (Fig. 17.4-2) confirms the need for surgical repair.

■ Postoperatively the thumb is immobilized in a thumb spica case for 4 to 6 weeks.

Suggested Treatment

■ The management of finger dislocations is summarized in Table 17.4-1.

TABLE 17.4-1 SUGGESTED TREATMENT OF JOINT DISLOCATIONS

Dislocation Type	Treatment
Reducible and stable	Closed reduction. Early motion
Reducible and unstable	Closed reduction. Splinting
Irreducible	Open reduction and splinting K-wiring may be necessary

SUGGESTED READING

Adolfsson L, Lindau T, Arner M. Acutrak screw fixation versus cast immobilisation for undisplaced scaphoid waist fractures. J Hand Surg (Br) 2001;26:192–195.

Ashkenaze DM, Ruby LK. Metacarpal fractures and dislocations. Orthop Clin North Am 1992;23:19–33.

Bhandari M, Hanson BP. Acute nondisplaced fractures of the scaphoid. J Orthop Trauma 2004;18:253–255.

Fusetti C, Meyer H, Borisch N, et al. Complications of plate fixation in metacarpal fractures. J Trauma 2002;52:535–539.

Ford DJ, Ali MS, Steel WM. Fractures of the fifth metacarpal neck: is reduction or immobilisation necessary? J Hand Surg (Br) 1989;14:165–167.

Green DP, O'Brien ET. Classification and management of carpal dislocations. Clin Orthop 1980;149:55–72.

Herbert TJ, Fisher WE. Management of the fractured scaphoid using a new bone screw. J Bone Joint Surg (Br) 1984;66:114–123.

Horton TC, Hatton M, Davis TR. A prospective randomized controlled study of fixation of long oblique and spiral shaft fractures of the proximal phalanx: closed reduction and percutaneous Kirschner wiring versus open reduction and lag screw fixation. J Hand Surg (Br) 2003;28:5–9.

Jupiter JB, Axelrod TS, Belsky MR. Fractures and dislocations of the hand. In: Browner BD, Jupiter JB, Levine AM, et al., eds. Skeletal trauma, 3rd ed. Philadelphia: WB Saunders, 2003.

Lamb DW, Abernethy PA, Raine PAM. Unstable fractures of the metacarpals. The Hand 1973;5:43–48.

Ring D, Jupiter J, Herndon J. Acute fractures of the scaphoid. J Am Acad Orthop Surg 2000;8:255–231.

Stern PJ. Fractures of the metacarpals and phalanges. In: Green DP, Hotchkiss RN, Peterson WC, eds. Green's operative hand surgery, 4th ed. New York: Churchill Livingstone, 1999.

Soyer AD. Fractures of the base of the first metacarpal: current treatment options. J Am Acad Orthop Surg 1997;7:403–412.

Trumble T, ed. Carpal fracture dislocations. Rosemont, Illinois: American Academy of Orthopaedic Surgeons, 2000.

18 CERVICAL SPINE FRACTURES

CHRISTOPHER M. BONO

Injuries of the cervical spine are relatively uncommon, but their effect may be devastating. As with other fractures, most were treated nonoperatively until relatively recently. The introduction of anterior and posterior plating techniques and screw fixation for upper cervical spine fractures has changed their management. The considerable problems associated with spinal cord injury still exist, unfortunately, but modern imaging techniques and advances in fracture management have advanced the assessment and treatment of these difficult injuries. The controversies in the assessment and treatment of cervical spine fractures are listed in Box 18-1. The anatomy and treatment of C1 and C2 fractures is somewhat different from that of the subaxial spine (C3-C7), and the two areas are considered separately.

SURGICAL ANATOMY

The anatomy of the upper cervical spine is unique at each level (Fig. 18-1). The bony restraints of the occipitocervical junction involve the convex occipital condyles, which articulate with the lateral masses of the atlas (C1). The posterior arch of C1 provides a bony limit to occipital extension. Ligamentous restraints are mainly formed by the alar ligaments, which run from the superolateral aspect of the odontoid process to the medial occipital condyle. Motion at

this segment is approximately 21 degrees of extension, 3 degrees of flexion, 7 degrees of rotation to each side, and 5 degrees of lateral bending to each side.

The atlas relies on two lateral masses for weight bearing. Embryologically, the caudal part of the C1 somite joins with the cranial C2 somite to form the odontoid process. By 3 to 6 years of age, the dens fuses with the body. In the absence of a disc between the occiput and C1, the anatomical relationship is maintained by ligaments. The atlanto-occipital membrane attaches to a tubercle at the base of the skull and is confluent with the anterior longitudinal ligament (ALL). The apical ligament joins the tip of the dens to the foramen magnum. The posterior longitudinal ligament (PLL) continues superiorly as the tectorial membrane. The most important ligamentous restraint to anterior translation of the

BOX 18-1 CURRENT CONTROVERSIES IN THE INVESTIGATION AND TREATMENT OF CERVICAL SPINE FRACTURES

Nonoperative or operative treatment for odontoid fractures?
Facet dislocations: How useful is a prereduction MRI scan?
Management of facet dislocations: anterior or posterior approach?
Does early spinal stabilization improve neurological outcome?
What is the role of steroids in spinal cord injury?
How should cervical spine injuries be detected?

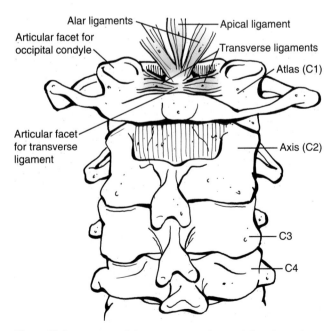

Figure 18-1 Anatomy of the upper cervical spine. The odontoid peg is secured to the anterior C1 ring by the transverse ligaments. The alar and apical ligaments secure the odontoid page to the anterior foramen magnum (basion).

C1-C2 complex is the transverse ligament, which traverses posterior to the odontoid to attach to the C1 lateral masses. Secondary restraint comes from the alar ligaments that arise along the medial aspect of the occipital condyles and lateral masses of C1 and insert onto the lateral aspect of the odontoid. Approximately 15 degrees of flexion and extension occurs at the occipitoatlantal junction. The muscular attachments to the cervical spine include the longus colli, which attaches to the anterior and inferior portions of the arch of C1. The rectus capitus medialis and lateralis and the trapezius insert posteriorly.

Although the atlantoaxial joint (50%) and subaxial spine (50%) contribute equally to rotation, most flexion and extension in the cervical spine occurs between C3 and C7. Up to 17 degrees of sagittal plane motion occurs at each motion segment of the subaxial spine. Coronal motion ranges from 4 to 11 degrees per motion segment in this region.

C2 represents a transition zone between the upper and lower cervical spine. The superior articular facets of C2 are anterior within the same coronal plane as the vertebral body. In contrast, the inferior articular facets of C2, which articulate with C3, lie within the posterior elements, similar to the arrangement seen in the lower cervical levels. The pars interarticularis, the column of bone that spans between these articular facets, is particularly prone to fracture with axial compressive loads, such as occurs with traumatic spondylolisthesis (Hangman fractures).

In the subaxial spine (C3-C7), each vertebral body is roughly cylindrical (Fig. 18-2). In each vertebral body the coronal diameter is greater than the sagittal diameter. The uncinate processes articulate with the rounded inferolateral borders of each superior vertebral body. This articulation, called the uncovertebral joint, is a useful surgical anatomical landmark that signals proximity to the lateral aspect of the vertebral body. It is believed to limit posterior translation of the upper vertebra. The annulus fibrosis of the disc is intimately related to the anterior and posterior longitudinal ligaments. The longus colli muscles lie directly over and insert onto the anterolateral aspects of each cervical vertebra. The sympathetic plexus lies on top of the lateral muscle belly, placing it at risk from overly aggressive dissection or retraction, which may lead to a Horner syndrome. The prevertebral (deep) and alar (superficial) fascial layers separate the spine from the overlying esophagus.

The transverse processes project from the lateral aspects of the vertebral body. The vertebral artery ascends to the head through the C6 to C1 transverse foramina. It enters the C7 transverse foramen in only 5% of the population. Fractures that enter or displace the transverse processes may cause injury or occlusion of the vertebral artery. The transverse process also guides the cervical spinal nerves as they exit from the spinal canal. The spinal nerves lie posterior to the vertebral artery.

The facet joints, also known as the zygoapophyseal articulations, are highly mobile diarthrodial joints formed by the superior and inferior articular processes. The articular surfaces are angled approximately 45 degrees in relation to the transverse axis of each segment. The pillar of bone between the superior and inferior articular processes is commonly referred to as the lateral mass. It is a useful site for posterior screw or wire stabilization of the cervical spine.

The laminae arise from the posteromedial border of the lateral masses to form bifid spinous processes (C2-C6). An elastic yellow ligament, called the ligamentum flavum, spans the interlaminar spaces. Strong interspinous and

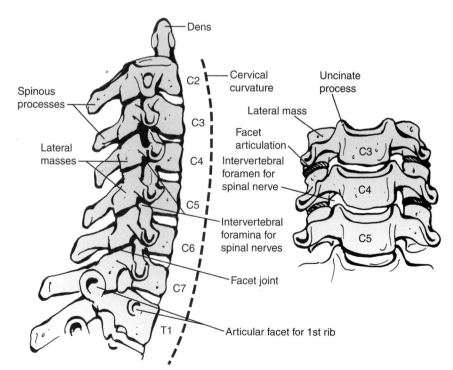

Figure 18-2 Anatomy of the lower cervical spine. This is relatively uniform in contrast to the upper cervical spine.

TABLE 18-1 BORDERS OF THE SPINAL CANAL

Location	Border
Anterior	Vertebral body, intervertebral disc, posterior longitudinal ligament
Posterior	Laminae, ligamentum flavum
Lateral	Pedicles, medial aspect of the facet joints.

supraspinous ligaments (ligamentum nuchae) together form a posterior ligamentous complex (PLC). Disruption of this complex results in mechanical instability.

Spinal Canal

The borders of the spinal canal are summarized in Table 18-1. The spinal canal can be compromised by bony fragments, which are usually retropulsed vertebral body fragments, disc prolapse, and translational malalignment as occurs with facet joint dislocations.

Spinal Cord

Injury to the cervical spinal cord can be caused by ischemia, compression, distraction, penetration, or various combinations of these. Knowledge of spinal cord and nerve root anatomy is useful in determining the level and type of spinal cord injury.

The lateral spinothalamic tract is an afferent (ascending) tract located within the anterolateral aspect of the cord that transmits pain and temperature sensation (Fig. 18-3). It is somatopically arranged; representation of more cephalad levels is within its anteromedial aspect and that for

more caudal levels within its posterolateral aspect. Pain and temperature nerve fibers decussate at the level they exit the spinal cord. Injury to the lateral spinal thalamic tract therefore, results in pain and temperature loss of the contralateral side of the body.

The dorsal columns comprise the fasciculi gracilis and fasciculi cuneatus. They transmit non-noxious (not pain and temperature) sensory input to the brain. This includes proprioception, vibratory sense, pressure, and tactile discrimination (touch). The dorsal columns are also arranged somatopically. However, more cephalad innervation is located within the lateral regions of the tract. Tract fibers decussate above the foramen magnum before the spinal cord is formed. Injury therefore causes ipsilateral deficits.

Spinal cord gray matter (cell bodies) has a butterfly or H-shaped appearance in cross section and as such has been divided into dorsal and anterior horns. The dorsal horns contain sensory nerve cell bodies that transmit pain, temperature, and touch. The anterior horns contain motor nerve cell bodies. Gray matter is topographically arranged so more cephalad innervation is located within its central aspects. This helps explain why patients with central cord syndrome have greater upper extremity than lower extremity involvement.

CLASSIFICATION

A number of classifications are used for cervical spine fractures.

Occipital Condyles

These have been classified by Anderson and Montesano (1988). The classification is shown in Figure 18-4. There are three types. Type I fractures are comminuted fractures caused by impaction of the occipital condyle onto the lateral mass of the atlas. Type II fractures are associated with a basal skull fracture and usually caused by a direct blow, and type III fractures are avulsion fractures caused by a distraction force through the alar ligaments.

Occipitocervical Instability

The classification system for occipitocervical instability is based on the direction of displacement. It is shown in Figure 18-5. There are three types. Type I fractures present with anterior displacement of the occiput with respect to the atlas. This type is common in children. In type II fractures, distraction occurs at the occipitoatlantal level in IIa lesions and at the atlantoaxial level in IIb lesions. In the rare type III lesion, there is posterior displacement of the occiput with respect to the atlas.

Odontoid Fractures

Anderson and D'Alonzo (1974) defined the three types of odontoid fractures (Fig. 18-6). Type I fractures are avulsion fractures of the tip of the dens. These are usually stable, although they can occur with occipitocervical instability. Type II fractures occur at the base of the dens, and type III fractures occur through the body of C2.

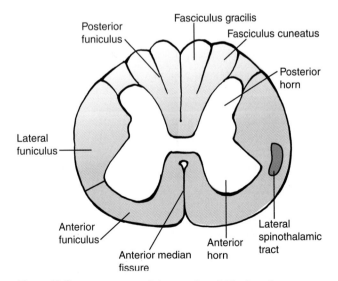

Figure 18-3 Cross section of the spinal cord. The lateral spinothalamic tract transmits pain and temperature. It decussates at the level it innervates; therefore an injury causes a contralateral deficit. The dorsal columns (fasciculus gracilis and cuneatus) transmit non-noxious sensation. The gray matter (cell bodies) appears as an "H" or butterfly on cross section. It is divided into posterior horns (sensory) and anterior horns (motor).

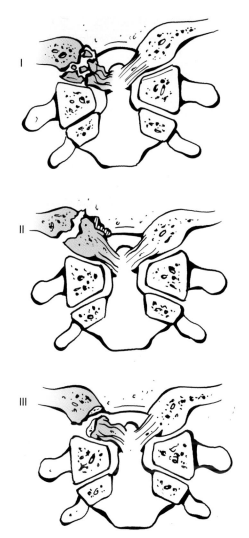

Figure 18-4 The Anderson and Montesano (1988) system for classification of occipital condyle fractures.

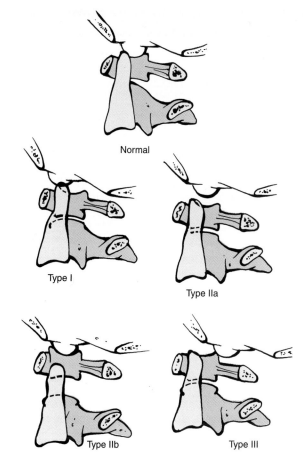

Figure 18-5 Classification of occipitocervical instability.

Traumatic Spondylolithesis of the Axis (Hangman Fracture)

Hangman fracture was classified by Levine and Edwards (1992). There are four types, which are shown in Figure 18-7. In type I fractures, the fracture is through the isthmus near the base of the pedicle. There is less than 3 mm of displacement and no angulation. They result from hyperextension or axial loads. In a type Ia variant, the fracture line is more oblique and difficult to see on a conventional lateral radiograph. The C2 isthmus appears elongated. In type II fractures, there is more than 3 mm of translation and significant angulation. These are caused by initial hyperextension and axial loading, followed by hyperflexion. There may be some compression of the anterosuperior portion of the body of C3, and disruption of the C2-3 disc often occurs. The fracture line is usually vertical and close to the junction of the body and pedicle. The anterior longitudinal ligament is stripped off the superior one third to one half of the body of C3 but is still in continuity. Type IIA fractures show significant angulation (>15 degrees) and minimal translation. They occur as an outcome of flexion

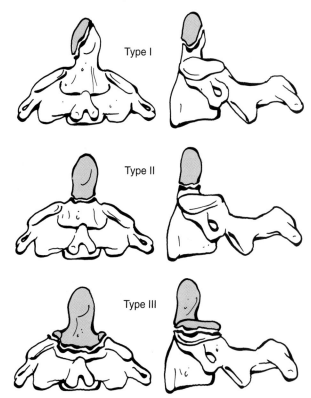

Figure 18-6 Odontoid fractures are classified by the location of the fracture line (Anderson and D'Alonzo, 1974). Type II fractures have the poorest healing potential.

TABLE 18-2 DESCRIPTIVE CLASSIFICATION OF SUBAXIAL CERVICAL INJURIES

Classification	Description
Vertebral body fractures	
Compression fractures	Anterior wedge fractures with no posterior vertebral body involvement
Teardrop fractures	A fracture that extends obliquely from the anterosuperior vertebral body to the inferior endplate
	The degree of endplate involvement varies
Burst fractures	Extensive vertebral body comminution with height loss and retropulsion of bone fragments into the spinal canal
Facet injuries	
Isolated facet fractures	Can be associated with ligamentous injury leading to subluxation and instability that is usually rotational
Facet subluxations	Associated with capsule and posterior ligament disruption
	Some of the facets still in apposition
Facet dislocations	May be unilateral or bilateral
	Often described as perched or locked
Facet fracture-dislocations	Unilateral or bilateral facet dislocations associated with fracture
Pedicle and laminar fractures	
Isolated unilateral pedicle fractures	Can suggest rotational instability
	Pedicle and facet fractures often referred to as lateral mass fractures
Laminar and pedicle fractures	This fracture combination negates the stabilizing effect of the adjacent facet joint
	Referred to as a floating lateral mass fracture
	Can destabilize two motion segments
Anterior tension band disruption	The anterior longitudinal ligament and disc fail in tension
	X-rays show widening of the disc space suggestive of significant instability
	There may be small avulsion fractures of the vertebral body; these are referred to as extension-type teardrop fractures
	More common in elderly patients

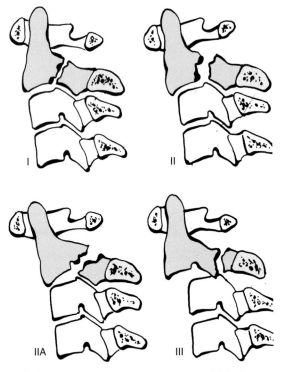

Figure 18-7   Classification of traumatic C2 spondylolisthesis (Hangman fracture) by Levine and Edwards (1992). The types are separated according to angulation and displacement. Type III injuries should be not be placed in cranial traction.

distraction, resulting in failure of the posterior disc. In type III fractures, there is a C2-3 facet dislocation in addition to the displaced pars fractures and a higher rate of neurological injury than with other fracture types.

Subaxial Fractures

Allen et al. (1982) devised a classification system based on the mechanism of injury. They divided fractures into six groups, shown in Figure 18-8. The injury mechanisms are compression flexion, vertical compression, distraction flexion, compression extension, distraction extension, and lateral flexion.

Descriptive Classification

Cervical fractures and dislocations can be described using identifiable injury characteristics thought to influence mechanical stability and the method of treatment. A descriptive classification is listed in Table 18-2.

EPIDEMIOLOGY

The basic epidemiology of cervical spine fractures is given in Table 18-3. The overall spinal distribution shows a type H curve with a bimodal distribution in men and women (see Chapter 1).

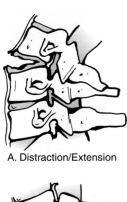
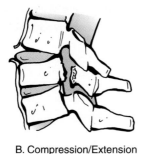
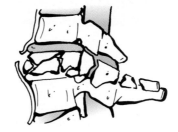
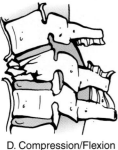
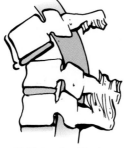
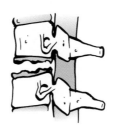

A. Distraction/Extension   B. Compression/Extension   C. Compression

D. Compression/Flexion   E. Distraction/Flexion   F. Lateral flexion

Figure 18-8 Classification of subaxial fractures proposed by Allen and Ferguson (1982).

Fractures of the atlas represent about 10% and odontoid fractures 18% of all cervical spine fractures. Fractures of C6 and C7 account for 40% of cervical spine injuries. Spinal cord damage is more commonly associated with lower cervical spine fractures and dislocations. Motor vehicle accidents account for most of the fractures in younger patients, with falls causing most injuries in older patients.

Associated Injuries

As with all fractures with a bimodal distribution, young patients who present with high-energy cervical spine injuries tend to have other musculoskeletal injuries. In the patients analyzed in Table 18-3, 37% had other musculoskeletal injuries, with an equal distribution between upper limb and lower limb injuries. In older patients, cervical spine fractures tend to follow low-energy injuries, such as a fall, and be isolated injuries.

TABLE 18-3 EPIDEMIOLOGY OF CERVICAL SPINE FRACTURES

Proportion of all fractures	0.3%
Proportion of spinal fractures	52.5%
Average patient age	43.4 y
Men/women	58%/42%
Distribution	Type H
Incidence	$3.6/10^5$/y
Open fractures	0%
Most common cause	
Motor vehicle accident	47.4%
OTA (AO) classification	
Type A	64.3%
Type B	28.6%
Type C	7.1%
Most common subgroup	
A3	42.9%

DIAGNOSIS

Clinical History and Examination

■ A complete examination should be undertaken in the awake, alert patient.
   ▨ If the patient has been injured in a motor vehicle accident or a fall from a height, multiple injuries are likely, and an examination according to ATLS principles is mandatory.
   ▨ The patient should be questioned about previous injuries, the nature of the current injury, and where he or she is feeling pain.
   ▨ Concomitant injuries, such as extremity or pelvic fractures, can decrease a patient's awareness of pain associated with a spinal injury. This highlights the importance of performing both an initial and secondary examination.
   ▨ The direction of impact, such as in a motor vehicle collision, can yield clues about the possible mechanism of spinal injury.
   ▨ In the unconscious, nonalert patient, eyewitnesses or emergency medical technicians present at the scene may be questioned about the mechanism of injury.
■ The spine should be examined in a systematic manner.
   ▨ The spinous processes should be palpated individually noting tenderness, crepitus, or step-off.
   ▨ Bruising or laceration, as well as penetrating wounds, should be noted and marked.
   ▨ Swelling and fullness in the anterior neck can suggest prevertebral hematoma, which may be a clue to significant trauma to the spine.
   ▨ Rotation of the head and neck should be noted because patients with C1-C2 rotatory subluxation or occipitocervical dislocations may present with a cock-robin spine.

TABLE 18-4 MYOTOMES, DERMATOMES, AND REFLEXES OF THE UPPER AND LOWER LIMBS

Nerve Root Level	Motor	Sensory	Reflex
C5	Deltoid (shoulder abduction)	Lateral shoulder and arm	Biceps
C6	Biceps/wrist extension	Lateral forearm, thumb and index finger	Brachioradialis
C7	Triceps/wrist flexors	Middle finger	Triceps
C8	Finger flexors	Ring and little finger, medial forearm	—
T1	Hand intrinsics (abduction)	Medial arm	—
T12	—	Inguinal crease	—
L2-3	Iliopsoas (hip flexion)	Anterior thigh	—
L4	Quadriceps (knee extension)	Medial ankle	Patella tendon (knee jerk)
L5	Anterior tibialis, EHL (dorsiflexion)	First web space foot	—
S1	Gastrocnemius (plantar flexion)	Lateral foot	Achilles tendon (ankle jerk)
S2-4	—	—	Bulbocavernosus
S4-5	Anal sphincter	Perianal	Anocutaneous

■ Areas of ecchymosis on the face or scalp might be the result of direct impact and may suggest the direction of injury.
■ A detailed neurological examination is performed in the awake, alert patient.
  ■ This should include motor, sensory, and reflex testing in all myotomes and dermatomes (Table 18-4).
  ■ Muscle strength should be graded from 0 to 5.
  ■ Perianal sensation is a sign of sacral nerve root sparing and can be a positive prognostic sign for neurological recovery in patients who otherwise would be classified as having a complete spinal cord injury (no other motor or sensory function below the level of injury).
  ■ In the nonalert patient, the neurological examination is limited, but key components can still be performed.
  ■ If the patient has not been paralyzed pharmacologically, rectal tone should be evaluated and graded.
  ■ The presence or absence of a bulbocavernosus (BC) reflex should also be noted and documented.
  ■ The return of the BC reflex marks the end of spinal shock, which usually resolves within 48 hours of injury.

Radiologic Examination

Upper Cervical Spine

■ A lateral cervical radiograph is a standard component of the general trauma series.
  ■ This view is useful in detecting up to 85% of cervical spine injuries.
■ Although plain films are traditionally considered the standard initial imaging technique for the cervical spine, CT scans have become more widely used in recent years because they are better than plain radiography at visualizing the craniocervical junction.
■ A number of important measurements and relationships in the upper cervical spine can be noted on a plain lateral film (Fig. 18-9).
■ Harris described the basion-dens interval (BDI) and basion-axis interval (BAI) for detection of occipitocervical dissociation or dislocation.

■ Measurements of 12 mm or more should be considered highly suspicious of instability.
■ The Power ratio is also useful.
  ■ The ratio of a line drawn from the basion to the posterior arch of the atlas over the line from the opisthion to the anterior arch of the atlas should be less than 1.0.
  ■ A ratio greater than 1.0 is suggestive of an anterior occipitoatlantal dislocation.
■ The atlantodental interval (ADI) is used to determine the stability of the atlantoaxial segment.
  ■ A value greater than 3 mm in an adult and 4 mm in a child is suggestive of rupture of the transverse ligament.

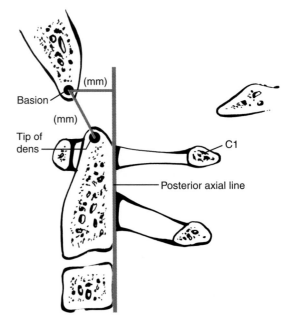

Figure 18-9 Harris's lines, or the rule of twelves, are an effective means of assessing craniocervical dissociation. A line is drawn from the tip of the dens to the basion (BDI). Normal, this should measure less than 12 mm. A posterior vertebral body tangent line is drawn behind C2. Normally, the transverse distance from this line to the basion (BAI) should also measure less than 12 mm.

Plain Radiographs

- A number of radiographic injury characteristics can be assessed and measured on a lateral cervical film.
- The atlantodens interval (ADI) is defined as the measurement between the posterior aspect of the anterior C1 ring and the anterior aspect of the odontoid process.
- Odontoid fracture angulation can be measured by drawing a line along the anterior aspect of the dens fragment and C2 vertebral body.
- Sagittal displacement of the fracture can also be measured on this view.
- Angulation of C2 on C3 is best measured using a posterior vertebral body tangent method.
  - This is helpful in evaluating and classifying Hangman fractures.
- The posterior vertebral body tangent can be used to measure translational displacement (Fig. 18-10).
- Open-mouth views are important in evaluating the amount of lateral overhang after C1 burst (Jefferson) fractures.

Computed Tomography

- Axial CT images should be studied systematically in each case to help detect subtle fractures of the occipital condyles, C1 ring, or odontoid process.
- Sagittal and coronal reconstructions can aid in the understanding of the three-dimensional nature of spinal injuries.
- Parasagittal slices through the occipitoatlantal joints can help determine if there is anterior or posterior displacement.
  - Widening of the joints can suggest the presence of a distraction injury, which is highly unstable.
- Midsagittal reconstructions can help visualize dislocations, subluxations, or fracture fragment size.

Magnetic Resonance Imaging

- The role of MRI continues to be defined in spinal trauma.

- Its superiority in visualizing the spinal cord, intervertebral disc, and spinal ligaments gives it some advantages over CT.
- Specifically, in the upper cervical spine, an MRI can demonstrate high signal intensity within the atlantodens articulation after transverse and alar ligament disruption.
- Similarly, it can reveal discontinuity of the tectorial membrane (the proximal continuation of the posterior longitudinal ligament that normally inserts onto the basion).

Subaxial Cervical Spine

- Plain radiographs are useful in diagnosing lower cervical injuries.
- A standard cervical series includes lateral, anteroposterior, and open-mouth views.
- Between 83% and 99% of injuries can be detected using these three views.
- A radiographic series that does not allow visualization of the entire cervicothoracic junction should be considered inadequate.
- Traction on the patient's arms can facilitate imaging.
- A swimmer's view entails placing one arm in a fully abducted position while leaving the other arm at the patient's side.
  - This view is particularly useful in visualizing the lower cervical spine and the cervicothoracic junction.
- Prevertebral swelling can be detected on a lateral radiograph by assessing the soft tissue shadow thickness anterior to the vertebral bodies (Fig. 18-11).

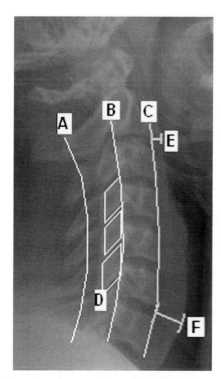

Figure 18-11 Lines and landmarks on a normal lateral cervical spine film. The spinolaminar line (**A**), posterior vertebral body line (**B**), and anterior vertebral body line (**C**) are normally unbroken. On a perfect lateral view, the facet joints should appear as stacked parallelograms (**D**). The prevertebral soft-tissue shadow is measured at the C2-3 (**E**) and C6-7 (**F**) disc spaces. More than 7 mm at the C2-3 and 21 mm at the C6-7 disc is strongly suggestive of an underlying spinal injury.

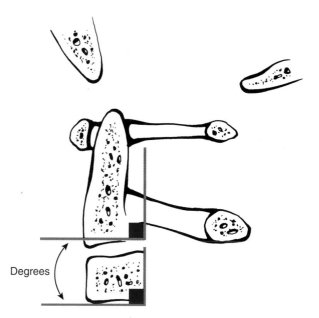

Figure 18-10 C2 angulation, as can occur with Hangman fractures, can be measured using the posterior vertebral body tangent method.

- If this measures more than 7 mm in front of the C2-3 disc space or more than 21 mm at the C6-7 disc space, there is a high likelihood of a cervical spinal injury.
    - The absence of prevertebral (retropharyngeal) soft tissue swelling does not reliably rule out an occult cervical spine injury, however, because its reported sensitivity is only 65%.
- Normally the spinolaminar line, posterior vertebral body line, and anterior vertebral body line should appear unbroken on the lateral cervical radiograph (see Fig. 18-11).
    - The spinolaminar line is perhaps the most useful because it is not usually affected by spondylotic changes such as osteophytes, which may be present along both the posterior vertebral and anterior aspects of the vertebral bodies.
- The lateral view is also useful in judging the distance between the interspinous processes.
    - Substantial widening at one level suggests disruption of the PLC.
- The facet joints normally appear as stacked parallelograms on the lateral cervical radiograph (see Fig. 18-11).
- In a perfect lateral view, the joints on either side should overlie each other, facilitating assessment of joint congruity.

Plain Radiographs

- A number of radiographic injury characteristics can be assessed and measured on a lateral cervical film.
- Segmental kyphosis can be measured by the Cobb method or posterior vertebral body tangent method.
- Kyphosis more than 11 degrees (or greater than 3.5 mm of translation) is strongly suggestive of posterior ligamentous injury and potential instability.
- Anteroposterior translational deformity can be assessed and measured on the lateral view.
- The distance between the posterior vertebral body tangent lines at the level of the disc space can be used to measure the absolute distance in millimeters.

- Vertebral body height is measured at the injured and adjacent uninjured levels to calculate the percentage height loss.
- Primary fracture lines, present with so-called tear-drop fractures, should be outlined.

Computed Tomography

- Axial CT images should be studied systematically.
- First, the vertebral bodies and pedicles should be labeled according to level so fractures or dislocations can be located accurately.
- CT is particularly useful for detecting sagittal vertebral body fracture lines that are usually less obvious on plain films.
- Fracture fragment retropulsion is readily appreciated on axial CT slices, as is the degree of vertebral body comminution.
- Pedicle fractures are often undetectable on plain films but easily seen on axial CT images.
- Facet and laminar fractures are also easily detected on CT images.
- Sagittal and coronal reconstructions can aid the understanding of the three-dimensional nature of spinal injuries.
- Parasagittal slices through the facet joints can help visualize dislocations, subluxations, or fracture fragment size (Fig. 18-12).

Magnetic Resonance Imaging

- MRI is superior to CT in visualizing the spinal cord, intervertebral disc, and spinal ligaments.
- MRI can detect subtle bone edema associated with vertebral body fractures, but its visualization of the bony architecture is inferior to CT, making it unsuitable as a stand-alone modality for fracture description.
- The most useful applications of MRI are in detecting traumatic disc herniations, epidural hematomata, spinal cord edema or compression, and posterior ligamentous disruption.
- An additional application of MRI is the ability to visualize vascular structures.

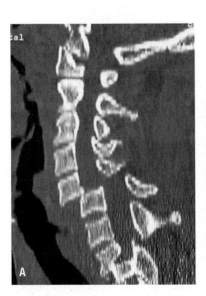

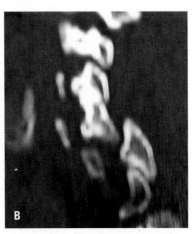

Figure 18-12 (A) Sagittal reconstructions can demonstrate the extent of canal compromise. In this case, bilateral facet dislocation was associated with a complete spinal cord injury. (B) Parasagittal reconstructions can help visualize facet dislocations.

■ MR arteriograms can be used to assess the patency of the vertebral arteries.

Prereduction MRI for Facet Dislocations

■ The role of prereduction MRI for facet dislocations remains controversial.
■ Closed reduction may result in increased neurological damage.
  ■ It is believed that intervertebral disc herniations, pulled back into the spinal cord during reduction, are a major contributing factor.
■ Because of this, some surgeons advocate MRI prior to reduction to exclude disc herniation.
■ In an awake, alert, and examinable patient, however, a prereduction MRI may not be necessary.
■ Two recent clinical reports have demonstrated that closed reduction of facet dislocation can be performed safely, provided that serial neurological examinations can be performed adequately.
■ Ultimately, the relative advantages and disadvantages of early reduction and anatomical alignment versus the increased complexity of performing anterior decompression and reduction on a dislocated spine are still not clearly established and likely to remain controversial.

TREATMENT

Initial Management

■ The initial management of a patient with a potential cervical spine injury begins in the field.
■ Manual immobilization of the head and neck should be maintained until a hard cervical collar can be applied.
■ Various types of cervical orthoses are available (see Chapter 31).
  ■ Ideally they should contain an anterior window to accommodate a tracheostomy tube or facilitate an emergency cricothyroidotomy.
■ Airway security and hemodynamic resuscitation are crucial to the overall survival of the patient.
  ■ With intubation, manipulation of the neck can potentially displace unstable cervical fractures or dislocations.
  ■ Manual in-line stabilization should be maintained throughout the intubation process.
■ If an unstable spine is suspected, a cricothyroidotomy may be the safest method of controlling the airway.
■ Helmets, like those used for sports or motorcycling, should be kept in place during initial evaluation and medical stabilization.
■ The face mask or visor can be removed to access the eyes, nose, and mouth.

Hospital Resuscitation

■ It is recommended that an arterial oxygen partial pressure of at least 100 Torr be maintained.
■ Neurogenic shock, as apposed to hemorrhagic shock in which compensatory tachycardia is usually present, should be treated with a combination of postural maneuvers (Trendelenburg position), appropriate fluid infusion, and vasopressor administration.
■ If neurogenic shock is treated as purely hypovolemic shock, fluid overload can quickly ensue, leading to pulmonary edema or other systemic complications.

Steroids

■ The role of steroids remains controversial. There is currently no consensus as to whether methylprednisolone (MP) should be administered to patients with acute spinal cord injury. Supportive data from large multicenter trials suggests it may have modest beneficial effects on neurological recovery.
■ Current recommendations for the administration of MP are based on the drug regimens used in these studies (Box 18-2).
■ Children less than 13 years of age and patients who sustained penetrating injuries were not included in these studies, and therefore these recommendations do not apply to these groups.
■ In subsequent studies steroid administration has not demonstrated neurological benefit in patients with penetrating spinal cord injury, although it has led to an increase in gastrointestinal and pulmonary complications.
■ It is recommended that steroids be used in adults who have spinal cord injury following blunt trauma.

Nonsurgical Treatment

■ The design and use of cervical braces, cervicothoracic braces, spinal traction, and halo-body casts and braces is discussed in Chapter 31.

Surgical Treatment

■ The optimal time to perform surgery, particularly in patients with neurological deficits, still remains unclear.
■ The two most commonly proposed benefits of early surgery are improved rates of neurological recovery and improved patient mobilization without the risk of spinal displacement.
■ Animal studies have suggested a significant benefit from early decompression after acute spinal cord injury.
■ Little human clinical evidence is available to support the belief that early surgical decompression and

---

BOX 18-2 CURRENT RECOMMENDATIONS FOR THE ADMINISTRATION OF METHYLPREDNISOLONE (MP)

■ Bolus dose of 30 mg/kg of MP to be administered over 15 to 30 minutes to patients presenting within 8 hours from injury
■ A maintenance dose of 5.4 mg/kg/hr of MP to be administered for 23 hours to patients presenting within 3 hours from injury
■ A maintenance dose of 5.4 mg/kg/hr of MP to be administered for 48 hours to patients presenting within 8 hours from injury

stabilization improves neurological recovery rates, however.

- In the only randomized, prospective, controlled trial found in the literature, surgery performed for cervical spinal cord injuries less than 72 hours versus more than 5 days after the injury demonstrated no significant difference in motor scores at final follow-up.
- Other nonrandomized prospective studies have demonstrated similar findings.
- In one report, only 10% of surgery could be performed within 8 hours of injury.

Upper Cervical Spine

- A synopsis of the commonly used surgical techniques for the upper cervical spine follows.
- The advantage of rigid internal fixation for cervical spinal injuries is that the need for postoperative external immobilization is reduced and may be eliminated.
- However, this should be evaluated on a case-by-case basis, mainly determined by the quality of fixation achieved.
- If indicated, postoperative antiembolic chemoprophylaxis can be started on day 4 or 5 to avoid an epidural hematoma.
- Prophylactic antibiotics are continued for 48 hours.

Odontoid Screw Fixation

- Anterior odontoid screw is used for type II and III odontoid fractures.
- Fracture lines that are anteroinferior to posterosuperior are not suitable.
- One or two screws are used.
- Anterior cervical approach at the C5-C6 level is used to gain proper trajectory for screw insertion.
- A barrel chest may make screw insertion difficult.

Occipitocervical Junction

- Occiput can be stabilized to the axis by a variety of methods.
- An early method involved wiring iliac crest autograft to the bone.
- Plate-rod systems have now been developed.
- A plate is secured to the external occipital protuberance and then connected to rods or plated secured to C2.

Atlantoaxial Junction

- The C1-C2 joint can be secured using simple wiring techniques using structural iliac crest autograft (Gallie or Brook fusion).
- Alternatively, transarticular screws may be placed across the C1-C2 facet joints.
- This technique may be contraindicated in patients with high C2 vertebral artery foraminae.

Subaxial Spine

- Subaxial fractures are surgically treated by anterior or posterior stabilization.

Anterior Surgery

- A left-sided incision is made, using the interval between sternocleidomastoid and the anterior strap muscles.
- Exposure is deepened between the carotid sheath laterally and the esophagus and trachea medially.

- Care should be taken not to damage the recurrent laryngeal nerve.
- Decompression is undertaken via discectomy or vertebrectomy, a decision based on the extent of the bony injury and degree of neural compression as determined by preoperative imaging.
- If there is a herniated cervical disc associated with dislocated facet joints, an anterior discectomy and decompression should be performed prior to reduction.
- After decompression the superior and inferior end plates of the defect are flattened and burred until there is punctate bleeding.
- Autograft or allograft strut grafts are then used to reconstruct the anterior column.
- Anterior cervical plates should be used to span discectomy or vertebrectomy defects.
- Fixed-angle locking screw-plate systems provide better biomechanical stability than nonfixed bicortical screw-plate systems.

Posterior Surgery

- A midline dissection is undertaken within the avascular plane of the ligamentum nuchae, which separates the right and left paraspinal muscles.
- Subperiosteal dissection is performed on each side of the spinous processes to the spinolaminar junction, and then laterally over the laminae.
- Lateral dissection should be undertaken only at the levels to be fused, and only the facet joints that will be fused should be exposed, along with their corresponding lateral masses.
- In the majority of acute traumatic subaxial spinal injuries, posterior decompression via laminectomy is not necessary.
  - This is not true, however, in cases of acute spinal cord injury associated with multilevel spondylotic stenosis or ossification of the posterior longitudinal ligament, in which a posterior decompressive procedure might be considered the procedure of choice if cervical lordosis has been maintained.
- Open reduction of dislocated facet joints can be performed using a posterior approach.
- If the spinous processes are intact, they can be grasped with towel clips near their base to flex and distract the injured joint.
- If they are fractured, an elevator can be placed over the top of the superior articular process at the lower level.
- If these maneuvers fail, the tip of the superior articular process of the lower vertebra can be resected using a burr or small rongeur.
- The simplest form of posterior instrumentation is interspinous process wire stabilization.
- Facet wiring has also been advocated to stabilize cervical spine injuries.
- Lateral mass screw fixation has become more popular in recent years.
- Both plate and rod systems are currently available.
- The newest systems include variable-angle titanium screws connected to longitudinal rods.
- The advantages of these systems over lateral mass plates are that they are more forgiving of minor variations in

screw position, and they enable optimal screw placement to be determined by the patient's anatomy or injury rather than the location of the holes in the plate.
- For fusion, the exposed bony surfaces should be decorticated using a high-speed burr.
- Cancellous bone harvested from the posterior iliac crest is used.

Treatment of Specific Fractures

Upper Cervical Fractures

- The suggested treatment of upper cervical fractures is shown in Table 18-5.

Subaxial Fractures

Compression Fractures

Nonsurgical Treatment
- Patients with cervical compression fractures without posterior ligamentous injury can be treated nonoperatively (Fig. 18-13).

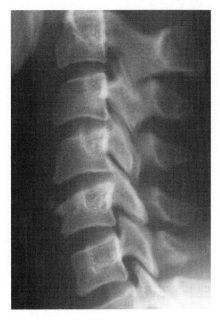

Figure 18-13 Simple compression fractures in the cervical spine are uncommon. In this case the posterior ligaments were intact, as evidenced by an unchanged kyphosis. The patient was successfully treated in a rigid cervical collar for 12 weeks.

TABLE 18-5 SUGGESTED TREATMENT OF UPPER CERVICAL FRACTURES

Injury	Treatment
Occipital condyle fractures (see Fig. 18-4)	
Type I	Cervical collar
Type II	
Stable	Rigid cervical collar
Unstable	Posterior occipitocervical fusion
Type III	Posterior occipitocervical fusion
Occipitocervical instability (see Fig. 18-5)	
Type I	Traction reduction. Halo immobilization
Type II	Posterior occipitocervical fusion
Type III	Traction reduction. Halo immobilization
C1 ring fractures	
Isolated posterior arch fracture	Cervical collar
Anterior and posterior ring fractures	
<7 mm displacement of C1 on C2	Rigid cervical collar
>7 mm displacement of C1 on C2	Halo traction. Halo immobilization
Odontoid fractures (see Fig. 18-6)	
Type I	Cervical collar
Type II	
Minimally displaced	Halo vest
Displaced	Screw fixation or C1-C2 fusion
Type III	
Minimally displaced	Cervical collar
Displaced	Halo vest
C1-C2 ligamentous instability	
Atlantodental interval <5 mm	
No neurological deficit	Collar
Neurological deficit	Posterior C1-C2 fusion
Atlantodental interval >5 mm	Posterior C1-C2 fusion
Traumatic spondylolisthesis of the axis (see Fig. 18-7)	
Type I	Rigid cervical collar
Type II	Traction reduction followed by halo vest
Type III	Open reduction and posterior C2-C3 fusion

- For injuries of C3 to C6, a rigid cervical collar usually suffices.
- For injuries of C7 or T1, a cervicothoracic brace offers better control.
- If the injury is stable, the orthosis minimizes motion at the fracture site, which can decrease pain and facilitate resolution of muscular spasm.
- A lateral radiograph should be obtained with patient sitting or standing prior to discharge because this can sometimes demonstrate instability.
- The fracture is usually healed by 3 months, at which time flexion extension views under the patient's own control should be obtained to rule occult instability, either at the level of the injury or at a distant site.

Surgical Treatment

- Surgical stabilization should be considered for patients with evidence of posterior ligamentous injury.
  - This is suggested by a segmental kyphosis greater than 11 degrees or significant vertebral body wedging.
  - MRI evidence of ligamentous injury should also be considered.
- Prior to surgery, cervical traction with slight extension can be used to realign the fracture.
  - This is best performed in the awake patient.

Burst Fractures

- Cervical burst fractures are usually high-energy injuries.
- Radiographic signs are vertebral body comminution that involves the posterior vertebral body, usually with retropulsed fragments that result in spinal canal compromise (Fig. 18-14).
- Spinal cord injury is common.
- Immediate realignment with cranial traction can help clear the canal to some degree, provided the PLL is intact.
  - It will also provide temporary stabilization until surgery.
- MRI and CT scans can be useful in detecting spinal cord edema and the location of retropulsed bony fragments.

Nonsurgical Treatment

- Nonoperative treatment can be considered in neurologically intact patients with little vertebral body comminution and only the mildest degree of canal compromise.
- There should be minimal kyphotic deformity and no indication of posterior ligamentous injury.
- Because of the potential for vertebral body collapse, a halo vest or rigid cervicothoracic orthosis should be used.
- Prior to discharge, radiographs should be obtained with the patient standing or sitting and compared to supine films.

Surgical Treatment

- Patients with neurological deficit, regardless of the integrity of the PLC, should be stabilized surgically.
- Retropulsed vertebral body fragments are most easily accessed through a direct anterior approach.
- The fractured vertebral body should be resected and the spinal canal decompressed.
- Intraoperative traction can help realign the spine if significant deformity exists.
- The anterior column should be reconstructed with a strut graft.
- An anterior cervical plate is then applied to restore anterior stability.
- If the PLC appears disrupted, a supplementary posterior instrumented fusion should be undertaken either during the same operation or at a later time.

Flexion-Type Teardrop Fractures

- The characteristic pattern of teardrop fractures has already been described.
- They often have a sagittal split within the posterior vertebral body and may be confused with burst fractures.
- These fractures typically occur in younger patients with high-energy trauma.
- Posterior ligament disruption is suggested by more than 11 degrees of kyphosis or posterior vertebral body translation.

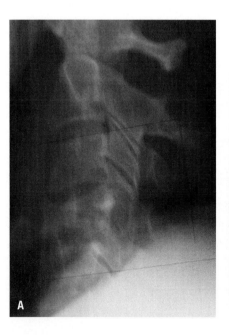

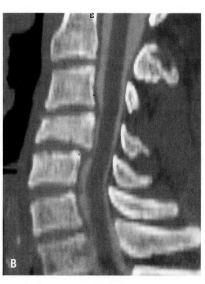

Figure 18-14 **(A,B)** Burst fractures are higher energy injuries. The proposed injury mechanism is an axial load, with or without flexion. Involvement of the posterior vertebral body, often with retropulsed fragments, is the radiographic hallmark. It is more easily assessed with CT.

- MRI can be confirmatory.
- Patients often present with a neurological deficit.

Nonsurgical Treatment
- There is a definite role for nonoperative treatment of cervical teardrop fractures.
- Minimally displaced fractures with little kyphosis and no PLC injury are stable.
  - They can be treated in a rigid cervical collar or cervicothoracic orthosis, depending on the level of injury.
- Halo treatment should be used for unstable fractures.
  - It can help realign fractures, which aids canal clearance in patients with spinal cord injury.
  - Halo treatment for unstable teardrop fractures results in inferior radiographic results compared to anterior surgery, although neurological and clinical outcome scores appear comparable.
  - The halo should be kept in place for 3 months, provided acceptable alignment has been maintained.
  - After it has been removed, a flexion extension radiograph should be obtained to confirm stability has been achieved.

Surgical Treatment
- In patients with a neurological deficit, anterior vertebrectomy is usually performed to remove the retropulsed bone fragments.
- This is followed by anterior strut grafting and rigid plating (Fig. 18-15).
- In some cases, an unstable teardrop fracture can occur in a neurologically intact patient.
  - In these cases, anterior surgery can include a nondecompressive vertebrectomy, which entails resection of the majority of the vertebral body back to, but not through, the posterior wall.
  - This is best reserved for injuries without a retrolisthesis.

- Some surgeons prefer to perform a single-level discectomy or partial vertebrectomy.
- If there is an extensive endplate fracture, there is a risk of failure of anterior fixation.
- Posterior surgery occasionally can be used.
  - This should be reserved for patients who are neurologically intact and have minimal vertebral body height loss with less than 30% of inferior endplate involvement.
  - A potential advantage of this approach is that the fusion can be limited to a single motion segment.

Facet Fractures Without Dislocation

- There is considerable disagreement concerning the management of facet fractures without dislocation.
- The majority of fractures initially present as minimally displaced fractures and can be treated nonoperatively with a rigid cervical collar without significant late displacement.
- In some cases, however, the fracture itself is not the essential lesion.
- Occult ligamentous disruption can be present.
- MRI has found an increasingly important role in differentiating so-called stable and unstable facet fractures and may be an important tool in treatment decision making.

Nonsurgical Treatment
- Most facet fractures are minimally displaced and can be considered mechanically stable.
- Such patients can be treated in a rigid cervical collar for a period of 6 to 12 weeks, monitored by frequent radiographic examination.
- Despite being minimally displaced, they can be associated with occult unstable ligamentous injury, however.
- Many authors recommend routine MRI examination to rule out significant ligamentous damage.

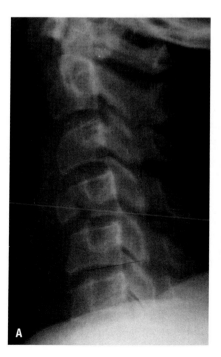
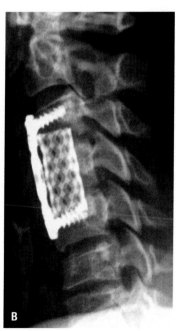

Figure 18-15 (**A**) Teardrop fractures usually occur from a flexion-compression-type mechanism. Shear forces result in the classic oblique teardrop fragment. The fracture line extends from anterosuperior to posteroinferior. (**B**) Anterior corpectomy, fusion, and plate stabilization is the usual treatment for unstable injuries.

- Disruption of the ALL and intervertebral disc are thought to play in important role in late displacement, although PLC injury can also occur.
- Neurological injury associated with the fracture is rare, and if present is usually limited to a mild single root radiculopathy that often resolves without formal decompression.
- Flexion extension views should be obtained after the application of a collar to confirm stability.
- Although late displacement is considered an indicator of instability by most surgeons, it has been observed that the spine can stabilize with time.
- The long-term consequences of residual deformity on the overall clinical outcome are unclear, however.

Surgical Treatment

- Because of the inconsistency of ligamentous instability, some surgeons have recommended operative treatment for nearly all facet fractures.
- Others have focused the indications by making use of flexion extension views or MRI scans.
- A study of the predictive value of MRI on displacement of facet fractures has yet to be published.
- Either anterior or posterior surgery can be performed to treat facet fractures.

Facet Subluxation/Dislocations

- The treatment of facet subluxations and dislocations (Fig. 18-16) is not differentiated in the literature, probably because they represent stages of the same traumatic process from facet capsule disruption to complete bilateral locked facets.
- Unilateral dislocations can occur without catastrophic PLC disruption, however, whereas bilateral facet subluxation, without frank dislocation, is usually associated with PLC disruption.

Nonsurgical Treatment

- There is little role for nonoperative treatment for facet dislocations.
- If used it should be reserved for unilateral facet dislocations in patients without any signs of neurological injury or for those who are too sick to undergo surgery.

- Cervical orthoses do not provide adequate treatment, and it has been shown that more than 50% of patients have persistent instability after treatment with a halo vest.
- Frequent radiographic examination is important.
- Evidence of fusion of the dislocated facet joint, or, less frequently, the disc space, is a sign of healing.
- After a course of about 3 months of halo immobilization, the device should be removed and flexion extension views should be obtained to confirm stability.
- Surgical fusion should be considered if instability is present.

Surgical Treatment

- The optimal treatment of unilateral or bilateral facet dislocations remains contentious.
- Closed reduction and the role of MRI have already been discussed.
  - Closed reduction is safe in the awake cooperative patient who can be serially examined.
  - In other patients, and particularly in the incomplete spinal cord injured patient, a prereduction MRI is required to look for a herniated disc.
- Once the facet dislocations have been reduced, anterior or posterior surgery can be performed.
- No clear evidence indicates which is better, although posterior stabilization more directly treats the instability caused by PLC disruption.
- A postreduction MRI is usually performed prior to surgery (see Fig. 18-16).
- Few surgeons use posterior surgery alone in the presence of a herniated disc after reduction in a neurologically intact patient.
- Anterior surgery can be performed to remove the herniated disc.
- Combined anterior and posterior surgery may also be performed, although this is usually reserved for patients with more severe or missed injuries with fixed deformities.

Pedicle and Lamina Fractures

- Unilateral pedicle fractures are usually considered rotational injuries, so their evaluation and treatment is similar to that of unilateral facet fractures.

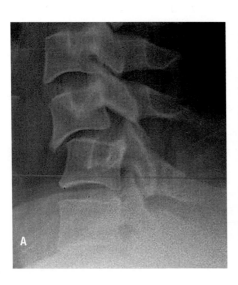
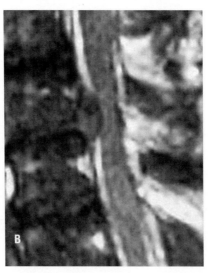

Figure 18-16 (**A**) If the patient is awake, closed reduction of facet dislocations is preferred. A postreduction MRI is usually obtained. (**B**) In this case, a large herniated disc was seen, although the patient remained neurologically intact. Most surgeons would elect to perform an anterior discectomy and fusion.

- Bilateral pedicle fractures may be a sign of a more serious injury.
  - In these injuries, the possibility of an unstable ligamentous injury should be considered.
- Isolated laminar fractures are usually benign, but they are frequently associated with other more significant fractures or dislocations.
- Multilevel laminar fractures can suggest a hyperextension mechanism of injury.
- Careful inspection of the uniformity of the disc spaces and the integrity of the ALL on a MRI help detect occult anterior tension band disruption.

Anterior Tension Band Injuries

- Disruption of the ALL can be associated with vertebral body avulsion fractures near the anterior endplate.
- Abnormal widening of the disc space is the clue to diagnosis.
- They can be associated with posterior fractures or gross PLC disruption, in which case sagittal and coronal malalignment is present.
- Anterior tension band injuries should be considered unstable.

Nonsurgical Treatment

- These injuries are usually highly unstable, and nonoperative treatment is usually only in cases in which the patient is too ill to undergo surgery.
- A halo device can be applied, and providing the PLC and facet capsules are intact, a flexion moment can reapproximate the vertebral bodies.
- If reduction can be maintained, bony ankylosis of the disc space can occur.
- Flexion extension views must be obtained to confirm adequate stability.

Surgical Treatment

- Anterior tension band disruption, consisting of discontinuity of the ALL, intervertebral disc, and possibly the PLL, is an ideal indication for anterior surgery.
- An anterior discectomy and plating with fusion can restore the tension band just as posterior fixation address PLC disruption with bilateral facet dislocations.
- Extension-type cervical teardrop fractures can be successfully treated with anterior or posterior surgery.
- The suggested treatment of subaxial cervical spine fractures is given in Table 18-6.

TABLE 18-6 SUGGESTED TREATMENT OF SUBAXIAL CERVICAL FRACTURES

Injury	Treatment
Compression fractures	
Intact posterior ligaments	
C3-C6	Cervical collar
C7, T1	Cervicothoracic orthosis (CTO)
Posterior ligament damage	Posterior fixation and fusion
Burst fractures	
Minor burst, intact neurology	Cervical collar or CTO
Little canal compromise	CTO or halo vest
Major burst, abnormal neurology	
Canal compromise	Anterior decompression and fusion
With posterolateral corner (PLC) disruption	Supplementary posterior fusion
Flexion teardrop fractures	
Minimally displaced, PLC intact	
C3-C7	Cervical collar
C7, T1	CTO
Abnormal neurology	Anterior decompression and fusion
PLC damaged	Supplementary posterior instrumentation and fusion
Neurologically intact	
Extensive endplate damage (>30%)	Anterior stabilization and fusion
Minimal endplate involvement	Posterior instrumentation and fusion
Facet fractures (No dislocation)	
Undisplaced	Cervical collar
Late displacement	Anterior discectomy and fusion or posterior instrumentation and fusion
Facet dislocations	
Awake reduction successful	
Postreduction MRI scan	
Prolapsed disc	Discectomy, anterior fusion, plate
no prolapsed disc	Anterior or posterior surgery
Not awake	
Prereduction MRI scan	
Prolapsed disc	Anterior discectomy. Open anterior or posterior reduction and fixation
no prolapsed disc	Closed reduction. Anterior or posterior surgery

COMPLICATIONS

Mortality

- The mortality rate tends to increase with age. Overall mortality rate in patients over 65 years is 23% to 26%.
  - In this age group the mortality in nonoperatively treated type II odontoid fractures is quoted as 27% to 42%, although it is lower in surgically treated patients.

Spinal Cord Injury

- This is more common with subaxial fractures and dislocations.
- The treatment of spinal cord injured patients is complex and beyond the scope of this book.
- In 1% to 5% of patients, there is deterioration of neurological function after surgery.
- This should be investigated by immediate X-ray and CT scan.
- If this is negative or inconclusive, MRI is required.

Nonunion

- The nonunion rate in C1-C2 fusions treated by screw fixation is 3% to 15% (average 4%).
  - The rate is higher if posterior wiring techniques are used (19% to 61%).
- The incidence of nonunion in nonoperatively treated type II odontoid fractures is 15% to 85% depending on the degree of displacement.
- Screw fixation is associated with an incidence of 10% to 12%.
- The rate of nonunion in type III odontoid fractures is 9% to 13%.
- The treatment of nonunion is refixation and bone grafting.

Deep Venous Thrombosis

- In quadriplegic patients, the incidence of DVT can be as high as 25%. This condition is discussed further in Chapter 41.

Other Complications

- Dural tears, whether traumatic or iatrogenic, should be repaired primarily.
- Prior to closure of an anterior neck wound, the esophagus should be inspected for tears.
- Unrecognized tears, whether caused by the initial trauma or by surgery, should be repaired primarily to avoid deep infection.
- The rate of wound infection does not appear to be significantly higher in patients undergoing anterior cervical surgery who have a preexisting tracheostomy.
- In general, posterior surgery appears to have a slightly higher rate of infection than anterior cervical surgery.

SPECIAL CIRCUMSTANCES

Ankylosing Spondylitis and Diffuse Idiopathic Skeletal Hyperostosis

- Bridging osteophytes, whether marginal as in ankylosing spondylitis (AS) or nonmarginal and flowing as in diffuse idiopathic skeletal hyperostosis (DISH), are the radiographic hallmarks of these diseases.
- They effectively fuse the spine into a solid, continuous piece of bone.
- Thus fractures in patients with DISH or AS are almost universally unstable and should be treated as such.
- The diagnosis is often missed, unfortunately, resulting in a very high rate of neurological deficits in previously intact patients.
- In cervical fractures, AS has been demonstrated to be a significant risk factor for neurological deterioration after fracture.
- Patients should be immobilized as soon as the diagnosis is made, admitted to the hospital, and placed on strict log-roll precautions until definitive management has been decided.

Spinal Cord Injury Without Instability in the Spondylotic Spine

- Patients often present with complete or incomplete spinal cord injury without radiographic signs of a frank injury, fracture, or ligamentous instability.
- Underlying cervical stenosis is often present, which can arise from degenerative changes or a congenitally narrow canal (Fig. 18-17).
- There is little information about optimal treatment.
- Nonoperative treatment will result in nearly complete resolution of their neural deficits in many patients.
- Long-term treatment is influenced by the presence of persistent signs or symptoms or myelopathy.

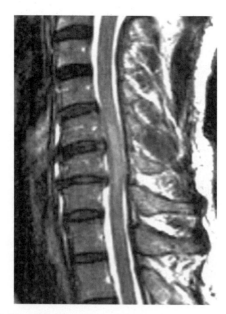

Figure 18-17   MRI scan showing a degenerative cervical stenosis.

- The role and timing of surgery is controversial.
- In a retrospective study, early surgery for patients with incomplete spinal cord injuries resulted in earlier neurological recovery, with better motor scores at 1 month and 6 months.
- However, at 2 years, there was no statistically significant difference between the operative and nonoperative groups.

Transverse Process Fractures

- The vertebral artery runs through foramina in the transverse processes and may be injured in transverse process fractures.
- Magnetic resonance arteriograms are an effective means of diagnosing vertebral artery occlusion or narrowing following cervical trauma.
- The incidence of vertebral artery injury following lower cervical spine trauma has been reported to be as high as 25% to 46%.
- The vast majority of injuries are unilateral, which fortunately have a very low rate of clinical sequelae.
- In most cases, no specific treatment is necessary.
- Bilateral vertebral artery injuries can be devastating, leading to cerebellar infarction.
- This has been reported in patients with severe dislocations of the subaxial cervical spine.

SUGGESTED READING

Allen B, Ferguson R, Lehmann T, et al. A mechanistic classification of closed, indirect fractures and dislocations of the lower cervical spine. Spine 1982;7:1–27.

Anderson LD, D'Alonzo RT. Fractures of the odontoid process of the axis. J Bone Joint Surg (Am) 1974;56:1663–1674.

Anderson PA, Montesano PX. Traumatic injuries of the occipitocervical articulation. In: Camins M, Oleary P, eds. Disorders of the cervical spine. Baltimore: Williams and Wilkins, 1992.

Blahd WH, Iserson KV, Bjelland JC. Efficacy of the posttraumatic cross table lateral view of the cervical spine. J Emerg Med 1985; 2:243–249.

Chen TY, Dickman CA, Eleraky M, et al. The role of decompression for acute incomplete cervical spinal cord injury in cervical spondylosis. Spine 1998;23:2398–2403.

Colterjohn NR, Bednar DA. Identifiable risk factors for secondary neurologic deterioration in the cervical spine-injured patient. Spine 1995;20:2293–2297.

Eismont FJ, Arena MJ, Green BA. Extrusion of an intervertebral disc associated with traumatic subluxation or dislocation of cervical facets. Case report. J Bone Joint Surg (Am) 1991;73:1555–1560.

Esses S, Langer F, Gross A. Fracture of the atlas associated with fracture of the odontoid process. Injury 1981;12:310–312.

Faerber EN, Wolpert SM, Scott RM, et al. Computed tomography of spinal fractures. J Comput Assist Tomogr 1979;3:657–661.

Farmer J, Vaccaro A, Balderston R, et al. The changing nature of admission to a spinal cord injury center: violence on the rise. J Spinal Disord 1998;11:400–403.

Fielding JW, Cochran GB, Lawsing JF, et al. Tears of the transverse ligament of the atlas. J Bone Joint Surg (Am) 1974;56: 1683–1691.

Finkelstein JA, Chapman JR, Mirza S. Occult vertebral fractures in ankylosing spondylitis. Spinal Cord 1999;37:444–447.

Fisher CG, Dvorak MF, Leith J, et al. Comparison of outcomes for unstable lower cervical flexion teardrop fractures managed with halo thoracic vest versus anterior corpectomy and plating. Spine 2002;27:160–166.

Garfin SR, Botte MJ, Waters RL, et al. Complications in the use of the halo fixation device. J Bone Joint Surg Am 1986;68:320–325.

Levine A, Edwards C. Treatment of injuries in the C1-C2 complex. Orthop Clin North Am 1986;17:31–44.

Levine A, Edwards C. Fractures of the atlas. J Bone Joint Surg (Am) 1991;73:680–691.

Levine AM, Edwards CC: The management of traumatic spondylolisthesis of the axis. J Bone Joint Surg (Am) 1985;67:217–226.

Sears W, Fazl M. Prediction of stability of cervical spine fracture managed in the halo vest and indications for surgical intervention. J Neurosurg 1990;72:426–432.

Spence K, Decker S, Sell K. Bursting atlantal fracture associated with rupture of the transverse ligament. J Bone Joint Surg (Am) 1970;52:543–549.

Swenson TM, Lauerman WC, Blanc RO, et al. Cervical alignment in the immobilized football player: radiographic analysis before and after helmet removal. Am J Sports Med 1997;25:226–230.

Vaccaro AR, Daugherty RJ, Sheehan TP, et al. Neurologic outcome of early versus late surgery for cervical spinal cord injury. Spine 1997;22:2609–2613.

Vaccaro AR, Falatyn SP, Flanders AE, et al. Magnetic resonance evaluation of the intervertebral disc, spinal ligaments, and spinal cord before and after closed traction reduction of cervical spine dislocations. Spine 1999;24:1210–1217.

Vale FL, Burns J, Jackson AB, et al. Combined medical and surgical treatment after acute spinal cord injury: results of a prospective pilot study to assess the merits of aggressive medical resuscitation and blood pressure management. J Neurosurg 1997;87:239–246.

Vertullo CJ, Duke PF, Askin GN. Pin-site complications of the halo thoracic brace with routine tightening. Spine 1997;22:2514–2516.

Wertheim SB, Bohlman HH. Occipitocervical fusion: indications, technique, and long-term results in thirteen patients. J Bone Joint Surg (Am) 1987;69:833–836.

Woodring JH, Lee C. The role and limitations of computed tomographic scanning in the evaluation of cervical trauma. J Trauma 1992;33:698–708.

THORACOLUMBAR FRACTURES AND DISLOCATIONS

CHRISTOPHER M. BONO
MARIE RINALDI

Thoracolumbar fractures and fracture dislocations were usually treated nonoperatively until the 1970s when posterior rodding, using the techniques developed for scoliosis surgery. became popular. In the 1980s, this technique gave way to posterior techniques employing intrapedicular screw fixation. The subsequent evolution of devices designed for anterior spinal stabilization resulted in surgeons using anterior decompression and stabilization techniques, and there is still debate about whether anterior or posterior approaches give better results. In recent years there has been renewed interest in the treatment of osteoporotic vertebral fractures, and the techniques of vertebroplasty and kyphoplasty are becoming popular.

The thoracolumbar junction represents a biomechanical transition zone between the rigid thoracic and more mobile lumbar spine. It also marks a sagittal alignment transition zone between the kyphotic thoracic spine and the lordotic lumbar region. With these features, large forces can be concentrated at the thoracolumbar spine during abrupt and dramatic acceleration changes, like those produced during motor vehicle accidents. Injuries can range from isolated minor vertebral body compression fractures to fracture-dislocations with circumferential osteoligamentous disruption, although burst fractures, secondary to axial loading of the spine, are one of the most common injuries. The likelihood of neurological injury is greater with higher energy lesions. There are a number of controversies in the management of thoracolumbar fractures, which are listed in Box 19-1.

SURGICAL ANATOMY

Thoracic vertebral bodies are roughly heart shaped in axial cross section; lumbar vertebral bodies are more cylindrical. Bony dimensions are relatively small in the upper thoracic spine and progressively increase from cranial to caudad to sustain increasing proportions of body weight. Likewise, the spinal canal is smaller in the thoracic spine than the lumbar spine. Among other factors, these dimensional constraints make the spinal cord much more susceptible to small amounts of thoracic canal compromise than the conus medullaris or cauda equina at the thoracolumbar junction or lumbar spine.

BOX 19-1 CONTROVERSIES IN THE TREATMENT OF THORACOLUMBAR FRACTURES

Should burst fractures with no neurological involvement
   be treated surgically?
Is anterior or posterior surgical stabilization better?
When should surgery be performed?
Does spinal stabilization improve neurological outcome?
How important is spinal canal clearance?
How useful are vertebroplasty and kyphoplasty?

Subtle wedging of the vertebral bodies collectively produces about 20 to 40 degrees of physiological thoracic kyphosis. The intervertebral discs and adjacent endplates are relatively parallel and contribute little to normal thoracic kyphosis. This is different than the lumbar spine in which physiological lumbar lordosis, ranging from 40 to 60 degrees, is produced primarily by wedging of the intervertebral discs, with larger anterior versus posterior heights. The transition between thoracic kyphosis and lumbar lordosis occurs between the T11 and L2 levels, the thoracolumbar junction. This area of the spine is normally straight in both the sagittal and coronal planes. Thus any degree of measured kyphosis after burst fracture is considered abnormal. This is not true, however, for the upper and middle thoracic spine and lower lumbar spine, where preinjury alignment must be considered when assessing kyphotic deformity.

The posterior ligamentous complex (PLC) is comprised of the interspinous ligaments, supraspinous ligaments, ligamentum flavum, and facet capsules. Combined, these structures act as a posterior tension band that limits the amount of flexion that can be safely tolerated by the neural elements. The PLC can be disrupted by fractures in which a flexion or translational vector is imparted. At the current time, PLC integrity is considered the most important determinant of mechanical stability of a fracture.

CLASSIFICATION

Many classification systems for thoracolumbar injuries have been proposed, each with unique advantages and disadvantages. Currently, there is no universally accepted system. The McAfee (1983) and OTA (AO) (1994) systems are two of the more popularly used classifications.

The McAfee system is an adaptation of the classification proposed by Denis (1983), based on dividing the spine into three distinct columns. Its development was based on analyzing multiplanar CT and plain radiographic images of 100 consecutive thoracolumbar injuries. The focus was to determine, or, more accurately, postulate, the mechanism of failure of the all-important middle column. McAfee et al. found that the middle column could fail by axial compression, axial distraction, or translation in the transverse

plane. They used sagittal CT reconstructions to determine if the posterior column had failed.

Magerl et al. (1994) introduced the more comprehensive OTA (AO) classification for thoracolumbar spine fractures. The system was based on analysis of CT and plain radiographic examination of over 1,400 consecutive injuries at five trauma centers. Injuries are divided into three general groups: A (compression), B (distraction), and C (torsion) injuries. These groups are further divided into subgroups based on fracture morphology, distinguishing between primarily bone or ligamentous failure and the direction of displacement (Fig. 19-1). Type A fractures are divided into A1,

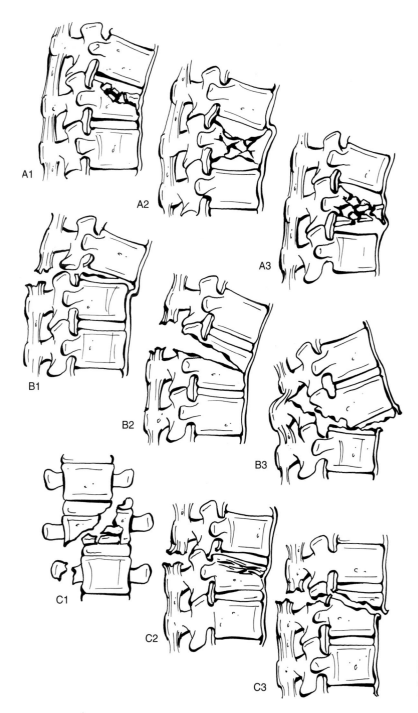

Figure 19-1 The OTA (AO) classification system divides injuries into type A (compression), type B (distraction), and type C (rotation) injuries.

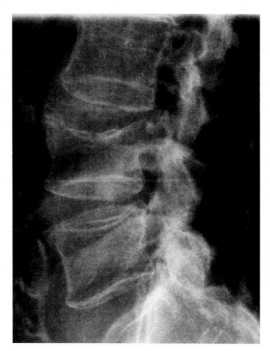

Figure 19-2 Compression fractures are usually stable injuries. The fracture does not extend to the posterior vertebral body wall.

impaction fractures; A2, split fractures; and A3, burst fractures. B1 and B2 fractures are flexion-distraction injuries, and B3 injuries are hyperextension shear injuries through the disc. Type C fractures are rotational injuries with C1 containing wedge, split, and burst fractures; C2, the flexion subluxation injuries; and C3, the rotational shear injuries. The OTA (AO) system is more inclusive than the McAfee system, but it is also much more complex. Its interobserver reliability has been found to be inversely proportional to its complexity.

Although not all inclusive, most thoracic and lumbar injuries can be described as one of the following: (1) compression fracture, (2) burst fracture, (3) flexion-distraction injury, or (4) fracture-dislocation. By convention, compression fractures include those that lead to some degree of vertebral body height loss without involvement of the posterior vertebral body (Fig. 19-2). Burst fractures contain fracture lines that extend into the posterior wall of the vertebral body without translation or dislocation (Fig. 19-3). Pure dislocations at the thoracolumbar junction are rare and usually occur from a flexion-distraction-type mechanism. The classic example is a lap-belt injury in which the facet joints can be subluxed, perched, or jumped (Fig. 19-4). Fracture-dislocations refer to those injuries with a translational component in addition to varying fracture patterns (Fig. 19-5). Importantly, fracture-dislocations can exhibit posterior vertebral body fractures that, on CT alone, may appear to be a burst pattern. However, translation on plain radiographs or CT reconstructions helps distinguish the injury types.

EPIDEMIOLOGY

The basic epidemiology of thoracolumbar fractures is shown in Table 19-1. As discussed in Chapter 1, the complete epidemiology of thoracolumbar fracture is impossible

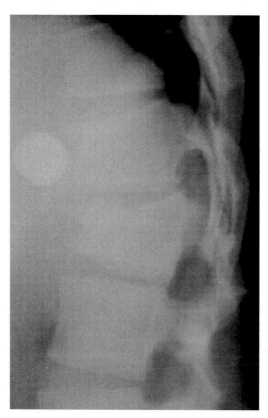

Figure 19-3 Burst fractures, by definition, demonstrate posterior vertebral body wall involvement without any significant translational deformity.

to determine because many osteoporotic fractures never present to hospital or even to a doctor! The fractures detailed in Table 19-1 follow a defined injury. Posttraumatic thoracolumbar fractures have a type B distribution (see

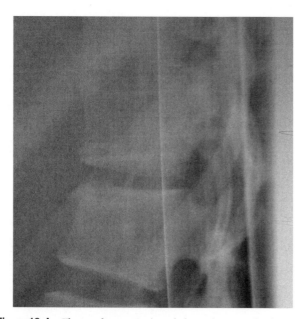

Figure 19-4 Flexion-distraction (seat-belt type) injuries lead to posterior ligament disruption by forceful flexion about an axis of rotation anterior to the spine. In this case, posterior interspinous and facet joint widening was associated with a mild amount of superior endplate compression.

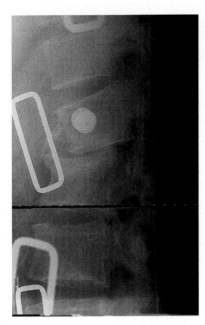

Figure 19-5 Fracture-dislocations demonstrate substantial translational deformities. This is usually a sign of gross ligamentous instability.

Chapter 1) mainly affecting young men. If osteoporotic vertebral fractures are also included, there is a type A distribution curve affecting younger men and older women.

Approximately 90% of all thoracic and lumbar injuries occur at the thoracolumbar junction. Table 19-1 shows that the burst (A3) fracture configuration is most common. Although many fractures follow a fall from a height, a recent study has demonstrated that the incidence of severe and multiple-level spinal injuries is higher with motorcycle versus automobile accidents. Within the military population, the incidence of thoracolumbar fractures in army pilots has been demonstrated to be about 13%; helicopter crashes and parachuting accidents were the most common associated traumatic event, accounting for 73% of cases.

TABLE 19-1 THE EPIDEMIOLOGY OF POSTTRAUMATIC THORACOLUMBAR FRACTURES

Proportion of all fractures	0.3%
Proportion of spinal fractures	47.5%
Average age	43.5 y
Male/women	63%/32%
Distribution	Type B
Incidence	$3.6/10^5$/y
Open fractures	0%
Most common cause	
Fall from height	68.4%
OTA (AO) classification	
Type A	73.7%
Type B	5.3%
Type C	21.0%
Most common group	
A3	63.2%

Associated Injuries

Because most posttraumatic spinal injuries in younger patients follow falls from a height or an MVA, multiple injuries are frequent. Significant lower limb fractures are common as are fractures of the pelvis and lower limb long bones. Frequently there are multiple spinal fractures. Osteoporotic thoracolumbar fractures are usually isolated.

DIAGNOSIS

History and Physical Examination

■ The patient and/or eyewitnesses should be questioned regarding the circumstances of the accident in order to determine the direction of force and mechanism of injury.
■ The physical examination begins with inspection.
    ■ A transverse band of ecchymosis across the abdomen can suggest a flexion-distraction type of injury caused by a seat belt.
    ■ If this is the case, a thorough examination of the abdomen is essential because flexion-distraction injuries are associated with a high incidence of intra-abdominal injury.
    ■ Similar bruising along the rib cage may suggest a thoracic fracture-dislocation.
■ The spine must be palpated systematically for tenderness, step-off, or interspinous process gapping.
■ A detailed neurological examination, including motor, sensory, and reflexes, should then be performed.
■ A rectal examination is also performed to assess rectal tone and the bulbocavernosus (BC) reflex.
■ The patient's neurological status should be assessed according to the ASIA (modified Frankel) system (Table 19-2).
■ All multiply injured patients should be examined according to ATLS guidelines, particularly bearing in mind that there may be significant injuries to the lower limbs in particular.

Radiologic Examination

■ If a thoracic or lumbar injury is detected, complete radiographs of the entire spine should be obtained because the incidence of concomitant, noncontiguous spinal injury can be as high as 12%.
■ Anteroposterior and lateral thoracic and lumbar views should be obtained.
■ Dedicated x-rays centered at the T12-L1 junction are invaluable in any patient with a suspected thoracolumbar injury.
■ Overall alignment can be assessed using lateral radiographs.
■ Kyphosis can be measured using the Cobb method.
    ■ This measures the angle between the superior endplate of the nearest uninjured cranial vertebra and the inferior endplate of the nearest uninjured caudal vertebra.
■ The percentage height loss of the injured vertebral body is a useful calculation.

TABLE 19-2 AMERICAN SPINAL INJURY ASSOCIATION (ASIA) IMPAIRMENT SCALE

ASIA Grade	Description	Criteria
A	Complete	No motor or sensory function below level of injury, including terminal sacral segments (S4-5)
B	Incomplete	Sensory function preserved below injury, including terminal sacral segments (S4-S5); no motor below injury level
C	Incomplete	Motor and sensory function preserved below level of injury; muscle strength is less than grade 3/5 (cannot overcome gravity)
D	Incomplete	Motor and sensory function preserved below level of injury; muscle strength is grade 3 or higher (can at least overcome gravity)
E	Normal	Motor and sensory function is normal

- This is based on comparing values of the injured segment to those of adjacent cranial and caudal uninjured vertebrae.
- Although not a constant rule, loss of greater than 50% of height is suggestive of posterior ligamentous complex (PLC) disruption.
- Coronal and rotational alignment of the spine can be assessed using the anteroposterior (A-P) radiograph.
  - The relative distance between the spinous processes and the pedicles is a reflection of rotation.
  - Coronal angulation or translation suggests high-energy trauma.
- Interpedicular width should also be noted.
- In general, width should successively increase from caudal to cranial.
  - Abnormal widening suggests lateral displacement of the pedicles, which is often associated with burst fractures.

Computed Tomography

- Thin CT slices should be obtained through both the level of injury and normal adjacent levels.
- Fracture lines extending to the posterior vertebral body distinguish burst from compression fractures.
- The dimensional effects of retropulsed bone fragments on the spinal canal are easily appreciated.
- Posterior element injuries, such as facet, pedicle, and laminar fractures, are also clearly visualized.
- Laminar fractures that occur concomitantly with a burst fracture are often associated with posterior dural tears and nerve root entrapment, which should be considered during treatment planning.
- The so-called naked facet is an indication of complete facet dislocation (Fig. 19-6).
- In the absence of this sign, translational deformities can be easily overlooked because they are in the same plane as axial CT images.
- High-quality sagittal and coronal CT reconstructions can facilitate diagnosis of even subtle distraction or translational injuries.
- Numerous methods for quantifying canal compromise have been described.

- Sagittal canal diameter is among the more simple measurements. This is the distance between the posterior aspect of the most posteriorly displaced wall fragment and the anterior aspect of the lamina.
- Canal compromise from translational deformity (as in fracture-dislocations) can be underestimated by axial CT images.
- Sagittal reconstructions are particularly helpful in assessing the spinal canal in these situations.
- Rotational deformity is best detected by an overlay technique of consecutive axial CT images.

Magnetic Resonance Imaging

- Magnetic resonance imaging (MRI) is the best method for evaluating the neural elements, the intervertebral discs, and the spinal ligaments.
- It may also show edema within the spinal cord and, rarely, cord transection.
- Nerve root entrapment within a laminar fracture can be seen on axial MR images.
- Intervertebral disc herniation can lead to canal compromise that is not easily appreciated with CT.

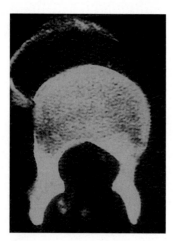

Figure 19-6 The so-called naked facet sign.

- The use of MRI to assess the integrity of the spinal ligaments is becoming more commonplace.
  - It can be used to assess the integrity of the posterior longitudinal ligament (PLL) or posterior ligamentous complex (PLC) (Fig. 19-7).
  - Findings may vary from mild increased signal between spinous processes on T2-weighted images (indicative of benign ligament sprain) to bright and expansive signal extending from the tip of the spinous process to the interlaminar interval (indicative of gross PLC disruption).

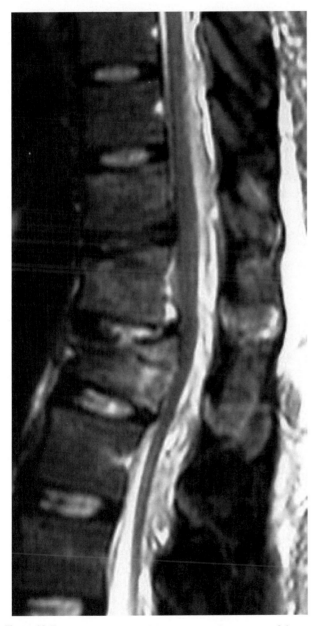

Figure 19-7 A MRI can be useful in assessing the integrity of the spinal ligaments after thoracolumbar injuries. In this case, a small amount of edema is present within the posterior soft tissues. However, the overall continuity of the ligaments was not disrupted. This neurologically intact patient was successfully treated in a brace.

TREATMENT

Burst and Compression Fractures

Nonsurgical Management

- Most thoracic and lumbar fractures can be treated nonoperatively.
- The clinical challenge is correctly analyzing the injury characteristics and then predicting which fractures can be successfully and safely treated in this manner.
- Clear-cut treatment recommendations do not exist, which is partially a result of inconsistent injury description in the literature that makes extrapolation of data difficult.
- Various forms of nonoperative management can be employed (see Chapter 31).
- Progressive mobilization and observation without an external support device may be used for some minor injuries.
- External orthoses can be used for more substantial fractures.
- Hyperextension braces such as a Jewett brace (see Fig. 31-20 in Chapter 31) are useful in counteracting sagittal flexion moments but offer minimal resistance to rotation or lateral flexion.
- Custom-fit clamshell devices, such as a thoracolumbar sacral orthosis (TLSO), provide multiplanar support (see Fig. 31-19 in Chapter 31).
- In rare circumstances, patients with mechanically unstable fractures are treated nonoperatively by extended bed rest and continued spinal precautions.
- Some complications of prolonged recumbency, such as decubitus ulcers and pulmonary compromise, can be mitigated with the use of a rotating bed.
- An intact posterior ligamentous complex (PLC) should be considered a prerequisite for nonoperative treatment.
- Anterior vertebral height loss of more than 50%, interspinous process gapping, or more than 30 to 35 degrees of kyphosis are suggestive of PLC disruption at the thoracolumbar junction.
- A higher index of suspicion is required for thoracic injuries where more than 30% height loss should cause the surgeon to consider operative treatment.
- An MRI is often useful to analyze the integrity of the posterior ligamentous complex.
- Burst fractures are higher energy injuries.
- As with compression fractures, an intact PLC should be considered a prerequisite for nonoperative care.
- Some experts feel that more than 50% canal compromise is an indication for surgical decompression and/or stabilization, but few data support this practice routinely in a neurologically intact patient with an intact PLC.
- A kyphosis more than 25 to 30 degrees and/or anterior height loss of greater than 50% are highly suggestive of posterior ligament injury.
  - Again, less deformity should be accepted in the upper and middle thoracic spine.
- Nonoperative treatment of burst fractures usually includes a custom-made form-fitting TLSO (see Fig. 31-19 in Chapter 31).

■ Before ambulation is begun, standing radiographs in the brace should be obtained.
  ■ The kyphotic angle and height loss should be measured and compared to initial values.
■ If kyphosis or height loss increases, the integrity of the posterior ligaments should be more closely evaluated.

Nonsurgical Versus Surgical Treatment of Burst Fractures

■ The results of surgical and nonsurgical treatment have been compared in select groups of patients with clearly defined thoracolumbar injuries.
■ An analysis of the literature comparing nonoperative management with posterior instrumentation using transpedicular screw systems in patients presenting with normal neurology is shown in Table 19-3.
■ These studies strongly suggest that the results of nonoperative management, consisting of bracing and early mobilization, are equivalent to those of an operative treatment method for thoracolumbar burst fractures without posterior ligamentous injury.
■ Surgery initially improves the posttraumatic kyphosis, but the final results for both kyphosis and canal encroachment, as measured by CT scans, are very similar.
■ Pain relief is also similar, but the return to work seems to be quicker with nonoperative treatment.
■ Unfortunately, none of the studies of either method of treatment give guidelines as to how to determine the integrity of the PLC.

Surgical Treatment

■ The indications for surgical treatment in thoracolumbar fractures are becoming more uniform (Box 19-2).

Compression Fractures

■ In the unusual situation that a compression fracture is associated with posterior ligament injury, posterior stabilization is usually preferred.
■ The surgical goal is to realign the spine by correcting the kyphosis until solid fusion is achieved.
■ Posterior pedicle screw or hook constructs can both be useful.

BOX 19-2 INDICATIONS FOR SURGICAL TREATMENT OF VERTEBRAL FRACTURES

■ Fracture dislocations
■ Flexion-distraction injuries (particularly if not pure fractures)
■ Complete paraplegia
■ Burst fractures
  ■ Progressive neurological deficit
  ■ Progressive kyphotic deformity
  ■ PLC disruption
      Progressive kyphotic deformity
      Kyphosis >25–30 degrees
      Vertebral body height loss >50%
      Neurological deficit >25% canal compromise
■ Painful metastatic involvement

■ Posterior instrumentation is rarely required, however.
■ In recent years considerable interest has been expressed in the use of vertebroplasty and kyphoplasty to treat osteoporotic compression fractures.
■ Vertebroplasty refers to the operation of injecting PMMA bone cement into a vertebra through a pedicle to stabilize the osteoporotic fracture and reduce pain.
■ In kyphoplasty a balloon is inserted into the vertebral body through a pedicle. It is then inflated and the height of the vertebral body is thereby partially restored.
  ■ The restored height is maintained by cement injection.
■ Vertebroplasty can be used in vertebrae in which pain is secondary to osteoporotic fracture, metastatic tumor (see Chapter 9), myeloma, or hemangioma.
■ The literature suggests 53% to 78% pain relief in patients with osteoporotic compression fractures with a 6% incidence of minor complications. A comparative study of vertebroplasty versus nonoperative treatment showed a 53% reduction in pain scores and 29% improvement in physical function after vertebroplasty, compared with nonoperative treatment immediately after treatment.

TABLE 19-3 COMPARISON OF NONOPERATIVE AND OPERATIVE TREATMENT OF BURST FRACTURES IN PATIENTS PRESENTING WITH A NORMAL NEUROLOGICAL EXAMINATION

Parameter	Nonoperative		Operative	
	Range	Average	Range	Average
Kyphosis (degree)				
Initial	11.3–20	16.5	10.1–17	14.9
Postoperative	—	—	0–10	5.2
Final	13.8–24	20.1	9.7–16	14.0
Canal encroachment (%)				
Initial	34–37	35.9	39	39
Final	14.5–19	16.1	22	22
No or minimal pain (%)	48.8–84.2	64	61.5	61.5
Same or equivalent work (%)	63–76	71	33–73	59
Surgical complications (%)	—	—	2.1–29.2	11.8

■ After 6 weeks the results were similar for both methods, however.

■ The literature shows that kyphoplasty is associated with more than 90% pain relief and 35% to 68% restoration of vertebral height.

■ Adverse effects vary between 0% and 1.5%.

■ Both procedures are technically demanding, and the exact indications for their use remain to be defined.

Burst Fractures

■ There is significant controversy regarding the indications and optimal method of surgical treatment of thoracolumbar burst fractures, particularly for patients without neurological deficit.

■ Some advocate posterior surgery alone; others believe anterior or combined anterior and posterior surgery is preferred.

■ In patients with neurological deficit, and particularly those with incomplete deficits, most surgeons agree that surgery is warranted.

■ Indirect reduction of displaced vertebral body fragments can be achieved through distraction and realignment with posterior instrumentation. This appears to be more effective if the PLL is intact and surgery is performed within 2 to 4 days of injury.

■ Direct fragment removal through an anterior approach offers better anatomical decompression, although the neurological benefits have not been established conclusively.

■ Others have developed techniques to remove vertebral body fragments and perform interbody fusion through a posterior approach.

■ Various anterior and posterior instrumentation options are available.

■ An analysis of results from the literature of posterior instrumentation and anterior decompression and instrumentation is presented in Table 19-4, which appears to show improved neurological improvement with anterior decompression and instrumentation, although there is some debate about this.

■ This depends on the degree of neurological damage in the patients included in the studies.

■ A study specifically comparing the two techniques in similar patient groups showed about 85% neurological improvement in both techniques.

■ The difference in the results in Table 19-4 is at least partially accounted for by the different degree of neurological compromise in different patients.

■ Patients who are ASIA grade A (see Table 19-2) will not show any neurological improvement, whereas grades B through D usually do.

■ Canal clearance is clearly better with anterior decompression, but no evidence indicates that canal clearance correlates with neurological improvement.

■ Final kyphosis is similar, but the incidence of nonunion and surgical complications is higher with anterior surgery.

Posterior Surgery

■ The role of posterior surgery is mainly for stabilization of burst fractures in neurologically intact patients, although Table 19-4 shows it is used in patients with abnormal neurology.

■ Stabilization can be effected using a variety of constructs.

■ Pedicle screws are among the more popular methods of fixation.

■ Screws enable short-segment fusion with the theoretical advantage over hook constructs of providing three-column stability.

■ At a minimum, the level above and below the fracture should be included in the fusion (short segment instrumentation), with some authors advocating two levels above and below.

■ Some surgeons have reported the rates of pedicle screw breakage or failure with short-segment instrumentation to be as high as 50%.

■ This is thought to be the result of continued cyclic loading amplified by anterior column deficiency.

■ Transpedicular intracorporeal bone grafting was introduced in an attempt to reconstitute the vertebral body

TABLE 19-4 RESULTS FROM THE LITERATURE COMPARING POSTERIOR TRANSPEDICULAR SCREW FIXATION WITH ANTERIOR DECOMPRESSION AND INSTRUMENTATION

Parameter	Anterior		Posterior	
	Range	Average	Range	Average
Abnormal neurology (%)	25–100	80.0	13.6–100	44.2
Neurological improvement (%)	44.4–100	81.4	26.3–100	48.2
Kyphosis (degrees)				
Initial	18.7–31	19.8	16.5–20	17.2
Postoperative	2.2–12	6.6	3–8	4.7
Final	8–18.5	9.2	6.7–14.5	12.7
Canal encroachment (%)				
Initial	47–58.1	48.2	36.3–44.5	39.3
Final	2–4.1	2.2	4.6–16.5	8.9
Nonunion (%)	0–6.7	4.1	0–4.3	0.2
Surgical complications (%)	11.1–27.6	18.7	1.2–10	4.2

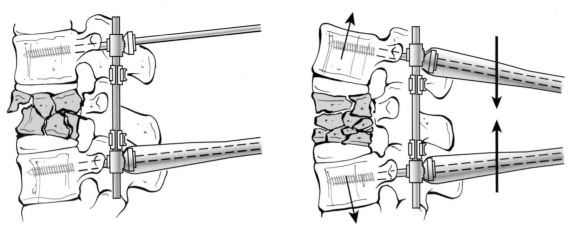

Figure 19-8 Posterior pedicle screw instrumentation can be used to stabilize burst fractures. Distraction can be applied through pedicle screws to help acutely reduced canal compromise and restore vertebral body height.

height, but this has not diminished the rate of hardware failure with short-segment pedicle screw stabilization.

- Although a useful option, posterior stabilization using hooks and rods has lost its popularity because it requires inclusion of at least two to three segments above and below the injury.
- Sublaminar wire constructs have little role in the stabilization of unstable burst fractures.
- Simple decompressive laminectomy has fallen out of favor because it causes further posterior destabilization and can lead to progressive kyphotic deformity.
- Indirect reduction, a concept that relies on longitudinal distraction along the fractured segment, works through ligamentotaxis of the displaced posterior vertebral fragments (Fig. 19-8).
- With distraction, an intact PLL and/or posterior annulus are thought to pull the fragments back into place.
- One study reported this technique in 22 junctional (T11 to L2) burst fractures, reporting an average 28% improvement in canal compromise; however, the rate of neurological recovery or injury could not be predicted based on the amount of canal clearance.
- A cadaveric study found a relationship between measured vertebral height loss or kyphosis and spinal canal compromise with simulated burst fractures.
- Indirect reduction for decompression has not been uniformly endorsed, however, because disruption of the PLL appears to compromise its effectiveness.
- One group documented an average improvement in canal compromise of only 19% (57% preoperatively to 38% postoperatively) after posterior distractive instrumentation in 30 patients.
  - Independent of canal clearance, incomplete (ASIA grades B through D) injuries improved one or more grades.
  - Although the authors felt disruption of the PLL was a contributing factor to the modest effects on canal clearance, they did not perform MRIs to assess the PLL.
  - From these findings, they inferred that more than 50% canal compromise might be indicative of PLL

disruption, and decompression should be performed through an anterior approach in these cases.

- A greater delay from injury to operation is thought to compromise the efficacy of indirect canal clearance.
  - One study found that operation performed within 1 week led to an average of 33% improvement of canal compromise.
  - Surgery done 1 or 2 weeks after injury resulted in 24% and 0% improvements.
  - As with other reports, all incomplete injuries improved by one or more Frankel grades regardless of canal clearance.
  - Others have found modestly better canal clearance in patients stabilized within 4 days (56% to 38%) compared to those fixed more than 4 days from injury (52% to 44%).
- Methods of anterior canal decompression through an all-posterior approach have been developed.
- One group used a posterolateral approach to reduce the displaced vertebral body segments to clear the spinal canal in 31 patients.
  - The technique included removal of the facet joint and/or pedicle to gain access to the posterior vertebral body.
- Supplementation with a pedicle screw construct is recommended.
- The combination of a concomitant laminar fracture with a burst fracture can be associated with a dural tear or entrapped nerve roots.
- One group of investigators demonstrated a high rate of dural lacerations with this injury pattern and subsequently recommended posterior laminectomy for exploration and dural repair prior to any planned anterior procedure.
- Another group reported a variant of this injury pattern in which nerve roots were entrapped in the laminar fractures.
  - They recommended freeing the roots through a posterior approach prior to any planned anterior decompression and stabilization.

Anterior Surgery

■ Anterior decompression is the most effective method of clearing the spinal canal after a burst fracture (see Table 19-4).

■ The majority of the injured vertebral body along with the adjacent discs can be removed.

■ Retropulsed fragments are carefully removed to relieve pressure on the spinal cord or cauda equina.

■ The highest rates of neurological recovery have been reported after anterior decompressive surgery for burst fractures in patients with incomplete neural injuries (see Table 19-4), but not all studies have confirmed these findings.

■ A median improvement of two Frankel grades in patients undergoing anterior decompression within 48 hours has been reported, however.

■ After decompression the vertebral body defect must be replaced with a supportive strut that will also eventuate bony fusion.

■ Structural bone graft, such as autograft rib, fibula, or iliac crest, or allograft struts can be used.

■ More recently, titanium mesh cages have become popular.

◾ These devices can be filled with harvested morcellized cancellous autograft iliac crest or salvaged bone from the excised vertebral body.

■ Anterior column strut grafting should be stabilized by anterior instrumentation, posterior instrumentation, or both.

■ Numerous constructs have been used for anterior stabilization.

■ In vitro biomechanical studies have compared various anterior devices.

◾ Among the more rigid devices are plates with fixed-angle vertebral body screws and cross-linked rod-screw-staple designs, such as the Kaneda system.

■ In general, anterior instrumentation and fusion leads to better maintenance of alignment than stand-alone procedures.

■ In one report, anterior surgery was performed for thoracolumbar burst fractures in 35 patients with neurological injury.

◾ High rates of neurological recovery were documented with incomplete injuries; complete neural damage showed no improvement. Of 21 patients with incomplete loss of bowel or bladder function initially, 19 showed some improvement.

◾ Twelve of 13 cases that presented within 10 days of injury recovered useful bladder function.

◾ Five of eight cases presenting more than 10 days after injury gained useful bladder function without incontinence.

■ Similarly, another group of surgeons used anterior plating techniques in conjunction with anterior decompression and strut grafting for a variety of thoracolumbar fractures, documenting excellent maintenance of alignment and rates of neural recovery.

■ In the largest series reported so far, 150 consecutive patients with thoracolumbar burst fractures were treated with a single-stage anterior decompression, strut grafting, and instrumentation using the Kaneda rod-sleeve-staple device.

◾ Canal clearance was nearly 100%. A 93% fusion rate was reported.

◾ Cases of pseudarthroses were successfully treated by posterior instrumentation and fusion.

◾ Ninety-five percent improved at least one Frankel grade.

Combined Anterior and Posterior Surgery

■ In some cases, combined anterior and posterior surgery can be performed.

■ The specific indications and benefits of this maneuver remain unclear.

■ Theoretical advantages include maximization of canal clearance, immediate stability, and fusion rates.

■ The added morbidity of the combined procedures is a potential disadvantage.

■ Although it probably does not offer a neurological benefit, combined anterior and posterior surgery may result in better maintenance of kyphosis correction.

■ Some surgeons advocate combined anterior and posterior techniques to maximize canal decompression and overall construct stability.

■ PLC disruption is an important factor for some surgeons in determining the requirement for this procedure.

Neurological Outcomes and Canal Compromise

■ The relationship between canal compromise and neurological involvement has been extensively investigated.

■ The severity of neurological deficit does not appear to correlate with the degree of residual canal stenosis.

■ The extent of neurological deficit is mainly influenced by the instantaneous canal compromise that occurs at the time of impact, which is substantially more than what is detectable on initial imaging.

■ The presence or absence of PLC disruption may more accurately predict neurological injury.

Flexion-Distraction Injuries

■ In contrast to the cervical spine, flexion-distraction injuries of the thoracolumbar spine are rare.

■ The most common mechanism is thought to be from wearing lap seat belts during motor vehicle trauma.

■ With head-on collision, an improperly worn high-riding lap belt can concentrate forces along an apex that is anterior to the thoracolumbar junction.

■ This potentiates distractive forces along the entire vertebral segment.

■ These injuries should be distinguished from flexion-compression injuries in which the axis of flexion is about the spinal canal, resulting in anterior compressive and posterior tensile forces.

■ Flexion-distraction injuries can have varying fracture patterns in the vertebral body and posterior elements.

■ They are distinguished from fracture-dislocations by the absence of translation, although these injuries are often confused in the literature.

■ Flexion-distraction injuries can be purely ligamentous, osteoligamentous, or purely osseous.

■ Fractures are typically transverse.

■ In some cases, a fracture line can be noted from the tip of the spinous process, through the laminae, and exiting the midanterior aspect of the vertebral body.

- In pure ligamentous injuries, the facet joints can be subluxed or, in some cases, frankly dislocated (perched or locked).
- Nearly two thirds of patients present with a neurological deficit, presumably from distraction of the neural elements.
- A commonly associated nonspinal injury is a perforated viscus, thought to be secondary to sudden increases of pressure within the intestines from abdominal compression.
- In some cases, the abdominal injury is discovered first, and the spine injury can be missed.
- An ecchymotic region along the abdomen is suggestive of this injury pattern.
- There is little role for nonoperative treatment of thoracolumbar flexion-distraction dislocations.
- In purely bony flexion-distraction injuries, hyperextension casting or bracing might be an option.
- This should be continued until bony union is radiographically and clinically confirmed, usually at about 3 to 4 months.
- Most other flexion-distraction injuries should be treated operatively.
- Because the spine flexes about an anterior axis of rotation, the anterior longitudinal ligament (ALL) is usually intact, and there is little, if any, vertebral body comminution.
- In most cases, anterior surgery necessitating resection of the ALL further destabilizes the spine. Therefore, posterior compressive instrumentation and fusion is the most common treatment.
- Because the intervertebral disc can be ruptured with severe injuries, care must be taken not to overcompress the construct for fear of expelling loose disc fragments into the spinal canal.
- Short-segment pedicle screw or hook constructs are effective means of stabilizing these injuries (Fig. 19-9).

Fracture-Dislocations
- Thoracolumbar fracture-dislocations are high-energy injuries with a high rate of complete neurological deficit.
- In patients with complete neural deficits, surgery is indicated to stabilize the spine, which can facilitate patient transfers, mobilization, and pulmonary care.
- Injuries can occur from a variety of mechanisms including flexion, shear, and extension forces.
- Fractures can be realigned through postural reduction in the prone position in the operating room.
- Occasionally misaligned fractures require open reduction and direct manipulation.
  - In the neurologically intact or incompletely injured patient, this must be performed carefully so as not to cause further neural injury.
- In the majority of cases, posterior instrumentation and fusion is sufficient for fracture-dislocations.
- In those cases with extensive vertebral body comminution, compression, or fragments displaced into the spinal canal, a combined anterior and posterior approach might be used; pure anterior procedures should be avoided, however.

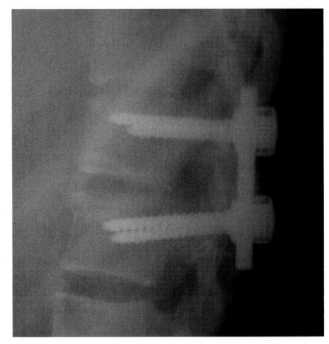

Figure 19-9 Flexion-distraction injuries are usually adequately stabilized with a single-level posterior instrumented fusion.

- A recent report demonstrated excellent maintenance of alignment in 15 cases stabilized by short-segment pedicle screw instrumentation.

Surgical Timing

- Surgical timing is an important consideration, in particular when dealing with polytraumatized patients.
- In one retrospective study, patients with injuries fixed within 3 days of injury had a lower rate of pneumonia and shorter hospital stay than those fixed after more than 3 days postinjury.
- It may also influence neurological recovery.
- Anterior decompression performed within 48 hours of injury appears to offer better neurological recovery than surgery after this interval.
- For a variety of reasons, not all patients undergo early decompressive surgery, and patients with residual canal stenosis may present months or even years after injury.
- In these cases, data suggests that substantial improvements in motor, sensory, and bladder and bowel function can be expected with decompression performed up to 2 years from the initial injury.

Suggested Treatment

- The suggested treatment of thoracolumbar fractures is given in Table 19-5.

COMPLICATIONS

- There are a number of relatively unusual complications of anterior thoracolumbar surgery including pneumothorax,

TABLE 19-5 SUGGESTED TREATMENT OF THORACOLUMBAR FRACTURES

Injury	Treatment
Compression fractures	Nonoperative
Burst fractures	
Normal neurology	Nonoperative
Abnormal neurology	Posterior intrapedicular screw fixation
Flexion-distraction fractures	Posterior instrumentation
Fracture dislocations	Posterior instrumentation

hemothorax, chylothorax, diaphragmatic rupture or herniation, ureteric damage, and great vessel injury.
- There are, however, a number of more common complications.

Nonunion

- The quoted ranges and the average incidence of nonunion associated with anterior and posterior instrumentation are given in Table 19-4.
- The usual symptom of nonunion is pain, although implant failure and a change of more than 5 degrees at a single functional spinal unit both suggest nonunion.
- The incidence of nonunion increases with age, malnutrition, obesity, tobacco use, and the use of nonsteroidal anti-inflammatory medication.
- Treatment is by posterior instrumentation and grafting.

Instrument Failure

- Pedicle screw fixation is associated with a number of complications.
- Too medial a screw may violate the spinal canal and cause dural or neurological damage.
- Too long a screw may damage the great vessels.
- In experienced hands, 0.2% nerve root irritation from pedicle screws has been reported, with a 0.5% incidence of screw breakage.

Late Deformity

- Table 19-3 and Box 19-2 show that late deformity can be expected after surgical stabilization of spinal fractures.
- The immediate postoperative correction is rarely maintained, although the loss of correction is rarely a clinical problem.

- Significant late deformity may cause severe back pain, progressive neurological deficit, or failure of an existing deficit to improve.
- The treatment is usually refixation and bone grafting.

Other Complications

- Dural tears, whether traumatic or iatrogenic, should be repaired primarily.
- The infection rate is difficult to separate from that of nontraumatic spinal surgery but is probably about 2% to 3%.

SUGGESTED READING

Alanav A, Acaroglu E, Yazici M, et al. Short-segment pedicle instrumentation of thoracolumbar burst fractures: does transpedicular intracorporeal grafting prevent early failure? Spine 2001;26: 213–217.

Croce MA, Bee TK, Pritchard E, et al. Does optimal timing for spine fracture fixation exist? Ann Surg 2001;233:851–858.

Dai LY. Remodeling of the spinal canal after thoracolumbar burst fractures. Clin Orthop 2001;382:119–123.

Denis F. The three-column spine and its significance in the classification of acute thoracolumbar spinal injuries. Spine 1983;8:817–831.

Diamond TH, Champion B, Clark WA. Management of acute osteoporotic vertebral fractures: a nonrandomized trial comparing percutaneous vertebroplasty with conservative therapy. Am J Med 2003;114:257–265.

Garfin SR, Yuan HA, Reiley MA. Kyphoplasty and vertebroplasty for the treatment of painful osteoporotic compression fractures. Spine 2001;26:1511–1515.

Kaneda K, Taneichi H, Abumi K, et al. Anterior decompression and stabilization with the Kaneda device for thoracolumbar burst fractures associated with neurological deficits. J Bone Joint Surg (Am) 1997;79:69–73.

Kim NH, Lee HM, Chun IM. Neurologic injury and recovery in patients with burst fracture of the thoracolumbar spine. Spine 1999;24:290–294.

Magerl F, Aebi M, Gertzbein SD. A comprehensive classification of thoracic and lumbar injuries. Eur Spine J 1994;3:184–201.

McAfee PC, Yuan HA, Fredrickson BE. The value of computed tomography in thoracolumbar fractures: an analysis of one hundred consecutive cases and a new classification. J Bone Joint Surg (Am) 1981;65:461–473.

Rechtine GR, Cahill D, Chrin AM. Treatment of thoracolumbar trauma: comparison of complications of operative versus nonoperative treatment. J Spinal Disord 1999;12:406–409.

Shen WJ, Shen YS. Nonsurgical treatment of three-column thoracolumbar junction burst fractures without neurologic deficit. Spine 1999;24:412–415.

Transfeldt E, White D, Bradford D, et al. Delayed anterior decompression inpatients with spinal cord and cauda equina injuries of the thoracolumbar spine. Spine 1990;15:953–957.

Wessberg P, Wang Y, Irstam L, et al. The effect of surgery and remodelling on spinal canal measurements after thoracolumbar burst fractures. Eur Spine J 2001;10:55–63.

Wood K, Butterman G, Mehbod A, et al. Operative compared with nonoperative treatment of a thoracolumbar burst fracture without neurological deficit. J Bone Joint Surg (Am) 2003;85:773–781.

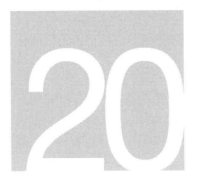

PELVIC AND ACETABULAR FRACTURES

Fractures of the pelvis and acetabulum that require active treatment are generally high-energy injuries in young patients. The epidemiology of pelvic and acetabular fractures shown in Table 20-1, however, indicates a high average age and a type E distribution (see Chapter 1). This is because about 75% of pelvic and acetabular fractures are in fact pubic rami fractures that occur in the elderly after a simple fall and do not require treatment beyond rest, analgesia, and assessment of their social circumstances. This chapter focuses on the other pelvic and acetabular fractures that frequently require surgical treatment. The management of these injuries must be individualized to the patient and based on his or her age, functional level, comorbidities, and associated injuries.

PELVIC FRACTURES

The management of pelvic ring injuries has evolved considerably over the past two decades. Injury patterns are better understood, and the identification of associated injuries has been aided by better understanding of the mechanism of pelvic injury. Improved approaches to fixation have diminished the incidence of posttraumatic deformity reported in earlier series, and nonunion is now uncommon. The aggressive treatment of hemorrhage with external stabilization and angiography has improved survival, and algorithms for the treatment of open pelvic fractures have resulted in mortality being lowered to less than half of the level of 20 years ago. Patient-based outcomes are now being reported, giving direction to future work that will improve on our current treatment strategies. Current controversies in the management of pelvic ring injuries center around issues of resuscitation, operative indications, and operative techniques. They are listed in Box 20-1.

SURGICAL ANATOMY

The pelvis is made up of the sacrum and the two innominate bones, held together by a complex array of ligaments. Anteriorly, the symphyseal bodies are held together by the symphyseal cartilage, a thick fibrocartilaginous structure

TABLE 20-1 EPIDEMIOLOGY OF PELVIC AND ACETABULAR FRACTURES

Proportion of all fractures	1.5%
Average age	69.6 y
Men/women	30%/70%
Distribution	Type E
Incidence	$17/10^5$/y
Open fractures	0.9%
Most common causes	
Fall	63.7%
Motor vehicle accident	14.3%
Fall from height	11.0%
Pelvic fractures	92.3%
Acetabular fractures	7.7%

BOX 20-1 CURRENT CONTROVERSIES IN THE INVESTIGATION AND TREATMENT OF PELVIC FRACTURES

What are the indications for external fixation versus external immobilization?

Should external stabilization or angiography be the first step in controlling pelvic bleeding in the hypotensive patient?

Is operative management of minimally displaced sacral fractures helpful or dangerous?

Is open reduction and neurological decompression an advantage in displaced sacral fractures?

What is an acceptable reduction of the anterior and posterior pelvic ring?

Is percutaneous reduction and fixation preferable to open reduction and internal fixation?

What is the role of lumbosacral fixation?

What are the indications for caval filter placement?

What is the best treatment for extraperitoneal bladder rupture?

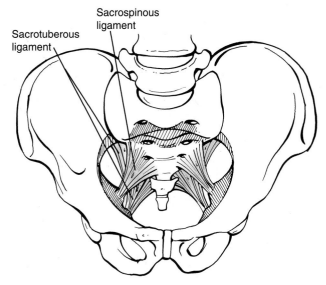

Figure 20-1   Diagram of the pelvis demonstrating the sacrospinous and sacrotuberous ligaments that support the pelvic ring.

that permits very little motion between the bodies. The symphysis is further supported by the sacrospinous ligaments and pelvic floor, which restrict external rotation of one hemipelvis with respect to the other, and the sacrotuberous ligaments, which help to restrict motion in the sagittal plane (Fig. 20-1). The inguinal ligaments, running from the anterior superior iliac spines (ASIS) to the pubic tubercles, and the obturator membrane help support the anterior ring, particularly in cases of pubic rami fracture.

The posterior pelvis is a complicated anatomical region. The sacrum is the base of the spine, and its shape is important because it relates to the location of fractures traversing it and to the methods of fixation for posterior ring injuries. The sacrum extends laterally into the sacral ala. The alae slope inferiorly and forward with the L5 nerve roots lying immediately on the periosteum approximately 1 cm

medial to the sacroiliac joints. The sacroiliac joints are shaped as an inverted L with a relatively small articular surface area. Each of the innominate bones is held to the sacrum by the anterior and posterior sacroiliac ligaments (Fig. 20-2). The posterior ligamentous complex is among the strongest anywhere in the body because it must support weight bearing by load transfer from the extremities to the spine.

The pelvis houses hollow viscera, reproductive organs, and the bladder (which sits in the space of Retzius immediately behind the symphysis). The area anterior to the iliac pelvic brim is known as the false pelvis, separated from the true pelvis by the iliopectineal fascia. There is a large vascular plexus anterior to the sacrum and sacroiliac joints, and in this region, the common iliac arteries divide into the internal and external iliac arteries. The internal iliac artery gives rise to the superior gluteal artery, which courses through the greater sciatic notch and is vulnerable in posterior ring injuries. The obturator artery also takes its origin from the internal iliac artery and runs along the quadrilateral surface of the pelvis, exiting through the obturator foramen. The external iliac artery travels medially to the iliopectineal fascia and emerges from under the ilioinguinal ligament as the femoral artery. Connections between the external iliac and obturator systems are common, and, when arterial, they are called the corona mortis. This may be one or more vessels that run over the superior ramus approximately 3 cm lateral to the symphysis and must be sought out when dissecting in that area.

CLASSIFICATION

Pelvic ring injuries are classified by several methods. The most basic is the anatomical classification of Letournel (1980), which divides anterior and posterior ring injuries into four types based on the location of the injury (Box 20-2). Sacral fractures can be subdivided by their location as described in Table 20-2. Sacroiliac dislocations can be anterior disruptions that do not compromise vertical

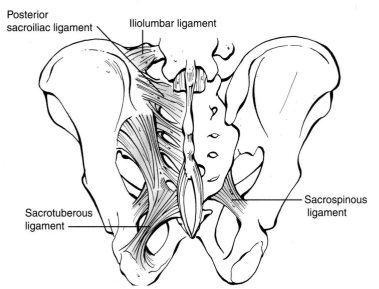

Figure 20-2   Diagram of the sacroiliac complex from posteriorly demonstrating the sacroiliac ligament, the strongest ligament in the body.

posterior ligamentous stability or complete disruptions that lead to multidirectional posterior instability. This difference highlights the findings of Bucholz (1981), who described instability of the pelvis by dividing it into three types. Type 1 is stable rotationally and vertically, type 2 is unstable in rotation but stable vertically (for instance, a sacroiliac [SI] injury with anterior opening and an intact posterior hinge), and type 3 is completely unstable in all planes. Fracture dislocations of the SI joint occur when a portion of the joint is intact and the rest is dislocated with the displaced hemipelvis. This may occur by avulsion of a portion of the sacrum but is usually a fracture through the iliac wing that extends into the SI joint, leaving an intact posterior portion of the ilium still attached to the sacrum via the posterior SI ligaments (Fig. 20-3). The most important system of classification is shown in Figure 20-4, based on the mechanism of injury. Its value is in its ability to predict associated injuries and the potential for bleeding. There are three main components described, as follows.

Anterior Posterior Compression (APC) Injuries

APC injuries occur from an anterior or posterior force vector and cause external rotation of the hemipelvis. They can also occur from forceful abduction of the leg, which is common in motorcycle accidents. The anterior ring injury is typically a symphyseal separation and the posterior injury an SI joint dislocation (Fig. 20-4B).

TABLE 20-2 CLASSIFICATION OF SACRAL FRACTURES

Type	Description
1	Lateral to the foramen
2	Through the foramen
3	Medial to the foramen (including horizontal fractures)

From Denis F, Davis S, Comfort T. Sacral fractures: an important problem: retrospective analysis of 236 cases. Clin Orthop 1988;227:67–81.

These are subdivided into three types. In APC1 injuries, there is minimal opening of the symphysis and near anatomical posterior anatomy. In APC2 injuries, there is an anterior separation of >2.5 cm with an opening of the SI joint or much less commonly a sacral fracture. These are rotationally unstable and vertically stable. The final stage of an APC injury is the APC3, in which the posterior tension band (the posterior SI ligaments) is lost, permitting complete instability of the hemipelvis rotationally and vertically.

Lateral Compression (LC) Injuries

These injuries are the most common type of pelvic injury. The hemipelvis is internally rotated, such as seen in a driver involved in a T-bone accident, with the impact vector coming from the patient's side. Rami fractures that are horizontal on the inlet view are characteristic of this injury type. The posterior ring injury is either a sacral fracture (mostly impacted types) or a fracture dislocation (Fig. 20-4A).

LC fractures are also subdivided into three types. In an LC1 injury there is no significant instability. Typically they are minimally displaced rami fractures and an impacted sacral fracture. An LC2 injury includes rotational instability of one hemipelvis, and in the LC3 injury one hemipelvis is driven across the midline opening up the other side (similar to an APC on that side). This represents the "windswept pelvis."

Vertical Shear (VS) Injuries

The third type is called vertical shear (VS) and results from a fall from a height. This is always completely unstable, and most often there is a posterior SI dislocation in conjunction with a symphyseal dislocation or rami fractures (Fig. 20-4C).

Combined Mechanical Injuries (CMI)

It should be understood that force vectors in pelvic injuries can be complex, and therefore some fractures do not fit neatly into the Young and Burgess classification. These are referred to as combined mechanical injuries.

EPIDEMIOLOGY

The overall epidemiology of pelvic fractures (see Table 20-1) does not represent the spectrum of pelvic fractures that present to specialist centers because about 75% of fractures are uncomplicated pubic rami fractures. This fact skews the epidemiology considerably and explains why the overall distribution is type E (see Chapter 1). The epidemiology of patients with pelvic fractures presenting to a major U.S. level 1 trauma center is shown in Table 20-3.

Table 20-3 shows that significant pelvic injuries are predominantly seen in young men. The vast majority present as LC1 patterns and are stable. Open fractures are rare, occurring in less than 5% of cases. There is a separate subgroup of up to 5% of severely injured patients, however, who are hypotensive at initial presentation. These patients must be dealt with differently than the group who present with stable vital signs.

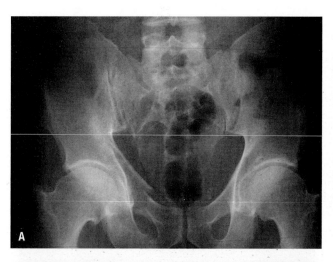

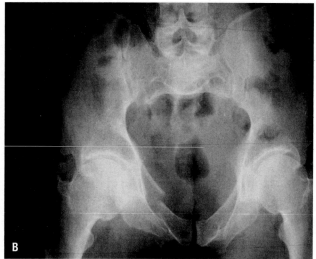

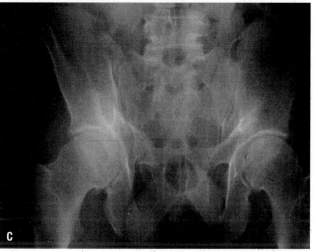

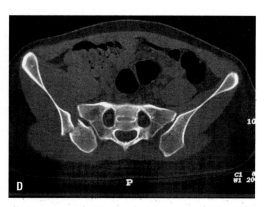

Figure 20-3   Anteroposterior (**A**), inlet (**B**), and outlet (**C**) radiographs of a fracture dislocation pattern demonstrating the intact fragment of the posterior ilium and the displaced hemipelvis. (**D**) A CT demonstrates the intact fragment to be the most posterior portion of the ilium (3D).

TABLE 20-3 EPIDEMIOLOGY OF 327 PELVIC FRACTURES PRESENTING TO A U.S. LEVEL I TRAUMA CENTER OVER A 3-YEAR PERIOD	
Average age	38 y
Men/women	78%/22%
Open fractures	2.1%
Fracture distribution	
LC	84
LC1	69
LC2	11
LC3	4
APC	9
APC1	2
APC2	5
APC3	2
VS	7

Associated Injuries

As opposed to most fractures, injuries to the pelvic ring are commonly associated with nonorthopaedic as well as other musculoskeletal injuries. As stated earlier, the mechanism of the fracture (APC, LC, VS) helps predict associated organ system injury. APC injuries are associated with injuries to the hollow viscera and with pelvic bleeding. The pelvic floor is torn, allowing for blood loss without a good tamponade. With increasing energy the risk of bleeding is higher, with APC3 injuries resulting in the highest blood loss and transfusion requirements.

Lateral compression fractures have a close association with head and chest injury, presumably from those parts of the body struck by the car during a side impact. When one hemipelvis is injured (LC1 and 2), the risk of arterial injury is low. However, in LC3 injuries, because the opposite hemipelvis is externally rotated and the pelvic floor is torn, there is a higher incidence of pelvic bleeding (similar to APC patterns).

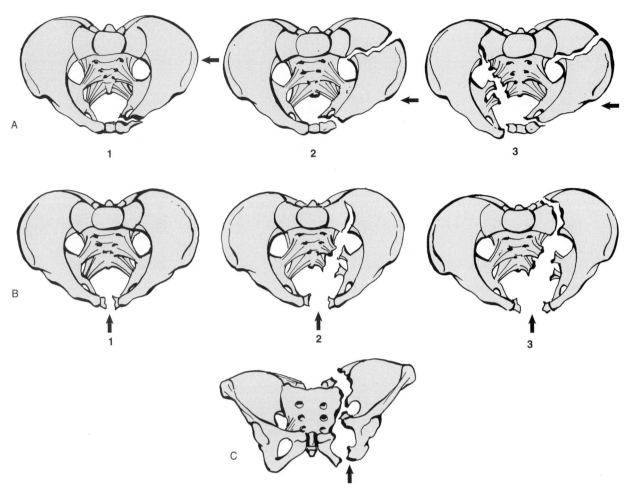

Figure 20-4   The Young and Burgess classification is the most commonly used classification for pelvic ring injuries. It is mechanistic in its approach. (**A**) Lateral compression (LC) injuries; (**B**) anterior posterior compression (APC) injuries; (**C**) vertical shear (VS) injury.

Urological injury is relatively common, reported in up to 15% of pelvic fractures. This must be carefully assessed as outlined earlier. Urological injury can be in the form of a bladder injury or urethral tear. Urethral tears primarily affect men and can lead to significant problems if not identified early. Bladder rupture can be intraperitoneal, requiring emergency repair, or extraperitoneal, in the space of Retzius. Although there is some debate about the need for repair of extraperitoneal ruptures, it is clear early repair should be performed if the pelvic injury requires anterior reduction and fixation.

Other fractures are present in up to 80% of patients. The lower extremities, acetabuli, and spine are the most commonly injured. A careful secondary survey must be performed after the initial resuscitation is complete to avoid missed injury.

DIAGNOSIS

History and Physical Examination

- In addition to a standard medical history, it is important to obtain details of the accident because most cases of pelvic injury come directly from the scene of the accident.

- Details of the accident will help assess the energy of the injury. Information from the emergency rescue team is valuable.
  - Was it a motorcycle or car accident? Was a second vehicle involved? Were there any fatalities at the scene?
  - The most important pieces of information are the blood pressure at the scene and during transport, the amount of fluid given, and the neurological status if known.
- Many patients will not be alert or responsive upon arrival, so a careful examination of the entire patient in addition to the extremities and pelvis according to ATLS guidelines is needed to identify musculoskeletal and other injuries.
- The examination specific to the pelvis includes a gentle examination with the hands pushing internally on the iliac crests.
- Because most instability patterns will be diagnosed from the radiographs and CT, only one person (the most senior) should physically manipulate the pelvis. Multiple examinations may dislodge a clot and cause increased bleeding.
- A thorough examination of the perineum and rectum should be performed to rule out an open injury (tension

failure of the skin in an APC pattern is the most devastating).

- Lateral compression fractures may also be open, with the rami violating the skin from the inside out.
  - This can be seen on the very high anterior thigh or near the anterior skin over the symphyseal region.
- In men, the penis should be examined for signs of blood at the meatus and a rectal exam performed.
- In women, examination of the vaginal vault and rectum will rule out injuries in these areas.
- Finally, in alert patients, a meticulous neurological examination of the lower extremities is performed to find any subtle deficits and establish baseline function.

Radiologic Examination

- The standard A-P pelvic radiograph performed on all trauma patients should allow for the identification and general classification of any pelvic injury.
- This should be followed by the additional four views of the standard five-view workup.
- The pelvis is evaluated using the AP, inlet (caudad), and outlet (cephalad) views (Fig. 20-5).
- The inlet view is the best to demonstrate posterior ring displacement, and it is easiest to see sacral impaction and coronal plane rotation on this view.
- The outlet view gives the best representation of sagittal plane deformity.
- Judet views, or 45-degree oblique views, complete the radiograph series.
  - These views are helpful to screen for associated acetabular fractures and iliac wing injuries.
- A CT scan will clarify the specific anatomy of posterior ring injuries and is required if surgical intervention is considered.
- The trauma CT scan typically is sufficient to diagnose the posterior ring injury, but a fine cut exam might be needed to plan surgical procedures.
- Three-dimensional reconstructions produce nice pictures but add nothing to the evaluation.
- Because of the high incidence of associated urological injury, a retrograde urethrogram should be performed in male patients prior to catheterization.
- A cystogram or CT cystogram is indicated if there is frank blood or more than 30 red blood cells in the urine.

TREATMENT

Surgical Treatment

- The treatment of a patient with a pelvic ring injury begins with resuscitation.
- Mortality is highest in patients who are hypotensive upon presentation.
- A standard trauma workup is needed to rule out other sources of bleeding and hypotension.
  - Bleeding may occur in the abdomen, chest, or extremities. The workup must include all of these areas.

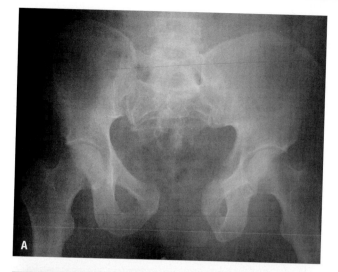

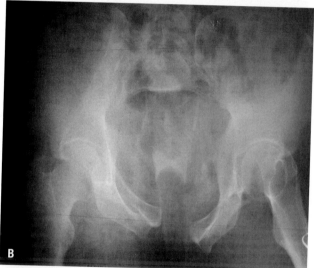

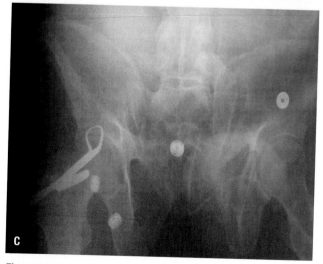

Figure 20-5 Anteroposterior (**A**), inlet (**B**), and outlet (**C**) radiographs of an APC type 3 pelvic ring injury. Note that the posterior displacement of the pelvis is best seen on the inlet view.

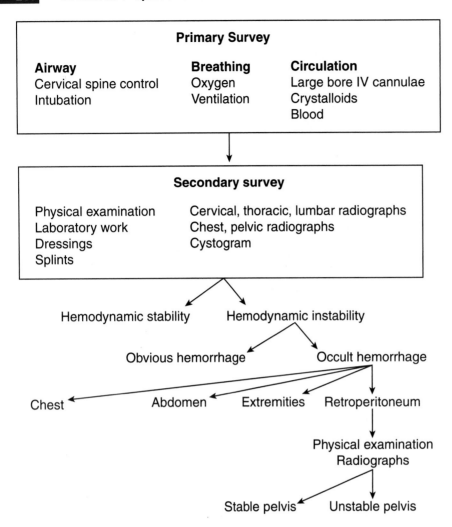

Primary Survey

Airway	**Breathing**	**Circulation**
Cervical spine control	Oxygen	Large bore IV cannulae
Intubation	Ventilation	Crystalloids
		Blood

Secondary survey

Physical examination Cervical, thoracic, lumbar radiographs
Laboratory work Chest, pelvic radiographs
Dressings Cystogram
Splints

Hemodynamic stability   Hemodynamic instability

Obvious hemorrhage   Occult hemorrhage

Chest   Abdomen   Extremities   Retroperitoneum

Physical examination
Radiographs

Stable pelvis   Unstable pelvis

Algorithm 20-1 The initial resuscitation of patients with pelvic fractures.

- In addition to bleeding, hypotension may occur from spinal injury (and subsequent spinal shock) and cardiogenic shock.
- If no other source of bleeding is found, the pelvis may be the cause.
- The CT typically will demonstrate blood in the pelvis in these cases, and a contrast-enhanced CT can locate pelvic arterial bleeding accurately.
- An outline of the initial resuscitation of a patient with a pelvic fracture is shown in Algorithm 20-1.
- Management of the pelvic ring injury begins with the resuscitation of the patient.
- If the pelvic volume is increased with tearing of the pelvic floor, such as APC2 or 3 and LC3 patterns, the pelvis should be mechanically stabilized.
  - Current methods include anteriorly placed C-clamps (Fig. 20-6), a sheet or binder wrapped around the pelvis close to the level of the greater trochanters, or an anterior external fixator (see Fig. 35-7 in Chapter 35).
- Regardless of the method chosen, any patient presenting with an increased pelvic volume should be externally stabilized if there is any question of hypotension, either on presentation or at the scene.

- If associated abdominal or urological injury requires operative intervention, skeletal stabilization should be performed prior to the laparotomy to avoid further displacement of the pelvis because the abdominal wall may be maintaining a tamponade.
- This is typically accomplished with either an anterior external fixator (see Fig. 35-7 in Chapter 35) or anteriorly placed C-clamp.
- Once the laparotomy is complete, fixation of the anterior ring is usually performed through the same incision but can be deferred depending on the comfort of the surgeon with this procedure.
- The initial management of the unstable pelvis is given in Algorithm 20-2.
- Definitive fixation of the pelvis is needed only if there is instability or unacceptable deformity.
- Recommendations for management of the different types of pelvic fractures outlined in the Young and Burgess classification are shown in Table 20-4.
- Nonoperative management is indicated for the vast majority of pelvic ring injuries.
- One series of over 70 patients with LC1 injuries showed healing without displacement even if full self-regulated weight bearing was allowed.

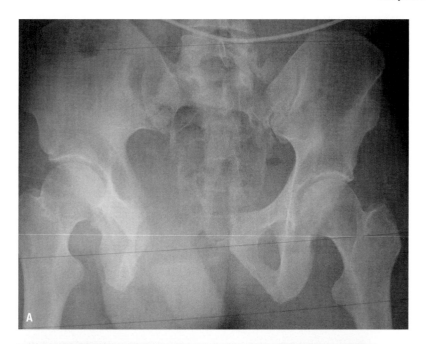

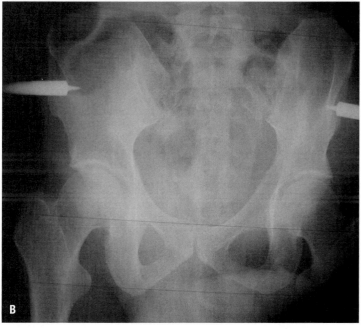

Figure 20-6 An example of an APC type 2 pelvic ring injury (**A**) with an anteriorly placed C-clamp to reduce the displacement (**B**).

- Unstable injuries are typically treated with reduction and internal fixation if the patient can tolerate it.
- Indications for anterior and posterior fixation differ, but there are some generally accepted tenets.
  - Ligamentous injuries do not heal as well as bony injuries, thus close opposition and stabilization are an advantage.
  - Symphyseal disruptions with greater than 2 cm of displacement have better outcomes with open reduction and internal fixation than nonoperative treatment.
  - Thus APC2 and 3 injuries with symphyseal disruption are good candidates for ORIF.
  - Well-performed single-plate fixation with more than two screws on each side yields predictable healing.

- In contradistinction to symphyseal disruptions, fractures of the rami rarely require fixation unless they are a component of an injury with posterior instability and remain widely separated after posterior fixation.
- Rami fractures have some inherent stability because the inguinal ligament and obturator membrane span them. They are most common in lateral compression injuries and are therefore unlikely to gap as the initial displacement is shortening.
- Reduction and fixation of the posterior ring is required only in Bucholz type 3 injuries in which the posterior ring is vertically unstable.
  - Thus in an APC2 injury with a symphysis separation and anterior SI widening but no vertical instability, it

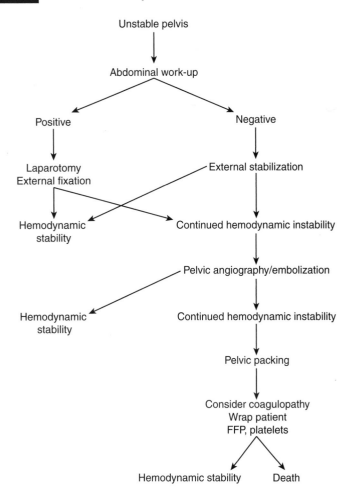

Unstable pelvis

↓

Abdominal work-up

Positive   Negative

↓   ↓

Laparotomy   External stabilization
External fixation

Hemodynamic   Continued hemodynamic instability
stability

↓

Pelvic angiography/embolization

↓

Hemodynamic   Continued hemodynamic instability
stability

↓

Pelvic packing

↓

Consider coagulopathy
Wrap patient
FFP, platelets

Hemodynamic stability   Death

Algorithm 20-2 The treatment of the patient with an unstable pelvis.

is clear that anterior fixation results in predictable healing and good results.

- Only if the SI joint is completely disrupted and vertically unstable does it require fixation.

- Vertically unstable posterior injuries, whether they be sacral fractures, SI joint dislocations, or SI joint fracture dislocations, should be reduced and fixed.
- The method of reduction and fixation are controversial.

TABLE 20-4 RECOMMENDED DEFINITIVE TREATMENT FOR PELVIC FRACTURES

Injury Pattern	Treatment of Anterior Ring	Treatment of Posterior Ring
APC 1	Nonoperative	Nonoperative
APC 2	ORIF, plate	Nonoperative
APC 3	ORIF symphysis	Iliosacral screws (SI joint, sacrum).
	ORIF rami if wide after posterior fixation	Consider lumbosacral fixation
LC 1	Nonoperative	Nonoperative
LC 2	Nonoperative rami	Iliosacral screws (SI joint or small fragment SI fracture dislocation)
	ORIF symphysis (rare)	ORIF fracture dislocation
LC 3	Nonoperative rami	ORIF widened side
	ORIF rami wide after posterior fixation	Consider ORIF internally rotated side
VS	ORIF symphysis	Iliosacral screws (SI joint, sacral fracture)
	Nonoperative rami	Consider lumbosacral fixation in comminuted sacral fracture

- Most authors agree that open reduction and fixation with plates and lag screws is the treatment of choice for fracture dislocations.
- In certain special cases in which the posterior intact fragment is small, iliosacral screw fixation is needed to improve the stability of fixation.
- Sacroiliac joint dislocations may be reduced closed or open.
- Regardless of the method chosen, the reduction should be anatomical.
- Fixation with iliosacral screws or plates placed on the superior surface of the SI joint have both been successful.
- Decision making in sacral fractures is more challenging because instability is not always obvious early and the neural elements may be at risk from compression.
  - If stability is difficult to determine, serial radiographs may reveal increasing displacement, indicating instability.
  - Intraoperative stress examination under fluoroscopic control has also been shown to demonstrate vertical displacement.
  - In either case, if instability is present, reduction and fixation are indicated to prevent deformity.
  - Some authors believe that if the fracture is through the foramen in zone 2 (see Table 20-2), an open technique should be used for nerve root decompression prior to fixation.
  - Others argue that if an acceptable reduction can be obtained closed, percutaneous fixation is preferred to avoid the risks of open surgery, such as infection.
  - One small series reported several nerve root injuries from compression of displaced sacral fractures treated several weeks after injury, although most were done open.
  - Advocates of the percutaneous approach believe the small risk of nerve injury is outweighed by the risk of infection using open techniques.
- Attention has been focused recently on the ability of the fixation to resist vertical displacement.
- Two modifications of standard iliosacral screw placement have been described.
  - The strongest is the addition of lumbosacral fixation. This is typically combined with either iliosacral fixation or intrasacral fixation. The addition of an L5 pedicle screw with spinopelvic fixation to the ilium may be strong enough to allow early weight bearing. This technique adds the risk of nerve injury from the pedicle screw(s), the increased risk of infection from a larger open procedure and bigger implants, and it requires implant removal.
  - The other method is to use much longer iliosacral screws, attempting to go across the sacrum to the opposite ala adjacent to the SI joint. This effectively increases the mechanical advantage of the screws to resist vertical displacement because there is a longer lever arm in the intact sacrum.
  - In either case, accurate reduction and compression of the fracture should be the rule.
- The outcome of pelvic ring injury is determined by many factors: the initial injury pattern, the quality of the reduction, the associated injuries, and social factors.

- Among these, the surgeon has control only of the accuracy of reduction and the stability of fixation.
- The associated neurological, urological, and other skeletal system injuries probably have a greater effect on outcome than does the pelvic fracture, provided it heals in an acceptable position.
- Vertically stable injuries fare much better then unstable ones.
- Well-fixed APC2 injuries have good to excellent results in over 90% of cases as compared with only 60% to 70% of APC3 injuries.
- The reduction of ligamentous injury is paramount, especially at the SI joint.
- Inaccurate reduction leads to significantly more pain than accurate reduction, likely because the joint stability is generated by scar tissue after healing.
- In general, about two thirds of patients with type 3 (posteriorly unstable) injuries have good or excellent outcomes when looking at any physical variable such as gait, pain, or sitting ability (Fig. 20-7).
- All pelvic ring injuries have the potential for long-term problems.
  - Validated summed outcome tools have demonstrated differences in physical function and mental subscores in this patient population.
  - The effect of associated injuries on the outcome scores has not been well delineated.
  - For example, a patient with a stable pelvic injury and a significant neurological injury whose pelvis has healed in a good position but still has a foot drop and impotence would be expected to have a low score primarily because of the associated injuries, not the pelvic ring fracture.

Nonsurgical Treatment

- Nonoperative management is indicated for the vast majority of pelvic ring injuries because they are stable (Table 20-4).
- For LC1 fractures, progressive weight bearing with repeat radiographs at a week or if there is more than expected pain identifies subtle instability and allows for reduction and fixation within an appropriate time frame.

COMPLICATIONS

Nerve Injury

- Complications of pelvic ring injuries may be from the injury or the related operative procedures.
- Most neurological injuries caused by the accident resolve to some degree.
- The more dense the sensory and motor injury, the worse is the prognosis.
- The L5 nerve root is the least likely to recover and may require brace treatment for the foot to allow for normal walking.
- The L5 root is also most susceptible to iatrogenic nerve injury.
- If there are neurological signs after iliosacral fixation, the posterior fixation should be assessed by CT scan to

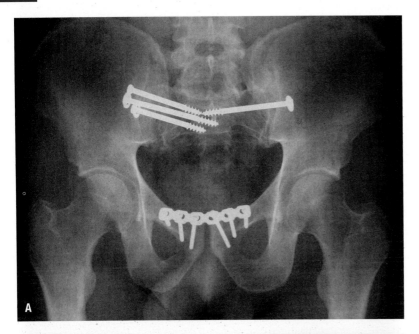

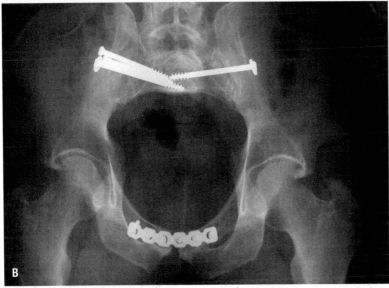

Figure 20-7 Follow-up anteroposterior (**A**) and inlet (**B**) radiographs at 2 years of the patient shown in Figure 20-5. The patient had an excellent outcome and returned to sporting activities.

look for its proximity to the nerve and be removed or replaced if impingement is possible.

■ Intraoperative stimulus-evoked motor potentials may diminish the risk of incorrect screw placement and therefore the risk of iatrogenic nerve injury.

Infection

■ The infection rate for anterior pelvic procedures is approximately 1% to 4%.

■ For posterior ring injuries treated with open techniques, the infection rate is variable.

■ The older literature reported the infection rate as high as 25%, but most of these series included patients treated without the currently recommended gluteal-sparing approaches.

■ Using this approach, a multicenter study reported an infection rate of lower than 4% for open procedures.

■ The infection rate for percutaneous fixation is negligible.

Malunion and Nonunion

■ Malunion is common after nonoperative treatment of unstable injuries, but nonunion is rare.

■ Malunion most commonly affects gait, sleeping, and sexual function. Sitting imbalance is also common.

■ The heights of the ischia on the A-P radiograph most accurately predicts sitting imbalance.

■ Nonunion is uncommon and usually seen in sacral or SI joint injuries that are not reduced and stabilized.

■ Pelvic non- and malunions are not simple problems and should be managed by a surgeon very familiar with the management of acute injuries.

Deep Venous Thrombosis (DVT) and Pulmonary Embolus (PE)

- Pelvic clots have been reported on MRI venography in as many as 60% of patients with pelvic and acetabular fractures.
- Most surgeons use some sort of chemical and physical method of prophylaxis for patients who will not be quickly mobilized.
- Using mechanical compression devices preoperatively and mechanical and chemical prophylaxis postoperatively yields a low rate of clinically symptomatic DVT and a very low rate of PE.
- The use of caval filters has become more common, especially with the advent of temporary removable filters.
- Patients with any significant risk of bleeding or other contraindications to chemical prophylaxis (such as brain injury, etc.) are candidates for early filter placement.
- DVT and PE are discussed in Chapter 41.

ACETABULAR FRACTURES

Acetabular fractures are considered among the most challenging orthopaedic injuries to manage. This is in part due to the complexity of the anatomy, the fracture patterns, and the highly concentric nature of the hip joint. Although operative management of displaced acetabular fractures is the mainstay of treatment, the indications for nonoperative management have become clearer in recent years. Longer term outcome studies have demonstrated the need for an anatomical reduction of the roof with a stable joint in diminishing the risk of osteoarthritis. The several areas of controversy are listed in Box 20-3.

SURGICAL ANATOMY

The osseous anatomy of the acetabulum is that of the innominate bone itself. The articular surface of the joint is horseshoe shaped, with a central depression called the fovea from which the ligamentum teres attaches to the femoral head. The hip joint has no meniscus or intervening

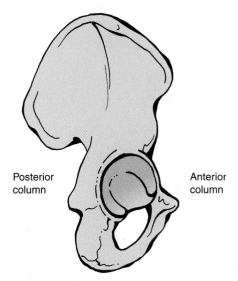

Figure 20-8 A diagram of the acetabulum viewed from the lateral aspect demonstrating the anterior and posterior supporting columns.

structures to relieve stress and as a sphere is the most constrained joint in the body. The innominate bone has some elasticity and during loading allows some accommodation of the acetabulum to the femoral head. Loading studies have demonstrated that the initial loading of the acetabulum is peripheral and with increasing load becomes more central.

The acetabulum, when viewed from the lateral side, is an inverted Y (Fig. 20-8). There is bony support anteriorly and posteriorly. These regions are called the columns of the acetabulum, and their extensions to the outer aspect of the joint, or rims, are called the anterior and posterior walls. The hip capsule is very strong and maintains its integrity at the peripheral aspect of the joint in fractures without dislocation. This finding is important in determining treatment and understanding fracture displacement. The most important region of the joint is the "roof," or superior surface, that bears the burden of gait. The posterior wall is also an area of high stress when the hip is loaded in flexion. This area is also loaded more during normal gait than the anterior areas of the joint. The acetabular labrum adds depth to the joint and helps maintain joint stability.

From a surgical perspective, the anterior acetabulum extends to the superior ramus and includes the iliac wing, brim of the pelvis, and anterior wall. The posterior acetabulum extends to the ischium, made up of the sciatic notch and posterior wall. The iliopectineal fascia separates the false pelvis from the true pelvis through its attachment to the pelvic brim. Deep behind this is the quadrilateral surface, or the medial wall of the acetabulum. This bony area is critical in the operative repair of fractures because it is manipulated to accomplish an indirect reduction of the column on the far side of the approach in many cases. The external iliac artery lies medial to the iliopectineal fascia and psoas gutter. Lateral to the fascia lies the tendon of the iliacus and psoas with the femoral nerve. The obturator artery and nerve run against the quadrilateral surface medial to the obturator internus. The superior gluteal artery and nerve and the sciatic nerve exit the pelvis posteriorly through the sciatic notch. The sciatic nerve is typically located

BOX 20-3 CURRENT CONTROVERSIES IN THE MANAGEMENT OF ACETABULAR FRACTURES

What are the indications for nonoperative management?
What is the optimal treatment for the elderly patient with a displaced acetabular fracture?
Are there any indications for percutaneous reduction and fixation of acetabular fractures?
What is the best method of prophylaxis against heterotopic ossification?
What are the indications for extensile approaches?

posteriorly to the obturator internus tendon and anterior to the piriformis, but in approximately 15% of patients the nerve or a portion of it may pass through the piriformis.

CLASSIFICATION

In contradistinction to almost all other fractures, the classification system for acetabular fractures is agreed on by all experts in the field. The system of Letournel (1974) is both descriptive and predictive. It is based on the areas of the joint that support the hip. Recent studies have demonstrated excellent intra- and interobserver agreement. In addition, the classification aids in determining the type of surgery and also predicts outcome. There are five "elemental" fractures and five associated (combinations of the elemental types) fractures (Fig. 20-9 and Table 20-5).

Young patients have injuries that are determined by the force vector of the blow. Side impacts result in TR, T, BC, ACH, and TR+PW fractures. Central dislocation or more commonly subluxation may occur, particularly in TR and T fractures. If the vector is angled more anteriorly, an anterior column fracture may occur. Fractures of the posterior joint occur primarily from a posteriorly directed force transmitted via the femoral shaft resulting in PW, PC, or combined PC+PW or TR+PW fractures. Associated posterior dislocations may be present. In older patients, the mechanism of injury is usually a fall from a standing height, and

TABLE 20-5 INCIDENCE OF THE DIFFERENT TYPES OF ACETABULAR FRACTURES

Type of Fracture	Incidence (%)
Elemental fractures	
Anterior wall (AW)	1.9
Anterior column (AC)	4.1
Posterior wall (PW)	23.7
Posterior column (PC)	3.2
Transverse (TR)	7.4
Associated fractures	
T shaped (T)	7.0
Posterior column + posterior wall (PC+PW)	3.4
Transverse + posterior wall (TR+PW)	19.4
Anterior column + posterior hemitransverse (ACH)	6.9
Both column (BC)	22.7

From Letournel E, Judet R. Fractures of the acetabulum, 2nd ed. Berlin: Springer-Verlag, 1993.

the pattern of fracture is most commonly an ACH or BC fracture. Due to the weaker bone stock, marginal impaction of the roof is more common in elderly patients. This is a difficult problem, and the prognosis is worse.

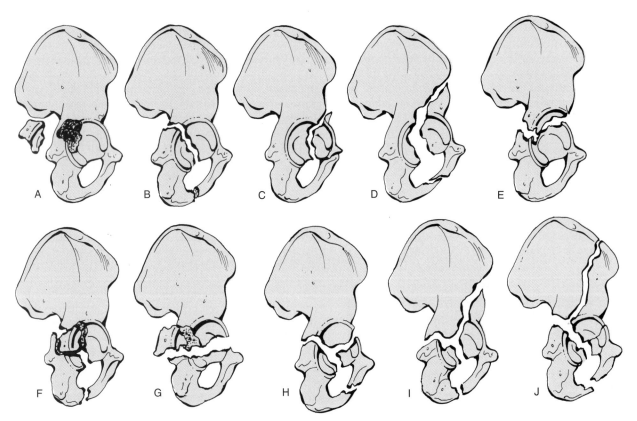

Figure 20-9   The Letournel classification. It separates the acetabular fractures into ten distinct types: posterior wall (**A**), posterior column (**B**), anterior wall (**C**), anterior column (**D**), transverse (**E**), posterior column and posterior wall (**F**), transverse and posterior wall (**G**), T-shaped (**H**), anterior column and posterior hemitransverse (**I**), and both columns (**J**). (See Table 20-5.)

EPIDEMIOLOGY

Acetabular fractures are rare, and few surgeons accumulate a large series. The data shown in Table 20-5 is from the 940 fractures documented by Letournel (1993). The men/women ratio is 66% to 34%, and 65% of the patients were between 20 and 49 years of age, suggesting the epidemiology is similar to pelvic fractures that present to specialist centers (see Table 20-3).

Associated Injuries

Other musculoskeletal injuries may occur in association with acetabular fractures. A list of the associated skeletal injuries is shown in Table 20-6. It can be seen that other musculoskeletal injuries are common. Vascular disruption may occur as may damage to the superior gluteal artery when the posterior column is very displaced because this occurs through the sciatic notch. The obturator artery may be injured in fractures that affect the quadrilateral surface and cause significant medial displacement.

Table 20-6 shows that both types of femoral head fracture (see Figs. 21.2-1 and 21.2-2 in Chapter 21) may occur. Although marginal impaction of the articular surface is evident on the CT by virtue of the impacted subchondral bone, scuffing and shear injury will not be seen until the area is directly inspected.

DIAGNOSIS

History and Physical Examination

The history and examination of the patient with an acetabular fracture is similar to that of a pelvic fracture patient as described earlier in this chapter. Because the mechanism of posterior injury is frequently the bent knee striking the dashboard, hip fracture dislocations are common (see Chapter 21) as are associated knee ligament injuries (see Chapter 26). These should be identified on the initial examination. The neurological status of the lower extremity needs to be determined prior to any attempt to reduce a dislocation. The peroneal nerve is at most risk from posterior

TABLE 20-6 INJURIES ASSOCIATED WITH ACETABULAR FRACTURES

Associated Skeletal Injury	Incidence (%)
Other fractures	45.2
Sciatic nerve lesion	12.2
Pubic symphysis diastasis	4.1
Anterior SI ligament damage	3.7
Ipsilateral femoral fracture	3.9
SI dislocation	2.6
Femoral head impaction fracture	2.1
Femoral head shear fracture	1.9
Ipsilateral hip fracture	1.2

From Letournel E, Judet R. Fractures of the acetabulum, 2nd ed. Berlin: Springer-Verlag, 1993.

hip dislocation, and foot eversion must not be overlooked. In elderly patients, reasons for falling, such as arrhythmia. must be ruled out in the same way as in a patient with a hip fracture.

Radiologic Examination

- The same radiographic series described for pelvic ring injuries needs to be performed in cases of acetabular fracture, including the A-P, inlet, outlet, and both Judet (45-degree oblique) views (see Fig. 20-11).
- Subtle pelvic ring injuries may exist with acetabular fractures (Table 20-6).
  - Specifically, an anterior SI joint opening is associated with BC and AHC fractures, and symphyseal separations are associated with TR and T fractures.
- In high-energy injuries, pelvic and acetabular fractures may be present in any combination.
  - The management of the acetabular fracture is different in the presence of a pelvic fracture, so these injuries must be identified.
- In addition to the standard radiographs, a fine cut CT (usually 2 mm) through the affected region of the acetabulum is obtained.
- Three-dimensional reconstructions may help one to understand the overall direction of the displacement, but they are not helpful in determining the type of surgery required because they may average out fractures that are important to the method of reduction.
- The CT is extremely helpful in recognizing marginal impaction, which is very common in any injury affecting the posterior wall.
- Understanding the radiographic landmarks of the acetabulum on the A-P radiograph and Judet views requires considerable experience.
  - The lines examined on the A-P include the ilioischial line (representation of the posterior column), the iliopectineal line (representation of the anterior column), the teardrop (a summary of lines that overlap), the roof, the anterior and posterior walls, and the iliac wing (Fig. 20-10).
  - The obturator oblique (45-degree internal rotation Judet view) profiles the posterior wall and the anterior column at the level of the joint (Fig. 20-11A).
  - The superior portion of the anterior column is the iliac wing and seen on the iliac oblique along with the anterior wall and posterior column (Fig. 20-11B).
  - To understand the radiography of acetabular fractures fully, it is recommended that the surgeon review many fractures while referring to a pelvic model.
  - Most acetabular surgeons have used model pelvises to draw out the fractures as part of the standard preoperative planning.

TREATMENT

- The goal of treatment for all acetabular fractures in young patients is a stable and congruent joint.
- Several specific fractures require separate discussion and are addressed individually.

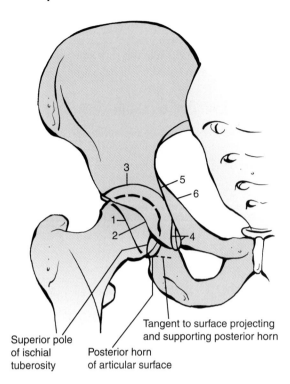

Superior pole
of ischial
tuberosity

Posterior horn
of articular surface

Tangent to surface projecting
and supporting posterior horn

Figure 20-10   A diagram of the pelvis with the ilioischial, iliopectineal, teardrop, roof, anterior, and posterior walls highlighted. 1, Posterior border of acetabulum; 2, anterior border of acetabulum; 3, roof; 4, teardrop; 5, ilioischial line; 6, brim of true pelvis.

■ Posterior wall fractures are more prone to instability and need to be assessed.
■ Both-column fractures, because the entire articular surface is separated from the intact pelvis, have better results than other patterns with displacement through the roof, warranting consideration of nonoperative management.
■ Elderly patients may be candidates for immediate or delayed total hip replacement.
■ Nondisplaced fractures are discussed in the nonoperative section.
■ An algorithm for the treatment of both column fractures is shown in Algorithm 20-3 and for other fractures in Algorithm 20-4.

DISPLACED FRACTURES (EXCEPT BOTH COLUMN)

Surgical Indications

■ The outcome of displaced acetabular fractures depends on the stability and congruence of the joint.
■ Any subluxation of the hip joint is an indication for operative reduction and fixation in a healthy patient.
■ Subluxation of the hip is demonstrated by a difference in the relationship of the head to the roof on any of the three standard radiographs (A-P and Judet views) when compared to the contralateral normal hip.
■ If the hip is congruent on all three views, the location of the fracture becomes important.
  ■ Posterior wall and both-column fractures are discussed later.
■ All other fractures must be assessed in relationship to the roof.

■ Displacement in the roof, particularly a step-off, leads to a higher rate of arthrosis.
■ Matta et al. (1986) described the use of roof arcs, initially as a tool to determine if the hip would be stable or not. This concept has evolved and is now used as a measure of roof integrity.
■ These measurements are made *only* in cases of displaced fractures in which the head is congruent with the intact roof segment on all three views.
■ Otherwise, the hip is subluxed (as described earlier) and operative management is indicated.
■ The method of measuring "roof arcs" is simple and performed on all three views.
  ■ A line is drawn vertically from the center of the femoral head. A second line is drawn from the center of the head to the fracture line medial to the vertical line where the fracture enters the joint (Fig. 20-12). This angle is the roof arc.
■ The weight-bearing surface is affected if this angle is less than 45 degrees on any of the three views.
■ Olson and Matta (1993) later reported on the CT correlation of the roof arc measurements. They demonstrated that the CT cut of the joint 1 cm below the subchondral bone, called the CT subchondral ring, was the arc subtended by the 45-degree roof arcs on the three views.
■ Thus if a high-quality CT is available, it can substitute for the roof arc measurements.
■ Subluxation or roof displacement is considered a relative indication for surgery, depending on the patient, institution, and surgeon (see Algorithm 20-4).
■ In cases that have no roof involvement, stability is important.
  ■ Some surgeons perform routine stability testing in the operating room to confirm that the joint does not sublux as indicated in Algorithm 20-4.

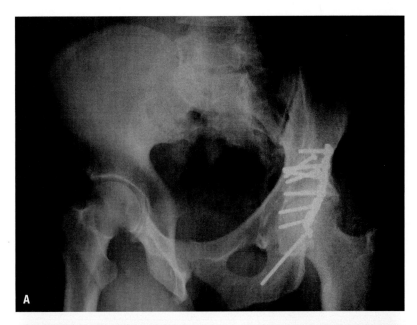

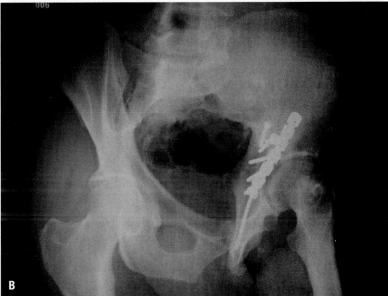

Figure 20-11 (A) Obturator oblique view demonstrates the posterior wall in profile and the anterior column at the level of the joint. (B) Iliac oblique view depicts the anterior column in the anterior wall best.

■ Fractures with instability are reduced and fixed, assuming that if instability can be demonstrated by an intraoperative stress exam, repeated subluxation might occur with normal function and cause arthrosis.

■ This concept has not been fully proven because no series of patients with congruent hips, intact roofs, and instability have been followed to determine the incidence of osteoarthritis.

Surgical Treatment

■ The goal of operative treatment is to reduce the joint as anatomically as possible and stabilize it in that position until union.

■ Although many surgeons consider the fixation challenging, it is in fact the reduction that is the difficult part of acetabular fracture surgery.

■ Letournel developed a system of approaches to deal with each fracture pattern.

■ With complex patterns, multiple options exist.

■ Treatment of posterior injuries (PW, PC, and PC+PW) is always performed through the Kocher-Langenbeck approach.

　■ Unlike the posterior approach for joint arthroplasty, in fracture work this approach is best performed with the patient in the prone position with the hip extended and knee flexed on a fracture table.

　■ This allows access to the posterior column and wall as well as the hip joint via the fracture.

　■ Anterior exposure can be aided by a trochanteric slide or osteotomy.

■ Fractures with anterior column components (AC, ACH, and BC) are typically reduced and fixed via the ilioinguinal approach.

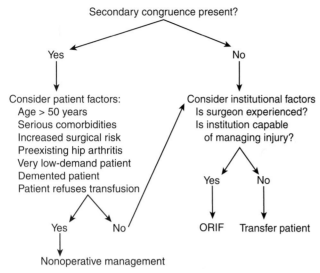

Secondary congruence present?

Yes — No

Consider patient factors:
Age > 50 years
Serious comorbidities
Increased surgical risk
Preexisting hip arthritis
Very low-demand patient
Demented patient
Patient refuses transfusion

Consider institutional factors
Is surgeon experienced?
Is institution capable
of managing injury?

Yes — No

Yes — No

Nonoperative management

ORIF   Transfer patient

Algorithm 20-3 The management of displaced BC acetabular fractures.

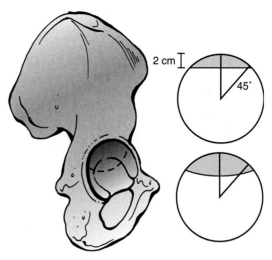

Figure 20-12 Radiographs demonstrating roof arc measurements. A line is drawn vertically from the center of the femoral head and a second line from the center of the femoral head to the fracture. The arc subtended is called the roof arc.

- This approach allows access to the entire inner aspect of the innominate bone and can be extended past the midline for symphyseal and rami injuries as well as to the anterior SI joint and external aspect of the ilium as needed.
- Fractures that affect both the anterior and posterior portions of the joint (TR, T, TR+PW) may be addressed via multiple approaches, depending on the level of the fracture, its direction, and timing.

- Extended approaches have been described to allow access to the entire external aspect of the innominate bone and the inner aspect of the joint via a capsulotomy.
- The extended iliofemoral approach was initially described by Letournel and involves elevating and reflecting the entire gluteus musculature off the ilium from both its origin and insertion on its vascular pedicle.
- This appears to be a safe method, but some authors have questioned its safety in cases where the superior

Is the femoral head congruent with the acetabular roof on A-P and Judet radiographs?

Yes — No

Evaluate radiologic factors:
Intact 45° roof arc
10mm CT subchondral ring intact
> 50% of posterior wall intact
    on all CT sections

Evaluate whether
fracture pattern can be
improved with ORIF

Consider patients factors:
Age > 60 years
Serious comorbidities
Increased surgical risk
Preexisting hip arthritis
Very low-demand patient
Demented patient
Patient refuses transfusion

Yes — No

No — Yes

Yes — No

Stable hip on flouroscopic
stress view under anesthesia?

Consider nonoperative treatment,
with THA as salvage if painful
arthritis develops

Consider institutional factors:
Is surgeon experienced?
Is institution capable of
managing injury?

Yes — No

Nonoperative management

Yes — No

ORIF   Transfer patient

Algorithm 20-4 The management of displaced acetabular fractures (except BC fractures). ORIF, open reduction and internal fixation. THA, total hip arthroplasty.

gluteal artery is damaged and have modified the approach to include iliac crest and other osteotomies in an attempt to preserve the circumflex anastomoses.

■ In either case, the dissection is much more aggressive than the Kocher-Langenbeck or the ilioinguinal and should be used only when absolutely required.

■ The indications are roof impaction, a segmental posterior column as part of a more complex injury, a fracture that extends into the SI joint, and fractures that have united to the extent the surgeon cannot achieve an indirect reduction of one area (usually more than 3 weeks).

■ Other fractures can be managed without extended approaches.

■ The treatment of transverse fractures is based on their location and direction.

■ The higher they are (transtectal) and more vertically oriented, the more they lend themselves to an anterior approach.

■ The lower and more horizontal, the easier they are to reduce from a posterior approach.

■ Likewise, the pattern of T fractures determines the approach.

■ Generally, one approaches the fracture from the side with less quadrilateral surface attached as an indirect reduction of the far column is performed using the quadrilateral surface.

■ If an indirect reduction cannot be accomplished, the nearside column is reduced and fixed, then the patient is turned for reduction and fixation of the far column through the other approach.

■ For instance, if the vertical limb is close to the pelvic brim, an anterior approach is chosen to reduce and fix the anterior column.

■ An indirect reduction of the posterior column is attempted and if obtained, fixation from the brim to the posterior column is performed.

■ If the posterior column cannot be accurately reduced, the anterior approach is closed and the patient is turned over for reduction and fixation of the posterior column via a Kocher approach.

■ Some surgeons combine a Kocher approach with a more limited Smith Peterson or ilioinguinal approach to handle TR and T fractures in the lateral position.

■ Postoperative management includes toe touch weight bearing for a minimum of 8 weeks, and most surgeons prefer 3 months.

■ Active assisted motion is permitted at 6 weeks, but resistive exercises are deferred for 10 to 12 weeks.

■ The outcome of acetabular fractures and the incidence of posttraumatic osteoarthritis is clearly related to the accuracy of the reduction.

■ Other factors such as marginal impaction and femoral head injury play a role, but the only factor that can be controlled by the surgeon is reduction.

■ If the reduction is excellent, one can expect a good or excellent result in approximately 80% of cases.

■ The results deteriorate as displacement increases.

■ Fractures with posterior wall components (TR+PW, PC+PW, and PW) and T fractures tend to have worse outcomes than the other patterns.

■ This is probably due to the significant cartilage injury that is common in these patterns.

POSTERIOR WALL FRACTURES

■ Posterior wall fractures are the most common type seen in automobile accidents.

■ As with other injuries, the indications for surgery are congruence and stability.

■ As opposed to column injuries, posterior wall fractures do not usually affect the roof and are not easily characterized on plain films.

■ CT evaluation is critical, demonstrating the amount of posterior wall affected as well as marginal impaction (Fig. 20-13). Associated dislocation at the time of fracture is an indication of instability but is not specific.

■ Several studies have examined the percentage of posterior wall required to maintain a stable hip.

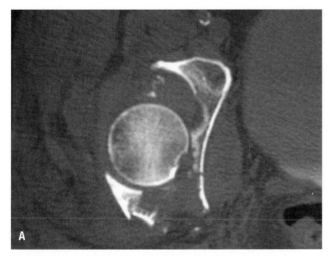
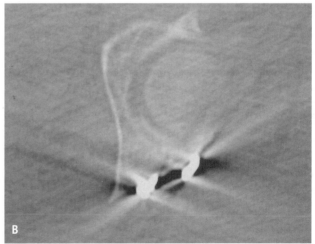

Figure 20-13 (A) CT scan of complex posterior wall injury demonstrating considerable chondral damage. (B) Postoperative CT scan demonstrating repositioning of impacted articular surface against the femoral head and support with bone graft.

- Unfortunately, different definitions were used, and no specific recommendations have been agreed on.
- When measuring the percentage of the joint surface that is affected, impacted cartilage is considered displaced.
- In general, if 20% or less of the posterior wall is affected, the hip will be stable.
- If more than 40% is affected, it will be unstable.
- Fractures comprising between 20% and 40% of the posterior wall may be stable or unstable, depending on the anatomy of the fracture and damage to the capsule and labrum.
- Narrow fractures that go from the top to the bottom of the joint may allow for instability, whereas wider fractures that affect only a small portion of the vertical height of the joint may be stable.
- For this reason, stability testing can be very helpful in these cases.
- In young individuals, loss of more that 30% of the posterior articular surface is an indication for surgery because the joint reaction forces probably increase if these are not reduced and fixed anatomically.
- Cadaveric models have shown that even if the fracture is reduced and well fixed, the loading pattern of the joint may not return to normal.
- Operative treatment of posterior wall fractures is always through the posterior approach and requires buttress plate fixation in all cases after reduction.
- Screw-only fixation is not as predictable in resisting displacement even in larger fragments, and no additional stripping or risk is added by using a buttress plate.
- The buttress plate should be placed toward the periphery of the bone, next to the rim for best support.
- Fractures that extend very anteriorly may require an additional superior antiglide plate.
- Impacted cartilage must be repositioned against the head and supported with graft or graft substitute (see Fig. 20-13).
- Despite plain films demonstrating an anatomical reduction in more than 95% of pure PW cases, the outcomes of posterior wall fractures, with regard to osteoarthritis, are among the worst of any type.
- Moed and colleagues (2000) have correlated this with step-offs and displacements that were seen only on postreduction CT scans, further supporting the need for anatomical reduction.

BOTH-COLUMN (BC) FRACTURES

- BC fractures are different than other patterns (with the one rare exception of a specific TR+PW pattern) in that the entire articular surface of the joint is no longer attached to the intact ilium.
- This means the segments of articular surface can displace from one another (typically though the intercolumn fracture) but remain congruent to the joint.
- This is called secondary congruence and has a far better outcome (65% excellent or good results) than any other displaced fracture / treated nonoperatively.

- For this reason, older patients and those with significant comorbidities may be best served by nonoperative management.
- A different algorithm is used for patients with BC fractures than any of the other types (Algorithm 20-3).
- If surgical treatment if chosen, most BC fractures are treated through the ilioinguinal approach.
- The anterior column is reduced and fixed first, followed by an indirect reduction and fixation of the posterior column.
- Rarely is a second approach needed.
- BC fractures may have associated anterior SI widening, which can be addressed through the same incision.
- Similarly, superoanterior posterior wall fractures can usually be addressed by a minor extension to the outside of the pelvis.
- Roof impaction, extension into the SI joint, and fractures after 3 weeks may be better suited to an extensile approach.
- The outcomes of BC fractures are among the best if accurately reduced.

ELDERLY PATIENTS

- Because avoidance of osteoarthritis is the primary reason for operative treatment of acetabular fractures, elderly patients differ from younger patients in that total hip arthroplasty (THA) is a management option.
- This can be performed acutely or after a planned delay allowing for fracture union.
- The loosening rate of THA done for failed acetabular surgery is reported as high as 40%, even with early and intermediate follow-up.
- Thus some surgeons recommend treatment of high-risk fractures with immediate THA.
- Fractures that fit these criteria include fractures in older patients with roof impaction, posterior wall fractures with very significant cartilage injury, and those that appear to be nonreconstructable due to osteopenia.
- Acute THA in these patients allows for earlier rehabilitation and better short- and intermediate-term results than fixation that fails and needs to be converted to a THA.
- Elderly patients with BC fractures may benefit from nonsurgical treatment and be considered for THA only if they become symptomatic, which is uncommon.

NONSURGICAL TREATMENT

- The first category of fracture that should be treated nonoperatively is undisplaced fractures, with the exception of transtectal transverse fractures, which may displace.
- All other patterns have been shown not to displace over time if weight bearing is delayed.
- Displaced fractures are different. As opposed to most other injuries in orthopaedics, where one evaluates a problem looking for operative indications, displaced fractures of the acetabulum are considered differently.

BOX 20-4 CRITERIA FOR NONOPERATIVE MANAGEMENT OF ACETABULAR FRACTURES

- Congruent hip (no subluxation) on the three views of the pelvis (A-P and both Judet views)
- Intact 45-degree roof arcs and subchondral CT ring
- Stable hip on stress testing

■ They are considered to be operative problems unless they meet specific criteria for nonoperative management.

■ If they do, the expected outcomes will be equal to or better than operative management for the same injury because operative risks are avoided.

■ As already discussed, the main criterion for a good outcome is a stable and congruent joint with respect to the weight-bearing area and posterior wall (Algorithm 20-4).

■ The specific criteria for nonoperative treatment are listed in Box 20-4.

■ The management of acetabular fractures that meet these criteria is exactly the same as for a postoperative patient.

■ Toe touch weight bearing for 10 to 12 weeks, continuous passive movement, and then strengthening exercises are recommended.

■ Approximately 80% good to excellent results can be expected in cases meeting these criteria.

COMPLICATIONS

Osteoarthritis

■ Osteoarthritis is by far the most common complication after acetabular fractures. Its avoidance is the primary reason for operative management.

■ Despite this, up to 40% of patients with displaced acetabular fractures have radiographic osteoarthritis in 15 to 20 years. This is not different from the rate of osteoarthritis in pure hip dislocations without fracture and probably occurs because of cartilage injury.

■ The incidence of osteoarthritis is inversely proportional to the quality of the reduction.

■ The presence of osteoarthritis is not always predictive of a poor outcome, however.

■ Posttraumatic osteoarthritis may be well tolerated by some patients for many years without surgery being needed.

Infection

■ The incidence of infection after acetabular surgery is in the range of 1% to 4%.

■ Perioperative antibiotics, appropriate preoperative workup for infection including a chest X-ray and urine analysis, the use of drains, and early removal of urinary catheters all help avoid infection.

■ The sequelae of infection are different depending on the type of fracture and the surgical approach used.

■ Infection after anterior approaches have fewer long-term complications than after posterior and extended approaches.

■ Because the joint is not directly visualized during the anterior approach, most infections in this area are extra-articular, and the joint may survive the infection.

■ In posterior approaches, the joint is almost always involved and early deterioration is common.

Heterotopic Ossification

■ Heterotopic ossification (HO) is common in posterior and extensile approaches.

■ It occurs in approximately 60% of patients but is clinically important in less then 10%.

■ Factors that correlate with the development of HO include male gender, posterior injury, trochanteric osteotomy, T fractures, extended approach, and significant gluteal injury.

■ Prophylaxis is indicated for patients who have a posterior approach, and indomethacin is most commonly used.

■ This should be used cautiously in patients with concomitant long-bone injury because nonunion of femur fractures is more common in these patients.

■ Low-dose gluteal radiation is very effective in eliminating clinically significant HO even in extended approaches.

■ 700 Gy in a single dose within the first few days of surgery is the current recommendation.

■ If HO occurs, it can lead to restricted painful motion and even extra-articular ankylosis.

■ Treatment is excision of the HO followed by radiation to avoid recurrence if the joint appears to be healthy and well preserved.

■ Care must be taken to find the sciatic nerve and free it up from the notch distal to the HO prior to removal.

Nerve Injury

■ Nerve injury may occur at the time of the injury or at surgery.

■ The sciatic nerve is most at risk.

■ Recovery is poor if occurring at the time of injury and better if occurring after surgery.

■ Intraoperative injury occurs from retraction.

■ Procedures that require dissection through the notch from the posterior approach put the nerve at most risk.

■ Nerve monitoring has been suggested as a method to diminish this complication, but little evidence indicates the incidence of nerve damage is increased if it is not used.

Avascular Necrosis

■ Avascular necrosis (AVN) occurs in approximately 5% of patients who have a posterior dislocation as a component of their injury.

■ It usually presents by 1 year, although it may been seen as long as 5 years after the initial accident.

- Most cases of AVN are not complete, and only one third of patients who develop AVN require surgery.
- It is also important to consider femoral head wear in the differential diagnosis of AVN after acetabular fracture.
- If the reduction is poor or there is instability of the hip, wear may mimic AVN.

Deep Venous Thrombosis and Pulmonary Embolism

- DVT and PE are also risks with acetabular fractures.
- See earlier discussion in pelvic fracture section.
- These are discussed in the pelvic fracture section and in Chapter 41.

SUGGESTED READING

Denis F, Davis S, Comfort T. Sacral fractures: an important problem. Retrospective analysis of 236 cases. Clin Orthop 1988;227:67–81.

Letournel E. Acetabulum fractures: classification and management. Clin Orthop 1980;151:81–106.

Letournel E, Judet R. Fractures of the acetabulum, 2nd ed. Berlin: Springer-Verlag, 1993.

Matta JM, Mehne DK, Roff R. Fractures of the acetabulum: early results of a prospective study. Clin Orthop 1986;215:241–250.

Moed BR, Carr SE; JT Watson. Open reduction and internal fixation of posterior wall fractures of the acetabulum. Clin Orthop 2000;377:56–67.

Montgomery KD; Potter HG; Helfet DL. The detection and management of proximal deep venous thrombosis in patients with acetabular fractures: a follow up report. J Orthop Trauma 1997;11: 330–336.

Norris BL, Hahn DH, Bosse MJ, et al. Intraoperative fluoroscopy to evaluate fracture reduction and hardware placement during acetabular surgery. J Orthop Trauma 1999;13:414–417.

Olsen SA, Matta JM. The computerized tomography subchondral arc: a new method of assessing acetabular articular congruity after fracture (a preliminary report). J Orthop Trauma 1993;7:402–413.

Reilly MC, Olson SA, Tornetta P III, et al. Superior gluteal artery in the extended iliofemoral approach. J Orthop Trauma 2000;14: 259–263.

Saterbak AM, Marsh JL, Nepola JV, et al. Clinical failure after posterior wall acetabular fractures: the influence of initial fracture patterns. J Orthop Trauma 2000;14:230–237.

Tornetta P III. Nonoperative management of acetabular fractures. The use of dynamic stress views. J Bone Joint Surg (Br) 1999;81:67–70.

PROXIMAL FEMORAL FRACTURES AND HIP DISLOCATIONS

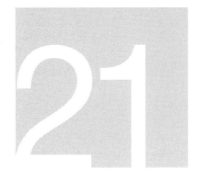

21.1 Hip Dislocation

21.2 Proximal Femoral Fractures

21.1 HIP DISLOCATION

SURGICAL ANATOMY

The anatomy of the hip joint is shown in Figure 21.1-1. The joint is essentially a ball and socket joint with the acetabulum being deepened by the labrum. Further stability is gained from the capsule which arises circumferentially around the acetabulum and inserts circumferentially at the

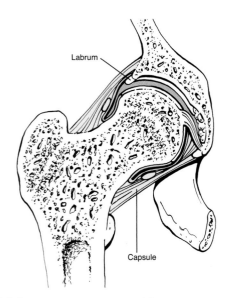

Figure 21.1-1   Anatomy of the proximal femur.

base of the femoral neck. Femoral head and neck fractures occur proximal to the capsule insertion and intertrochanteric fractures distal to it. Basicervical fractures may be intracapsular or extracapsular but are considered with the extracapsular fractures.

The vascular supply to the area is crucial in determining the incidence of avascular necrosis and nonunion of intracapsular fractures. The main arterial supply of the femoral head arises from the medial and lateral circumflex vessels (Fig. 21.1-2). These are branches of the profunda femoris artery which in turn is a branch of the femoral artery. The femoral artery enters the leg under the inguinal ligament together with the femoral nerve. The profunda femoris branch leaves the femoral triangle behind adductor longus. After giving off the lateral and medial circumflex arteries the profunda femoris and the other branch of the femoral artery, the superficial femoral artery, pass into the thigh.

The lateral and medial circumflex vessels form an extracapsular vascular ring at the base of the femoral neck. Ascending branches supply the trochanteric area and the cervical neck. The femoral head is also supplied through the ligamentum teres, usually by a branch of the obturator artery, although by itself this will not provide an adequate blood supply to the femoral head. Sub-capital fractures damage the ascending vessels, thereby causing avascular necrosis and nonunion.

The main nerve in the area is the sciatic nerve, which is formed from the lumbosacral plexus and exits the pelvis through the greater sciatic foramen deep to the muscle

259

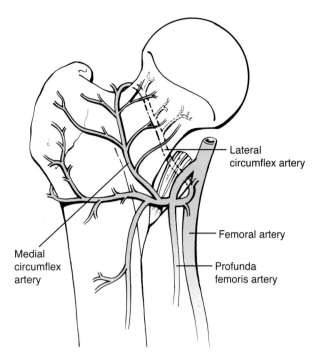

Figure 21.1-2 Vascular supply of the proximal femur.

belly of the piriformis. It therefore passes behind the hip joint and is at risk of damage from posterior dislocation, the usual cause of femoral head fracture. The femoral nerve runs with the femoral artery anterior to the hip joint and is rarely damaged in proximal femoral fractures.

EPIDEMIOLOGY

The hip joint is inherently stable, and subluxation or dislocation is usually associated with high-energy trauma. Hip dislocations are usually caused by motor vehicle accidents and are more common in unrestrained passengers or drivers. They can also occur in falls from a height, industrial accidents, and sports injuries. Hip dislocations are either posterior or anterior. Central dislocation is the name is given to the displacement of the femoral head into the pelvis through a complex acetabular fracture. This is discussed in Chapter 20 on acetabular fractures.

Posterior Dislocation

Posterior dislocations account for 85% to 90% of hip dislocations (Fig. 21.1-3). They are usually caused by axial loading on the knee with both knee and hip flexed. The type of injury varies with the degree of abduction or adduction of the hip. In adducted hips, axial force along the femur tends to cause a pure dislocation. With increasing abduction there is an increasing incidence of acetabular or femoral

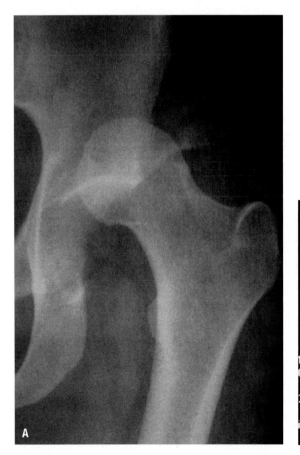

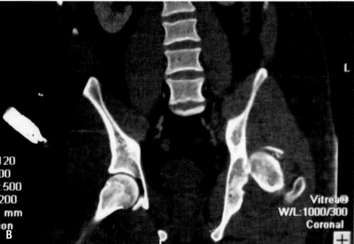

Figure 21.1-3   **(A)** Posterior hip dislocation with associated acetabular fracture. **(B)** A CT scan shows comminution of the posterior wall fragment.

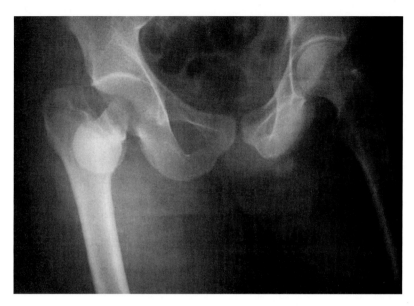

Figure 21.1-4 A posterior dislocation associated with a femoral neck fracture. This is a very rare fracture combination.

head fractures. A major axial load to the knee may also be associated with posterior knee dislocation, posterior cruciate injury, patellar fracture and femoral diaphyseal fracture. The posterior displacement of the femoral head is associated with impaction and shear fractures of the femoral head, acetabular fractures, femoral neck fractures (Fig. 21.1-4) and sciatic nerve damage.

Anterior Dislocation

These account for 10% to 15% of all hip dislocations (Fig. 21.1-5) and have a different mechanism of injury from posterior dislocation. They are caused by hyperabduction and extension of the hip joint and may follow lower energy injuries than posterior dislocations. Any injury causing the legs to straddle may cause anterior dislocation and they may therefore occur in sports injuries, assaults, or simple falls. Inferior dislocations account for

over 70% of anterior dislocations with superior dislocations, obturator dislocations, and the very rare pelvic dislocation comprising the remaining 30%. Associated injuries tend to be less common and less severe than in posterior dislocation, but impaction and shear femoral head fractures and femoral neck fractures may occur. Dislocation may rarely cause damage to the femoral nerve and vessels.

CLASSIFICATION

Posterior Dislocation

There are a number of classifications of posterior hip dislocations. All are somewhat similar and merely stress the possibility of damage to the femoral head, neck, and acetabulum. The classification of Thomson and Epstein (1951) is shown in Table 21.1-1.

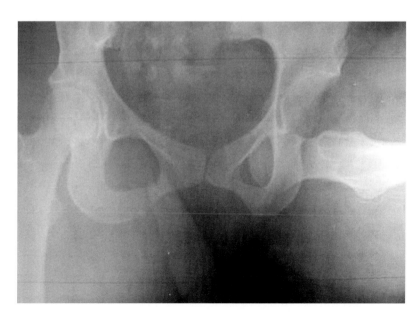

Figure 21.1-5 An anterior hip dislocation.

TABLE 21.1-1 CLASSIFICATION OF POSTERIOR HIP DISLOCATION

Type	Description
I	Dislocation with or without minor fracture
II	Dislocation with single large fracture of the posterior rim of the acetabulum
III	Dislocation with comminuted fracture of the rim, with or without a large major fragment
IV	Dislocation with fracture of the acetabular floor
V	Dislocation with fracture of the femoral head

From Thompson VP, Epstein HC. Traumatic dislocation of the hip. J Bone Joint Surg (Am) 1951;33:746–778.

Anterior Dislocation

Classifications of anterior dislocations are descriptive, drawing attention to the direction of dislocation and the association with other injuries. The Epstein (1973) classification of anterior dislocation is shown in Table 21.1-2.

DIAGNOSIS

History and Physical Examination

Posterior Dislocation

■ About 95% of patients with posterior hip dislocations have other injuries, and a thorough examination according to ATLS principles is mandatory.
■ Intraabdominal, head, chest, and pelvic injuries are relatively common.
■ There may also be a number of other musculoskeletal injuries, of which damage to the knee ligaments, patella, femoral diaphysis, proximal femur and acetabulum are the most common. There may be damage to the ipsilateral foot or lower leg.
   ■ All these areas should be carefully examined to exclude injury.
■ In posterior dislocation, the leg is held in flexion, adduction, and internal rotation.

TABLE 21.1-2 CLASSIFICATION OF ANTERIOR HIP DISLOCATION

Group	Description
A	Pubic (Superior)
1	No fracture
2	Fracture of femoral head
3	Acetabular fracture
B	Obturator (inferior)
1	No fracture
2	Fracture of femoral head
3	Acetabular fracture

From Epstein HC. Traumatic dislocations of the hip. Clin Orthop 1973; 92:116–142.

■ There may be sciatic nerve dysfunction, which must be carefully examined.
■ Vascular compromise is unusual.

Anterior Dislocation

■ As with posterior dislocation, many patients present having been involved in a motor vehicle accident or a fall from a height.
■ Thorough clinical examination must be undertaken, bearing in mind that there may be injuries to the abdomen, chest, and head.
■ The leg tends to assume an extended and externally rotated position.
■ Severe soft tissue damage may be associated with damage to the femoral nerve and vessels, and thus a complete neurological and vascular examination should be undertaken.

Radiologic Examination

■ Both anterior and posterior dislocations can be diagnosed on anteroposterior and lateral radiographs of the pelvis.
■ Oblique views may be helpful.
■ If there is an associated acetabular fracture, Judet views may be required.
■ Other imaging techniques are rarely required prior to treatment, although a CT scan may delineate the direction of displacement and associated acetabular damage (see Fig. 21.1-3) better than lateral or oblique radiographs.
■ After reduction, a CT scan can be used to check the congruency of reduction and an MRI scan will diagnose avascular necrosis of the femoral head at a later stage.

TREATMENT

■ Emergency closed reduction of hip dislocation is mandatory unless the patient's overall condition precludes this.
■ The only associated injury that should prevent an attempted closed reduction is a femoral neck fracture (see Fig. 21.1-4), in which case an open reduction and fixation should be undertaken.
■ Anterior dislocations are usually treated by traction and internal rotation.
■ Posterior dislocations are best treated by the Bigelow maneuver.
   ■ With the patient supine an assistant applies downward pressure over the anterior superior iliac spine of the pelvis and the surgeon applies traction in the direction of the deformity.
   ■ The leg is adducted and internally rotated.
   ■ A number of other techniques have been reported.
■ Two to 15% of dislocations are irreducible. The common causes of irreducibility are listed in Box 21.1-1.
■ Irreducible dislocations are treated as an emergency by open relocation.
■ A posterior approach is used for a posterior dislocation and an anterior approach for anterior dislocation.
■ Once the joint has been reduced anteroposterior and lateral radiographs should be obtained to assess the

BOX 21.1-1 CAUSES OF IRREDUCIBLE HIP DISLOCATION

Anterior Dislocation
Interposition of the following:
Rectus femoris
Iliopsoas
Anterior hip capsule
Labrum
Buttonholing through anterior capsule
Bony impingement in obturator foramen

Posterior Dislocation
Interposition of the following:
Piriformis
Gluteus maximus
Ligamentum teres
Labrum
Large bone fragments
Femoral neck fracture
Buttonholing through posterior capsule

congruency of a joint reduction and the position of any associated femoral head or acetabular fracture.
- The management of femoral head fractures is discussed later in this chapter, and acetabular fractures are discussed in Chapter 20.
- When possible, a postoperative CT scan should be obtained to look for intra-articular bone fragments. If present, these should be removed.
- Careful assessment of sciatic nerve function after reduction is important.
- If relocation of the joint causes sciatic nerve dysfunction, exploration of the nerve should be undertaken immediately.

RESULTS AND COMPLICATIONS

- The common complications of hip dislocations are listed in Table 21.1-3.
- Anterior hip dislocations cause less morbidity than posterior dislocations.
- Analysis of the excellent and good results following posterior dislocation shows that they average 84% in pure dislocations, 62% if there is a posterior acetabular rim fracture, and only 19% if there is a severe acetabular fracture.

- The common problems that occur after dislocation are avascular necrosis of the femoral head, osteoarthritis, heterotopic ossification, and sciatic nerve damage.

Avascular Necrosis

- The incidence of avascular necrosis correlates with the severity of the injury, occurring in about 6% of pure dislocations, 8% of posterior acetabular rim fractures, and close to 100% of severe acetabular or femoral neck fracture dislocations.
- The incidence also correlates with the time to reduction with rates of 0% to 10% reported if reduction is undertaken within 6 hours.
- Radiologic signs of avascular necrosis are usually present within 2 years.
- The avascular necrosis may be segmental or global and if symptomatic is usually treated by arthroplasty, although a rotational osteotomy of the femoral head may be used if there is symptomatic segmental avascular necrosis of the femoral head.

Osteoarthritis

- The incidence of osteoarthritis correlates with the severity of the fracture dislocation and averages about 25%.
- It worsens with time, with 100% being reported 30 years after dislocation.
- The treatment of symptomatic osteoarthritis is arthroplasty.

Heterotopic Ossification

- Heterotopic ossification is common after posterior fracture dislocations, particularly after open reductions.
- It is often asymptomatic but the incidence may be reduced by the use of Indomethacin or radiation therapy.

Nerve Damage

- Sciatic nerve damage is usually a neuropraxia, but the nerve can be lacerated or punctured by acetabular fragments or even trapped within an acetabular fracture.
- The peroneal branch is more commonly affected than the tibial branch, and it is reported that muscle weakness tends to be more common than dysesthesia, although both may occur.

TABLE 21.1-3 RESULTS OF THE MANAGEMENT OF HIP DISLOCATION

Result/Complication	Anterior (%)		Posterior (%)	
	Range	Average	Range	Average
Excellent/good	75–100	80.9	47.4–92.3	65
Avascular necrosis	0–3.4	2.1	11.4–34.4	20
Severe/moderate osteoarthritis	0–8.3	4.8	12.9–49.3	26.2
Heterotopic ossification	0	0	3.1–9.8	6.7
Sciatic nerve damage	?	?	5–20	10

■ Treatment should be nonoperative, although if there is no recovery between 1 and 3 weeks after the injury many authorities suggest exploration.

■ Complete recovery has been documented in 14% to 83% (average, 51%) of patients with partial recovery in 43% to 100% (average, 70%).

21.2 PROXIMAL FEMORAL FRACTURES

Proximal femoral fractures are the most common fractures to require surgical treatment. They usually occur in the less fit elderly population who have coexisting medical co-morbidities and not infrequently, the proximal femoral fracture marks the end of an independent existence. The mortality is considerable, and the expense involved in the rehabilitation and re-housing of these patients has made the proximal femoral fracture a social and political issue in many countries.

In this chapter the proximal femoral fracture is defined as occurring above or at the level of the lesser trochanter. A number of proximal femoral fractures extend into the subtrochanteric area and these are also often defined as proximal femoral fractures. (Subtrochanteric fractures are considered separately in Chapter 22.) There are six types of proximal femoral fracture: two are intracapsular and four are extracapsular. The intracapsular fractures are those of the femoral head and femoral neck, the latter often known as subcapital fractures. The extracapsular fractures occur in the basicervical area, the intertrochanteric area, the greater trochanter and the lesser trochanter. Chapter 1 shows that proximal femoral fractures account for 11.6% of all fractures. Further analysis shows that 46.3% are intracapsular and 53.4% are extracapsular.

Box 21.2-1 summarizes the current controversies in the management of proximal femoral fractures.

BOX 21.2-1 CURRENT CONTROVERSIES IN THE MANAGEMENT OF PROXIMAL FEMORAL FRACTURES

How should femoral head fractures be treated?
Internal fixation or arthroplasty for displaced femoral neck fractures?
Which arthroplasty should be used?
Should hemiarthroplasty prostheses be cemented?
Are bipolar prostheses superior to unipolar prostheses?
When should total hip replacement be used?
DHS or reconstruction nails for intertrochanteric fractures?
How common is refracture after proximal femoral fracture?
What is the incidence of fracture of the contralateral proximal femur?

INTRACAPSULAR FRACTURES

Femoral Head Fractures

There are two types of femoral head fracture. These are the *impaction* fracture, which is not dissimilar to the Hill-Sachs lesion of the proximal humerus, and the *cleavage* or *shear* fracture. The shear fracture has received more attention in the literature, but both are important and can cause considerable morbidity.

Chondral or osteochondral impaction fractures of the femoral head are relatively common after hip dislocation (Fig. 21.2-1). The older literature documented an incidence

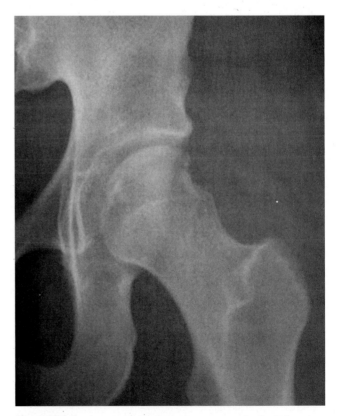

Figure 21.2-1   A superior impaction fracture seen in the dislocation shown in Figure 21.1-5 after reduction.

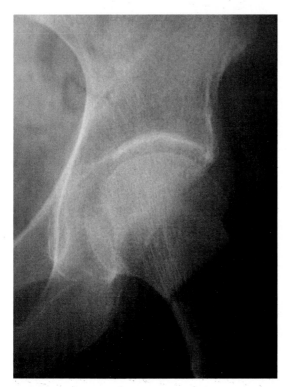

Figure 21.2-2   A Pipkin type I shear fracture of the femoral head.

TABLE 21.2-2 DISTRIBUTION OF FEMORAL HEAD FRACTURES[a]

Pipkin Type	Range (%)	Average (%)
I	7.7–62.5	28.8
II	18.7–60	40.5
III	0–13.3	10.2
IV	10–40.9	20.5

[a]In view of the rarity of this fracture, the data relating to the Pipkin type are taken from the world literature.

*Shear or cleavage fracture*s of the femoral head (Fig. 21.2-2) have been well documented but are very rare, accounting for 0.3% of the proximal femoral fractures shown in Table 1-1 in Chapter 1. They occur as a result of hip dislocation and are usually seen in unrestrained drivers or passengers involved in motor vehicle accidents, although they have been recorded in falls from a height, snowboarding, and skiing. Because about 85% of hip dislocations are posterior, most femoral head fractures follow posterior hip dislocation. The epidemiology and distribution of femoral head fractures are shown in Tables 21.2-1 and 21.2-2.

Hip dislocations and femoral head fractures are high-energy injuries, and 95% of patients will have other musculoskeletal injuries or significant injuries to other body systems, with injuries to the central nervous system, chest, and abdomen frequently reported. Other musculoskeletal injuries to the ipsilateral limb are common, with fractures of the patella, femoral diaphysis, and acetabulum often associated with femoral head fractures. Approximately 25% of patients with femoral head fractures have ipsilateral knee ligament injuries.

CLASSIFICATION

The AO classification of proximal femoral fractures is shown in Figure 21.2-3 and used for all proximal femoral fractures. Type C fractures involve the femoral head. The most commonly used classification of femoral head fractures is the Pipkin classification (1957). This is shown in Figure 21.2-4. There are four types of femoral head fracture. In type I injuries, the fracture is inferior to the fovea, and in type II injuries, the fracture line extends superiorly to the fovea. Type III fractures consist of coexisting head and neck fractures, and type IV fractures are associated with an acetabular fracture. Table 21.2-2 shows that types I and II fractures account for about 70% of femoral head fractures, and type III fractures are very rare.

DIAGNOSIS

History and Physical Examination

■ A complete history should be taken from the conscious patient or from a companion if the patient is unconscious, uncooperative, or unable to communicate.

of 7% to 16%, but with a heightened awareness of the problem and better imaging, it seems that impaction fractures actually occur in about 60% of hip dislocations. About 75% of the impaction fractures occur close to the fovea.

There is evidence that the incidence of posttraumatic hip osteoarthritis relates to the severity of the impaction fracture, with an incidence of 100% osteoarthritis reported in patients whose impaction fracture is deeper than 4 mm. Impaction fractures must always be considered when treating patients with a hip dislocation, and an MRI scan should be used to diagnose the condition. Treatment may be difficult. Minor impaction fractures are best left untreated, but surgeons should consider elevation and packing with bone graft or bone substitutes in more severe lesions in younger patients. There are no published results of the success of these procedures, however. All older patients with severe impaction fractures are best treated by hip arthroplasty.

TABLE 21.2-1 EPIDEMIOLOGY OF FEMORAL HEAD FRACTURES

Proportion of all fractures	0.03%
Age	40.5 y
Male/female	73%/27%
Distribution	Type B
Incidence	$0.4/10^5$/y
Most common causes	
Motor vehicle accidents	
Falls from height	
Open fractures	0%

- The main purpose of the history is to investigate the cause of the injury and to determine whether associated musculoskeletal injuries may be present.
- Because 95% of patients with femoral head fractures are multiply injured, a careful physical examination according to ATLS principles is mandatory.
- Surgeons should be aware that a hip dislocation may accompany any knee or femoral injury that has occurred in a motor vehicle accident or a fall from a height, and a thorough examination of the complete lower limb must be taken.
- Neurovascular examination of the affected limb is essential because patients with a femoral head fracture associated with a posterior dislocation may present with sciatic nerve dysfunction and patients with anterior dislocation may have damage to the femoral nerve and vessels.

Radiologic Examination

- Anteroposterior and lateral radiographs of the hip should be supplemented by 45-degree oblique Judet views to allow better visualization of the femoral head.
- A CT scan best defines the location and extent of femoral head fracture and also indicates the presence of intra-articular bone fragments, which should be removed.
- Vascular injuries are unusual, but angiography or Doppler examination may be used if indicated.
- Later electromyographic studies of the sciatic or femoral nerves or an MRI scan to look for avascular necrosis of the femoral head may be required.

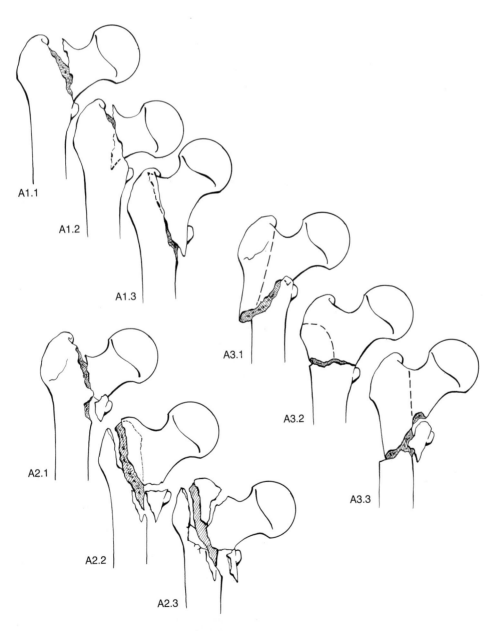

Figure 21.2-3   OTA (AO) classification of proximal femoral fractures.

TREATMENT

- The treatment of hip dislocations has already been described.
- There is debate whether closed hip reduction is appropriate in patients who have associated femoral head fractures.
- Gentle closed reduction can be undertaken in Pipkin type I, II, or IV fractures, but should not be undertaken in Pipkin type III fractures because an undisplaced femoral neck fracture may well displace.
  - Open reduction should be undertaken in these fractures.
- Once a successful reduction has been undertaken, radiographs or a CT scan should be used to examine the adequacy of the fracture reduction and to look for the presence of bone fragments in the hip joint.
- As with many fractures, there has been increasing use of open reduction and internal fixation for femoral head fractures in the last 20 years.

- The decision as to how to treat the fracture depends on the fracture type, its residual displacement after reduction, and the age of the patient.
- Small head fragments can be excised, but larger Pipkin type I fractures are best treated with closed reduction and nonoperative management if postreduction radiographs or a CT scan show a step-off of less than 1 mm.
- If closed reduction is impossible or results in poor reduction of the femoral head fracture, open reduction is required with intrafragmentary screw fixation of the fracture.
- In Pipkin type II fractures in younger patients, the same approach is followed, although the fracture is generally less stable than the type I fracture and internal fixation is usually required.
- In older patients, hip arthroplasty should be used.
- The prognosis for Pipkin type III and IV fractures is worse.
- A closed reduction of a type III undisplaced femoral neck fracture may cause displacement, and open reduction is required.

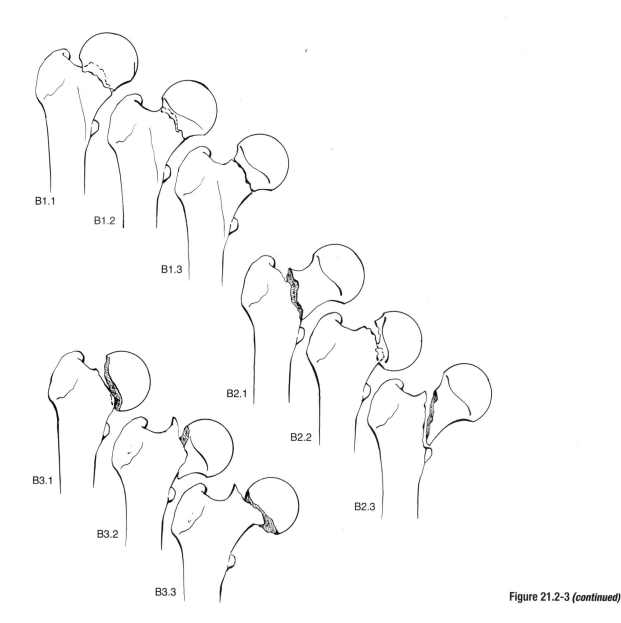

B1.1
B1.2
B1.3
B2.1
B2.2
B2.3
B3.1
B3.2
B3.3

Figure 21.2-3 *(continued)*

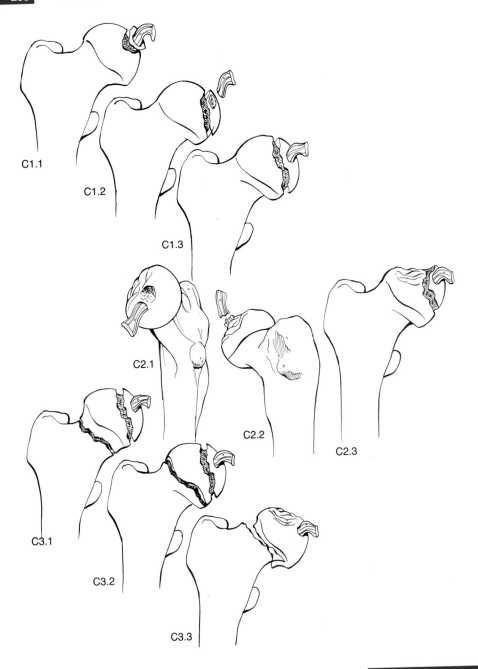

C1.1

C1.2

C1.3

C2.1

C2.2

C2.3

C3.1

C3.2

C3.3

Figure 21.2-3 *(continued)*

- In younger patients, screw fixation of both head and neck fracture should be undertaken, but in older patients, primary arthroplasty is indicated.
- In type IV fractures, internal fixation of both acetabular and femoral head fractures should be undertaken.
- The suggested treatment of femoral head fractures is given in Table 21.2-3.

COMPLICATIONS

- The literature indicates 75% excellent or good results in Pipkin type I and II fractures and about 50% excellent or good results in type III and IV fractures.
- Recent studies, however, indicate that about 50% of patients eventually require a hip arthroplasty after a femoral head fracture.

TABLE 21.2-3 MANAGEMENT OF FEMORAL HEAD FRACTURES

Pipkin Type	Younger Patients (<60 y)	Older Patients (>60 y)
I and II	Open reduction Internal fixation	Open reduction Internal fixation
III	Open reduction Internal fixation both fractures	Arthroplasty
IV	Open reduction Internal fixation both fractures	Open reduction Internal fixation both fractures Probable secondary arthroplasty

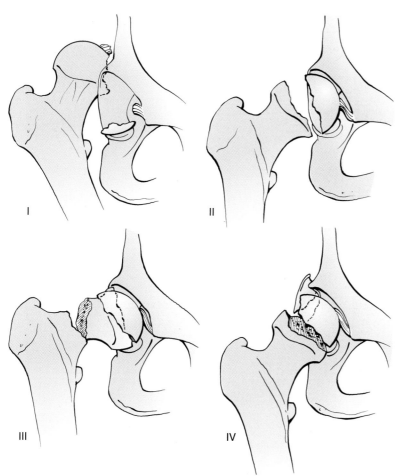

Figure 21.2-4   The Pipkin classification of femoral head fractures.

- Evidence indicates that an anterior Smith-Peterson approach for fixation is better than a posterior approach because the incidence of avascular necrosis and sciatic nerve damage is less, although there is a higher incidence of heterotopic ossification.
- The common complications and their incidence are listed in Table 21.2-4.
- There are wide variations in the incidence of the common complications, mainly because of differences in definition but the incidences of avascular necrosis and post-traumatic osteo-arthritis are consistently high.
- Type I and II fractures have a lower incidence of osteoarthritis, and the incidence is even lower if internal fixation rather than nonoperative management is used.

TABLE 21.2-4 COMMON COMPLICATIONS ASSOCIATED WITH FEMORAL HEAD FRACTURES

Complication	Range (%)	Average (%)
Avascular necrosis	10–36.6	23.4
Osteoarthritis	15.4–75.7	29.4
Heterotopic ossification	2.1–64	14.7
Sciatic nerve palsy	6.6–19	11.1

Femoral Neck Fractures

These fractures occur within the neck of the femur (Fig. 21.2-5). They predominantly affect the elderly population. Not infrequently, the patients have a significant number of medical comorbidities and are demented and live in residential care. In these patients, morbidity and mortality is high. Femoral neck fractures usually present with either posterior or valgus displacement of the femoral head on the neck, although varus displacement does occasionally occur. Conventionally more than 10 degrees of displacement in any direction is regarded as significant displacement (see Fig. 21.2-5). Fractures that show less than 10 degrees of displacement are regarded as undisplaced or minimally displaced (Fig. 21.2-6). Approximately 26% of femoral neck fractures are undisplaced, the range varying from 15% to 33%. Treatment of femoral neck fractures depends on the degree of displacement of the fracture and the age and general health of the patient.

CLASSIFICATION

The Garden classification is often employed. This is shown in Figure 21.2-7. Type I is an impacted valgus fracture and type II is an undisplaced fracture. Types III and IV are displaced fractures, with type III incompletely displaced such that the bone trabeculae are not parallel. In type IV

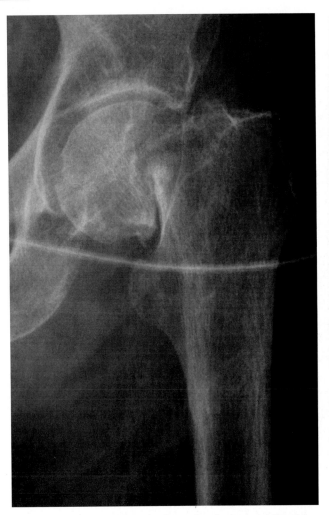

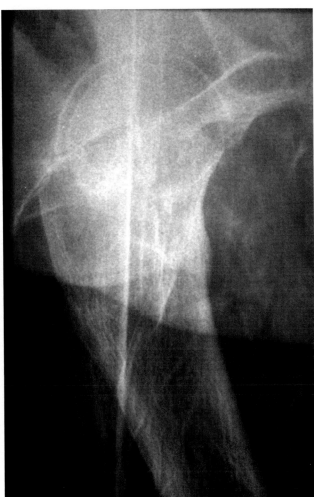

Figure 21.2-5   A-P and lateral radiographs of a displaced (B3.3) femoral neck fracture.

fractures, the displacement is complete and the trabeculae are parallel. Conventionally, types I and II are considered as undisplaced fractures, and types III and IV as displaced fractures.

The AO classification is shown in Figure 21.2-3. Femoral neck fractures are all contained in the type B subgroups. The B1 subgroups contain the impacted valgus or undisplaced fractures, with the B1.1 fractures in at least 15 degrees of valgus and the B1.2 fractures in less than 15 degrees of valgus. B1.3 fractures are undisplaced. The B2 fractures consist of basicervical fractures (B2.1), adducted femoral neck fractures (B2.2), and shear femoral neck fractures (B2.3). The B3 subgroups contain all the nonimpacted displaced fractures. B3.1 fractures show moderate varus displacement and external rotation. B3.2 fractures show moderate vertical translation and external rotation, and B3.3 fractures show marked displacement.

EPIDEMIOLOGY

Virtually all subcapital fractures occur in older patients. The literature suggests that about 1% to 3% occur in patients less than 50 years of age. Because these are

treated differently from fractures in older patients, the epidemiology shown in Table 21.2-5 has been separated between older and younger patients. It is apparent that most subcapital fractures are isolated fractures occurring in elderly patients after a fall.

The incidence of femoral neck fractures is increasing worldwide at a rate that cannot be explained just by population aging. The age-specific incidence of femoral neck fractures doubles every 5.6 years after 30 years of age in women and correlates with increasing age-related osteopenia which in turn correlates with improved medical treatment and increasing longevity. Falls are the most common cause of femoral neck fractures. The risk of falling also increases with age, the rate of falls doubling between 65 and 85 years. Many of the medications prescribed to the elderly increase the likelihood of falling. Other factors that increase the risk of subcapital fracture are alcohol intake, smoking, and low body weight. The causes of osteopenia and osteoporosis are listed in Chapter 8. Patients with femoral neck fractures are physiologically younger and more independent than patients with intertrochanteric fractures.

In younger patients subcapital fractures occur more commonly in men (see Table 21.2-5). In adults less than

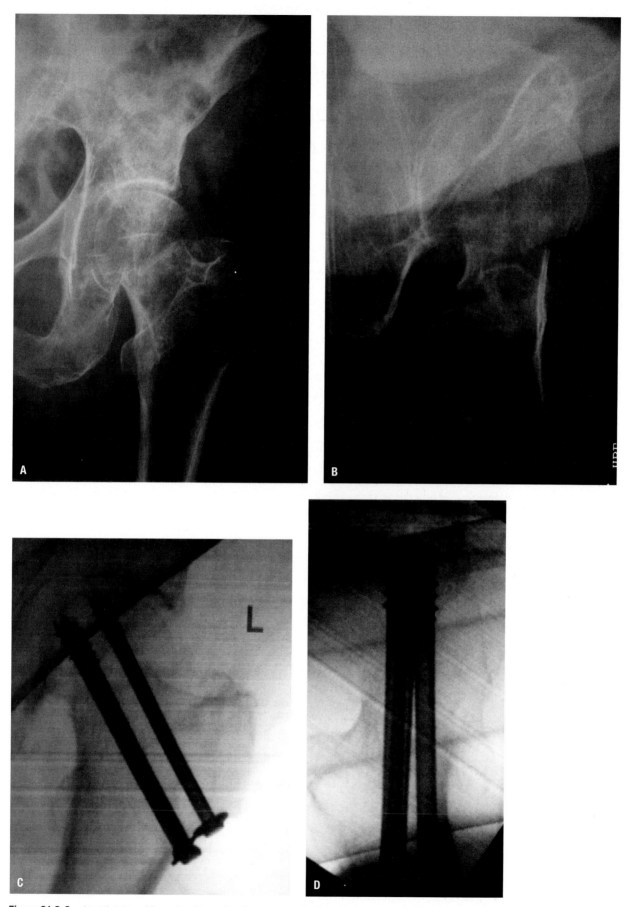

Figure 21.2-6 (A, B) A-P and lateral radiographs of an impacted valgus fracture. (C, D) Fluoroscopic views of cancellous fixation.

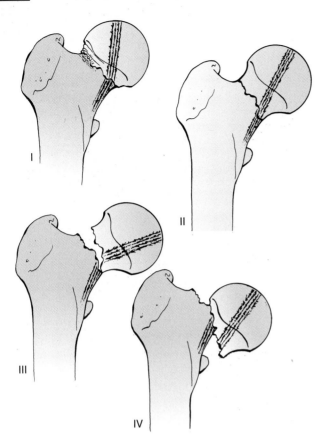

Figure 21.2-7   Garden (1961) classification of femoral neck fractures.

40 years of age, it has been shown that 77% occur in men and 87% are high-energy injuries. Between 40 and 50 years of age, 59% occur in women and 94% are caused by simple falls. In this age group, medical comorbidities such are neuromuscular disorders, arthritis, and cardiorespiratory problems are common, with over 90% of patients on medication.

High-energy fractures may be associated with other musculoskeletal injuries or damage to other body systems, but the most common injuries associated with subcapital fractures are fractures of the distal radius and proximal humerus, which occur in about 4% of cases.

DIAGNOSIS

History and Physical Examination

- In view of the frequency of associated medical comorbidities, a thorough clinical history must be obtained from the patient, companion, or caregiver.
- The patient's domicile must be investigated because frequently the fracture signifies the patient can no longer live alone and requires residential or supervised care.
- About 90% of patients have at least one comorbid condition, and over 33% have at least three comorbid conditions.
  - Most commonly involved are the cardiovascular and respiratory systems, although assessment of renal and hepatic function is important, and the diabetic status of the patient must be checked.
- A complete drug history is essential.
- Many patients are on anticoagulants, and a coagulopathy must be reversed prior to surgery.
- A careful assessment of the patient's mental function is essential.
- About 25% to 30% of patients with proximal femoral fractures have impaired mental function and consequently a very poor prognosis.
- Physical examination may show a shortened, externally rotated leg if the fracture is displaced, but painful, restricted hip function may be the only clinical finding if the fracture is undisplaced.
- A proximal femoral fracture must be considered in any elderly patient who presents after a fall.

TABLE 21.2-5 EPIDEMIOLOGY OF FEMORAL NECK FRACTURES

	Patients 12–50 y	Patients >50 y	All Fractures[a]
Proportion of fractures (%)			5.4
Proportion of femoral neck fractures (%)	1.1	98.9	
Age			77.9 y
Male/female (%)	75/25	26/74	27/73
Distribution			Type F
Annual incidence	$0.7/10^5$	$59.1/10^5$	$59.8/10^5$
Open fractures	0	0	0
Most common causes (%)			
Fall from height	50		
Fall	25	89.7	89.8
Pathological	25		
Most common subgroups (%)			
B3.1			26.1
B3.2			20.1
B3.1			15.5
B1.2			13.4

[a]For information about fracture distribution curves see Chapter 1.

Radiologic Examination

■ Anteroposterior and lateral radiographs are usually sufficient to diagnose a femoral neck fracture.

　■ About 8% of patients have false-negative x-rays.

■ There is little evidence that further plain radiographs 12 to 24 hours later increase sensitivity, and if the patient is thought to have a femoral neck fracture, an isotope bone scan, CT scan, or MRI scan should be undertaken.

　■ MRI scans have the highest sensitivity.

TREATMENT

Undisplaced Femoral Neck Fractures

■ Management of undisplaced or minimally displaced subcapital fractures (see Fig. 21.2-6) is independent of the patient's age.

■ There are two possible treatment methods—nonoperative management and internal fixation using three cannulated screws or pins (see Figure 21.2-6).

■ No good evidence indicates that the type of screw or pin matters, but there is evidence that three screws are preferable to two.

■ The complete results of operative and nonoperative management of undisplaced subcapital fractures are shown in Table 21.2-6, which illustrates that internal fixation gives better results than nonoperative management.

■ About 15% of undisplaced or impacted fractures will displace if treated nonoperatively, the incidence of secondary displacement rising with increasing age and in patients with comorbid conditions.

■ Nonoperative management also confines elderly patients to bed for a prolonged period and should not be used.

■ The only indications for nonoperative treatment is if patients are moribund on admission or have presented late with evidence that the femoral neck fracture is uniting.

Displaced Femoral Neck Fractures

Young Patients

■ The definition of what constitutes a young patient with a femoral neck fracture is difficult.

■ Most of the literature has concerned the 1% to 3% of patients who are less than 50 years of age.

■ Many surgeons, however, accept 65 years as an appropriate cutoff between young and older patients, probably because it is a reasonable age at which to perform a hip arthroplasty if necessary.

■ Most surgeons believe that in younger patients the femoral head should be conserved, and internal fixation using multiple screws or pins is the universally accepted treatment method.

■ The results from the literature are given in Table 21.2-7.

■ Nonunion is rare, and many of the patients who have avascular necrosis are asymptomatic.

■ The results are good and there is no indication for primary arthroplasty in younger patients with displaced subcapital fractures unless comorbid conditions suggest the patient might be "physiologically older."

Older Patients

■ In older patients, the choice of treatment for displaced subcapital fractures lies between internal fixation using multiple screws (Fig. 21.2-6) or pins and arthroplasty.

■ Three different types of arthroplasty are in routine use—unipolar hemiarthroplasty (Fig. 21.2-8), bipolar hemiarthroplasty (Fig. 21.2-9), and total hip replacement (Fig. 21.2-10).

　■ Unipolar hemiarthroplasties have a metallic head that articulates directly with the acetabulum.

　■ Bipolar arthroplasties use a standard femoral stem and head that articulates with a second larger head which, in turn, articulates with the acetabulum. Theoretically, movement can occur between the smaller and larger femoral heads giving improved function compared with a unipolar hemiarthroplasty.

　■ In total hip replacement, both the proximal femur and acetabulum are replaced.

TABLE 21.2-6　RESULTS OF NONOPERATIVE AND OPERATIVE MANAGEMENT OF UNDISPLACED AND MINIMALLY DISPLACED FEMORAL NECK FRACTURES

Result/Complication	Nonoperative (%)		Operative (%)	
	Range	Average	Range	Average
Excellent/good	79	79	96	96
Union	86–92	87.3	96.5–100	97.2
Avascular necrosis	2.1–19.6	10.2	2.3–15	4.6
Fracture displacement	7.5–31	15	0–4.3	0.9
Secondary fracture	0	0	0–2.3	1.8

TABLE 21.2-7 RESULTS OF INTERNAL FIXATION OF DISPLACED FEMORAL NECK FRACTURES IN YOUNGER PATIENTS

Result	Range (%)	Average (%)
Excellent/good	86.6–89.3	87.4
Union	93–100	98.6
Avascular necrosis	6.6–18.7	10.9
Infection	0–3.4	2.0

- Until recently, many surgeons believed internal fixation was preferable to primary arthroplasty because the femoral head was conserved and if nonunion, avascular necrosis, or failure of fixation occurred secondary arthroplasty could easily be performed.
- The results from the literature strongly suggest, however, that internal fixation is associated with poorer results. The comparative results of internal fixation, hemiarthroplasty, and total hip replacement are given in Table 21.2-8.

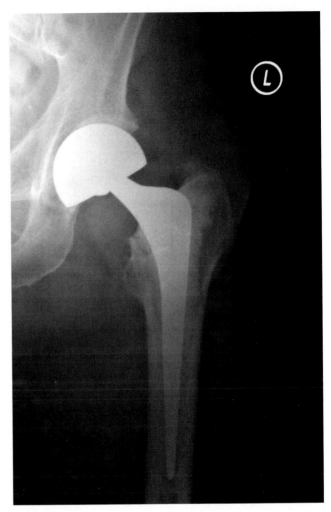

Figure 21.2-9   A bipolar cemented hemiarthroplasty.

- This shows that the mortality is similar, but the reoperation rate following internal fixation is very high.
- It also indicates that the functional outcome following total hip replacement is superior to the other two treatment methods.
- A number of meta-analyses and multicenter prospective studies have investigated the treatment of displaced femoral neck fractures.
  - These have clearly shown that total hip replacement is associated with a lower incidence of reoperation and better functional outcome.
  - A careful cost analysis has also shown that the decreased incidence of reoperation means that hip replacement is in fact cheaper than both hemiarthroplasty and internal fixation.
- There are several current debates regarding the use of hemiarthroplasty prostheses:
  - Do bipolar prostheses perform better than unipolar prostheses?
  - Should hemiarthroplasty prostheses be cemented or uncemented?
  - Which hemiarthroplasty should be used in the very elderly or infirm where the mortality is high?

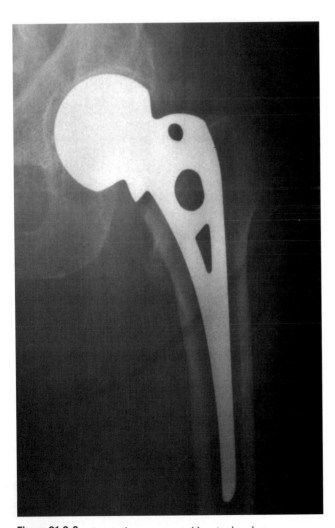

Figure 21.2-8   A unipolar uncemented hemiarthroplasty.

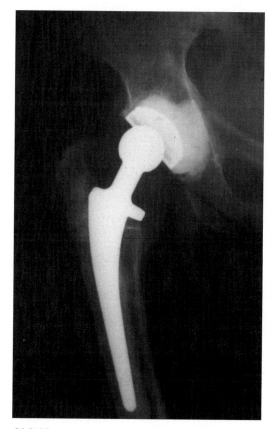

Figure 21.2-10   A total hip arthroplasty.

- It is obvious that the results of the use of unipolar and bipolar prostheses are remarkably similar, which prospective comparative studies have confirmed.
- The two disadvantages of bipolar prostheses are that they are more expensive and open reduction is often required if dislocation occurs.
- Table 21.2-10 contains information from the literature about the use of cemented and uncemented unipolar hemiarthroplasty.
  - Information is relatively sparse but unquestionably favors cemented fixation.
  - The main disadvantage of cemented fixation is if an infected prosthesis needs to be removed, but this is relatively uncommon and outweighed by the functional benefits that accompany the use of cemented prostheses.
- Although Table 21.2-8 indicates that the results of total hip replacement are better than those of internal fixation and hemiarthroplasty, many patients are very old, debilitated, or demented at the time of presentation.
  - Their life expectancy is poor, and if total hip replacement is used, surgeons can reasonably expect higher complications than shown in Table 21.2-8.
  - The literature suggests that in this group the results of hemi-arthroplasty are not dissimilar to those shown in Table 21.2-8 and cemented hemiarthroplasty is the treatment of choice for many of the very elderly, demented or infirm who present with displaced subcapital fractures.
- No good evidence indicates that the posterior, anterior, or anterolateral approach is associated with better results for either hemiarthroplasty or total hip arthroplasty.
  - Surgeons should use whichever approach is most familiar and comfortable.
- A number of conditions commonly present with femoral neck fractures. The treatment of these is listed in Table 21.2-11.

- There is also debate about the best surgical approach.
- Fluoroscopic studies of the movement of bipolar prostheses have given conflicting results, but most studies have suggested that these prostheses function as unipolar prostheses and movement is between the prosthetic head and the acetabulum rather than between the smaller and larger heads.
  - This is borne out by the comparative results of the two devices shown in Table 21.2-9.

TABLE 21.2-8   RESULTS OF THE MANAGEMENT OF DISPLACED FEMORAL NECK FRACTURES

Result	Internal Fixation (%)		Hemiarthroplasty (%)		Arthroplasty (%)	
	Range	Average	Range	Average	Range	Average
Death	15–34	25	18–31	26	9–23	21
Reoperation	25–39	36	0–13	5.2	4–9	6.2
Infection	0–15	3.5	0–5.2	2.3	1.1–4	2.5
Dislocation	0	0	1.6–11	3.4	0–17.9	10.7
Avascular necrosis	4.9–18	8.8	0	0	0	0
Normal mobility	27–57	42.2	27.2–55.6	40.4	49–53	50.3
No pain	12–71.5	50.1	42–79.1	66.1	43–100	75
Normal self-care	71	71	69	69	83	83
Normal activities of daily living	38	38	38	38	46	46

TABLE 21.2-9 RESULTS OF UNIPOLAR AND BIPOLAR HEMIARTHROPLASTIES

Result/Complication	Unipolar		Bipolar	
	Range	Average	Range	Average
Death (%)	21–38.6	27.1	27.1–31	28.1
Infection (%)	2.3–7.6	4.4	1.1–3.4	2.1
Dislocation (%)	0.6–4.4	2.1	0–2.9	1.5
Acetabular erosion (%)	2.3–5	3.8	0–5.4	3.4
No pain (%)	53–74.1	61.3	55.1–82	64.3
Normal mobility (%)	28.8–35.2	31.3	39.8–43.8	41.1
Normal activities of daily living (%)	35.2	35.2	43.8	43.8
Hospital stay (days)	18–19.8	19	17–22	19.3

TABLE 21.2-10 RESULTS OF CEMENTED AND UNCEMENTED UNIPOLAR HEMIARTHROPLASTIES

Result	Uncemented (%)		Cemented (%)	
	Range	Average	Range	Average
Death	23.1	23.1	29.6	29.6
No pain	20–55	37.5	68.4–90	79.5
No walking aids	20–35	27.5	57.9–85	64.1

TABLE 21.2-11 MANAGEMENT OF FEMORAL NECK FRACTURES IN SPECIFIC CONDITIONS

Condition	Treatment	Comments
Metastatic fractures	Arthroplasty	X-ray femur for distal metastases
Previous irradiation		
Undisplaced	Cannulated screws	25%–30% bilateral fractures
Displaced	Arthroplasty	
Paget's disease		Femoral bowing may necessitate an osteotomy
Undisplaced	Cannulated screws	
Displaced	Arthroplasty	
Hyperparathyroidism	Arthroplasty	Amyloid deposition leads to nonunion
Spastic diplegia	Hemiarthroplasty or arthroplasty	High dislocation rate
Parkinson disease		
Undisplaced	Cannulated screws	High dislocation rate
Displaced	Hemiarthroplasty or arthroplasty	
Rheumatoid arthritis		
Undisplaced	Cannulated screws	
Displaced	Arthroplasty	

COMPLICATIONS

Death

- The mortality rate after femoral neck fractures is high and the published ranges are quoted in Tables 21.2-8 and 21.2-9.
- A number of factors have been shown to increase mortality (Box 21.2-2).
- At approximately 12 to 18 months after fracture the mortality rate for hip fracture survivors falls to the level expected for their age.

Nonunion

- Nonunion was a significant problem when internal fixation was the treatment of choice for displaced femoral neck fractures with incidences of up to between 50% and 70% reported.
- With increasing use of joint replacement techniques in recent years, nonunion and failure of fixation have tended to be combined in a figure for reoperation (see Table 21.2-8).
- The requirement for reoperation increases with increasing age and infirmity.
- The factors that cause increased mortality (see Box 21.2-2) also tend to be related to fixation failure.
- The treatment of nonunion and failure of fixation is joint replacement with a hemi-arthroplasty or arthroplasty used, depending on the age and overall medical condition of the patient.
- The results of secondary arthroplasty carried out to treat a complication are not as good as the results of primary arthroplasty.

Avascular Necrosis

- The incidence of avascular necrosis ranges from almost 5% to 18%.
- It should be suspected in any patient who presents with a painful hip after internal fixation of a femoral neck fracture.
- An MRI scan will confirm the diagnosis.

- Arthroplasty is the treatment of choice in symptomatic avascular necrosis, although a rotational osteotomy may be undertaken in younger patients.

Infection

- The management of osteomyelitis is detailed in Chapter 40.
- Infection after reduction and internal fixation of a femoral neck fracture often causes septic arthritis in patients who are already debilitated.
  - Aggressive debridement and drainage and the use of antibiotics may allow the prosthesis to be maintained, but not infrequently a Girdlestone excision arthroplasty is required.
  - This is a very debilitating procedure for an elderly patient and is associated with high morbidity and mortality rates.

Refracture

- A secondary femoral fracture may occur after fixation of a proximal femoral fracture no matter which implant is used (see Chapter 7).
  - The fracture usually occurs at the tip of the implant: the proximal end of cannulated screws, the distal end of the plate in a dynamic hip screw system or the tip of the stem of a prosthesis.
- The incidence of refracture was examined by Robinson et al. (2002). The different incidences of secondary fracture are shown in Table 21.2-12.
  - The treatment for a fracture at the proximal end of cannulated screws is to refix the fracture with a dynamic hip screw or reconstruction nail.
  - Fractures at the distal end of a dynamic hip screw plate are best treated by intramedullary nailing using a conventional nail or a reconstruction nail.
- The treatment of fractures around implants is discussed in Chapter 7.
- Patients who have a proximal femoral fracture are at risk of a second fracture in the contralateral hip.
  - Analysis has indicated that this occurs in about 3% of patients with the incidence increasing with time.

BOX 21.2-2 FACTORS ASSOCIATED WITH INCREASED MORTALITY IN PATIENTS WITH DISPLACED FEMORAL NECK FRACTURES

Male gender
Increasing age (particularly >90 y)
Admission from a long-term care facility
Living at home with social support
Preoperative delay
Higher ASA score
Lower mental test score
Low Barthel score (activities of daily living)
Malignancy
Malnutrition
Comorbid medical conditions

TABLE 21.2-12 INCIDENCE OF SECONDARY FRACTURE AFTER FIXATION OF FEMORAL NECK FRACTURE

Fixation Device	Incidence[a] (%)
Secondary arthroplasty	22.4
Reconstruction nail	18.7
Cementless hemiarthroplasty	11.7
Primary arthroplasty	6.2
Cannulated screws	4.5
Compression hip screw	4.5

[a]The figures are expressed per 1,000 person-years.
Data from Robinson CM, Adams CI, Craig M, et al. Implant-related fractures of the femur following hip fracture surgery. J Bone Joint Surgery (Am) 2002;84:1116–1122.

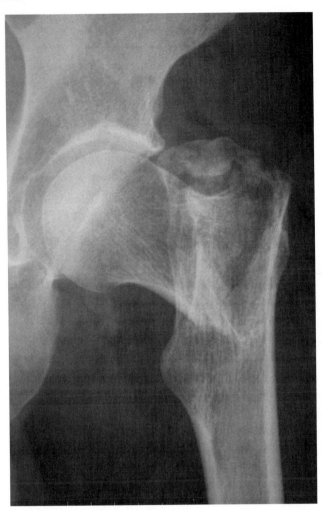 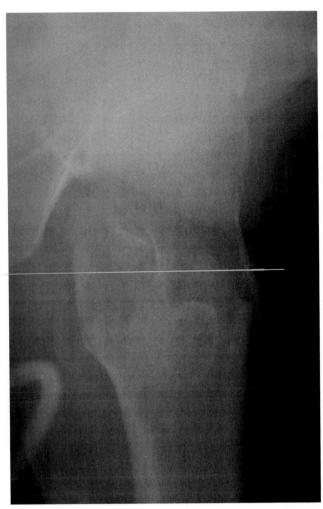

Figure 21.2-11 A-P and lateral radiographs of a basicervical (B2.1) fracture.

■ Thus 1% have the second fracture within 3 months, 2.8% by 1 year, and 7.3% by 3 years.

■ Increasing frailty is associated with an increasing incidence of second fracture. The incidence is greater in institutionalized and housebound patients.

■ In 70% to 75% of patients, similar fracture patterns occur in both hips.

EXTRACAPSULAR FRACTURES

There are four types of extracapsular proximal femoral fractures:basicervical fractures, intertrochanteric fractures, and isolated fractures of the greater and lesser trochanters.

Basicervical Fractures

Fractures at the base of the femoral neck (OTA [AO] B2.1) (Fig. 21.2-11) may strictly speaking not be extracapsular, with the exact definition of the fracture depending on its location in relation to the capsule that inserts close to the fracture site. The fractures are best treated as extracapsular fractures, however, because their lateral location means there is an increased varus moment at the fracture site and cancellous screws may not provide adequate fixation. Thus basicervical fractures are considered with intertrochanteric fractures.

Intertrochanteric Fractures

Intertrochanteric fractures occur between the greater and lesser trochanters of the proximal femur (Fig. 21.2-12). They may exit above or below the lesser trochanter, and the lesser trochanter may be a separate fragment. There may also be comminution of the greater trochanter. Some fractures may start above the lesser trochanter and pass laterally and distally into the femur. This will result in a reverse obliquity (OTA [AO] A3) fracture.

CLASSIFICATION

The Evans classification is often used for intertrochanteric fractures. It has five basic types depending on the position of the fracture line and the degree of comminution. The OTA (AO) classification is more extensive, however, and

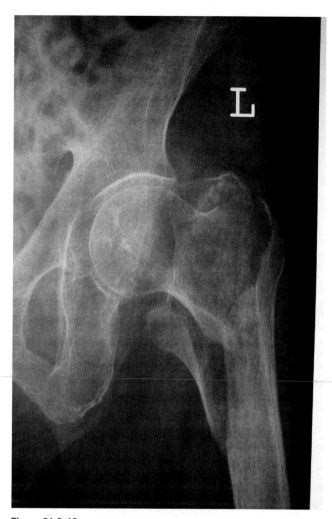 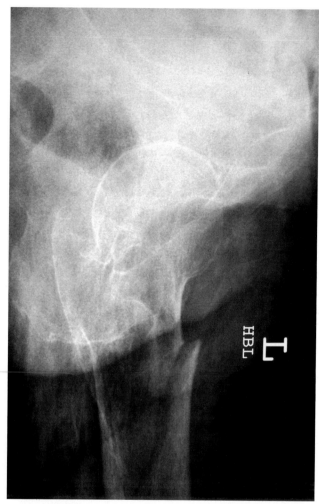

Figure 21.2-12 A-P and lateral radiographs of an intertrochanteric (A2.3) fracture.

provides improved definition of the different fracture types (see Figure 21.2-3). Type A fractures are intertrochanteric, with A1 and A2 fractures distinguished by the position of the fracture line and the degree of comminution. A1 fractures are simple fractures with A1.1 fractures occurring along the intertrochanteric line. A1.2 fractures occur through the greater trochanter, and A1.3 fractures exit below the lesser trochanter. The A2 fractures are multifragmentary intertrochanteric fractures, with A2.1 fractures having one intermediate fragment and A2.2 fractures several intermediate fragments. The A2.3 fractures extend more than 1 cm below the lesser trochanter. The A3 fractures are the reverse obliquity fractures, with the A3.1 fractures having a simple oblique configuration and the A3.2 fractures a simple transverse configuration. The A3.3 fractures are multi-fragmentary fractures.

EPIDEMIOLOGY

The epidemiology of patients who present with intertrochanteric fractures is shown in Table 21.2-13. Comparison with patients who present with femoral neck fractures indicates that the patients tend to be older. The female patients who present with intertrochanteric fractures tend to be more dependent and more likely to be restricted to their home or place of domicile. This is not true of male patients, however. Studies have indicated that osteoporotic women are more likely to sustain intertrochanteric fracture than a femoral neck fracture but this difference may be age related.

Because virtually all intertrochanteric fractures are caused by a simple fall, the most common associated injuries are fractures of the distal radius and proximal humerus, which occur in about 4% of patients.

TABLE 21.2-13 EPIDEMIOLOGY OF INTERTROCHANTERIC FRACTURES

Proportion of all fractures	6.2%
Age	81.2 y
Men/women	25%/75%
Distribution	Type F
Incidence	$69/10^5/y$
Most common cause	
Fall	87.1%
Open fractures	0%
Most common subgroups	
A1.1	40.1%
A2.1	23.3%
A1.2	12.5%

DIAGNOSIS

History and Physical Examination

■ History and physical examination are as for patients who present with femoral neck fractures.

Radiologic Examination

■ Anteroposterior and lateral radiographs are sufficient to diagnose an intertrochanteric fracture.

■ MRI and CT scans may be useful if there is an isolated greater trochanter and the surgeon wishes to see if there is an intertrochanteric extension.

   ■ They are also used in the diagnosis of lesser trochanter fractures to see if the fracture is associated with a metastasis.

TREATMENT

■ Many different implants have been used to treat intertrochanteric fractures, including flexible intramedullary pins, blade plates, fixed angle devices, sliding hip screws and sliding plates.

■ Currently, however, the choice of treatment is between a dynamic hip screw (Fig. 21.2-13) and a short reconstruction nail (Fig. 21.2-14).

■ If a dynamic hip screw or short reconstruction nail is used, it is important to position the tip of the lag screw as close to the apex of the femoral head as possible.

■ The tip-apex distance (TAD) correlates with the incidence of lag-screw cutout from the femoral head (Fig. 21.2-15). The TAD is the sum, in millimeters, of the distance from the tip of the lag screw to the apex of the femoral head in the anteroposterior and lateral radiographs.

■ A correction must be made for radiographic magnification, which is done by comparing the true and apparent diameters of the shaft of the lag screw.

■ Analysis has indicated that a TAD of less than 27 mm is not associated with lag-screw cutout, but if the TAD is more than 45 mm, the lag-screw cutout rate is 60%.

■ Surgeons still employ medial displacement or valgus osteotomies for comminuted intertrochanteric fractures, but little evidence indicates that they are effective, and it is usually preferable to reduce the fracture

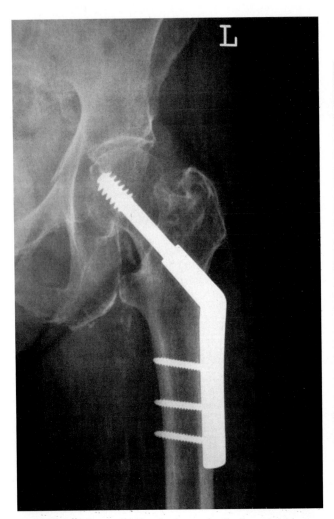
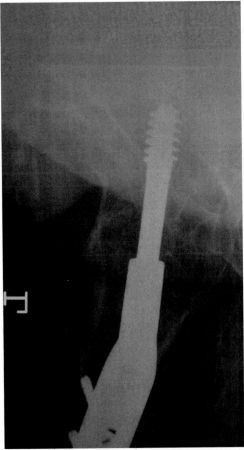

Figure 21.2-13   A-P and lateral radiographs of a dynamic hip screw.

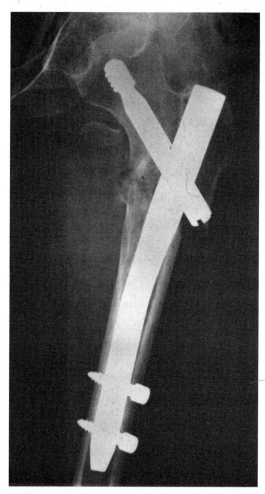

Figure 21.2-14 A short reconstruction nail.

and then apply a dynamic hip screw or a short reconstruction nail.

- Nonoperative management and external fixation have been used, but there are very few indications for these methods of management.
- A summary of the treatment of extracapsular proximal femoral fractures is given in Table 21.2-14.

TABLE 21.2-14 SUGGESTED TREATMENT OF EXTRACAPSULAR PROXIMAL FEMORAL FRACTURES

Type/Location	Treatment
A1 and A2 fractures	DHS or reconstruction nail
A3 fractures	Reconstruction nail
Basicervical fractures (B2.1)	DHS
Greater trochanter	
Undisplaced	Nonoperative management
Displaced	Interfragmentary screws or tension band wiring
Lesser trochanter	Consider neoplasia

RESULTS

Dynamic Hip Screw or Reconstruction Nail

- There have been a considerable number of prospective studies comparing dynamic hip screw systems with short reconstruction nails.
  - The results are shown in Table 21.2-15, which shows remarkably little difference between the two systems.
  - The two features of note in the reconstruction nails are the increased incidence of femoral fractures and the higher lag-screw cutout rate.
- The incidence of perioperative or postoperative femoral fracture following reconstruction nailing has decreased since the initial articles were published, probably because of improved operative technique, but reconstruction nails clearly are associated with a higher incidence of femoral fracture (see Table 21.2-12).
- The only technique with a higher incidence of secondary femoral fracture is secondary arthroplasty performed after failure of the initial proximal femoral fracture treatment.
- The higher incidence of lag-screw cutout is because placement of the lag-screw close to the apex of the femoral head is more difficult in reconstruction nails than in dynamic hip screw systems.

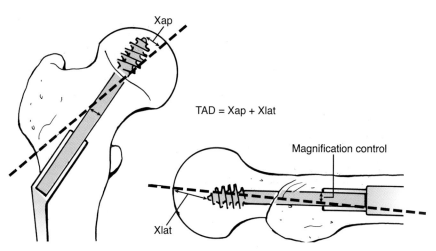

TAD = Xap + Xlat

Figure 21.2-15 The tip-apex distance (TAD).

TABLE 21.2-15 RESULTS OF THE USE OF RECONSTRUCTION NAILS AND DYNAMIC HIP SCREW SYSTEMS IN THE MANAGEMENT OF INTERTROCHANTERIC FRACTURES

Result/Complication	Reconstruction Nail (%)		Dynamic Hip Screw (%)	
	Range	Average	Range	Average
Death	16–38.8	24	12.2–31	22.3
Infection	0–4.1	1.3	0–3.2	0.9
Reoperation	1.4–7.6	3.6	0.9–4	2.2
Femoral fracture	2–6	13	0–2	0.5
Nonunion	0–1	0.1	0–2	0.1
Lag-screw cutout	2.1–8	4.6	1.1–2	1.8
Hip/thigh pain	23.6–26	25.3	10.5–34.4	26.5

■ Surgeons have noted a higher incidence of lag-screw placement in the superior part of the femoral head if reconstruction nails are used.

■ The literature clearly shows no significant difference in operating time, anesthetic time, blood loss, transfusion requirement, postoperative hemoglobin, or postoperative complications such as deep venous thrombosis, pneumonia, or sepsis between the two techniques.

  ▪ Postoperative mobility and hip function are also similar.

  ▪ Essentially there seems to be no significant difference between the two implants.

■ The only fracture in which there is evidence that a short reconstruction nail may be beneficial is in the reverse obliquity (A3) fracture.

■ In this configuration, the dynamic hip screw permits lateral displacement of the fracture, whereas the reconstruction nail does not.

Nonsurgical Treatment

■ Nonoperative management is rarely used for the treatment of intertrochanteric fractures.

■ The patients are elderly and infirm, and prolonged bed rest is associated with significant medical problems.

■ If nonoperative management is used, the average patient needs to be in traction for about 7 weeks but may be in traction for as long as 20 to 23 weeks.

■ Intertrochanteric fractures unite well, but varus displacement is common.

■ Nonoperative management confines the elderly and infirm patients to bed for a prolonged period and should not be used.

■ The only indication for nonoperative management is if the patient is moribund on admission or presents late and the fracture is already uniting.

External Fixation

■ External fixation is not in widespread use for the management of intertrochanteric fractures, but the technique has its proponents.

■ Published results are good, the stated advantages being a short surgical and anesthetic time, no blood loss and a shorter hospitalization.

■ External fixation is associated with a higher incidence of varus instability of the fracture, which is increased in older patients and unstable fracture configurations.

■ External fixation devices are said to be well tolerated, but more studies are required before this method of fixation can be advocated.

COMPLICATIONS

■ Complications associated with intertrochanteric fractures are less than with subcapital fractures (see Table 21.2-15).

■ The treatment of nonunion and infection are discussed in the relevant chapters and the incidence and management of femoral fractures is discussed in Chapter 23.

■ Despite the fact that the incidence of fixation failure is much less than with subcapital fracture it remains the main complication.

■ Lag-screw cutout may lead to coxa vara and significant disability.

■ Treatment is by refixation if the fracture has not united or by a valgizing osteotomy or total hip replacement if it has.

■ Refixation is very difficult because the bone is osteopenic and the original implant has already created a large void in the femoral neck and head.

■ A 95-degree blade plate can be used with insertion of the blade into the inferior part of the head.

■ The same implant is also useful for valgizing osteotomies (see Figure 39-11 in Chapter 39).

■ It is recommended that a valgizing osteotomy be used in younger fitter patients, with hip replacement reserved for the older patient.

Greater Trochanter Fractures

■ Isolated fractures of the greater trochanter are relatively rare.

  ▪ They usually occur in older patients after a fall.

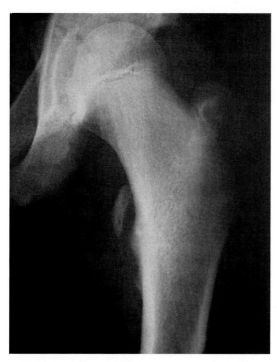

Figure 21.2-16   An avulsion fracture of the lesser trochanter.

- The greater trochanter is displaced superiorly and posteriorly.
- Anteroposterior and lateral radiographs are usually sufficient to diagnose a fracture, although a technetium bone scan, CT scan, or MRI scan can be used if a fracture is suspected and x-rays are negative.
- MRI scans often indicate that an apparently isolated greater trochanter fracture in fact has an intertrochanteric extension.
- Treatment is normally nonoperative, although in very displaced fractures in younger patients operative fixation may be indicated.
- Interfragmentary screw fixation or a tension band (see Chapter 34) can be used.
- Traumatic apophyseal avulsion of the greater trochanter has been reported in adolescence.
- This is extremely rare and best treated by internal fixation.

Lesser Trochanter Fractures

- Lesser trochanter fractures are also very rare. Their importance is that they are often pathological (see Figure 9-10 in Chapter 9).

- The subtrochanteric area is a common area for metastatic deposits, and an isolated lesser trochanteric fracture should be assumed pathological until proved otherwise.
- In younger patients they may be avulsion fractures (see Figure 21.2-16)
- The treatment is usually nonoperative.

SUGGESTED READING

Baumgaertner MR. Intertrochanteric hip fractures. In: Browner BD, Jupiter JB, Levine AM, et al., eds. Skeletal trauma, 3rd ed. Philadelphia: WB Saunders, 2003:1776–1816.

Baumgaertner MR, Curtin SL, Lindskog DM, et al. The value of the tip-apex distance in predicting failure of fixation of peritrochanteric fractures of the hip. J Bone Joint Surg (Am) 1995; 77:1058–1064.

Epstein HC. Traumatic dislocations of the hip. Clin Orthop 1973; 92:116–142.

Evans E. The treatment of trochanteric fractures of the femur. J Bone Joint Surg (Br) 1949;31:190–203.

Garden RS. Low-angle fixation in fractures of the femoral neck. J Bone Joint Surg (Br) 1961;43:647–663.

Holmberg S, Kalen R, Thorngren K-G. Treatment and outcome of femoral neck fractures; an analysis of 2418 patients admitted from their own homes. Clin Orthop 1987;218:42–52.

Lu-yao GL, Keller RB, Littenburg B, et al. Outcomes after displaced fractures of the femoral neck: a meta-analysis of one hundred and six published reports. J Bone Joint Surg (Am) 1994;76: 15–25.

Müller ME, Nazarian S, Koch P, et al. The comprehensive classification of fractures of long bones. Berlin: Springer-Verlag, 1990.

Ong BC, Maurer SG, Aharonoff GB, et al. Unipolar versus bipolar hemiarthroplasty: functional outcome after femoral neck fracture at a minimum of thirty-six months follow up. J Orthop Trauma 2002;16:317–322.

Parker MJ, Prior GA. Gamma versus DHS nailing for extracapsular femoral fractures. Meta-analysis of ten randomised trials. Int Orthop 1996;20:163–168.

Pipkin GJ. Treatment of grade IV fracture dislocation of the hip. J Bone Joint Surg 1957:1027–1042.

Robinson CM, Adams CI, Craig M, et al. Implant-related fractures of the femur following hip fracture surgery. J Bone Joint Surgery (Am) 2002;84:1116–1122.

Rogmark C, Carlsson A, Johnell O, et al. A prospective randomised trial of internal fixation versus arthroplasty for displaced fractures of the neck of the femur. Functional outcome for 450 patients at two years. J Bone Joint Surg (Br) 2002;84: 183–188.

Swiontkowski MF, Winquist RA. Displaced hip fractures in children and adolescents. J Trauma 1986;384–388.

Thompson VP, Epstein HC. Traumatic dislocation of the hip. J Bone Joint Surg (Am) 1951;33:746–778.

Tornetta P. Hip dislocations and fractures of the femoral head. In: Bucholz RW, Heckman JD, eds. Fractures in adults, 5th ed. Philadelphia: Lippincott Williams and Wilkins, 2001:1547–1578.

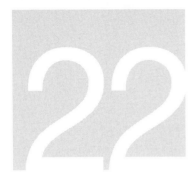

SUBTROCHANTERIC FRACTURES

Subtrochanteric fractures are considered more difficult to treat than proximal femoral fractures because the unopposed action of iliopsoas means the proximal femoral fragment tends to assume a flexed and varus position and closed reduction may be difficult. About 17% of subtrochanteric fractures are pathological. The most common cause is metastases from breast, prostate, renal, and lung carcinomas, or from multiple myeloma (see Chapter 9). The subtrochanteric area is also the most common site for pathological fractures from Paget's disease, with 20.5% of fractures occurring in this area compared with 17.5% in the subcapital area and 3.2% in the trochanteric area.

SURGICAL ANATOMY

The musculature of the subtrochanteric area of the femur is shown in Figure 22-1. It can be seen that a number of muscles span the subtrochanteric area but the clinically important muscle is that of iliopsoas which is formed by iliacus and psoas major and inserts into the lesser trochanter. In subtrochanteric fractures, the unopposed action of iliopsoas tends to cause the proximal fragment to flex, and the unopposed action of gluteus medius and minimus tends to cause it to abduct. The adductor muscles then pull the distal femoral shaft into varus.

The femoral artery enters the thigh within the femoral triangle. It gives off the profunda femoris branch, which leaves the femoral triangle behind the adductor longus close to the femur. The lateral and medial circumflex arteries arise from the profunda femoris near its origin. The sciatic and femoral nerves are the two major nerves of the thigh. The femoral nerve enters the thigh under the inguinal ligament and lateral to the femoral artery. It then divides into a number of muscular and cutaneous nerves. The sciatic nerve enters the thigh through the greater sciatic foramen and descends into the thigh under the long head of biceps femoris on the posterior surface of adductor magnus. The obturator nerve enters the thigh through the obturator groove and divides into anterior and posterior divisions. The anterior division descends between pectineus and adductor longus anteriorly and adductor brevis posteriorly to end in the sub-sartorial plexus on the medial side of the thigh. The posterior branch pierces obturator externus and descends between adductor brevis anteriorly and adductor magnus posteriorly to descend with the femoral artery into the thigh.

CLASSIFICATION

There are a number of classifications of subtrochanteric fractures. Classification is difficult because the definition of what constitutes a subtrochanteric fracture varies. Seinsheimer (1978) defined eight different subgroups, and Russell and Taylor (1992) separated subtrochanteric fractures into four types. Both classifications remain in use. It seems likely, however, that the OTA (AO) classification will be adopted by most surgeons, and it is used in this chapter. In this classification, subtrochanteric fractures are combined with femoral diaphyseal fractures. The full classification is shown in Figure 23-2.

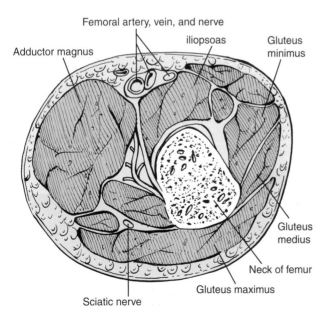

Figure 22-1   Anatomy of the proximal femur.

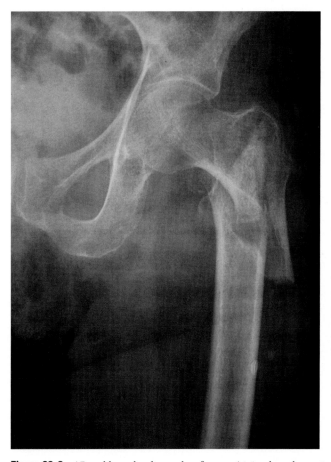 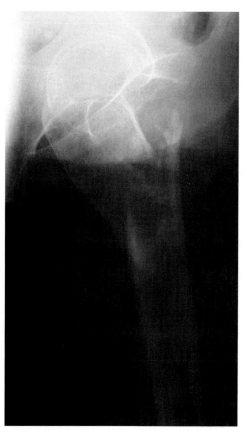

Figure 22-2 AP and lateral radiographs of a type A1.1 subtrochanteric fracture.

In type A and B fractures, the suffix 0.1 indicates a sub-trochanteric fracture, with spiral, oblique, and transverse fractures in the A1, A2, and A3 groups, respectively. Spiral, bending, and fragmented wedge subtrochanteric fractures are placed in the B1, B2, and B3 groups. It could also be reasonably argued that the OTA (AO) proximal femoral classification contains a number of subtrochanteric fractures, as the A1.3, A2.3, A3.1, and A3.3 fractures have extensions below the lesser trochanter.

EPIDEMIOLOGY

The epidemiology of subtrochanteric fractures is shown in Table 22-1. A review of the literature suggests the incidence of subtrochanteric fractures in the elderly is rising. The overall average age is about 76 years, and the average age of patients injured in a simple fall is 83 years, very similar to the average age of patients with proximal femoral fractures. Most fractures are caused by simple falls or falls from a height. Other causes are rare.

Associated Injuries

Young patients who present with high-energy sub-trochanteric fractures tend to be more seriously injured. In some series, between 21% and 51% of patients with subtrochanteric fractures have other injuries, mainly head, abdominal, and pelvic injuries in addition to other lower limb injuries. Ipsilateral patellar and tibial diaphyseal fractures are particularly associated with high-energy subtrochanteric

TABLE 22-1 EPIDEMIOLOGY OF SUBTROCHANTERIC FRACTURES	
Proportion of all fractures	0.3%
Proportion of femoral diaphyseal fractures	30.1%
Average age	76.5 y
Men/women	47%/53%
Distribution	Type F
Incidence	$3.2/10^5$/y
Most common causes	
Fall	64.7%
Fall from height	11.8%
Open fractures	5.9%
OTA (OA) classification	
Type A	64.7%
Type B	35.3%
Type C	0%
Most common subgroups	
A1.1	47.1%
B1.1	17.6%
B3.1	17.6%

fractures. Elderly patients usually have isolated injuries, but, as with proximal femoral fractures, patients may present with distal radial or proximal humeral fractures as a result of the fall. In the series detailed in Table 22-1, 17.6% were periprosthetic fractures (see Chapter 7)

DIAGNOSIS

History and Physical Examination

- The clinical history usually involves a high-energy injury in younger patients and a simple fall in the elderly.
- Most patients are unable to weight bear, and examination usually shows a shortened, externally rotated leg with a swollen thigh.
- Attempted hip movement is extremely painful, and palpation may reveal the flexed proximal femoral fragment in thinner patients.
- Neurological and vascular injuries are unusual unless the fracture has been caused by a gunshot injury.
- As with other proximal femoral fractures, elderly patients may present with a number of medical comorbidities.
- A thorough history of their social circumstances and place of domicile is important because the fracture may mean the end of an independent existence.
- In view of the association of subtrochanteric fractures with metastatic disease, it is important to take a history of renal, breast, prostatic, or pulmonary symptoms in particular.

Radiologic Examination

- Anteroposterior and lateral radiographs are usually sufficient to diagnose a subtrochanteric fracture (see Fig. 22-2).
- The hip and knee joints must be x-rayed to exclude adjacent dislocations or fractures.
- Further imaging with CT or MRI scans is rarely necessary to diagnose a fracture.
- Angiography or Doppler studies may be required if there is suspicion of a significant vascular injury.
- In view of the possibility of pathological fractures, a chest x-ray is recommended in older patients.
- If there is evidence of a pathologic fracture, it is important to x-ray the whole femur to see whether there are other metastatic deposits.
- Appropriate pulmonary, breast, or renal imaging may be required.

TREATMENT

Surgical Treatment

- The mainstay of the treatment of subtrochanteric fractures has been plating, although in recent years intramedullary nailing with reconstruction nails has become popular.
- External fixation is rarely indicated.

TABLE 22-2 RESULTS ASSOCIATED WITH THE USE OF 95-DEGREE BLADE PLATES

Result/Complication	Range	Average
Union time (wk)	13–24	16
Nonunion (%)	0–14	10
Infection (%)	0–7.5	6.2
Malunion (%)	0–16.6	4.2
Mechanical failure (%)	0–50	10

Plating

- Three plate types are commonly used to treat subtrochanteric femoral fractures: the 95-degree blade plate, the 95-degree dynamic condylar screw plate, and the 135-degree dynamic hip screw.

95-Degree Blade Plate

- The 95-degree blade plate (see Fig. 39-11 in Chapter 39) is now less commonly used to treat subtrochanteric fractures.
- It is technically the most difficult plate to insert but remains useful for complex fractures not suitable for nailing.
- The results given in Table 22-2 reveal a relatively high incidence of mechanical failure and nonunion.
- Improved results can be obtained by using indirect fracture reduction, thereby reducing the damage to the vasculature.
  - If this is done, the literature suggests that the incidence of infection and nonunion is significantly reduced.

95-Degree Dynamic Condylar Screw Plate (DCS)

- The 95-degree dynamic condylar screw plate (Fig. 22-3) is technically easier to use as the screw is inserted separately.
- The results shown in Table 22-3 appear very similar to those associated with the use of the 95-degree blade plate, with a relatively high incidence of malunion and nonunion.

135-Degree Dynamic Hip Screw (DHS)

- The 135-degree dynamic hip screw is commonly used for the treatment of intertrochanteric fractures (see

TABLE 22-3 RESULTS ASSOCIATED WITH THE USE OF THE 95-DEGREE DYNAMIC CONDYLAR SCREW PLATE

Result/Complication	Range	Average
Union time (wk)	17	17
Nonunion (%)	0–20	6
Infection (%)	?	?
Malunion (%)	0–26.6	12.5
Mechanical failure (%)	0–18	8

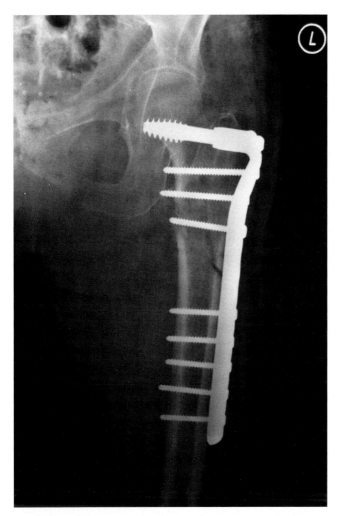

Figure 22-3 A dynamic condylar screw (DCS) used to treat a subtrochanteric fracture.

Figure 21.2-13 in Chapter 21) but if a longer side plate is attached it can be used for subtrochanteric fractures.

■ The results are better than those for the other two types of plates (Table 22-4).

■ The two significant problems associated with plating are the difficulty of maintaining non-weight-bearing status in elderly patients and the requirement for bone grafting if there is subtrochanteric comminution.

■ The literature clearly shows that failure of plate fixation is associated with failure to bone graft areas of extensive

comminution and extensive comminution is a contraindication for their use in the subtrochanteric area.

Intramedullary Nailing

■ Subtrochanteric fractures can be treated with conventional intramedullary nails provided the lesser trochanter is intact (Fig. 22-4).

■ Nowadays, however, most surgeons prefer to use a reconstruction nail, which allows them to place the proximal cross screw into the femoral neck and head (Fig. 22-5).

■ The operative technique and complications of reconstruction nails are discussed in Chapter 33.

■ Short reconstruction nails are not infrequently used to treat intertrochanteric fractures, and their use is discussed in Chapter 21.

■ The results of the use of standard interlocking femoral nails for the management of subtrochanteric fractures are given in Table 22-5.

■ The apparently prolonged union time is due to the fact that most series deal with higher energy injuries in younger patients.

■ The overall results are very good.

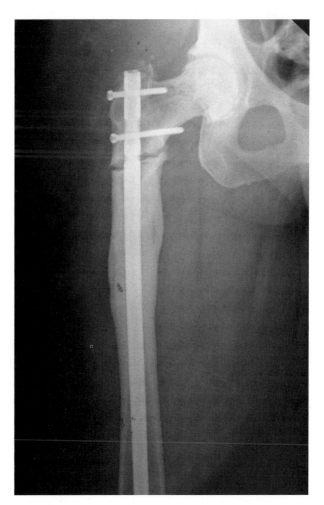

Figure 22-4 An interlocking nail used to treat an insufficiency fracture in a patient with osteopetrosis.

TABLE 22-4 RESULTS ASSOCIATED WITH THE USE OF THE 135-DEGREE DYNAMIC HIP SCREW

Result/Complication	Range	Average
Union time (wk)	10–18	16
Nonunion (%)	0–8	3
Malunion (%)	0–2	2
Infection (%)	0–2.1	2
Mechanical failure (%)	0–11	5

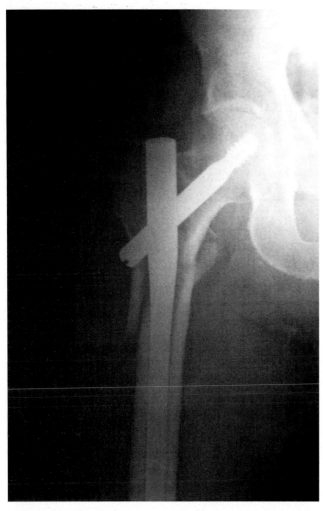

Figure 22-5   A reconstruction nail used to treat a subtrochanteric fracture.

Reconstruction Nails

■ Short reconstruction nails can theoretically be used for some subtrochanteric fractures, but surgeons now tend to use long reconstruction nails because of the lower incidence of perioperative or postoperative femoral diaphyseal fracture and the significant risk of a late femoral fracture in an osteoporotic femoral diaphysis.

TABLE 22-5 RESULTS ASSOCIATED WITH THE USE OF INTERLOCKING INTRAMEDULLARY NAILS

Result/Complication	Range	Average
Union time (wk)	18.2–25.5	21.9
Nonunion (%)	0–9.7	3
Infection (%)	?	?
Malunion (%)	3.2–6.3	5.5
Mechanical failure (%)	0–11	2
Knee flexion (%)	115–127	118

TABLE 22-6 RESULTS ASSOCIATED WITH THE USE OF LONG RECONSTRUCTION NAILS

Result/Complication	Range	Average
Union time (wk)	13–27	18.6
Nonunion (%)	3.8–9.3	6.3
Malunion (%)	0–7	3.1
Infection (%)	0	0

■ The results of the use of long reconstruction nails are given in Table 22-6.
■ There are as yet relatively few studies of this implant, but the results are encouraging.
■ The rate of mechanical failure is higher than in conventional nailing, but most reported failures involved locking screw breakages, which were associated with very low morbidity.
■ The nonunion incidence is low, and the studies report no infections.
■ Overall it is reported that 80% to 85% of patients returned to full function and the early ambulation permitted by the use of intramedullary nails is undoubtedly advantageous.
■ The requirement for bone grafting is lower than with plating.

External Fixation

■ There is no evidence that primary external fixation is indicated in the treatment of isolated subtrochanteric fractures.
■ It may be used in multiply injured patients for primary fixation with definitive secondary internal fixation carried out later.
■ There is little information about the success of external fixation of subtrochanteric fractures in civilian injuries but it has been examined with reference to wartime injuries, and an incidence of 12% osteomyelitis and 16% nonunion has been quoted.
■ In war conditions, however, these represent reasonable results.

Pathological Fractures

■ The treatment of pathological fractures is discussed in Chapter 9.
■ The choice of surgical stabilization lies between plates and intramedullary nails.
■ The mechanics of fracture fixation clearly favor nailing and if closed nailing techniques are used, supplementary PMMA may not be required as it frequently is with plating.
■ The choice is between standard locking nailing and reconstruction nailing, but with the introduction of long reconstruction nails these have become the implant of choice (see Figure 9-11 in Chapter 9).

Nonsurgical Treatment

- There are no indications for nonoperative management except in the patient who is moribund on admission.
- Nonoperative management requires prolonged bed rest and is associated with a high morbidity and mortality.
- Traction can be used, but the incidence of malunion and nonunion is relatively high.

Suggested Treatment

- All subtrochanteric fractures are best treated with a long reconstruction nail.
- In younger patients with good bone stock a conventional locked intramedullary nail may be used provided the lesser trochanter is intact.

COMPLICATIONS

- Tables 22-2 to 22-6 indicate that with the introduction of intramedullary nailing for the treatment of subtrochanteric fractures, the incidence of complications has decreased.
- The most common complications are nonunion, malunion, and loss of fracture fixation because of implant failure, nonunion, or failure to bone graft areas of comminution in plated fractures.
- The treatment of nonunion, malunion, and infection are discussed in the appropriate chapters in this book.
- Loss of fracture fixation is treated by refixation using an intramedullary nail.

SUGGESTED READING

Barquet A, Francescoli L, Renzi D, et al. Intertrochanteric-subtrochanteric fracture treatment with the long Gamma nail. J Orthop Trauma 2000;14:324–328.

Kinast C, Bolhofner BR, Mast JW, et al. Sub-trochanteric fractures of the femur. Results of treatment with the 95° condylar blade-plate. Clin Orthop 1989;238:122–130.

Müller ME, Nazarian S, Koch P, et al. The comprehensive classification of fractures of long bones. Berlin: Springer-Verlag, 1990.

Parker MJ, Dutta BK, Sivaji C, et al. Sub-trochanteric fractures of the femur. Injury 1997;28:91–95.

Rantanen J, Aro HT. Intramedullary fixation of high sub-trochanteric femoral fractures: a study comparing two implant designs, the Gamma nail and the intramedullary hip screw. J Orthop Trauma 1998;12:249–252.

Russell TA. Subtrochanteric fractures of the femur. In: Browner BD, Jupiter JB, Levine AM, et al., eds. Skeletal trauma. Philadelphia: WB Saunders, 2003:1832–1878.

Seinsheimer F. Subtrochanteric fractures of the femur. J Bone Joint Surg (Am) 1978:60;300–306.

Wiss DA, Brien WW. Subtrochanteric fractures of the femur. Results of treatment by interlocking nailing. Clin Orthop 1992;283:231–236.

FEMORAL DIAPHYSEAL FRACTURES

Femoral diaphyseal fractures have always challenged surgeons. They often occur in multiply injured patients, and until the introduction of modern operative treatment methods, the complication rate was high. The move to early fracture fixation revolutionized the management of the multiply injured patient, lowering mortality and morbidity. Plating was adopted initially as the optimal treatment method, but after the Second World War, unlocked intramedullary nailing became accepted. In the 1970s and 1980s, antegrade locked nailing became the treatment of choice, but more recently treatment methods have continued to change with the introduction of retrograde nailing. Controversies regarding the treatment of femoral diaphyseal fractures are summarized in Box 23-1.

SURGICAL ANATOMY

The femur is the largest and strongest bone in the body. It has an anterior bow that averages 12 to 15 degrees. Posteriorly, a thickened ridge, the linear aspera, gives rise to the medial and lateral intramuscular septae. There are three compartments in the thigh. The anterior compartment contains the knee extensors: the vastus lateralis, vastus medialis, vastus intermedius, sartorius, and rectus femoris. The posterior compartment contains the knee flexors: the semimembranosis, semitendinosis, and biceps femoris. The medial compartment contains the adductors: adductor

longus, adductor brevis, adductor magnus, and gracilis. A cross section of the middle third of the thigh is shown in Figure 23-1.

The femoral artery enters the thigh within the femoral triangle. It gives off the profunda femoris branch, which leaves the femoral triangle behind the adductor longus close to the femur. The lateral and medial circumflex arteries arise from the profunda femoris near its origin. The profunda femoris gives off three perforating branches close to the femur and ends as the fourth perforating artery. These are at risk in femoral plating or occasionally from external fixator pins. The femoral artery continues as the superficial femoral artery after giving off the profunda femoris. It passes through the hiatus in the adductor magnus and

---

BOX 23-1 CURRENT CONTROVERSIES IN THE TREATMENT OF FEMORAL DIAPHYSEAL FRACTURES

Is antegrade or retrograde intramedullary nailing more appropriate?
How should open femoral fractures be treated?
What is the role of primary nailing in multiply injured patients?
What is the role of external fixation?
How should combined neck and diaphyseal fractures be treated?

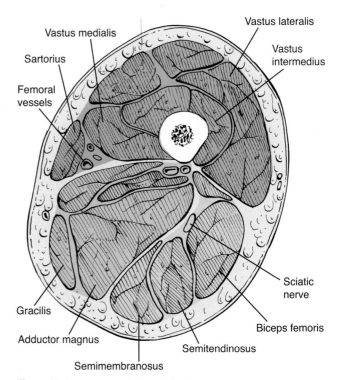

Figure 23-1 Anatomy of the midthigh.

enters the posterior compartment and then the popliteal fossa.

The sciatic and femoral nerves are the two major nerves of the thigh. The femoral nerve enters the thigh under the inguinal ligament and lateral to the femoral artery. It divides into a number of muscular and cutaneous nerves. The sciatic nerve enters the thigh through the greater sciatic foramen and descends into the thigh under the long head of biceps femoris on the posterior surface of the adductor magnus. It ends as the common peroneal and tibial nerves at a point above the popliteal fossa.

CLASSIFICATION

The OTA (AO) classification is widely used to classify femoral diaphyseal fractures. This is a morphological classification based on the initial anteroposterior and lateral radiographs (Fig. 23-2). Type A fractures are simple fractures and include spiral fractures (A1), oblique fractures (A2), and transverse fractures (A3). Type B fractures are wedge fractures and include spiral wedges (B1), bending wedges (B2), and fragmented wedges (B3). Type C fractures are complex fractures with the C1 group containing

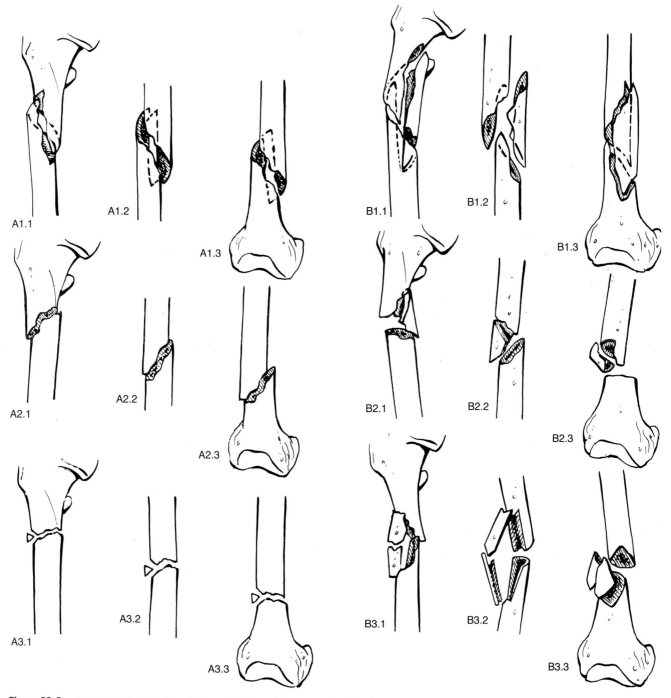

Figure 23-2 OTA (AO) classification of femoral diaphyseal fractures. *(continued)*

all spiral fractures, the C2 group all segmental fractures, and the C3 group all comminuted fractures. In type A and B fractures, the suffix 0.1 represents a fracture in the subtrochanteric zone, with 0.2 used for the middle zone and 0.3 for the distal zone. In type C fractures, the suffixes 0.1 through 0.3 represent increasing bone damage.

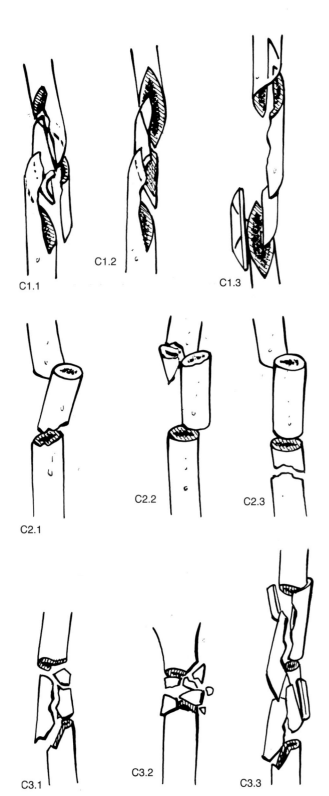

Figure 23-2 *(continued)*

EPIDEMIOLOGY

The epidemiological characteristics of femoral diaphyseal fractures are shown in Table 23-1. Femoral fractures exhibit a type A bimodal distribution (see Chapter 1) with higher incidences seen in younger men and older female patients. In young patients the fractures are usually related to high-energy injuries such as motor vehicle accidents, falls from a height, or gunshot wounds, whereas most femoral fractures in the elderly are insufficiency fractures that occur after a simple fall or after previous arthroplasty surgery. With improved road safety and workplace legislation, many countries now have a declining incidence of high-energy injuries in younger patients and an increasing number of fractures in the elderly, many of which are periprosthetic.

The epidemiological characteristics of femoral fractures caused by the most common types of injury are shown in Table 23-2. This shows the advanced average age in patients injured in a fall and the fact that most have type A fractures. Predictably, there is a higher incidence of more complex fractures after falls from a height and particularly after motor vehicle accidents and gunshot wounds. Sports-related fractures are rare, but femoral fractures are associated with sports such as skiing and with motorcycle and automobile racing.

Associated Injuries

The fact that many patients who present with femoral diaphyseal fractures sustain high-energy injuries means they commonly present with other injuries. Epidemiological studies suggest that 61.5% of femoral diaphyseal fractures are isolated fractures. In the group of patients who present with multiple injuries, 94% have other musculoskeletal injuries, 60% have a head injury, 16% have a facial injury, 62% have a thoracic injury, and 35% have an abdominal injury.

TABLE 23-1 EPIDEMIOLOGY OF FEMORAL DIAPHYSEAL FRACTURES[a]

Proportion of all fractures	0.6%
Average age	62.4 y
Men/women	32%/68%
Distribution	Type A
Incidence	$7.1/10^5$/y
Open fractures	7.9%
Most common causes	
Falls	57.9%
Motor vehicle accident	23.7%
OTA (AO) classification	
Type A	68.4%
Type B	15.8%
Type C	15.8%
Most common subgroups	
A1.2	23.7%
A3.2	18.4%
A1.3	15.8%

[a]Subtrochanteric fractures are excluded. These are reviewed in Table 22-2 in Chapter 22.

TABLE 23-2 EPIDEMIOLOGY OF FEMORAL DIAPHYSEAL FRACTURES ACCORDING TO MODE OF INJURY

	Age (y)	Open (%)	OTA (AO) Type (%)		
			A	B	C
Fall	82.5	0	81.8	9.1	9.1
Motor vehicle accident	23.2	33.3	22.2	33.3	55.5

Femoral diaphyseal fractures may be associated with a number of other musculoskeletal injuries. Some associated injuries, listed in Table 23-3, deserve particular attention. This shows that the principal associations are with injuries adjacent to the femoral diaphysis. The apparent incidence of femoral neck fractures has risen in recent years with the use of CT scanning, and arthroscopic evaluation of the ipsilateral knee has produced a more accurate estimate of the extent of knee ligament and meniscal damage. The incidence of meniscal injury can only be estimated because it is impossible to assess the incidence of preexisting meniscal damage. Ipsilateral femoral and tibial fractures, the floating knee complex, are relatively rare but difficult to treat and often associated with a poor outcome.

DIAGNOSIS

History and Physical Examination

- Patients who present with high-energy femoral fractures must be carefully examined according to ATLS guidelines because there a high incidence of associated injuries.
- Femoral fractures are usually easily detected, particularly in the conscious patient, because pain, deformity, and swelling are apparent.
- Surgeons should be aware of the possibility of a femoral diaphyseal fracture in all unconscious patients, particularly if they have been injured in a motor vehicle accident or a fall from a height.
- Clinical examination should include an assessment of any open wound in addition to a thorough neurological examination and assessment of the vascular status of the limb.

TABLE 23-3 INJURIES ASSOCIATED WITH FEMORAL DIAPHYSEAL FRACTURES

Injury	Prevalence[a] (%)
Femoral neck fractures	2.5–6
Hip dislocation	0–1.1
Distal femoral fractures	0–3.4
Knee ligament injuries	17–48
Meniscal injuries	25–32
Tibial fractures (floating knee)	0–2

[a]The incidences have been taken from the literature.

- This is particularly relevant if there has been a gunshot injury.
- If there is any suggestion of vascular compromise, Doppler studies and angiography should be undertaken.
- In elderly patients there may be a number of medical comorbidities, and a complete history should be taken from the patient or a companion.

Radiologic Examination

- Anteroposterior and lateral radiographs should be sufficient to diagnose a femoral diaphyseal fracture (Fig. 23-3).
- In view of the associated injuries documented in Table 23-3, it is mandatory to include the hip and knee in the radiographic series.
- Further imaging with CT or MRI scans may be required to diagnose associated injuries (Table 23-3), and angiography or Doppler studies may be used if there is concern about vascular damage.
- MRI scanning may be used to diagnose stress fractures of the femoral diaphysis (see Chapter 6).

TREATMENT

Surgical Treatment

- There is probably no other fracture in which there is such a strong consensus in favor of one treatment method.
- Locked intramedullary nailing is now accepted as the treatment method for virtually all femoral diaphyseal fractures, although there are some indications for other treatment methods.

Antegrade Intramedullary Nailing

- The surgical technique and complications of antegrade intramedullary nailing are discussed in detail in Chapter 33.
- The use of a locked antegrade intramedullary nail allows virtually any femoral diaphyseal fracture to be stabilized using a closed technique (Fig. 23-4).
- Conventional intramedullary nailing stabilizes any fracture between the lesser trochanter and a point about 5 cm above the distal femoral epiphysis.
- Both reamed and unreamed nailing are used, but the evidence indicates that reamed nailing is advantageous in terms of union time and the avoidance of secondary

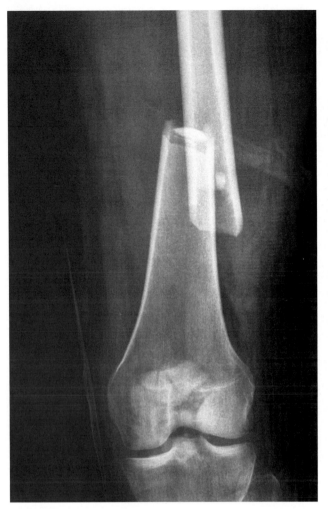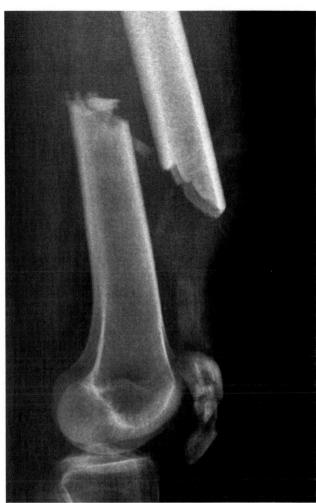

Figure 23-3   A-P and lateral radiographs of a femoral diaphyseal (A2.2) fracture in a multiply injured 22-year-old woman who presented with bilateral femoral and patellar fractures.

surgery, with meta-analyses indicating that reaming does not increase the incidence of malunion, infection, pulmonary embolus, or compartment syndrome.

■ Most surgeons now use interlocking intramedullary nailing for all grades of open fractures. The main indication for not treating a femoral fracture with an intramedullary nail is in multiply injured patients where primary external fixation and secondary intramedullary nailing may minimize the initial operative time, allowing

early intensive care and thereby reducing the complications associated with polytrauma (see Chapter 3).

■ The results of the use of reamed and unreamed antegrade nails for the treatment of open and closed femoral diaphyseal fractures are shown in Table 23-4.

■ The results indicate that the requirement for secondary surgery is less with reamed nails than with unreamed nails, although the differences are less obvious than in the tibia (see Chapter 27).

TABLE 23-4 RESULTS OF REAMED AND UNREAMED ANTEGRADE FEMORAL NAILING

Result/Complication	Reamed		Unreamed	
	Range	Average	Range	Average
Union time (wk)	12–32	17.0	15.6–39.4	19.3
Secondary surgery (%)	0–14	2.4	0–39	5.9
Malunion (%)	0–15	7.2	0–4.5	1.9
Infection (%)	0–2.4	0.4	0–2.9	0.8

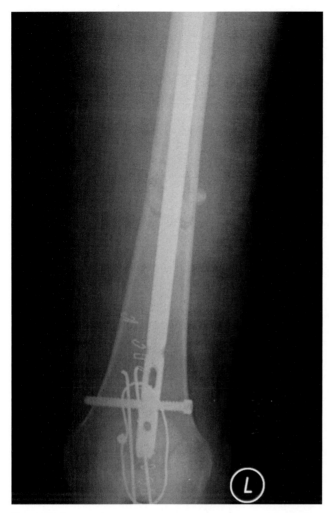
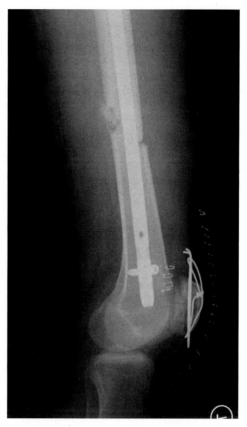

Figure 23-4 The fracture shown in Figure 23-3 has been treated with a statically locked antegrade intramedullary nail. The patella has been fixed with K-wires and cerclage wiring (see Chapter 25).

- The lower incidence of malunion in the unreamed series probably represents the greater experience that surgeons had with nailing by the time unreamed nails became popular.
- The incidence of infection is similar in both techniques.

Complications
- The complications of antegrade femoral nailing are discussed in Chapter 33 and summarized in Table 23-5.

- The most common complications are buttock or hip discomfort and heterotopic ossification (Fig. 23-5).
  - The two are related in that the severity of heterotopic ossification correlates with buttock or hip discomfort.
  - Buttock discomfort may also be caused by prominent nails and surgical scarring.
- It is worth noting that unreamed antegrade femoral nailing has a significantly lower incidence of heterotopic

TABLE 23-5 COMPLICATIONS OF ANTEGRADE FEMORAL NAILING

Complication	Range (%)	Average (%)
Femoral neck fractures	0–2.5	1
Femoral comminution	0–5	3
External rotation deformity	0–55	10
Neurological damage	0–6	1
Heterotopic ossification	60–68	65
Buttock/hip pain	0–41	40
Nail breakage	0–3	1
Avascular necrosis	Rare	<1

TABLE 23-6 RESULTS OF REAMED AND UNREAMED RETROGRADE FEMORAL NAILING

Result/Complication	Reamed		Unreamed	
	Range	Average	Range	Average
Union time (wk)	12.6–18.1	14.6	17–31.8	16.7
Secondary surgery (%)	0–8	5.1	12.6–19.9	8.3
Malunion (%)	1.7–33	12.6	0–4.5	1.9
Infection (%)	0	0	0	0

ossification compared with reamed nailing (9.4% and 35.7%, respectively).

Retrograde Femoral Nailing

■ Retrograde femoral nailing (Fig. 23-6) has become popular in the last 10 years.

■ Its indications, surgical techniques, and complications are discussed in Chapter 33.

■ A relatively straightforward procedure that does not require a nailing table, it is particularly useful in obese and pregnant patients and in patients who have proximal femoral pathology or implants, or acetabular fractures.

■ It is also used in the treatment of ipsilateral femoral and tibial diaphyseal fractures.

■ As with antegrade nailing, there has been debate about the use of reaming prior to the introduction of retrograde femoral nails. The results of both reamed and unreamed retrograde femoral nailing are shown in Table 23-6.

■ This indicates that, as with antegrade femoral nailing, the incidence of secondary surgery for nonunion is

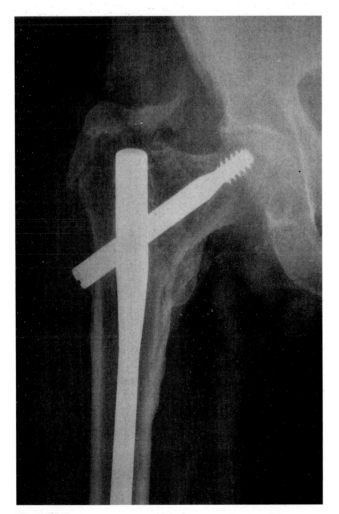

Figure 23-5   Heterotopic ossification after the insertion of a reconstruction nail.

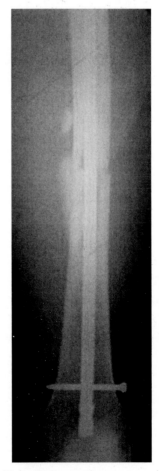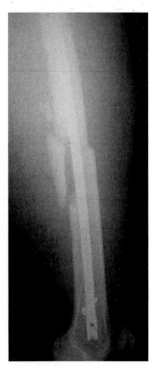

Figure 23-6   The use of a statically locked retrograde nail to treat a B3.2 femoral diaphyseal fracture.

slightly higher with unreamed nails and the malunion incidence is less.

Complications

■ Because retrograde nailing has only become popular in recent years, there is less information available about its complications than for antegrade nailing.

■ Understandable concern has been expressed about knee damage during retrograde nailing, and septic arthritis and heterotopic ossification have been sporadically reported, but there are no reports of the incidences of these complications.

■ Knee pain occurs in about 30% of patients, but the pain is usually mild.

■ Animal studies have shown decreased blood flow in both cruciate ligaments as a result of retrograde femoral nailing, but no clinical evidence indicates this is a problem in humans.

Antegrade or Retrograde Nailing?

■ Tables 23-4 and 23-6 suggest very little difference in the results of antegrade and retrograde femoral nailing.

■ Comparative studies have suggested that the incidence of knee pain is higher with retrograde nailing, and the incidence of hip and buttock pain is higher with antegrade nailing.

■ Studies also predictably suggest that proximal femoral diaphyseal fractures are controlled better with antegrade nailing, whereas distal diaphyseal fractures fare better with retrograde nailing.

■ Surgeons are understandably concerned about the possibility of iatrogenic knee pathology with retrograde nailing, but the incidence is low.

■ It seems, therefore, that both techniques are useful, and it is likely the use of retrograde nailing will increase.

Special Circumstances

Open Fractures

■ In the last 15 to 20 years, there has been a major change in the management of open femoral diaphyseal fractures.

■ External fixation was more popular in the past, but intramedullary nailing is now used for all grades of open fracture.

■ The results of the use of intramedullary nailing in open femoral fractures are given in Table 23-7.

■ This indicates that the results are extremely good, despite the fact that an average of 32% of the fractures were Gustilo type III in severity.

TABLE 23-7 RESULTS OF INTRAMEDULLARY NAILING OF OPEN FRACTURES[a]

Result/Complication	Range	Average
Gustilo III fractures (%)	19–51.7	32.0
Union time (wk)	16.5–22.5	21.4
Infection (%)	2.6–7.1	3.7
Nonunion (%)	0–4.8	2.4

[a]All studies used antegrade nailing.

■ Nonunion and infection rates are very low, reflected in the relatively short average union time.

■ The functional results of patients with nailed open femoral fractures are also good, with virtually all patients achieving at least 120 degrees of knee flexion.

Multiple Injuries

■ It has been accepted for about 20 years that the optimal treatment of multiply injured patients includes primary fixation of long-bone fractures.

■ A number of clinical studies in the 1980s clearly indicated that early femoral fracture fixation improved mortality and morbidity, with particular benefit noted in very severely injured patients and in older patients.

■ It was assumed that because nailing was the best method of treating femoral fractures, primary nailing was therefore the optimal treatment method for femoral fractures in multiply injured patients.

■ This view was challenged by surgeons in Hannover, Germany, who demonstrated that small-diameter unreamed nails were associated with lower mortality and ARDS than reamed nails in patients who had significant pulmonary trauma.

■ This work could not be reproduced in animal models or clinical studies, however, and it was concluded that pulmonary complications after femoral fractures occurred as a result of prolonged immobilization, massive blood transfusion, fluid overload, underlying illness, aspiration of gastric contents, or activation of the systemic inflammatory response (see Chapter 3).

■ A large retrospective study in two U.S. level 1 trauma centers compared the results of patients with thoracic injuries who were treated by reamed intramedullary nailing or plating.

■ There was no difference in the incidence of ARDS, pneumonia, pulmonary embolus, multiple organ failure (MOF), or mortality, suggesting that nailing was not a significant problem.

■ More recently, surgeons have examined the phenomenon of the so-called second hit, a secondary increase in inflammatory markers such as interleukin-I, -6 and -8 and elastase caused by the surgery required to stabilize femoral fractures in the multiply injured patients.

■ Reamed and unreamed nailing definitely increase the levels of various inflammatory markers, and it is possible this may be important in the pathogenesis of ARDS and MOF (see Chapter 3).

■ Prospective studies have indicated that primary external fixation and secondary intramedullary nailing are not associated with the same increase in inflammatory markers.

■ This has introduced the concept of damage control surgery with a more rapid, less invasive initial stabilization of long-bone fractures followed by secondary definitive surgery when the condition of the patient has improved.

■ There is as yet little evidence that a rise in inflammatory markers is associated with an increased incidence of ARDS or MOF, however, and it should be remembered there have been major advances in the intensive care of polytraumatized patients in the last few years, which may account for improved results.

- The superficial attraction of damage control surgery needs to be balanced by the possibility that a number of patients may not be fit for secondary surgery for a significant period, and pin tract sepsis may then prevent secondary intramedullary nailing.
- Surgeons should use intramedullary nailing for femoral fractures in multiply injured patients where possible but use damage control techniques when the patients' condition makes intramedullary nailing hazardous.
- An algorithm for the management of severely injured patients is shown in Algorithm 3-1 in Chapter 3.

Adolescent Patients

- The use of intramedullary femoral nailing in adolescent patients with open proximal femoral physes has been studied in some detail.
- Most surgeons have demonstrated good results, but there are sporadic reports of avascular necrosis of the femoral head.
- The incidence is unknown, but the condition undoubtedly occurs.
- The cause is not known, but it seems likely avascular necrosis is due to damage to the medial circumflex artery near the piriformis fossa that vascularizes much of the femoral head.

Elderly Patients

- There is an increasing incidence of femoral diaphyseal fractures in the elderly.
- The osteopenic nature of elderly bone means the use of plates and external fixation is ill advised and intramedullary nailing provides the best fixation.
- Even with intramedullary nailing and early mobilization, however, the complication rate for elderly patients has been estimated between 46% and 54% and the mortality between 17% and 20%.
- Age and mental status are the main determinants of survival.
- Elderly patients frequently have osteoarthritic hip joints, making the antegrade approach difficult.
- There may be a fixed flexion or abduction deformity, and retrograde nailing is indicated in these patients, provided the knee can be adequately flexed.
- Despite these problems, intramedullary nailing remains the best treatment option in the elderly.

Pathological Fractures

- Intramedullary nailing is a good option in patients with metastatic femoral fractures because they can mobilize

fully weight bearing after treatment, and the stability of fixation is superior to other treatment methods.
- Many metastatic fractures are subtrochanteric in location (see Chapters 9 and 22), and if the lesser trochanter is intact, a conventional interlocking antegrade nail may be used.
- If the metastasis is above the lesser trochanter, a reconstruction nail with a screw placed into the femoral neck and head is required.
- Studies indicate that about 90% of the patients are mobile postoperatively, and pain is abolished or tolerable in 90% to 95% of patients.
- In many series, the mortality rate after nailing of metastatic femurs approaches 10%, with no difference observed between reamed and unreamed nails.

Gunshot Fractures

- The results of femoral fractures caused by gunshot injuries are shown in Table 23-8.
- This indicates that the results are good, despite an average of 6.3% Gustilo type IIIc fractures that require vascular reconstruction.
- The nonunion rate is low and the rate of infection only 0.5%.
- These results are mainly from low-velocity gunshot injuries, however.
- In high-velocity gunshot injuries, the results are much worse and the amputation rate is high.
- In war injuries, damage control surgery is practiced and primary external fixation is usually used.
- Definitive treatment can be undertaken at a later time.

Floating Knee

- Ipsilateral femoral and tibial fractures usually occur in polytraumatized patients in whom there may well be injuries in other body systems.
- It has been estimated that between 52% and 67% of such patients have major trauma to the head, trunk, or other extremities.
- It has also been recorded that 21% to 29% of patients have significant vascular damage.
- Up to 80% of the fractures may be open, and over 50% of patients have been recorded as having a ligamentous injury to the knee.
- Under these circumstances the surgeon may choose to use damage control surgery with primary external fixation and secondary intramedullary nailing.
  - Either one long external fixator spanning both fractures or two separate external fixators may be used.

TABLE 23-8 RESULTS OF INTRAMEDULLARY NAILING IN THE TREATMENT OF OPEN FEMORAL FRACTURES CAUSED BY GUNSHOT INJURIES[a]

Result/Complication	Range	Average
Gustilo IIIc fractures (%)	15–21.4	6.3
Union time (wk)	14–23.8	19.1
Nonunion (%)	0–16.7	3.1
Infection (%)	0–2.6	0.5

[a]All studies used antegrade nailing.

- The advantage of using one fixator is that the potentially damaged knee is also immobilized. This is recommended in the acute situation.
- If definitive surgery is undertaken, it is recommended that both fractures be treated by intramedullary nailing through a single incision.
- The femoral fracture is nailed using a retrograde technique, with antegrade nailing used for the tibial fracture.
- This technique has been shown to be associated with good results, although the morbidity and complications related to the tibial fracture in particular remain high.
- Early mobilization is allowed, and most patients regain good knee function.

Bilateral Femoral Fractures

- The published literature suggests that between 5.8% and 9.6% of patients with femoral fractures have bilateral fractures, the incidence varying with the type of institution.
- Patients with bilateral fractures tend to be seriously injured and have a high incidence of open fractures.
- Treatment of bilateral fractures is the same as for unilateral fractures, although the high incidence of head injury, abdominal injury, and pelvic fractures associated with these patients means the surgeon may elect to use primary external fixation and secondary nailing if the clinical state of the patient suggests this is necessary.
- Studies indicate that the clinical risks of nailing bilateral femoral fractures are very similar to the risks of nailing unilateral femoral fractures.

External Fixation

- The only major indication for the use of external fixation for the treatment of femoral diaphyseal fractures is in damage control surgery where an external fixator can be used primarily followed by secondary intramedullary nailing.
- The excellent results associated with intramedullary nailing for isolated femoral fractures means that external fixation, with its accompanying problems of muscle tethering, joint stiffness, malunion, and pin tract infection, is not indicated for definitive management.
- Conversion from external fixation to intramedullary nailing is usually straightforward, but nailing should not be undertaken in the presence of discharging pin tracts.
- Thus care should be exercised in inserting the external fixator pins so as to minimize the risk of later infection.

- The duration of external fixation ideally should be relatively short to reduce the incidence of pin tract infection, and a one-stage conversion should be undertaken where possible.
- Good results have been reported that compare favorably with the use of primary nailing.

Plating

- Plating was used extensively for the treatment of femoral fractures until intramedullary nailing became popular in the 1980s.
- Table 23-9 shows the results from published series.
- Implant failure or loosening and refracture are significant complications, although the incidences of nonunion and infection are comparatively low.
- These figures do not include the relatively high incidence of bone grafting that is required to obtain good results.
- Bone grafting is indicated in all patients with cortical defects, unstable fracture fixation, or devascularized bone fragments.
- The results of plating osteoporotic bone are also poor. Although the new locking screw plate (LCP) systems will probably improve the results in elderly patients, it is unlikely they will be as good as the results of intramedullary nailing.
- Femoral plating is particularly useful in the management of periprosthetic fractures (see Figs. 7-6 and 7-9 in Chapter 7) and can be used in the rare combination of proximal femoral and femoral diaphyseal fractures (Fig. 23-7).

Nonsurgical Management

- Nonoperative management is rarely undertaken nowadays if the option of surgical fixation is available.
- Prolonged bed rest and the use of cast braces resulted in a high incidence of malunion, nonunion, and knee stiffness as well as in medical and psychological problems.
- The method is also expensive and time consuming.
- It is difficult to analyze much of the older literature, but malunion rates approach 50%, and knee flexion of 90 degrees was considered good!

Ipsilateral Femoral Diaphyseal and Hip Fractures

- As with bilateral femoral fractures and floating knee injuries, patients who present with the combination of proximal femoral and femoral diaphyseal fractures are usually multiply injured.

TABLE 23-9 RESULTS OF PLATING FEMORAL DIAPHYSEAL FRACTURES

Result/Complication	Range (%)	Average (%)
Infection	0–10	4.0
Implant failure/loosening	5–13	8.5
Nonunion	2.2–15	6.1
Refracture	1.6–8.7	3.2

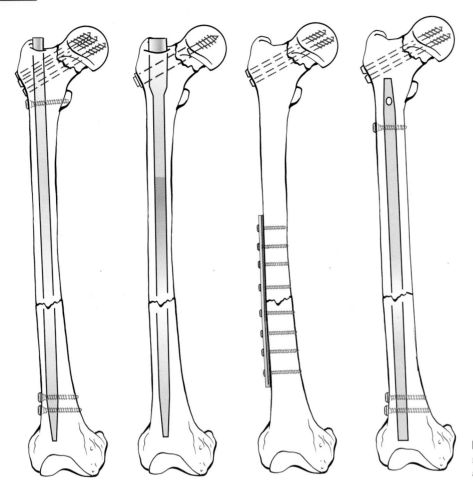

Figure 23-7 Different methods of management of combined femoral neck and diaphyseal fractures.

■ Up to 90% of patients have other musculoskeletal injuries.

■ The types of fracture, associated injuries, and complications are shown in Table 23-10.

■ On average, about 20% of proximal femoral fractures are missed.

■ Most fractures are subcapital in location, although the distribution of fractures varies among centers.

■ There is a high incidence of associated knee injury, particularly patellar fractures, and careful examination of the knee is essential.

■ Nowadays the outcome is usually good, although nonunion of either fracture or avascular necrosis of the femoral head may occur.

■ There are a number of treatment methods (Fig. 23-7; see Figs. 33-2 and 33-6 in Chapter 33). Most involve

TABLE 23-10 EPIDEMIOLOGY, ASSOCIATED INJURIES, AND RESULTS OF THE TREATMENT OF PROXIMAL FEMORAL AND FEMORAL DIAPHYSEAL FRACTURES

Result	Range (%)	Average (%)
Missed hip fracture	6–39	21
Subcapital fractures	31.2–100	68
Basicervical fractures	0–43.7	12.1
Intertrochanteric fractures	0–58	19.7
Ipsilateral knee damage	33.3–42.8	35.2
Patellar fracture	8.3–21.9	16.9
Proximal femoral nonunion	0–7.1	3.3
Diaphyseal nonunion	0–29.2	7.9
Avascular necrosis	0–13.3	1.3

TABLE 23-11 SUGGESTED TREATMENT OF FEMORAL DIAPHYSEAL FRACTURES

Injury	Treatment

Open and closed diaphyseal fractures.	Antegrade or retrograde nailing
	Antegrade
	  Proximal and middle third fractures
	Retrograde
	  Distal third fractures
	  Obese and pregnant patients
	  Patients with pelvic or acetabular fractures

Multiply injured	Consider primary external fixation and secondary intramedullary nailing in severely injured patients (see Table 3-4 in Chapter 3)
Pathological fractures	Antegrade nailing if lesser trochanter not involved. Reconstruction nailing if involved
Floating knee	Femoral and tibial nailing
Combined neck and diaphyseal fractures.	Retrograde nailing for diaphysis Cancellous screw fixation for femoral neck (see Figure 23-7)

antegrade or retrograde nailing, although the diaphyseal fracture can be plated.

■ Priority should be given to the femoral neck fracture, and it is recommended that this be treated with cancellous screws and a retrograde nail used for the diaphyseal fracture.

■ Antegrade nailing or reconstruction nailing can be used.

■ If an intertrochanteric fracture is present, either a reconstruction nail or a combination or a proximal hip screw and diaphyseal plate should be used.

Complications

■ With the advent of closed intramedullary nailing, complications following the management of femoral diaphyseal fractures are relatively unusual.

■ The common complications are aseptic nonunion, infection, bone loss, malunion, compartment syndrome, and knee stiffness.

■ The incidence of aseptic nonunion, infection, and malunion are given in this chapter and in the appropriate chapters dealing with complications.

■ About 7% of femoral diaphyseal fractures are Gustilo type IIIb or IIIc and associated with bone loss. The treatment of this condition is discussed in Chapter 39.

■ The incidence of thigh compartment syndrome is probably underestimated. The literature suggests an incidence of 1% to 1.4%, but the true incidence is probably higher.

■ The anterior compartment is always involved, and the condition should be diagnosed by using a pressure monitor placed into the anterior compartment.

■ Treatment is by fasciotomy.

■ Thigh compartment syndrome may be caused by a fracture but also by coagulopathy, vascular injury, or the use of military antishock trousers (MAST).

■ Thigh compartment syndrome is discussed in more detail in Chapter 38.

■ Knee stiffness is a particular problem with nonoperative management but can occur with any treatment method.

■ Physical therapy is usually sufficient treatment, but arthroscopic adhesion release, limited soft tissue release, or even quadricepsplasty may be required to restore adequate knee function.

Suggested Treatment

The suggested treatment of femoral diaphyseal fractures is given in Table 23-11.

SUGGESTED READING

Bone LB, Johnson KD, Weigelt J, et al. Early versus delayed stabilisation of femoral fractures. J Bone Joint Surg (Am) 1989;71:336–340.

Bosse MJ, MacKenzie EJ, Riemer BL, et al. Adult respiratory distress syndrome, pneumonia, and mortality following thoracic injury and a femoral fracture treated either with intramedullary nailing with reaming or with a plate. J Bone Joint Surg (Am) 1997;79:799–809.

Brumback RJ. Ellison TS, Poka A, et al. Intramedullary nailing of open fractures of the femoral shaft. J Bone Joint Surg (Am) 1989;71:1324–1330.

Christie J, Court-Brown C, Kinninmonth AWG, et al. Intramedullary locking nails in the management of femoral shaft fractures. J Bone Joint Surg (Br) 1988;70:206–210.

Clatworthy MG, Clark DI, Gray DH, et al. Reamed versus unreamed femoral nails. J Bone Joint Surg (Br) 1998;80:485–489.

Court-Brown CM. Femoral diaphyseal fractures. In: Browner BD, Jupiter JB, Levine AM, et al., eds. Skeletal trauma. Philadelphia: WB Saunders, 2003:1879–1956.

Giannoudis PV, Veysi VT, Pape HC, et al. When should we operate on major fractures in patients with severe head injuries? Am J Surg 2002;183:261–267.

Mileski RA, Garvin KL, Crosby LA. Avascular necrosis of the femoral head in an adolescent following intramedullary nailing of the femur. A case report. J Bone Joint Surg (Am) 1994;76:1706–1708.

Moed BR, Watson JT, Cramer KE, et al. Unreamed retrograde intramedullary nailing of the femoral shaft. J Orthop Trauma 1998; 12:334–342.

Müller ME, Nazarian S, Koch P, et al. The comprehensive classification of fractures of long bones. Berlin: Springer-Verlag, 1990.

Pape H-C, Hildebrand F, Pertschy S, et al. Changes in the management of femoral shaft fractures in polytrauma patients: from early total care to damage control orthopedic surgery. J Trauma 2002; 53:452–462.

DISTAL FEMORAL FRACTURES

Distal femoral fractures have always been difficult to treat. They often occur in older patients with osteopenic bone, and fixation is difficult. Surgeons traditionally have relied on a number of different plating systems, although in recent years retrograde femoral nailing has become popular. The introduction of locked plates is likely to improve the treatment of this difficult fracture. A list of current controversies associated with the treatment of distal femoral fractures is shown in Box 24-1.

SURGICAL ANATOMY

The lower end of the femur expands to form the medial and lateral condyles separated posteriorly by the intercondylar notch and united anterosuperiorly by the concave articular facet for the patella. The lateral and medial epicondyles give attachments to the medial and lateral ligaments of the knee. The anterior cruciate ligament attaches to the posterior part of the medial surface of the lateral condyle, and the posterior cruciate ligament attaches to the anterior portion of the lateral surface of the medial condyle. There are no muscle attachments anteriorly, but the vastus lateralis and medialis muscles arise posteriorly. The vasti insert into the upper border of the patella overlying the anterior aspect of the distal femur. Adductor magnus inserts posteriorly, and the two heads of gastrocnemius arise from the posterior aspects of the medial and lateral femoral condyles. The popliteal artery and vein run through the popliteal fossa, which also contains the tibial

nerve. The common peroneal nerve, the other terminal branch of the sciatic nerve, arises just above the popliteal fossa and descends along the lateral border of the fossa. It runs over the lateral head of gastrocnemius and around the neck of the fibula before it divides into the superficial and deep peroneal nerves. A cross section of the lower femur is shown in Figure 24-1.

CLASSIFICATION

As with other fractures of the femur, a number of different classifications have been developed for distal femoral fractures. The most popular classification in common use is

BOX 24-1 CURRENT CONTROVERSIES IN THE TREATMENT OF DISTAL FEMORAL FRACTURES

Is the epidemiology of distal femoral fractures changing?
Which plates should be used?
Is the LISS system useful?
Is antegrade or retrograde nailing better?
How useful is external fixation?
Should knee arthroplasty ever be used?

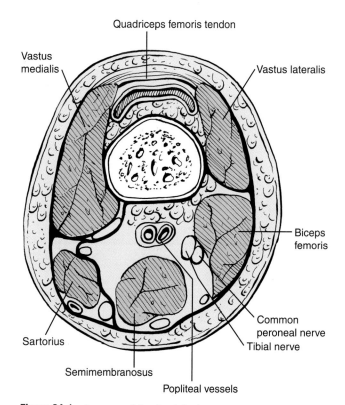

Figure 24-1 Anatomy of the distal thigh.

303

the OTA (AO) classification, which divides distal femoral fractures into 27 subgroups based on the direction of the fracture line, the involvement of the articular surface, and the degree of comminution (Fig. 24-2). Type A fractures are extra-articular including simple fracture patterns (A1), wedge fractures (A2), and metaphyseal comminution (A3). Type B fractures are partial articular fractures involving the lateral condyle (B1) or medial condyle (B2) in the sagittal plane or partial articular fractures in the frontal plane (B3). Type C fractures are severe articular fractures with a simple articular and metaphyseal morphology (C1), a simple articular morphology and metaphyseal comminution (C2), or severe articular comminution (C3). The suffixes 0.1 to 0.3 refer to the position of the fracture and the degree of comminution.

EPIDEMIOLOGY

Surgeons often assume that the distal femoral fracture has a bimodal distribution affecting young men and older women. The change in fracture epidemiology associated with an increasingly elderly population, however, means the distal femoral fractures now have a type E distribution (see Chapter 1). Despite this, surgeons working in level 1 trauma centers see a significant number of younger patients with high-energy fractures. As with subtrochanteric fractures, it is likely that the incidence of distal femoral fractures in the elderly is increasing rapidly, and Table 24-1 shows the average age is now 61 years.

The most common cause of distal femoral fractures in the elderly is a simple fall, and the average age of the group

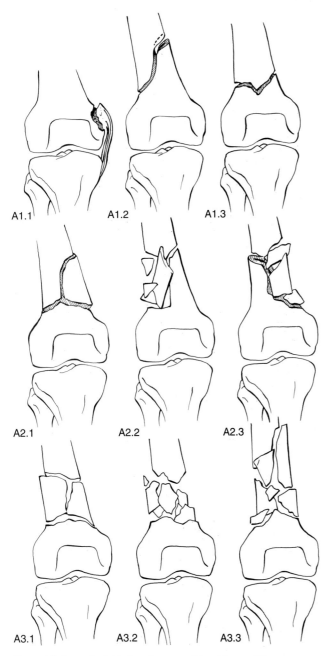

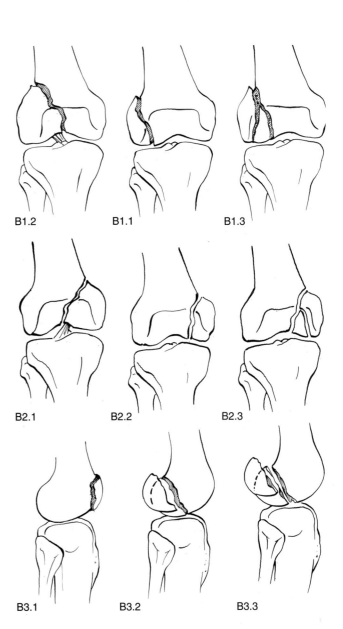

Figure 24-2 OTA (AO) classification of distal femoral fractures.

injured in this way is 77.8 years. Motor vehicle accidents and falls from a height are the common causes of these fractures in younger patients, with gunshot injuries also causing distal femoral fractures in a number of countries. The epidemiology of the different causes of these fractures is shown in Table 24-2. There is a higher incidence of OTA (AO) type C fractures in young patients following motor vehicle accidents than in the older group in which type A fractures usually follow a fall.

Associated Injuries

In older patients distal femoral fractures are usually isolated, but in younger patients there may be a number of associated injuries. The literature suggests that up to 60% of

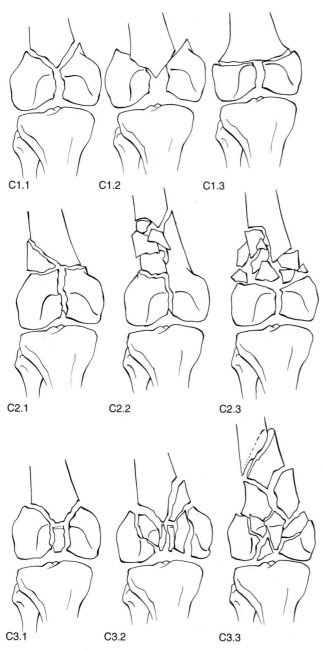

C1.1   C1.2   C1.3

C2.1   C2.2   C2.3

C3.1   C3.2   C3.3

Figure 24-2 *(continued)*

TABLE 24-1 EPIDEMIOLOGY OF DISTAL FEMORAL FRACTURES	
Proportion of all fractures	0.4%
Average age	61.0 y
Men/women	33%/67%
Distribution	Type E
Incidence	$0.2/10^5/y$
Open fractures	8.3%
Most common causes	
Fall	41.7%
Motor vehicle accident	16.7%
Height	8.3%
OTA (AO) classification	
Type A	50%
Type B	16.7%
Type C	33.3%
Most common subgroups	
C1.1	20.8%
A1.2	16.7%
A1.1	12.5%

younger patients may be multiply injured, presenting with head, abdominal, craniofacial, or chest injuries and other extremity fractures. There may be an ipsilateral hip dislocation or fracture dislocation, particularly following a motor vehicle accident when the flexed knee has struck the dashboard. There is also a relatively high incidence of other fractures in the ipsilateral leg, including fractures of the femoral and tibial diaphyses, proximal femoral fractures, and fractures of the tibial plateau. About 38% of high-energy distal femoral fractures are open, and an estimated 20% are associated with significant ligamentous injury to the ipsilateral knee.

DIAGNOSIS

History and Physical Examination

- The clinical history is usually that of a high-energy injury in younger patients and a simple fall in older patients.
    - Thus a careful history of the mode of injury in younger patients is important, bearing in mind the possibility of other injuries.
- In young patients with high-energy injuries, a thorough examination according to ATLS principles is essential.
- In older patients the history must include a careful evaluation of any medical comorbidities and an assessment of the patient's home circumstances or domicile.
- Examination usually shows a deformed, swollen distal femur.
- Care must be used in looking for an open wound, and a thorough examination of the vascular and neurological status of the limb must be undertaken.
- Unlike knee dislocation, vascular injury associated with distal femoral fractures is relatively uncommon but may follow motor vehicle accidents or gunshot wounds.

TABLE 24-2 EPIDEMIOLOGY OF DISTAL FEMORAL FRACTURE ACCORDING TO MODE OF INJURY

Cause	Age (y)	Open (%)	OTA (AO) Type (%)		
			Type A	Type B	Type C
Fall	77.8	0	70	0	30
Motor vehicle accident	41.7	25	0	25	75
Fall from height	36.0	50.0	0	0	100
Sport	17.5	0	0	100	0

Radiologic Examination

- As with most fractures, anteroposterior and lateral radiographs are usually sufficient to diagnose a distal femoral fracture (Fig. 24-3).
- CT scans may help if there is doubt about intra-articular involvement.
    - This may be important if retrograde nailing is proposed.
- CT scans may also show any associated chondral damage.
- It is mandatory to obtain good radiographs of the pelvis and proximal femur as well as of the femoral diaphysis in view of the incidence of ipsilateral fractures of the thigh and pelvis.
- Angiography or Doppler studies may be required to assess vascular damage, and a later MRI scan of the knee may be required if there is evidence of ligamentous injury.

TREATMENT

Surgical Treatment

The treatment of distal femoral fractures has changed in the last 10 to 15 years with the advent of retrograde nailing of the femur. Prior to the introduction of this technique, most distal femoral fractures were treated by internal fixation with a plate, but retrograde nailing improved the management of these fractures, particularly in the elderly where the osteoporotic nature of the bone means that successful plate fixation is more difficult. In the last few years, however, the introduction of the locking compression plate (LCP) and minimally invasive percutaneous plate osteosynthesis (MIPPO) has improved the usefulness of plate fixation, and it is likely the next 5 years will define whether modern plating techniques or retrograde intramedullary nailing is the best method of management for distal femoral fractures.

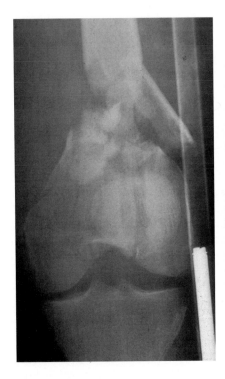
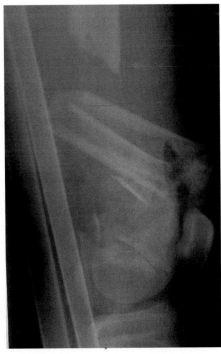

Figure 24-3 A-P and lateral radiographs of a distal femoral (C3.3) fracture.

TABLE 24-3 RESULTS OF THE USE OF THE 95-DEGREE BLADE PLATE

Result/Complication	Range	Average
Union time (wk)	12.5–13.6	13.5
Excellent/good (%)	52–100	70
Nonunion (%)	0–7.1	3.1
Malunion (%)	6.6–40	9.1
Infection (%)	0–4.7	2.3
Knee flexion (degree)	107–124	108

TABLE 24-5 RESULTS OF THE USE OF THE LISS PLATE

Result/Complication	Range	Average
Union time (wk)	11–14.3	12.4
Excellent/good (%)	74	74
Nonunion (%)	0–7.7	5.3
Infection (%)	3–3.4	3.2
Malunion (%)	4.3–19.8	14.7
Implant failure (%)	0–1.7	1.1
Knee flexion (degree)	103–104	103

Plating

- Plating remains a good method of treating distal femoral fractures of all types.
- Four basic plate types are used internally to fix supracondylar or intercondylar femoral fractures: the 95-degree blade plate, the 95-degree dynamic condylar screw plate, the condylar buttress plate, and the LISS plate, which incorporates LCP technology and a MIPPO approach.
- Plating is the treatment of choice for type B partial articular fractures.
  - These can be fixed with intrafragmentary screws, but it is advisable to supplement with a neutralization plate.
  - This can be a T-plate, blade plate, or dynamic condylar screw plate.
- Type A extra-articular fractures are relatively easy to plate, and type C complete articular fractures can be treated by intrafragmentary screw fixation and either a blade plate, dynamic condylar screw plate, or a LISS plate.
- Tables 24-3 to 24-5 suggest the results of the three plates are very similar, but the use of the LISS system is associated with less bone grafting than the two earlier plates, and it is likely that it will be more useful in osteoporotic distal femoral fractures.

95-Degree Blade Plate

- A 95-degree blade plate is a fixed angle neutralization plate that was designed for distal femoral fractures (Fig. 24-4).

- It is a relatively difficult implant to use because of the fixed angle and because the blade must be inserted correctly in all three planes simultaneously.
- It can be used for type A, B, and C distal femoral fractures, although it is more commonly used for type A extra-articular and type C complete articular fractures.
- The results of the use of blade plates in the distal femur are given in Table 24-3.
- This indicates a relatively high incidence of malunion because of the difficulty of plate insertion.
- Otherwise the results are good and comparable with other techniques, although it should be noted that the percentage of excellent and good results is less than for both antegrade and retrograde intramedullary nailing (Tables 24-6 and 24-7).

95-Degree Dynamic Condylar Screw Plate

- The dynamic condylar screw plate is a two-piece system consisting of a large cancellous screw and a 95-degree side plate (Fig. 24-5).
- The two-piece nature of the implant makes it easier to insert than a blade plate.
- The results of using the 95-degree dynamic condylar screw plate are given in Table 24-4.
- When compared with blade plating (Table 24-3), the only major difference is the incidence of malunion, highlighting the relative difficulty of insertion of the blade plate.
- Otherwise the clinical results are very similar.

TABLE 24-4 RESULTS OF THE USE OF THE 95-DEGREE DYNAMIC CONDYLAR SCREW PLATE

Result/Complication	Range	Average
Union time (wk)	11.3–18.6	15.3
Excellent/good (%)	75	75
Nonunion (%)	0–9.5	2.8
Malunion (%)	0–7.7	2.8
Infection (%)	0–4.3	1.4
Knee flexion (degree)	112–120	116

TABLE 24-6 RESULTS OF ANTEGRADE FEMORAL NAILING FOR DISTAL FEMORAL FRACTURES

Result/Complication	Range	Average
Union time (wk)	12–17.3	13.9
Excellent/good (%)	76–94	86
Nonunion (%)	0–5	3.4
Malunion (%)	10.9–12.1	11.7
Infection (%)	0–4.2	1.4
Implant failure (%)	0–4.2	1.9

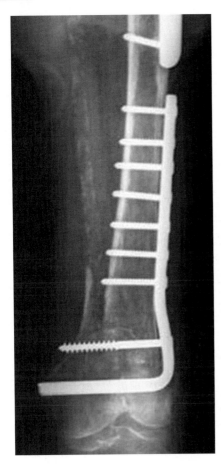

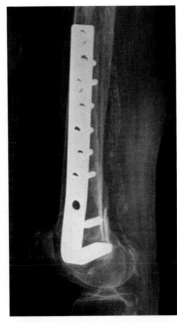

Figure 24-4 A-P and lateral radiographs of a distal femoral (A2.3) fracture treated with a 95-degree blade plate.

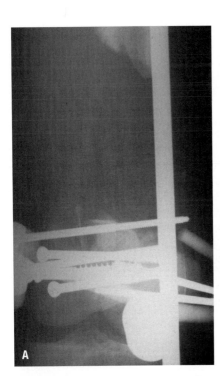

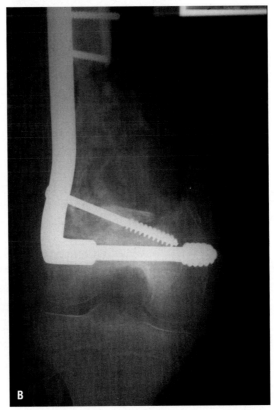

Figure 24-5 (A) The fracture shown in Figure 24-3 was initially treated with interfragmentary screw fixation and a temporary external fixator. (B) After 6 weeks a 95-degree dynamic condylar screw (DCS) was used together with allograft and autograft.

TABLE 24-7 RESULTS OF RETROGRADE FEMORAL NAILING FOR DISTAL FEMORAL FRACTURES

Result/Complication	Range	Average
Union time (wk)	13–15.6	14.1
Excellent/good (%)	85–94	88
Nonunion (%)	0–9.7	5.8
Malunion (%)	0–12.5	6.2
Infection (%)	0–3.2	1.2
Knee flexion (%)	90–130	101

Condylar Buttress Plate

■ The condylar buttress plate is a broad plate with a cloverleaf distal portion designed for the lateral aspect of the distal femur.

■ Fixation is gained by using cortical screws proximally and cancellous screws distally.

■ Supplementary interfragmentary screws may be used to fix a intercondylar fracture.

■ The implant is relatively easy to use and theoretically advantageous in that the angle of the distal cancellous screws can be altered according to the fracture morphology.

■ Several cancellous screws can be inserted to increase fracture stability.

■ Evidence indicates the implant is useful in nonunions of the distal femur, but when used to treat fresh fractures, studies have shown a high incidence of varus collapse, particularly in comminuted distal femoral fractures.

■ The varus malalignment is associated with a relatively high incidence of nonunion and knee arthrosis.

■ The results of the use of this implant do not appear to be as good as those of other plates.

LISS Plate

■ The latest plate to be introduced for the treatment of distal femoral fractures is the LISS (less invasive stabilization system) plate (Fig. 24-6).

■ This is a plate designed to be applied to the lateral aspect of the distal femur.

■ It is a locking compression plate with the screws locking into the plate.

■ Unicortical screws can be used, although bicortical screws are preferred in osteoporotic bone.

■ The plate is designed to be used with a minimally invasive percutaneous (MIPPO) technique, although an open technique can be used.

■ A small incision is made distally, and the plate and screws are inserted under fluoroscopic control.

■ Reduction is gained using indirect techniques.

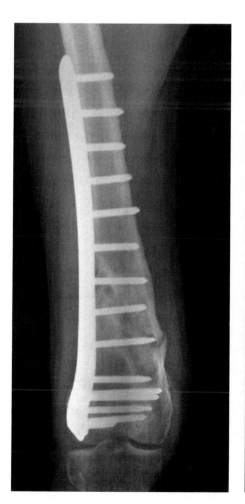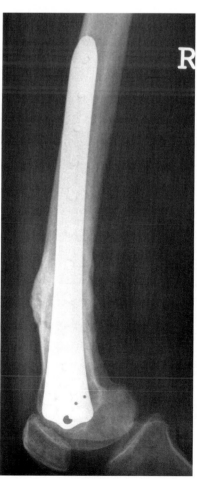

Figure 24-6 A-P and lateral radiographs of a LISS plate used to treat an A1.2 Gustilo IIIb open fracture in an 83-year-old woman.

- The results for the LISS plate are given in Table 24-5.
- The technique is considerably more difficult than the open technique used for the 95-degree blade plate and the 95-degree dynamic condylar screw plate, which probably accounts for the higher incidence of malunion.
  - Otherwise the results are very similar to the two earlier plates.
- One advantage of the LISS plate over the earlier plates is that only about 5% of the patients require bone grafting.

Intramedullary Nailing

- As with femoral diaphyseal fractures, both antegrade and retrograde nailing (Fig. 24-7) can be used to treat distal femoral fractures.
- The techniques and complications of both methods are discussed in Chapter 33.
- Antegrade nailing is most useful for type A supracondylar fractures, although it can be used for type C fractures that are not associated with significant comminution, the articular surface being reconstructed with intrafragmentary screws.
- Retrograde nailing is also easier to perform in type A fractures but can be used for type C fractures.
- If nailing is undertaken in type C fractures, care must be taken to position the interfragmentary screws in the femoral condyles so they do not interfere with the passage of the antegrade or retrograde nail.
- The results of antegrade and retrograde nailing of distal femoral fractures are given in Tables 24-6 and 24-7.

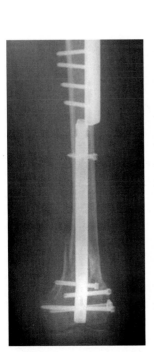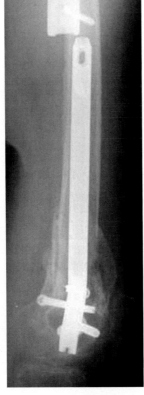

Figure 24-7   A-P and lateral radiographs of a retrograde nail used to treat an A3.3 distal femoral fracture.

- The results are very similar, although there is a higher malunion rate with antegrade nailing, indicating the difficulty of maintaining a good reduction if the fracture is very distal to the nail entry point.
- The proportion of excellent and good results is significantly higher than achieved with a plating system.
- Comparative studies of open and percutaneously inserted retrograde nails have shown better results with percutaneous nailing in the same way that indirect reduction techniques improved the results of plating of distal femoral fractures.
- Retrograde nailing is particularly useful for the treatment of periprosthetic fractures above a knee prosthesis.
- The treatment of these fractures is discussed in Chapter 7.
- If the design of the femoral component permits the passage of a retrograde nail, biomechanical studies have shown that a nail produces greater stability than a LISS plate, although good results can be obtained with a LISS plate (see Fig. 7-9 in Chapter 7).

External Fixation

- A few studies have investigated the role of external fixation in the treatment of distal femoral factures.
- The technique has been mainly used in younger patients and has the theoretical advantage of indirect fracture reduction, closed treatment, and speed of application.
- Pin tract sepsis and muscle tethering are particular problems, however.
- The results of external fixation in the management of distal femoral fractures are detailed in Table 24-8, which shows fewer excellent and good results compared with intramedullary nailing.
- Pin tract sepsis is clearly a problem, but it is rare for pin tract sepsis to cause osteomyelitis, although septic arthritis of the knee has been described.
- The results detailed in Table 24-8 suggest that external fixation should not be used as definitive primary management for distal femoral fractures, although it undoubtedly has a place in the management of the severely injured patient.
- In damage control surgery, primary external fixation can be undertaken with definitive secondary internal fixation carried out once the patient's condition improves.
- External fixation is particularly useful in wartime where damage control surgery is important.

TABLE 24-8 RESULTS FOR EXTERNAL SKELETAL FIXATION IN DISTAL FEMORAL FRACTURES

Result/Complication	Range	Average
Union time (wk)	11–16	13.3
Excellent/good (%)	64–71	68
Nonunion (%)	0–6.2	3.0
Malunion (%)	0–14.3	6.4
Infection (%)	0–7.1	3.2
Pin tract sepsis (%)	21–41	32

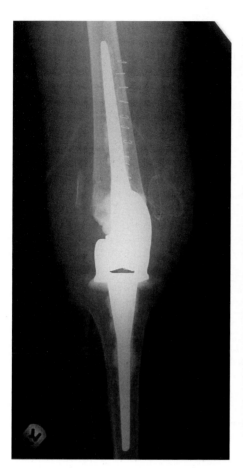
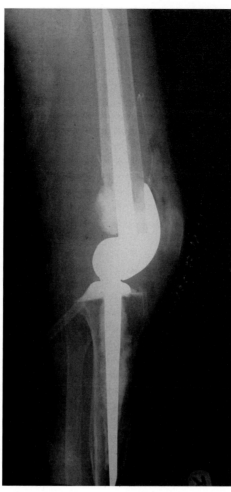

Figure 24-8 A-P and lateral radiographs of a hinged knee prosthesis used to treat a distal femoral fracture in an 86-year-old woman.

Knee Arthroplasty

- There are a number of case reports of the use of constrained knee arthroplasties for the primary treatment of supracondylar or intercondylar femoral fractures in the very elderly.
- Given the increasing incidence of these fractures in the very elderly and the relative difficulty of treating them, it seems likely that knee arthroplasty will be used more frequently in the future.
- Patients in this age group frequently have advanced osteoarthritis or rheumatoid arthritis, and the used of a prosthesis seems reasonable.
- In a larger study, 13 patients with an average age of 84 years were treated with a hinged knee arthroplasty (Fig. 24-8).
- All had type A or type C fractures.
- There were no infections or evidence of loosening after 6 months.
- Eleven patients returned to their original level of independence in the community within 12 weeks of surgery.
- Only one patient required revision surgery after 5 years.
- Arthroplasty would seem to be a good method of treatment for the very elderly, particularly if the knees are already osteoarthritic.

Nonsurgical Management

- Nonoperative management of distal femoral fractures is now rarely used if the facilities for surgical treatment exist.
- Comparative studies of operative and nonoperative treatment have all favored surgery.
- The best results for nonoperative management listed in the literature shows 67% excellent or good results, with a 9% delayed or nonunion rate.
- Better results were achieved with supracondylar rather than intercondylar fractures and where there was only minimal displacement.
- Nowadays nonoperative treatment should be reserved for the rare insufficiency fracture of the distal femur or for the occasional undisplaced fracture in the very elderly or infirm.

Suggested Treatment

The suggested treatment of distal femoral fractures is shown in Table 24-9.

TABLE 24-9 SUGGESTED TREATMENT OF DISTAL FEMORAL FRACTURES

Injury/Condition	Treatment
Type A supracondylar fracture	DCS, or LISS plating, or retrograde nailing
Type B partial articular fracture	Interfragmentary screws. with a neutralization DCS, T-plate, or LISS plate
Type C fracture	DCS or LISS plate
Very elderly and infirm	As above but consider hinged arthroplasty in low type A and type C fractures
Multiply injured	Consider temporary external fixation (see Chapter 3)
Periprosthetic fractures	Retrograde nail or LISS plate

COMPLICATIONS

- The incidences of nonunion, malunion, and infection for the different treatment methods are listed in Tables 24-3 to 24-8.
- The complications of plating, intramedullary nailing, external fixation, and nonoperative treatment are given in the appropriate chapters.
- Because the majority of distal femoral fractures occur in osteopenic or osteoporotic bone, nonunion may be caused by failure of fixation.
- Nonunions in this location are usually atrophic and should be treated by refixation, usually with an intramedullary nail supplemented by bone grafting.

SUGGESTED READING

Bell KM, Johnstone AJ, Court-Brown CM. Primary knee arthroplasty for distal femoral fractures in elderly patients. J Bone Joint Surg (Br) 1992;74:400–402.

Bolhofner BR, Carmen B, Clifford PH. The results of open reduction and internal fixation of distal femur fractures using a biologic (indirect) reduction technique J Orthop Trauma 1996;10: 372–377.

Butt MS, Krikler SR, Ali MS. Displaced fractures of the distal femur in elderly patients. J Bone Joint Surg (Br) 1996;77:110–114.

Dunlop DG, Brenkel IJ. The supracondylar intramedullary nail in elderly patients with distal femoral fracture. Injury 1999;30: 475–484.

Krettek C, Helfet, D. Fractures of the distal femur. In: Browner BD, Jupiter JB, Levine AM, et al., eds. Skeletal trauma. Philadelphia: WB Saunders, 2003:1957–2011.

Müller ME, Nazarian S, Koch P, et al. The comprehensive classification of fractures of long bones. Berlin: Springer-Verlag, 1990.

Rademakers MV, Kerkhoffs GM, Sierevely IN, et al. J Orthop Trauma 2004;18:213–219.

Ricci AR, Yue JJ, Taffet R, et al. Less invasive stabilisation system for treatment of distal femur fractures. Am J Orthop 2004;33:250–255.

PATELLA FRACTURES

There has been little progress in the treatment of patellar fractures over the last 30 years in that the use of K-wires and tension banding remains the most popular method of management. Until relatively recently, patellectomy was commonly performed, and a substantial body of surgeons believed this procedure was not only benign, but even beneficial for knee function. This is no longer the case, and open reduction and internal fixation is the preferred treatment method when possible. A number of areas of controversy are listed in Box 25-1.

SURGICAL ANATOMY

The patella is the largest sesamoid bone in the body. It increases the moment arm of the extensor mechanism, thereby facilitating knee extension. It contributes the extra 60% of torque needed to gain the last 15 degrees of knee extension.

The quadriceps mechanism is composed of four muscles: rectus femoris, vastus medialis, vastus lateralis, and vastus intermedius. All four muscles insert onto the proximal patella, with rectus femoris the most superficial and vastus intermedius the deepest. The patellar tendon arises mainly from fibers of the rectus femoris and inserts into the tibial tuberosity. The blood supply of the patella is derived from the geniculate arteries.

On the undersurface of the patellar are two facets that articulate with the distal femur. These vary in size but never occupy the whole of the undersurface (Fig. 25-1). Much of the patella is, in fact, extra-articular, which is why the relatively common distal pole avulsion fracture is generally benign and partial patellectomy can give good results.

BOX 25-1 CONTROVERSIES IN THE TREATMENT OF PATELLAR FRACTURES

Should undisplaced fractures be internally fixed?
What are the indications for partial patellectomy?
Should total patellectomy be performed?

PATELLAR DISLOCATION

Patellar dislocations usually occur in adolescents or young adults and often follow low-energy injuries. They are caused by a rotational injury with simultaneous contraction of the quadriceps. They are almost invariably lateral, although horizontal and superior dislocations have been described. Lateral dislocations are associated with a tear of the medial retinaculum, and about 5% have associated osteochondral fractures. A number of predisposing structural abnormalities can increase the likelihood of lateral patellar dislocation. These are listed in Box 25-2.

Patients present with a lateral swelling, hemarthrosis, and an inability to move the knee. The dislocation may have spontaneously relocated, and the patient may present with a significant knee effusion and tenderness over the medial retinaculum. Anteroposterior, lateral, and axial radiographs (Fig. 25-2) confirm the diagnosis and may show the presence of an osteochondral fracture.

Treatment is by aspiration of the hemarthrosis, which may show fat globules if an osteochondral fracture is present. An extension cast or brace is applied for 3 to 6 weeks. There is no evidence that soft tissue repair of the medial retinaculum is beneficial. If an osteochondral fracture is suspected, arthroscopic repair or excision is undertaken.

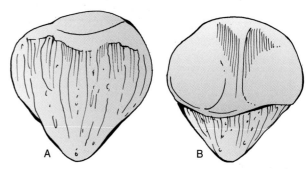

Figure 25-1 Anatomy of the patella. **(A)** Superior surface. **(B)** Inferior surface. Much of the inferior pole of the patella is extra-articular.

The most common complication is recurrent dislocation, which is usually seen in patients less than 20 years of age and may require surgery to stabilize the patella.

PATELLAR FRACTURES

CLASSIFICATION

There is no good classification of patella fractures. The early classifications were merely descriptive, and it could be argued that the OTA (AO) classification is overcomplicated. It does include all fractures types, however, and is shown in Figure 25-3. It follows the usual OTA (AO) classification

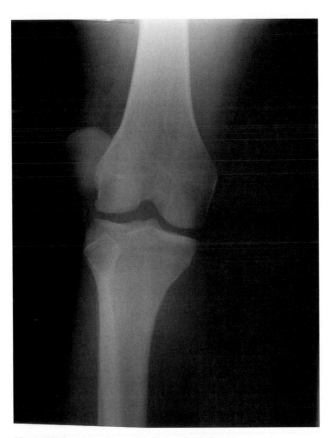

Figure 25-2   A-P radiograph of a patella dislocation.

with type A fractures extra-articular, type B partial articular, and type C complete articular fractures. There are two type A groups, with A1 fractures extra-articular avulsion fractures and A2 extra-articular body fractures. There are no A1 subgroups, and A2 fractures are divided into simple fractures (.1) and multifragmentary fractures (.2). The type B partial articular fractures are vertical fractures, with B1 fractures in the lateral part of the patella and B2 fractures in the medial patella. Simple fractures are again .1, and multifragmentary fractures are .2. B3 fractures are extra-articular stellate fractures.

Type C fractures are either transverse or complex. Simple transverse fractures are C1, divided into .1 to .3 by the location of the transverse fracture. Fractures of the middle of the patella are labeled .1, proximal fractures are .2, and distal fractures are .3. C2 fractures are transverse fractures with a third fragment. The suffixes .1 to .3 are used in the same way as for C1 fractures. C3 fractures are multifragmentary fractures with .1 denoting three fragments, .2 more than three fragments, and .3 unreconstructable.

EPIDEMIOLOGY

The basic epidemiology of patellar fractures is shown in Table 25-1. They usually occur in older patients and are caused by low-energy injuries. Open fractures are rare, but when they occur they are usually severe and may be associated with distal femoral or proximal tibial fractures (Fig. 25-4). About 25% of fractures are extra-articular, with type B vertical fractures less common. In the type C fractures, 47% are simple transverse fractures, 23.5% are complex transverse fractures, and 17.2% are multifragmentary.

Table 25-2 shows the causes of patellar fractures. Most are caused by falls in elderly patients. Type C fractures either occur in osteopenic bone after a low-energy injury or in younger patients after severe falls or motor vehicle accidents.

TABLE 25-1 EPIDEMIOLOGY OF PATELLAR FRACTURES

Proportion of all fractures	1.0%
Average age	56.5 y
Men/women	44%/56%
Distribution	Type F
Incidence	$10.7/10^5$/y
Open	3.5%
Most common causes	
Fall	71.9%
Fall from height	14.0%
Fall down stairs	7.0%
OTA (AO) classification	
Type A	24.6%
Type B	19.3%
Type C	56.1%
Most common subgroups	
A1	21.0%
C1.1	17.5%
C3.3	14.0%
B1.1	14.0%

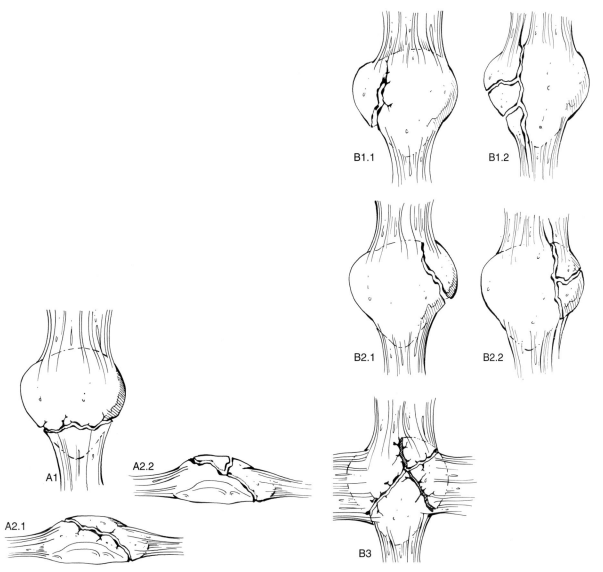

Figure 25-3 The OTA (AO) classification of fractures of the patella. *(continued)*

Associated Injuries

Most patellar fractures are isolated, but in high-energy injuries they may be associated with fractures to the ipsilateral femur or hip joint in particular. They may also be associated with a posterior hip dislocation or acetabular fracture, particularly if they occur in motor vehicle accidents. Occasionally a distal radial fracture may be caused by the same fall.

DIAGNOSIS

History and Physical Examination

■ Because most patellar fractures are isolated, the most common presentation is with a painful swollen knee associated with impaired or absent extension.

TABLE 25-2 EPIDEMIOLOGY OF PATELLA FRACTURES ACCORDING TO MODE OF INJURY

			OTA (AO) Type		
Cause	Age (y)	Open (%)	A	B	C
Fall	63.0	2.4	21.9	19.5	58.5
Fall from height	38.2	12.5	25.0	25.0	50.0
Fall down stairs	47.2	0	25.0	0	75.0

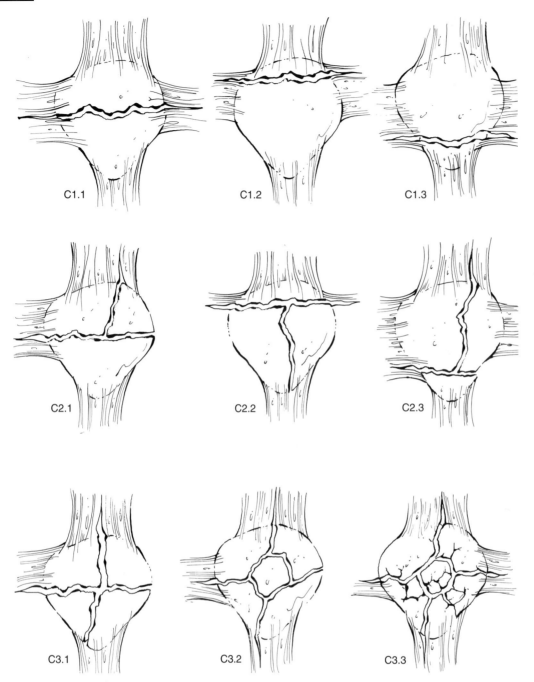

Figure 25-3 *(continued)*

■ In motor vehicle accidents or other high-energy injuries, a thorough examination according to ATLS principles must be undertaken and the ipsilateral femur and hip carefully examined.

■ Neurovascular injuries are very uncommon.

Radiologic Examination

■ Anteroposterior and lateral radiographs are sufficient to diagnose patellar fractures (Fig. 25-5), but care

must be taken to avoid diagnosing a bipartite patella as a fracture.

■ The condition is usually bilateral, and the other knee should be X-rayed if a bipartite patella is suspected.

■ CT scans and MRI scans are not required to diagnose patellar fractures, although an MRI scan or ultrasound may be useful to diagnose soft tissue injuries to the extensor mechanism.

■ An MRI scan may be used later if the patient complains of late pain and there is suspicion of chondral damage to the patella or distal femur.

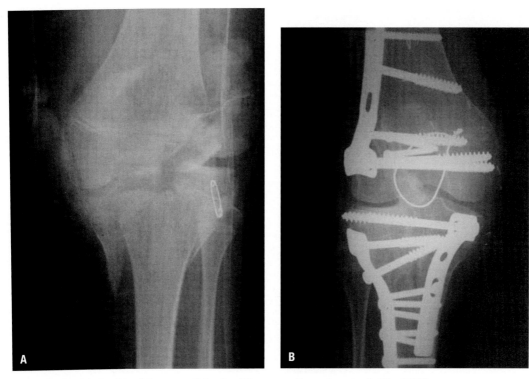

Figure 25-4   (A) Combined fractures of the distal femur, patella, and proximal tibia. (B) These were internally fixed, although patellar comminution meant a cerclage wire was all that could be used.

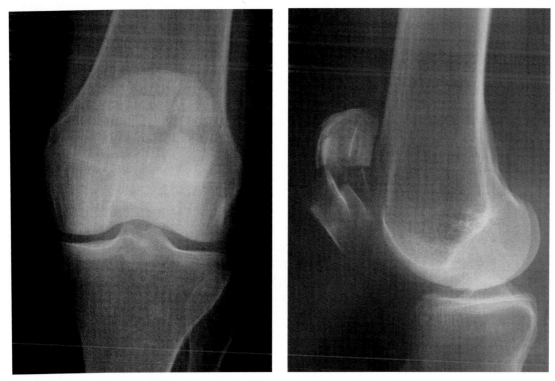

Figure 25-5   A-P and lateral radiographs of a (C2.1) fracture of the patella.

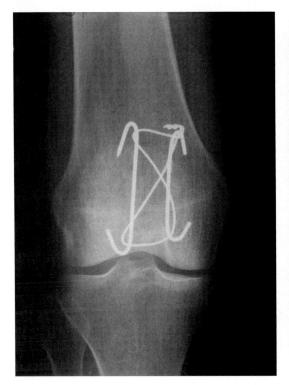
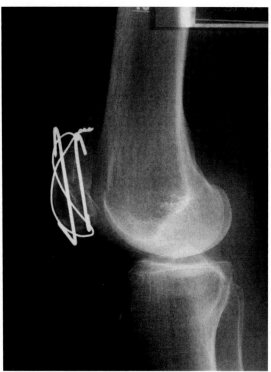

Figure 25-6   A-P and lateral radiographs of a patellar fracture fixed with K-wires and tension band wiring.

TREATMENT

■ There are four basic methods of treating patellar fractures: nonoperative, open reduction and internal fixation, partial patellectomy, and total patellectomy.

Nonsurgical Treatment

■ There is very little information in the current literature about the success of nonoperative management.

■ Results in the older literature cannot be successfully extrapolated because nonoperative management was not infrequently used for displaced fractures that nowadays would be treated operatively.
  ■ The implication is that undisplaced fractures treated nonoperatively do very well, and all surgeons accept that undisplaced fractures should be treated in a cast or brace for 6 to 8 weeks.

■ Weight bearing is allowed.

■ If nonoperative management is chosen, careful follow-up is essential because displacement of transverse and comminuted fractures may occur and secondary surgery becomes necessary.

Surgical Treatment

■ The literature clearly shows that if operative treatment is to be undertaken it should confer rigid fixation.
  ■ Nonrigid fixation is associated with poorer results.

■ The use of intraosseous suturing or tapes to secure fragments is associated with a higher incidence of nonunion.

■ Circumferential wiring without transosseous K-wires or screws is also associated with poorer results.

■ Surgical treatment should be undertaken using a tension band technique combined with either K-wires (Fig. 25-6) or cannulated screws (Fig. 25-7) to provide axillary fixation.

■ The use of intrafragmentary screws without a supplementary tension band wire should be restricted to the management of vertical (type B) fractures.

■ The results of tension band wiring using either K-wires or cannulated screws are shown in Table 25-3.
  ■ Overall the results are good with low complication rates except for the incidence of osteoarthritis, although the literature indicates that few patients get

TABLE 25-3 RESULTS OF THE USE OF TENSION BAND WIRING WITH K-WIRES OR CANNULATED SCREWS

Result/Complication	Range (%)	Average (%)
Excellent/good	50–85.7	71.7
Infection	0–2	<1
Septic arthritis	0–2	<1
Nonunion	0–2	<1
Loss of reduction	0–7.8	5.2
Hardware removal	0–65.7	42.5
Osteoarthritis	0–32.1	21.2

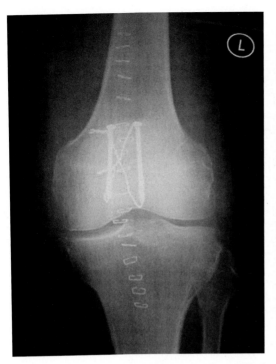
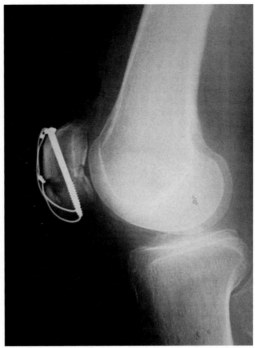

Figure 25-7 A-P and lateral radiographs of a patellar fracture fixed with cannulated screws and tension band wiring.

severe osteoarthritis and very few require patellectomy or other treatment because of symptomatic osteoarthritis.

- The older literature indicates a significant loss of quadriceps power in about 35% of patients, but Table 25-1 indicates these patients are usually older, and it seems unlikely this is a significant problem.

■ The most troublesome complication is discomfort from the hardware, and over 40% of patients require their hardware removed.

■ If adequate rigid fixation of the patellar fracture is achieved, early mobilization is allowed with graduated exercises undertaken.

■ If the fixation is felt to be inadequate, the patient should be placed in a supportive cast or brace for 3 to 4 weeks to allow union to commence prior to starting mobilization. This may be more important in older patients.

Partial Patellectomy

■ Partial patellectomy is reserved for fractures of the lower pole of the patellar (group A1, C1.3) where there is extensive comminution and internal fixation is impossible.

■ These are extra-articular, and if the patellar tendon is repaired to the remaining patella after excision of the lower pole, reasonable results can be expected.

■ The technique can be used in C2.3 fractures if the vertical component of the fracture is reconstructed using intrafragmentary screws.

■ Reconstruction of the patellar tendon is achieved with transosseous sutures or by the use of bone anchors.

■ The results associated with partial patellectomy are shown in Table 25-4.

- The overall results are not dissimilar to tension band wiring (see Table 25-3), but surgeons do report significant quadriceps power loss and loss of knee flexion.
- It has been reported that up to 73% of patients show osteoarthritic change, with up to 33% of patients complaining of significant pain.

■ If partial patellectomy is undertaken, care should be taken not to pull the proximal patellar down more than is necessary because this may increase the incidence of osteoarthritis.

■ The soft tissue repair should also be protected with a wire loop between the proximal patellar and the proximal tibia (Fig. 25-8).

- The tibial fixation can be through a drill hole or around a transosseous screw.
- The loop may be a figure-of-eight or simple loop.

TABLE 25-4 RESULTS OF PARTIAL PATELLECTOMY

Result/Complication	Range (%)	Average (%)
Excellent/good	42.8–100	66.6
Infection	0–1.5	<1
Septic arthritis	0–1.5	<1
Flexion loss (>30 degrees)	4–19	11.7
Significant quadriceps weakness	0–47.6	13.9

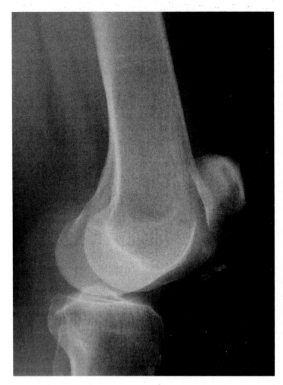 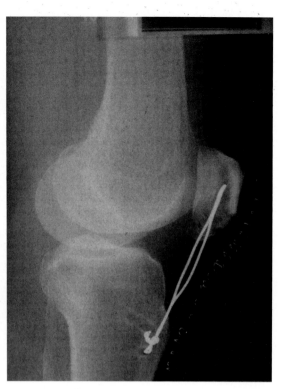

Figure 25-8   The use of a wire loop to stabilize the patella after a partial patellectomy.

- It is wise to protect the repair for 2 to 3 weeks with a cast or brace, even with a wire loop in position.
- Graduated knee movements can then be instituted.
- The wire loop should be left in place for at least 3 months.

Total Patellectomy
- Complete excision of the patella has been less popular in recent years.
- The literature results for patellectomy are summarized in Table 25-5, which shows a similar incidence of good and excellent results to other methods.
- Studies of patellectomized patients using more sophisticated outcome criteria have shown a greater loss of quadriceps power and knee flexion than is encountered in patients who have a partial patellectomy.
- Studies have also shown that only about 6% of patients are happy with the long-term outcome of patellectomy, and 90% complain of an ache and 60% of weakness.
- Patellectomy should be reserved for severe unreconstructable patellar fractures.

TABLE 25-5 RESULTS OF TOTAL PATELLECTOMY

Result/Complication	Range (%)	Average (%)
Excellent/good	30–85.7	72
Flexion loss (>30 degrees)	25	25
Significant quads weakness (%)	11.5–33.3	26
Osteoarthritis	25–50	34.7

Suggested Treatment

- The suggested management of patellar fractures is shown in Table 25-6.

COMPLICATIONS

- The incidence of nonunion is generally accepted to be about 5%, but most occur in nonoperatively managed vertical (type B) fractures.
  - Many are asymptomatic but if symptomatic can be treated by intrafragmentary screw fixation.

TABLE 25-6 SUGGESTED MANAGEMENT OF PATELLAR FRACTURES

Injury	Management
Undisplaced fractures (all types)	Cast or brace 6 to 8 weeks
Displaced fractures	
Noncomminuted lower pole	Tension band wiring with K-wires or cannulated screws
Transverse	Tension band wiring
Three or four fragment	Tension band wiring
Vertical fractures	Interfragmentary screws
Comminuted lower pole	Partial patellectomy
Unreconstructable	Total patellectomy

■ Infection is rare, and the major problems relate to loss of function secondary to quadriceps weakness, reduction in knee movement, and osteoarthritis.

■ Osteoarthritis is obviously fairly common, but most authorities agree that in many patients it is asymptomatic or gives rise to only minimal symptoms.

  ■ It is very slowly progressive, and few patients require secondary surgery.

■ Failure of fixation should be treated by early refixation using the techniques outlined in this chapter. If this is done, reasonable results can be expected.

SUGGESTED READING

Archdeacon MT, Sanders RW. Patella fractures and extensor mechanism injuries. In: Browner BD, Jupiter JB, Levine AM, et al., eds. Skeletal trauma, 3rd ed. Philadelphia: WB Saunders, 2003:2103–2144.

Carpenter JE, Kasman R, Matthews LS. Fractures of the patella. J Bone Joint Surg (Am) 1993;75:1550–1561.

Harris RM. Fractures of the patella. In: Bucholz RW, Heckman JD, eds. Rockwood and Green's fractures in adults, 5th ed. Philadelphia: Lippincott Williams and Wilkins, 2001:1775–1799.

Sutton FS, Thompson CH, Lipke J, et al. The effect of patellectomy on knee function. J Bone Joint Surg (Am) 1976;58:537–540.

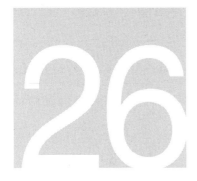

PROXIMAL TIBIAL FRACTURES AND KNEE DISLOCATIONS

Fractures of the tibial plateau have received considerable attention in the last few years. As with all fractures there has been a shift away from nonoperative management with a recognition that the best results are obtained by accurate reduction and rigid fixation of the fracture fragments. As with other metaphyseal and intra-articular fractures, there has been recent interest in periarticular external fixation and the Ilizarov ring fixator, and its hybrid variants have been used for high-energy bicondylar tibial plateau fractures in particular. There have also been studies of the use of bone substitutes to replace the use of autogenous bone graft. The number of controversies in the treatment of knee dislocations and proximal tibial fractures are listed in Box 26-1.

SURGICAL ANATOMY

Many tibial plateau fractures are high-energy injuries with often considerable damage to the adjacent soft tissues. There may be extensive damage to the cruciate ligaments, menisci, collateral ligaments and joint capsule, and supporting retinacular fibers. The popliteal vessels and common peroneal nerve are also at risk. The tibial plateau is formed from the medial and lateral plateaus separated by the intercondylar eminence (Fig. 26-1). The medial plateau is larger and concave in both sagittal and coronal planes. The lateral plateau is smaller and higher than the medial plateau and convex in both planes. The intercondylar eminence is nonarticular and contains the attachment of both cruciate ligaments. The posterior cruciate attaches to the posterior intercondylar area and the posterior surface of the tibial metaphysis. The anterior cruciate is attached anteriorly to the medial intercondylar tubercle. The medial and lateral menisci are attached peripherally to the appropriate plateau by meniscotibial ligaments. The fibular collateral ligament is attached to the fibula head, and the medial collateral ligament is attached to the proximal tibial metaphysis. There are deep and superficial components to the medial collateral ligament.

The popliteal artery is the continuation of the femoral artery. It runs behind the proximal tibia to divide into the anterior and posterior tibial arteries at the lower border of popliteus muscle. It is at risk in knee dislocations or occasionally in severe proximal tibial fractures. The tibial nerve passes across the popliteal fossa with the popliteal vessels to exit the popliteal fossa between the heads of gastrocnemius. The common peroneal nerve passes laterally in the popliteal fossa to terminate by dividing into the deep and superficial peroneal nerves lateral to the neck of the fibula. It is at risk in severe tibial plateau fractures and from external fixator pins or fine wires.

KNEE DISLOCATION

Knee dislocations (Fig. 26-2) are relatively uncommon but associated with considerable soft tissue injury. They are probably underdiagnosed because a number of patients present with a spontaneously relocating knee dislocation. In the early 1960s, the amputation rate associated with knee dislocation was reported as high as 89%, but improved vascular surgery has reduced the problems associated with popliteal artery disruption. In recent years better

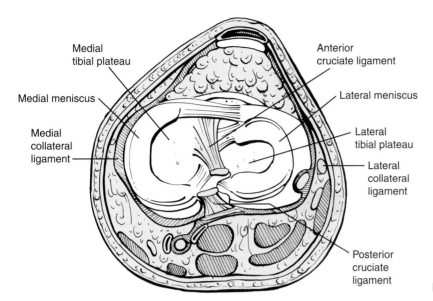

Medial tibial plateau

Medial meniscus

Medial collateral ligament

Anterior cruciate ligament

Lateral meniscus

Lateral tibial plateau

Lateral collateral ligament

Posterior cruciate ligament

Figure 26-1 The anatomy of the tibial plateau.

understanding of the problems associated with ligamentous instability and improved surgical techniques have greatly improved the outcome after this severe injury.

CLASSIFICATION

Classification systems of knee dislocation are based either on the direction of dislocation of the tibia in relation to the femur or on the injury pattern with the description of the actual ligamentous damage presented. The latter is more precise, but the former is in widespread use and shown in Table 26-1. Anterior, posterior, and lateral dislocations are more common than medial and rotatory dislocations.

ASSOCIATED INJURIES

Ligamentous Injuries

The incidence of damage to the different knee ligaments is shown in Table 26-2. Damage to both the anterior and posterior cruciate ligaments is usual, but dislocation

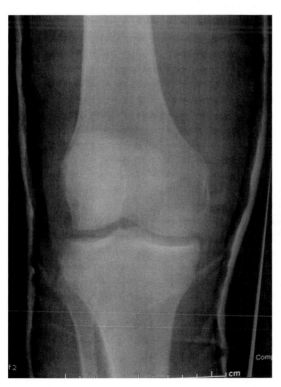
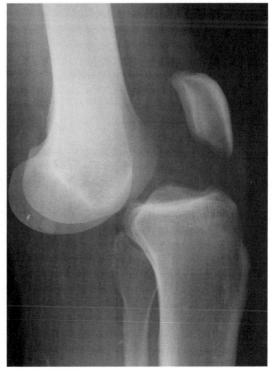

Figure 26-2 A-P and lateral radiographs of a knee dislocation.

TABLE 26-1 TYPES AND INCIDENCES OF DIFFERENT KNEE DISLOCATIONS[a]

Type	Incidence (%)
Anterior	30.6
Posterior	24.9
Lateral	13.5
Medial	3.3
Rotatory	3.7
Anteromedial	
Posteromedial	
Anterolateral	
Posterolateral	
Unspecified	24.1

[a]The classification is that of Kennedy (1963), and the incidences are from Green (1977).

associated with isolated ACL or PCL ruptures can occur. It is important to know the overall pattern of ligamentous injuries, and Table 26-2 shows that almost 50% of knee dislocations are associated with damage to the ACL, PCL, and MCL, with about 20% associated with damage to the ACL, PCL, and the posterolateral complex. In a minority of patients, all ligaments are ruptured. Unlike isolated cruciate injuries, knee dislocations have a high incidence of avulsion fractures at the ligament insertion. PCL avulsions have been reported in up to 80% of knee dislocations and ACL avulsions in up to 50%.

Other Injuries

The incidence of nonligamentous complications of knee dislocation is summarized in Table 26-3. There is a high incidence of both vascular and neurological damage with knee dislocations. Popliteal artery damage averages about 25% but has been reported as high as 40% in anterior and posterior dislocations, 25% in medial dislocations, and 3% in lateral dislocations, although it is virtually unknown in rotatory dislocations. The damage is often an intimal tear but can be more severe, and arterial transection can occur.

Nerve damage usually involves the common peroneal nerve, although tibial nerve involvement has been described. The damage may be a neuropraxia, axonotmesis, or neurotmesis. Meniscal injury is frequent, and the incidence of impaction fractures of the femoral condyles has been reported as high as 100%, although osteochondral fractures are less common. Other musculoskeletal injuries have been reported in 40% to 60% of patients. These are often other fractures of the ipsilateral leg.

DIAGNOSIS

History and Physical Examination

- Knee dislocations usually follow a high-energy injury such as a motor vehicle accident or a fall from a height, but about 20% occur in low-energy injuries.
- The patients are usually young and medically fit.
- A thorough examination of the vascular and neurological state of the limb is mandatory.
- It must be remembered that the knee may have spontaneously relocated. If there is any suspicion that a knee dislocation may have occurred, a Doppler examination of the limb should be undertaken.
- If there is any suggestion of vascular damage, either exploration or arteriography should be performed depending on the findings.
- Patients with high-energy injuries should be examined according to ATLS principles, with particular attention of the rest of the leg because there may be other injuries.

Radiologic Examination

- The diagnosis is usually determined by standard anteroposterior and lateral radiographs (see Fig. 26-2).
- Doppler and arteriography (Fig. 26-3) are used to examine the vascular supply to the limb, and MRI scans can be used to investigate ligamentous injuries.
- An MRI scan is also useful if there is a suspicion the dislocated knee has relocated spontaneously.
- It will confirm the degree of ligamentous injury.

TABLE 26-2 INCIDENCE OF DIFFERENT LIGAMENT INJURIES INCLUDING COMBINATION INJURIES[a]

Injury	Range (%)	Average (%)
ACL	80.7–106	95
PCL	84.6–100	96
MCL	57.7–60	59.4
LCL	28–50	39.6
ACL + PCL	65.4–100	91.1
ACL + PCL + MCL	45.4–48	47
ACL + PCL + posterolateral complex	16–27.3	20.5
All ligaments	12–15.3	13.9

[a]Data taken from recent literature (1997–2004).

TABLE 26-3 INCIDENCE OF OTHER INJURIES ASSOCIATED WITH KNEE DISLOCATION

Injury	Incidence (%)	
	Range	Average
Vascular damage	7.7–52.9	24.5
Neural injury	8–40	21.3
Meniscal damage	45–76	62.2
Osteochondral fracture	12–15.3	13.7

TREATMENT

■ The treatment of knee dislocation has improved markedly because of better vascular techniques and an appreciation of the importance of operative ligamentous repair.

■ The dislocation should be reduced as an emergency, and once reduced a further assessment of the neurovascular status of the limb should be undertaken.

■ Few dislocations are now treated nonoperatively.

■ Surgeons may choose to stabilize the knee with a temporary spanning external fixator and undertake secondary cruciate reconstruction and repair of the posterolateral complex.

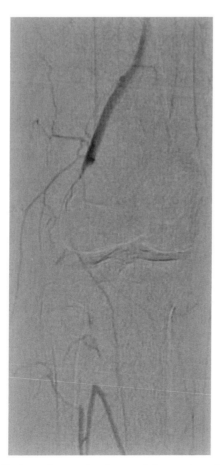

Figure 26-3 An angiogram showing vessel damage secondary to a knee dislocation. The knee has been relocated.

■ Vascular damage is treated by interpositional vein grafting, and nerve damage is treated expectantly, although full recovery does not always occur.

■ Good or excellent results have been reported in 53.8% to 100% (average 66.6%) of recent series.

■ Late complications include knee pain and stiffness, instability, and posttraumatic osteoarthritis.

PROXIMAL TIBIOFIBULAR DISLOCATION

This is a rare injury that occurs in high-energy trauma. It has been reported associated with posterior dislocation of the hip, open tibial fractures, and fractures of the knee. They can occur in sports injuries, however, and may be associated with a twisting injury to the knee. The patient presents with lateral knee pain, and X-rays classically show the proximal fibula lateral to the proximal tibia. In a normal anteroposterior knee X-ray, there is overlap between the fibula and the tibia. Views of the normal knee should be obtained for comparison. Treatment is by closed reduction. Common peroneal palsy has been reported in up to 5% of cases.

TIBIAL PLATEAU FRACTURES

CLASSIFICATION

The OTA (AO) classification is shown in Figure 26-4. Type A fractures are extra-articular fractures with A1 fractures avulsion fractures of the proximal fibula (.1), tibial tuberosity (.2), and tibial eminence (.3). The A2 fractures are simple metaphyseal fractures distinguished by different fracture morphology. The suffix .1 describes fractures that are oblique in the frontal plane, with .2 fractures oblique in the sagittal plane, and .3 fractures transverse. A3 fractures are comminuted metaphyseal fractures with .1 fractures having an intact wedge, .2 fractures having a fragmented wedge, and .3 fractures extensively comminuted.

The common type B fractures are partial articular fractures affecting one condyle. B1 fractures are simple split fractures with .1 fractures lateral, .2 fractures medial, and .3 fractures medial or lateral fractures that involve the tibial eminence. B2 fractures are depression fractures with .1 fractures lateral fractures with extensive depression, .2 fractures lateral fractures with limited depression, and .3 fractures medial depression fractures. B3 fractures are split depression fractures with the suffix .1 to .3 the same as for B1 fractures.

Type C fractures are bicondylar. C1 fractures are simple split fractures, with .1 containing minimally displaced fractures, .2 containing fractures showing displacement of one condyle, and .3 containing fractures with displacement of

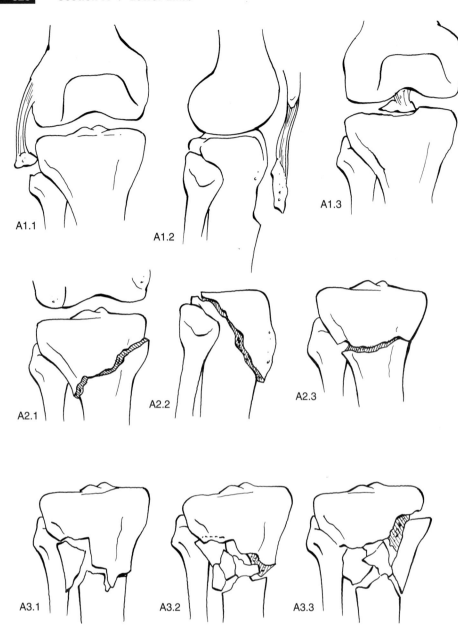

Figure 26-4 The OTA (AO) classification of proximal tibial fractures.

both condyles. C2 fractures are wedge fractures with .1 fractures having an intact wedge, .2 fractures a fragmented wedge, and .3 fractures complex. The C3 fractures contain fractures with extensive articular comminution. The .1 fractures are lateral, the .2 fractures are medial, and the .3 fractures are bicondylar.

The OTA (AO) classification was derived from the Schatzker classification, which divided tibial plateau fractures into six types and is still in use. Type I contains split fractures of the lateral plateau (OTA [AO] B1.1). Type II fractures are depression fractures of the lateral plateau (B2.1 and B2.2), and type III fractures are split depression lateral plateau fractures (B3.1). All medial plateau fractures are classified as type IV fractures (B1.2, B2.3, B3.2), and bicondylar fractures are classified as types V and VI (type C). Type V fractures are split bicondylar fractures, and type VI fractures contain all articular fractures associated with the separation of the metaphysis from the diaphysis.

EPIDEMIOLOGY

The basic epidemiology of the tibial plateau fractures is shown in Table 26-4. They are unusual fractures in that they have a type H distribution (see Chapter 1) with both men and women showing a bimodal distribution. The highest incidence is seen between the ages of 30 to 39 years (21%), and about 24% occur in patients aged 65 years or more. There is an almost equal gender distribution, and over 70% of fractures are OTA (AO) type B partial articular fractures. About 55% of tibial plateau fractures are B1.1, B2.1, or B3.1 fractures (Schatzker types I, II, and III). In older patients with osteopenic bone, about 60% of fractures involve significant depression of the lateral cortex (B2.1, B3.1, or C3.1), and 66% of the A2.3 transverse extra-articular fractures occur in the elderly as insufficiency fractures after a minor injury. Overall, open tibial plateau fractures are

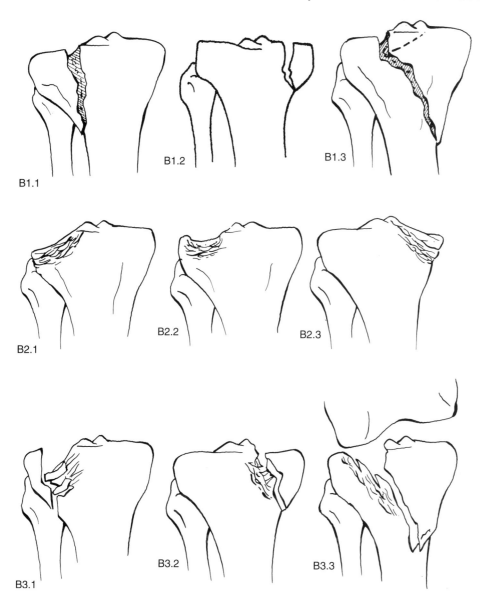

Figure 26-4 *(continued)*

relatively uncommon, but they are seen more frequently in level 1 trauma centers.

Table 26-5 shows the epidemiology of tibial plateau fractures according to the mode of injury. Motor accident pedestrians and patients injured in falls predictably are older, with most type C bicondylar fractures caused by motor vehicle accidents.

Associated Injuries

The proximity of the knee joint to the tibial plateau ensures a high incidence of associated intra-articular injury. The highest incidences are associated with high-energy bicondylar or medial plateau fractures. The ranges and mean values for damage to the different knee ligaments are shown in Table 26-6. It is likely that the incidence of combined ligament injuries is higher than shown in Table 26-6 because it has only been comparatively recently that surgeons have been aware of this problem. Table 26-6 shows that damage to the medial collateral and anterior cruciate ligaments is relatively common.

TABLE 26-4 EPIDEMIOLOGY OF TIBIAL PLATEAU FRACTURES

Proportion of all fractures	1.2%
Average age	48.9 y
Men/women	54%/46%
Incidence	13.3/10^5/y
Distribution	Type H
Open fractures	2.8%
OTA (AO) classification	
Type A	16.9%
Type B	70.4%
Type C	12.7%
Most common subgroups	
B2.1	21.1%
B3.1	18.3%
B1.1	18.3%

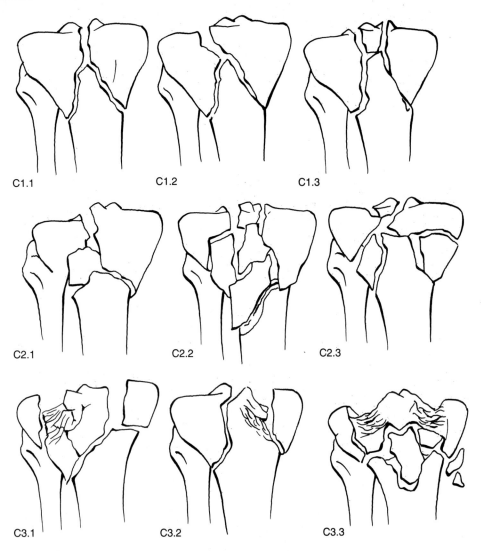

C1.1 C1.2 C1.3

C2.1 C2.2 C2.3

C3.1 C3.2 C3.3

Figure 26-4 *(continued)*

Table 26-6 shows that the incidence of meniscal injury is high, with the incidence in studies specifically looking for meniscal damage as high as 47%. The difference in incidence between lateral and medial menisci mirrors the difference between lateral and medial plateau fractures, and it is the meniscus related to the fracture that is almost exclusively damaged, although recent reports have detailed a higher incidence of bilateral meniscal injury. It should be remembered that cadaveric studies have shown that 5% to 18% of knees have meniscal lesions, but the association

with plateau fractures is such that arthroscopic examination should be considered if closed fracture treatment is undertaken. An analysis of the different incidences of meniscal tears in the common type B fracture has shown the same incidence of lateral meniscal damage in B1 and B2 fractures, but the B3 split depression fractures are associated with twice as many meniscal lesions (approximately 35%).

Other injuries around the knee joint are uncommon. Neuropraxia of the common peroneal nerve does occur but virtually always recovers. Popliteal artery damage occurs

TABLE 26-5 EPIDEMIOLOGY OF TIBIAL PLATEAU FRACTURES ACCORDING TO MODE OF INJURY

Cause	Age (y)	Open (%)	OTA (AO) Type (%)		
			A	B	C
Motor vehicle accident	50.2	4.2	12.5	58.3	29.2
Fall	58.7	6.2	31.2	68.7	0
Falls from height	46.7	0	20.0	60.0	20.0
Sport	36.7	0	11.1	88.9	—

TABLE 26-6 INCIDENCE OF LOCAL ASSOCIATED INJURIES

Injury	Incidence (%) Range	Incidence (%) Average
Ligament injuries	13.8–40	22.7
Anterior cruciate	0–27.6	8.5
Posterior cruciate	0–5.7	0.7
Medial collateral	0–56.4	13.9
Lateral collateral	0–20.5	2.3
Combined	0–53.8	4.4
Meniscal tears	12.5–50	30.6
Medial	10.2–50	21.0
Lateral	50–89.8	78.1
Common peroneal nerve palsy	0–8.3	1.1
Popliteal artery damage	0–2.1	0.7
Osteochondral fracture	0–6.1	0.8

more frequently in medial plateau or bicondylar fractures but is rare. Osteochondral fractures of the femoral condyles are probably much more common but have not been looked for in most series, hence the low incidences reported in Table 26-6.

Approximately 20% of patients have other fractures. The incidence obviously varies among different types of institutions. The most common associated fractures are fractures of the ipsilateral femur and tibia. Ipsilateral supracondylar femoral fractures occur in about 5% of cases, and about 3% of patients with tibial diaphyseal or plafond fractures have an associated plateau fracture.

DIAGNOSIS

History and Physical Examination

- Many older patients merely relate having fallen, but a careful history of the mode of injury should be obtained to distinguish between low-energy and high-energy injuries, the latter commonly associated with other musculoskeletal damage, particularly in the same limb.
- In older patients a complete medical and social history should be obtained.
- All patients should be asked about preaccident knee symptoms in view of the high incidence of knee injury associated with tibial plateau fractures.
- All patients injured in high-energy accidents should have a complete examination according to ATLS principles.
- A thorough examination of the affected limb should be undertaken.
- The literature suggests that about 12% of high-energy tibial plateau fractures have compartment syndrome, which should be checked out.
- Vascular and neurological examination may reveal common peroneal nerve and popliteal artery damage.
- If there is any indication of vascular injury, angiography or Doppler examination should be undertaken.
- The incidence of open proximal tibial fracture is relatively low, but any open wound should be examined.

- In the elderly population, degloving may be present after a motor vehicle accident.

Radiologic Examination

- Standard anteroposterior and lateral radiographs (Fig. 26-5) are usually all that is required to diagnose a tibial plateau fracture, but oblique radiographs in internal and external rotation may be useful in detailing the extent of articular or metaphyseal comminution.
- CT scans should be obtained in bicondylar or complex plateau fractures (Fig. 26-6).
- MRI scanning is undoubtedly very useful in the assessment of tibial plateau fractures.
  - With their use, the detection of meniscal and ligamentous injury has increased.
  - One study has shown that the treatment plan was altered in 23% of cases by the results gained by an MRI scan.
  - MRI scanning is particularly useful if closed management of the fracture is proposed.

TREATMENT

- The treatment for intra-articular tibial plateau fractures is accurate reduction of the articular surface and rigid fixation to maintain the reduced position and permit joint function.
- The three recent advances have been the use of arthroscopic and fluoroscopic techniques to allow closed reduction and fixation, the use of external fixation, usually ring fixation, and the use of bone substitutes instead of bone grafts to maintain the reduced position of the depressed plateau fragments.

Nonsurgical Treatment

- As with all fractures, nonoperative management was popular until 20 to 30 years ago, and it is still used for undisplaced fractures, particularly type A insufficiency fractures in the elderly.

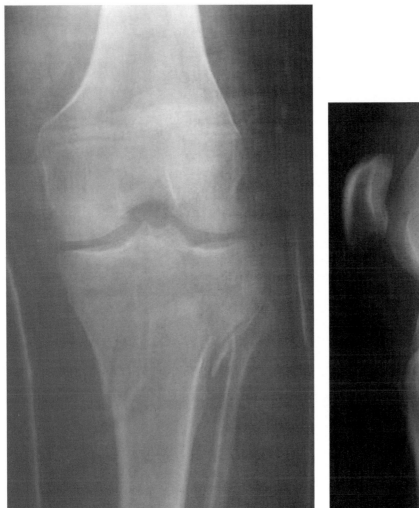
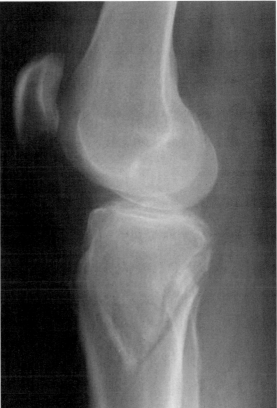

Figure 26-5   A-P and lateral radiographs of a C1.3 proximal tibial fracture.

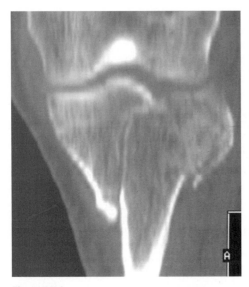
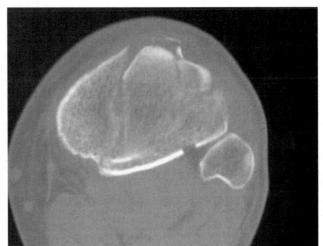

Figure 26-6   CT scans of proximal tibial fracture shown in Figure 26-5 illustrating the extent of the fracture.

TABLE 26-7 RESULTS OF NONOPERATIVE MANAGEMENT OF SPECIFIC TIBIAL PLATEAU FRACTURES

Fracture Type	Result/Complication (%)		
	Excellent/Good	Flexion	Severe Osteoarthritis
Split (B1)	61.5	125	9.1
Depression (B2)	41.2	118	40
Split depression (B3)	50	100	66
Bicondylar (C)	35.3	112	71.4

■ It is generally accepted there is little benefit in operating if there is no more than 3 mm of plateau depression. Nonoperative management should be used.

■ Nonoperative management usually involves the use of a knee brace for between 4 and 6 weeks.

■ Non-weight-bearing mobilization is encouraged, but in the elderly this is difficult.

■ The results of nonoperative management for more severe fractures are difficult to interpret, despite the fact that the method of assessment of excellent and good results is remarkably uniform throughout the literature.

■ Table 26-7 contains the results of nonoperative management for different types of displaced tibial plateau fractures.

■ There is insufficient data about medial plateau fractures to merit inclusion in the table.

■ It is obvious that the results are relatively poor for depressed and bicondylar fractures and only reasonable for split fractures.

Surgical Treatment

Lateral Plateau

■ The traditional method of open reduction and internal fixation of lateral tibial plateau fractures was to use interfragmentary screws or plates for split fractures and plates and supplementary autogenous bone graft for depressed and split depression fractures (Fig. 26-7).

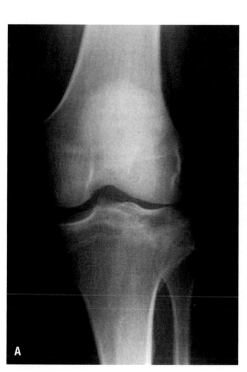
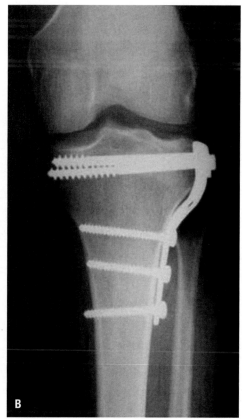

Figure 26-7   A split depression (B3.1) fracture (**A**) treated with a lateral plate (**B**).

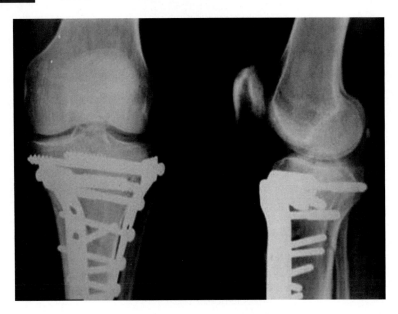

Figure 26-8 A bicondylar tibial plateau fracture treated with two plates.

- Bicondylar fractures were often fixed with medial and lateral plates (Fig. 26-8).
  - The results of this type of approach for lateral plateau fractures are shown in Table 26-8.
  - The results are better than nonoperative management, but the best results were in the management of B1 split fractures where no bone grafting is required.
  - In B2 and B3 lateral plateau fractures, the results are not as good, mainly because open bone grafting does not adequately maintain the reduced position of the bone fragments.
- Table 26-8 also shows the results of limited open reduction and internal fixation.
  - This is done either under arthroscopic or fluoroscopic control and consists of elevating depressed segments of bone percutaneously through a small lateral metaphyseal window.

- The articular reduction is undertaken using an arthroscope or a fluoroscope to check the position, and bone graft is then packed under the reduced articular cartilage.
- Intrafragmentary screws, or occasionally a plate, are then used to maintain the reduction.
- Studies of these techniques have generally been undertaken in lower energy injuries, but the results detailed in Table 26-8 are good with improved results for lateral depression and split depression fractures.
  - Comparison of the use of arthroscopy and fluoroscopy has shown no difference between the two techniques.
- More recently surgeons have attempted to dispense with bone graft and used bone substitutes such as Norian SRS, an injectable calcium phosphate cement (Fig. 26-9).
- Table 26-8 shows that overall the results are as good as those obtained from limited open reduction and internal fixation and bone grafting.

TABLE 26-8 RESULTS OF DIFFERENT TYPES OF INTERNAL FIXATION FOR LATERAL PLATEAU FRACTURES AND BICONDYLAR FRACTURES

Result/Complication	Open Fixation and Grafting (%)		Arthroscopically or Fluoroscopically Assisted fixation and Grafting (%)		Arthroscopically or Fluoroscopically Assisted Fixation and Bone Substitutes (%)	
	Range	Average	Range	Average	Range	Average
Good/excellent						
B1	87.5–100	90.1	93.3–100	95.2	—	—
B2	75–100	86.4	66.6–100	90.5	95.4–100	96.1
B3	77.2–100	85.9	86.6–100	93.1	78.9–92	86.4
C	52–100	75	50–77.4	74.3	66.6–100	80
Open	0–25	10.2	0–7.9	4.6	0	0
Nonunion	0	0	0	0	0	0
Infection	0–4.2	3.2	0–3.9	2.3	0–2.1	1.3
Septic arthritis	0	0	0	0	0	0
Malunion	0–6.6	4.2	0–15.8	4.6	0–7.7	2.7
Severe osteoarthritis	0–12.5	9.8	?	?	?	?

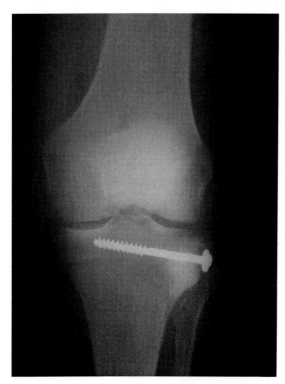

Figure 26-9 A depressed lateral tibial plateau fracture treated with calcium phosphate cement and interfragmentary screws.

- Studies have indicated that injection of calcium phosphate cement into the knee joint does not cause demonstrable damage and the material usually maintains the reduced position of the articular cartilage.
- Because the use of bone graft is not without complications, injectable calcium phosphate is recommended where possible for the treatment of lateral plateau depression and split depression fractures.
- Interest has been expressed recently in the use of percutaneous plating for both tibial plateau fractures and proximal tibial diaphyseal fractures.
- This technique utilizes the LISS system, and the results are given in Table 27-13 in Chapter 27.
- External fixation has been used to treat lateral plateau fractures.
- Bone graft is still required, and the data suggests that 86% of patients have good or excellent results.
- Because this is no better than the easier technique of limited open reduction and internal fixation using either bone graft or bone substitutes, there is no indication to use external fixation routinely for the management of lateral plateau fractures.

Bicondylar Fractures
- The principle of closed or limited open reduction with minimal soft tissue damage has been taken further in the treatment of bicondylar tibial plateau fractures.
- These are high-energy injuries with a significant incidence of associated soft tissue damage and open fracture.
- They are not particularly common, and information about their management comes from level 1 trauma centers in Europe and North America.

- Tables 26-7 and 26-8 indicate that the results of treating bicondylar fractures nonoperatively or with open or limited open reduction and internal fixation are relatively poor.
- With increasing interest in external fixation (Fig. 26-10) in the 1990s, surgeons used different types of external fixation to stabilize bicondylar type C fractures, usually combining external fixation with interfragmentary screws or occasionally a plate.
- Bone grafting or bone substitutes are used as required.
- As yet there is limited experience of the use of bone substitutes in type C fractures, with the results detailed in Table 26-8 associated with C3.1 lateral plateau fractures.
- Three types of external fixator have been used.
  - These are a conventional unilateral frame with proximal and distal half pins, a full Ilizarov ring fixator, and an intermediate hybrid frame consisting of a proximal ring secured with fine wires and distal half pins (see Fig. 26-10).
  - The results of all three types are given in Table 26-9.
- It can be seen that more information is available about the use of external fixation than regarding the use of internal fixation or nonoperative management!
- Comparison of Table 26-9 with Tables 26-7 and 26-8 shows that the bicondylar fractures detailed in Table 26-9 are more severe, having a much higher incidence of open fractures.
  - Overall, the results of the three different external fixators are very similar, although the percentage of good and excellent results with hybrid fixation tends to be higher.
- As with all external fixators, pin tract sepsis is a problem, and septic arthritis of the knee is unique to external fixation.
  - To minimize this, the half pins or fine wires should ideally be extracapsular, although this is not always possible.
- The results suggest that hybrid fixation (see Fig. 26-10) produces good results, and if this technique is used there is no requirement for distal muscle penetration with fine wires.
- In severe injuries, transarticular or joint spanning external fixation is used.
  - This is rarely used as definitive fixation but may be used primarily with periarticular or joint sparing fixation substituted after the soft tissues have healed.
- Evidence from the literature suggests the results of transarticular fixation are not as good as the results of periarticular fixation because of knee stiffness.
- Transarticular external fixation may be required, but preferably periarticular external fixation should be used.

Medial Plateau Fractures
- Fractures of the medial tibial plateau are relatively unusual.
- There is insufficient data in the literature to allow accurate analysis of the best treatment method. Extrapolation of the data relating to lateral and bicondylar fractures is useful, however.

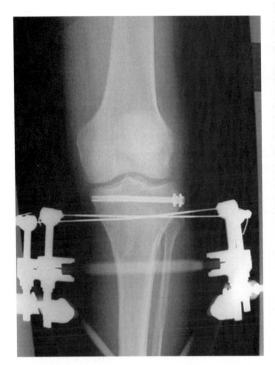
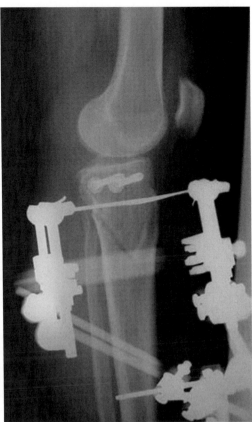

Figure 26-10 The fracture shown in Figure 26-5 fixed with interfragmentary screws and a hybrid external fixator.

- Low-energy medial plateau fractures can be treated by interfragmentary screws or a plate.
- High-energy fractures can be treated by medial plating or by external fixation, particularly if there is significant comminution.

Suggested Treatment

The suggested treatment of proximal tibial fractures is given in Table 26-10.

COMPLICATIONS

- Nonunion and infection are relatively uncommon and discussed in the appropriate chapters. A number of other complications may occur.

Compartment Syndrome

- In low-energy tibial plateau fractures in elderly patients, the incidence of compartment syndrome is low, but in

TABLE 26-9 RESULTS OF EXTERNAL FIXATION IN BICONDYLAR TIBIAL PLATEAU FRACTURES

Result/Complication	Ring Fixators		Hybrid Fixators		Unilateral Fixators	
	Range	Average	Range	Average	Range	Average
Excellent/good (%)	62.5–80	69.7	69.6–98	89	62.5–72.2	69.2
Open (%)	20.8–48.8	34.1	27.2–62.5	37.5	50–62.5	54.5
Nonunion (%)	0–1.7	0.8	0–4	2.3	0	0
Malunion (%)	0–10	6.5	0–4.5	3.4	0–4.8	3.4
Infection (%)	0–8.8	4	0–13.6	4.5	9.5–12.5	10.3
Pin sepsis (%)	33–100	70.5	4.5–38	27.3	12.5–42.8	34.5
Septic arthritis (%)	0–4.2	1.6	0–4	2.3	0–9.5	6.9
Severe osteoarthritis (%)	15–29.2	23.5	?	?	14.2	14.2
Knee flexion (degree)	103–112	105	107–120	116	125	125

TABLE 26-10 SUGGESTED TREATMENT OF TIBIAL PLATEAU FRACTURES

Injury	Management
Undisplaced (<3 mm)	Nonoperative
Displaced	
Type A extra-articular fractures	Hybrid periarticular external fixation or LISS plate
Type B partial articular fractures	
Split fractures (B1)	Interfragmentary screws. Neutralization plate in osteopenic bone. Fluoroscopic assistance.
Depressed fractures (B2)	Same as B1 fractures but with bone substitute to maintain joint reduction. Use graft if substitute unavailable.
Split-depression fractures (B3)	As for B2 fractures but plate usually required.
Type C complete articular fractures	Interfragmentary screws and hybrid external fixation. Bone substitute may be required to maintain joint reduction.
Multiple injuries	Primary transarticular external fixation. Secondary definitive treatment may be required.

high-energy fractures the incidence in the literature ranges from 6.6% to 33.3%, although on average an incidence of about 12% can be expected.

■ This is higher than in tibial diaphyseal fractures, and surgeons must be aware of this relatively common complication.

Osteoarthritis

■ Table 26-9 indicates that severe degenerative osteoarthritis is relatively common after high-energy tibial plateau fractures.

■ Less severe osteoarthritis is very common, and the literature indicates that about 50% of patients show radiologic changes suggestive of osteoarthritis after tibial plateau fractures.

■ Meniscectomy unquestionably increases the incidence of posttraumatic osteoarthritis and should be avoided where possible.

■ Residual knee instability, marked articular step-off, and septic arthritis are all associated with an increased incidence of posttraumatic osteoarthritis.

■ Most articles detail their results at 1 or 2 years after injury, but analysis of results 5 years after injury indicates that the progression of osteoarthritis is slow and few patients actually require knee arthroplasty.

■ If arthroplasty is required, the consensus is that the operation decreases pain and increases knee function, but there is an increased incidence of perioperative and postoperative complications compared with primary knee arthroplasty, and a failure rate of up to 33% has been quoted.

Osteochondral Defects

■ The high incidence of depressed tibial plateau fractures means there will be residual osteochondral defects in many patients.

■ In older patients knee arthroplasty may be undertaken, but this is inappropriate in younger patients, and a number of techniques have been used to fill the defects.

■ Osteochondral plugs and autologous chondrocyte transplantation have been used, but the best results are associated with the use of osteochondral allografts.

■ Analysis indicates that the 5-year survival rate is 95%, with 80% at 10 years, 65% at 15 years, and 46% at 20 years.

■ Survivorship seems to be increased if meniscal transplantation is undertaken along with the osteochondral graft.

■ The technique is associated with a 9% incidence of graft collapse in excess of 3 mm, and 40% of patients display moderate or severe degenerative change.

SPECIAL SITUATIONS

Elderly Patients

■ The majority of tibial plateau fractures in the elderly are caused by low-velocity injuries and usually follow a simple fall.

■ They are usually B2.1, B3.1 or A2.3 fractures, and the treatment depends on the mobility and overall health of the patient.

■ Nonoperative management is indicated for minor depression fractures in elderly patients, although percutaneously inserted locking plates may be useful for displaced extra-articular and intra-articular fractures (Fig. 26-11).

■ Many of the A2.3 extra-articular fractures are undisplaced insufficiency fractures that should be treated nonoperatively.

■ One analysis of plateau fractures in the elderly showed that 68% were treated nonoperatively, with 26% treated with internal fixation and 5% with external fixation.

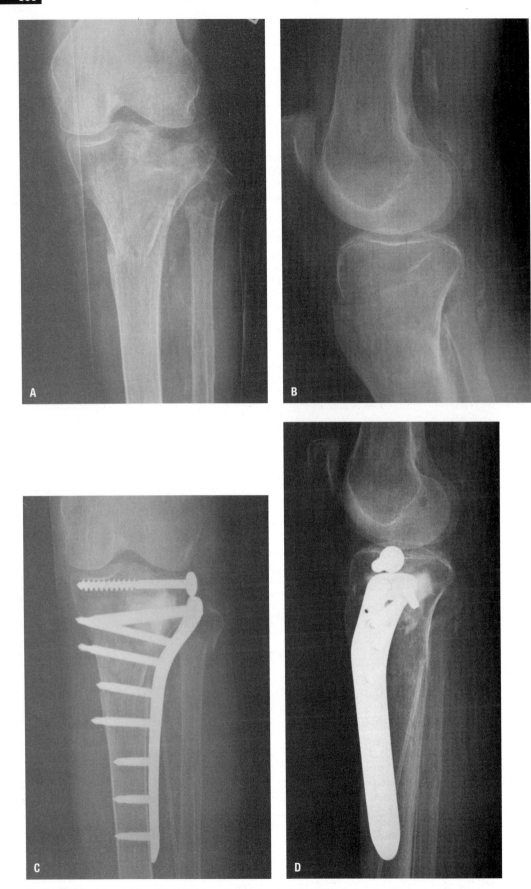

Figure 26-11 A bicondylar (C2.2) fracture (**A,B**) treated with a LISS plate and calcium phosphate cement (**C,D**).

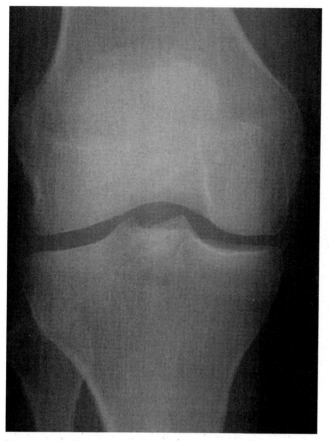
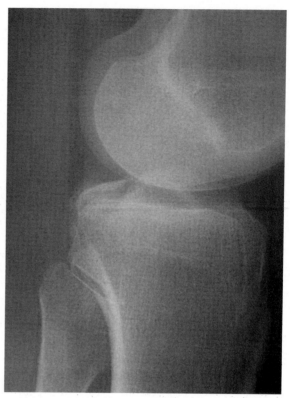

Figure 26-12 A-P and lateral radiographs of an A1.3 (Meyers and McKeever type I) tibial eminence fracture.

- Over 65% of patients showed evidence of osteoarthritis, but arthroplasty was rarely required.

Tibial Eminence Fractures

- Fractures of the tibial eminence (A1.3) tend to occur in children and young adults (Fig. 26-12), although they are probably more common in older patients than previously recognized.
- Displaced tibial eminence fractures are associated with cruciate instability.
- They have been classified by Meyers and McKeever (1970) into three types.
  - Type I lesions are undisplaced or minimally displaced.
  - In type II lesions the eminence fragment is elevated anteriorly, and in type III lesions it is separate.
- The literature suggests about 35% of adults with tibial eminence fractures have associated knee injuries, usually other tibial plateau fractures, meniscal lesions, or ligamentous injuries.
- Treatment consists of arthroscopy to lavage the joint, examine the menisci, and confirm the stability of the tibial eminence fracture. The knee joint should be checked for instability.
- Treatment depends on the age of the patient and the type of fracture.

- Type I lesions in younger patients can be treated non-operatively, assuming the joint is stable.
- Type II and III lesions should be treated operatively, with fixation using wire loops, screws, or pins.
  - This may be undertaken arthoscopically or through an arthrotomy.
- In adults, type I lesions are unusual and therefore surgery is usually required.
- The results for treatment are good, with an average of 130 degrees of flexion having been reported.

Segond Fracture

- The Segond fracture is an avulsion fracture of the lateral tibial plateau (Fig. 26-13).
- The fragment corresponds to the insertion of the lateral capsular ligament of the knee.
- Its importance is that the fracture usually indicates anterior cruciate ligament damage.
- Analysis shows that about 10% of patients with anterior cruciate ligament lesions have a Segond fracture compared with about 0.7% of other knee injuries.
- Treatment of the fracture is unnecessary, but investigation and treatment of any associated anterior cruciate ligament lesion must be undertaken.

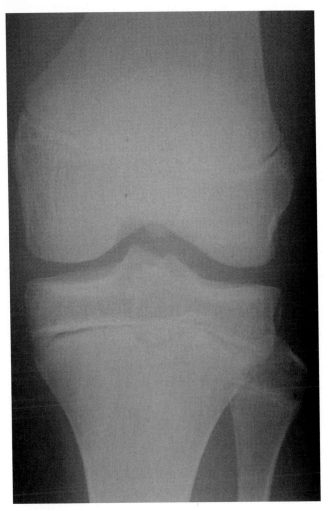

Figure 26-13 A Segond fracture.

Reverse Segond Fracture

■ Reverse Segond fractures are rare.
■ These are avulsion fractures of the medial side of the tibial plateau associated with avulsion of the deep portion of the medial collateral ligament.
■ As with Segond fractures the fracture itself is unimportant, but it may indicate damage to the posterior cruciate ligament and medial meniscus.
■ Further investigation with MRI scan should be undertaken and the ligament and meniscal injury dealt with appropriately.

Meniscal and Ligament Injuries

■ The treatment of meniscal and ligament injuries associated with tibial plateau fractures is not dissimilar from the treatment of isolated injuries, although the timing may be different.
■ It may prove difficult to reconstruct cruciate ligaments in the presence of a complicated plateau fracture.
■ Under these circumstances secondary reconstruction may be undertaken.
■ The decision requiring ligament reconstruction depends on the age of the patient, degree of knee instability, and type of fracture.
■ The menisci should not be sacrificed unless absolutely necessary because meniscal sacrifice is associated with poorer late functional results.
■ Thus meniscal repair, debridement, and partial meniscectomy should be undertaken as indicated.

SUGGESTED READING

Cole PA, Zlowodzki M, Kregor PJ. Less invasive stabilization system (LISS) for fractures of the proximal tibia: indications, surgical technique and preliminary results of the UMC clinical trial. Injury 2003;34(Suppl 1):16–29.

Egol KA, Su E, Tejwani NC, et al. Treatment of complex tibial plateau fractures using the less invasive stabilization system plate: clinical experience and a laboratory comparison with double plating. J Trauma 2004;57:340–346.

Honkonen SE. Degenerative arthritis after tibial plateau fractures. J Orthop Trauma 1995;9:273–277.

Hung SS, Chao EK, Chan YS, et al. Arthroscopically assisted osteosynthesis for tibial plateau fractures. J Trauma 2003;54:356–363.

Koval KJ, Polatsch D, Kummer FJ. Split fractures of the lateral tibial plateau. Evaluation of three fixation methods. J Orthop Trauma 1996;10:304–308.

Müller ME, Nazarian S, Koch P, et al. The comprehensive classification of fractures of long bones. Berlin: Springer-Verlag, 1990.

Myers MH, McKeever FM. Fracture of the intercondylar eminence of the tibia. J Bone Joint Surg (Am) 1970;52:1677–1684.

Schatzker J. Fractures of the tibial plateau. In: Schatzker J, Tile M, eds. Rationale of operative fracture care. Berlin: Springer-Verlag, 1987:279.

Simpson D, Keating JF. Outcome of tibial plateau fractures managed with calcium phosphate cement. Injury 2004;35:913–918.

Su EP, Westrich GH, Rana AJ, et al. Operative treatment of tibial plateau fractures in patients older than 55 years. Clin Orthop 2004;421:240–248.

Watson JT, Schatzker J. Tibial plateau fractures. In: Browner BD, Jupiter JB, Levine AM, et al., eds. Skeletal trauma, 3rd ed. Philadelphia: Saunders, 2003:2074–2130.

TIBIA AND FIBULA DIAPHYSEAL FRACTURES

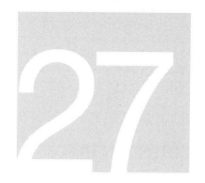

Fractures of the tibial diaphysis are the most common long-bone fractures treated by orthopaedic surgeons. They have always been regarded as difficult because until comparatively recently cast management was the treatment of choice, and the associated soft tissue defects could only be treated by basic plastic surgery techniques such as cross leg flaps. Nonunion was common, and complications such as compartment syndrome and infection were frequently devastating. Recent advances in intramedullary nailing, the detection of compartment syndrome, the management of nonunion and infection, and improved plastic surgery techniques, however, have resulted in improved management and results. A number of the controversies about the management of tibial diaphyseal fractures are listed in Box 27-1.

SURGICAL ANATOMY

The subcutaneous location of the anteromedial border of the tibia and the fact that the diaphysis becomes thinner distally makes the tibia susceptible to injury, particularly to open fractures and closed spiral fractures. The leg is divided into four compartments (Fig. 27-1) that contain all the muscles, nerves, and blood vessels. The anterior compartment contains four muscles: the tibialis anterior, extensor hallucis

longus, extensor digitorum longus, and peroneus tertius. It also contains the anterior tibial artery, with its vena comitantes, and the deep peroneal nerve that arises from the common peroneal nerve after it passes around the neck of the fibula. This nerve is at risk of damage from external fixator pins or proximal intramedullary cross screws. It may also be injured by fractures of the fibular neck.

The lateral compartment contains two muscles, peroneus longus and brevis. There are two posterior compartments, the superficial and deep. The three muscles in the superficial posterior compartment are the gastrocnemius, plantaris, and soleus. Gastrocnemius and soleus muscle flaps are frequently used to close soft tissue defects associated with proximal tibial diaphyseal fractures. The deep posterior compartment contains flexor digitorum longus,

BOX 27-1 CURRENT CONTROVERSIES IN THE TREATMENT OF TIBIA DIAPHYSEAL FRACTURES

Cast management or intramedullary nailing for closed fractures?
Intramedullary nailing or external fixation for open fractures?
Reamed or unreamed nailing?
How should proximal tibial diaphyseal fractures be treated?
What are the results of primary external fixation and secondary intramedullary nailing?
The management of isolated tibial fractures?
Who gets compartment syndrome after tibial fracture?

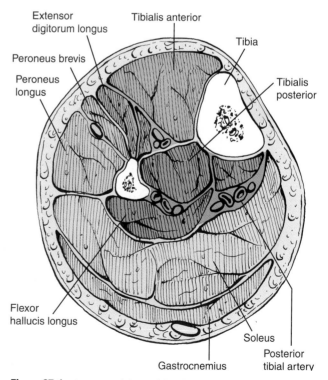

Figure 27-1 Anatomy of the middle of the leg.

flexor hallucis longus, and tibialis posterior muscles as well as the posterior tibial artery, its vena comitantes, and the posterior tibial nerve. Together with the anterior compartment it is often involved in compartment syndrome, and it is damage to the deep posterior muscles that causes the pes cavus and toe contractures commonly associated with missed compartment syndrome. Damage to the posterior tibial nerve may be of importance in determining the requirement for amputation after severe tibial fracture.

CLASSIFICATION

The OTA (AO) classification is widely used for fractures of the tibia and fibula diaphyses (Fig. 27-2). Type A fractures are unifocal and distinguished by the morphology of the fracture (A1 are spiral, A2 are short oblique, and A3 are transverse fractures) and the presence and location of a fibular fracture. The suffix .1 indicates an intact fibula, .2 a fibular fracture distant to the tibial fracture, and .3 a fibular fracture at the same level as the tibial fracture.

Type B fractures are bifocal wedge fractures with B1 containing intact spiral wedge fractures. B2 are intact bending wedge fractures, and B3 are comminuted wedge fractures. The suffix .1 to .3 is the same as for type A fractures. Type C fractures are complex multifragmentary, segmental, or comminuted fractures. C1 fractures are spiral wedge fractures, with the suffix .1 to .3 indicating the number of intermediate fragments. The C2 fractures are segmental, with the suffix .1 to .3 detailing the number of segments and degree of comminution. C3 fractures are comminuted, with .1 to .3 detailing the extent and severity of the comminution.

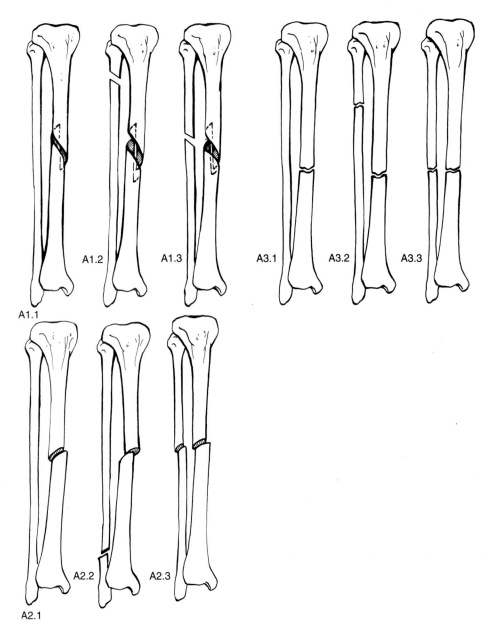

Figure 27-2 The OTA (AO) classification of tibial diaphyseal fractures.

EPIDEMIOLOGY

The basic epidemiology of tibial diaphyseal fractures is shown in Table 27-1. The highest incidence is seen in young men, and most are caused by motor vehicle acci- dents or sports injuries. Falls are the most common cause in the elderly. There is a high incidence of open in- juries compared with other fractures, and about 19% of all tibial fractures are isolated with no associated fibular fracture. Isolated tibial fractures occur in younger

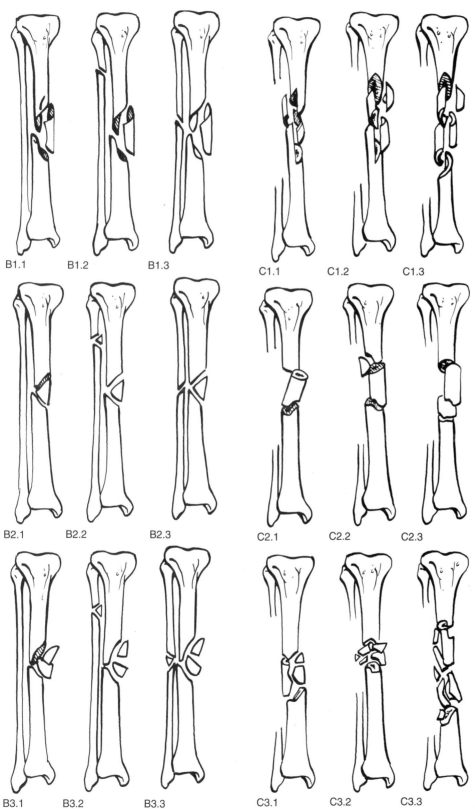

B1.1 B1.2 B1.3 C1.1 C1.2 C1.3

B2.1 B2.2 B2.3 C2.1 C2.2 C2.3

B3.1 B3.2 B3.3 C3.1 C3.2 C3.3 **Figure 27-2** *(continued)*

TABLE 27-1 EPIDEMIOLOGY OF FRACTURES OF THE DIAPHYSES OF THE TIBIA AND FIBULA

Poportion of all fractures	1.9%
Average age	40.0 y
Men/women	61%/39%
Distribution	Type A
Incidence	21.5/10^5/y
Open fractures	19.1%
Most common causes	
Motor vehicle accident	27.8%
Fall	27.8%
Sport	25.2%
OTA (AO) classification	
Type A	61.1%
Type B	16.8%
Type C	22.1%
Most common subgroups	
A1.2	23.0%
A3.3	10.6%
B2.3	8.0%
A2.1	8.0%

The table shows the importance of falls in causing fractures of the tibial diaphysis in the elderly and the severity of the fractures caused by falls from a height and motor vehicle accidents. Sports-related tibial fractures occur in younger patients and tend to be associated with a low incidence of soft tissue injury.

Associated Injuries

Because a significant number of tibial diaphyseal fractures are associated with high-energy injuries, patients may present with a wide range of musculoskeletal injuries and injuries to other body systems. The commonly associated injuries occur in the same limb, however. Analysis shows that about 15% of patients have other musculoskeletal injuries and 2% of patients present with bilateral tibial fractures. About 70% of associated injuries are in the lower limbs, and surgeons should be aware of the possibility of ipsilateral femoral fractures (floating knee) as well as other fractures of the femur, tibia, and foot. There may be damage to the ipsilateral knee ligaments or a knee dislocation. About 4% of tibial diaphyseal fractures are bifocal, with the occurrence of other fractures of the tibial plateau, plafond, or ankle in association with the diaphyseal fracture.

patients with an average age of 30 years. About 90% are OTA (AO) type A fractures, and only 7% are open. About 45% of isolated tibial fractures are caused by sports injuries.

Evidence indicates the epidemiology of tibial diaphyseal fractures is changing in many countries because of improved road safety and the increasing incidence of osteopenic fractures in the elderly. Analysis of tibial diaphyseal fractures in the elderly has shown considerable morbidity and mortality. The mortality at 4 months is about 17%, with 36% mortality in the 85- to 89-year group. Open tibial fracture mortality at 12 months is 33%. This compares with mortality after proximal femoral fractures. An analysis of tibial diaphyseal fractures according to the mode of injury is shown in Table 27-2.

DIAGNOSIS

History and Physical Examination

- Fractures of the tibial diaphysis are usually obvious, the patient presenting with local pain, swelling, and deformity.
- The possibility of a tibial fracture should be considered in all unconscious or severely injured patients, and a thorough physical examination should be undertaken.
- A complete history should be obtained from the patient, relative, or caregiver.
  - The cause of the fracture indicates the extent of the injury and the possibility of coexisting injuries.

TABLE 27-2 EPIDEMIOLOGY OF TIBIAL DIAPHYSEAL FRACTURES ACCORDING TO MODE OF INJURY

Cause	Age (y)	Open (%)	OTA (AO) (%)		
			A	B	C
Motor vehicle accident	35.5	34.4	35.5	22.6	41.9
Fall	55.7	6.2	71.9	12.5	15.6
Sport	23.2	6.9	79.3	17.2	3.5
Fall down stairs	57.7	11.1	77.8	0	22.2
Fall from height	30.6	62.5	25.0	37.5	37.5

- In the elderly the history should involve details about any comorbid conditions, the prefracture ambulatory status, and their domicile because these may alter the treatment and determine outcome.
- Physical examination should include a complete examination of the limb, looking for other injuries.
- The knee, ankle, and hindfoot must be carefully examined and the vascular and neurological status of the leg checked.
- There may be damage to the common peroneal nerve and its branches, the posterior tibial nerve, or the sural and saphenous nerves.
- Proximal diaphyseal fractures in particular may be associated with vascular injury.
- The possibility of compartment syndrome must be considered in all patients with tibial diaphyseal fractures.
  - It may occur within a few hours of the accident, and a thorough examination of the level of pain, sensory loss, muscle function, and pulses is mandatory.
  - Compartment monitoring ideally should be undertaken at this stage (see Chapter 38).

- The soft tissues around the tibial fracture should be examined, looking in particular for an open wound related to the fracture.
- Open fractures require emergency care.
- If there is evidence of skin crushing, the possibility of underlying myonecrosis should be considered.
  - Skin crushing may occur in motor vehicle accidents and in drug addicts, alcoholics, and the elderly, all of whom may lie on the ground or a floor for a prolonged period after fracture.

Radiologic Examination

- Anteroposterior and lateral radiographs should be sufficient to diagnose a tibial diaphyseal fracture (Fig. 27-3).
- The knee and ankle must be included to see if the fracture extends proximally or distally and to check for other musculoskeletal injuries.
- CT scans and MRI scans are not usually required, although MRI scans may be useful to diagnose a stress fracture or an associated ligamentous injury of the knee.

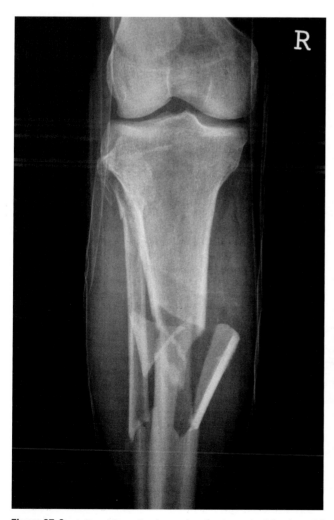
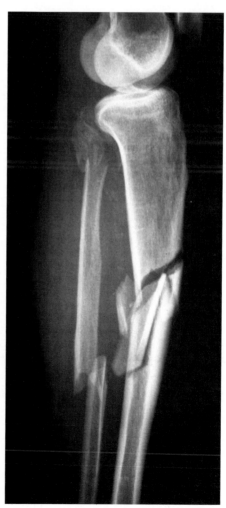

Figure 27-3   A-P and lateral radiographs of a C3.1 tibial diaphyseal fracture.

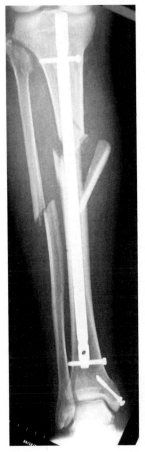
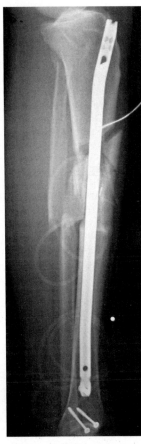

Figure 27-4 A-P and lateral radiographs the tibial diaphyseal fracture shown in Figure 27.3 treated with an antegrade nail. Note the medial malleolar fracture.

■ Arteriography or Doppler studies may be required if there is suspicion of vascular injury.

TREATMENT

Surgical Treatment

■ There are four major treatment methods for tibial diaphyseal fractures: intramedullary nailing, external fixation, plating, and nonoperative management.

■ Other methods are occasionally employed, but surgeons have tended to focus on intramedullary nailing in the last 10 to 15 years.

■ Plating is now less popular, and although nonoperative management is still used for less severe closed tibial diaphyseal fractures, it is now inappropriate to use it in the management of open fractures.

■ Traction should not be used for the management of tibial diaphyseal fractures because it is associated with increased intracompartmental pressure and the effects of prolonged bed rest.

Intramedullary Nailing

■ Both reamed and unreamed nails (see Chapter 33) are used to treat tibial diaphyseal fractures (Fig. 27-4).

■ An analysis of the results of both methods in the management of closed fractures is given in Table 27-3.

■ The table shows that reamed nails in particular give very good results, with a low incidence of infection, nonunion, and malunion.

■ Unreamed nails have a higher incidence of nonunion, indicating that reaming is beneficial in the management of closed tibial diaphyseal fractures.

■ The incidence of joint stiffness is low, regardless of which method is used.

■ In open fractures (Fig. 27-5), the benefit of reaming disappears presumably because of the effect of the considerable soft tissue damage on the prognosis.

■ Table 27-4 contains the results of the use of reamed and unreamed nails in open tibial diaphyseal fractures.

■ All grades of open fracture are included in Table 27-4, which accounts for the slight difference in results between the two procedures.

■ As would be expected, the union time and incidence of nonunion, infection, malunion, and joint stiffness are all higher in open than in closed fractures.

■ There has been considerable interest in the treatment of Gustilo IIIb open tibial fractures by intramedullary nailing, and Table 27-5 contains the results of Gustilo IIIb open tibial diaphyseal fractures treated by both reamed and unreamed nailing.

■ Again, the different fracture grades and definition of outcome account for most of the differences between the two techniques.

■ The results are very good given the severity of these fractures, and comparative studies have shown no

TABLE 27-3 RESULTS OF REAMED AND UNREAMED INTRAMEDULLARY NAILING IN CLOSED TIBIAL FRACTURES

	Reamed Nails		Unreamed Nails	
Result/Complication	Range	Average	Range	Average
Union (wk)	15.4–18	17.1	22.8–32	25.2
Infection (%)	0–2	1.4	0–5.2	1.7
Nonunion (%)	0–4	2.1	11–26.9	15.6
Malunion (%)	0–4	2.1	0–16	5.3
Joint stiffness (%)	7.2–13	8	Minor	Minor

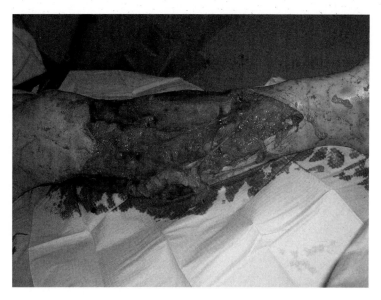

Figure 27-5 A Gustilo IIIb open tibial fracture in a 64-year-old patient. Note the skin degloving.

significant difference between the two nailing techniques.
- The complications of tibial nailing are discussed in Chapter 33.

External Fixation
- There has been considerable debate about the ideal type or configuration of external fixator and the ideal stiffness with which tibial diaphyseal fractures should be held by a fixator. There are three basic designs of external fixator: the uniplanar fixator (Fig. 27-6), applied to the subcutaneous border of the tibia; the multiplanar device, which can be constructed in many different configurations (Fig. 27-7); and the ring fixator, which is usually applied with fine wires rather than half pins (Fig. 27-8). Ring fixators have been used for the primary management of tibial diaphyseal fractures, but their use is usually confined to the management of tibial nonunion or infection. The results of the use of uniplanar and multiplanar external fixators in mixed series of both open and closed tibial diaphyseal fractures are given in Table 27-6, and the results of the use of external fixation in Gustilo type IIIb open fractures are given in Table 27-7.

- External fixation is usually used for treatment of open tibial fractures, which accounts for the prolonged union time and the higher incidences of infection and nonunion in Table 27-6.
  - The results of the two types of fixator are remarkably similar.
  - Studies of the use of the Ilizarov ring fixator have shown results that are also similar to those associated with the use of uniplanar and multiplanar external fixation.
  - Clinical studies show no evidence that one type or configuration of external fixator gives superior results to another type.
  - If external fixation is used to treat tibial fractures, it is suggested the simplest frame appropriate for the fracture morphology be applied.
- Precise comparison of external fixation and intramedullary nailing is difficult because of the problems of analysis of different fracture types and the adoption of different outcome criteria in different studies.
- Comparison of the results shown in Tables 27-3 to 27-7 suggests that external fixation is associated with a higher incidence of nonunion and malunion compared with intramedullary nailing, although there is a similar incidence of infection.

TABLE 27-4 RESULTS OF REAMED AND UNREAMED INTRAMEDULLARY NAILING IN OPEN TIBIAL FRACTURES

Result/Complication	Reamed Nails		Unreamed Nails	
	Range	Average	Range	Average
Union (wk)	30.2–33.2	32.3	26.4–31.1	29.3
Infection (%)	5.4–9.7	6.5	2.4–12	6.2
Nonunion (%)	8–36.3	14	4–48.3	21.4
Malunion (%)	4.2–6	5.5	0–49	9.2
Joint stiffness (%)	14–36.6	21.5	38	38

TABLE 27-5 RESULTS OF REAMED AND UNREAMED INTRAMEDULLARY NAILING IN GUSTILO IIIB TIBIAL FRACTURES

Result/Complication	Reamed Nails		Unreamed Nails	
	Range	Average	Range	Average
Union (wk)	39–50.1	43.4	23–40.3	32.4
Infection (%)	11–23.1	15.1	5.9–25	15.4
Nonunion (%)	17–69.2	36.4	17.6–80	30.8
Malunion (%)	5–15.4	9.1	0–41.2	13.2
Joint stiffness (%)	32–84.6	51.5	35.3	35.3

- Joint stiffness has not been adequately measured in papers dealing with external fixation, but clearly pin tract sepsis is relatively common.
- Studies directly comparing intramedullary nailing and external fixation have shown that intramedullary nailing of open fractures gives better results than external fixation.
- In particular, final function is better with patients treated by intramedullary nailing, showing improved hindfoot function and walking distance.
- Union tends to be faster and fewer secondary procedures are associated with intramedullary nailing than external fixation.
- There is still debate about the use of intramedullary nailing in Gustilo IIIb fractures, but most surgeons now accept its use in other open fracture grades.
- Primary external fixation and secondary intramedullary nailing is used in "damage control surgery" for the management of tibial diaphyseal fractures in severely injured patients (see Chapter 3).
- Results of the use of this technique are given in Table 27-8.

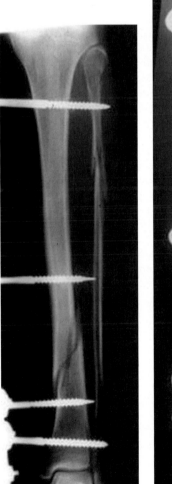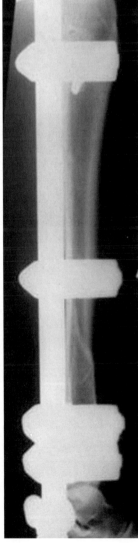

Figure 27-6 A-P and lateral radiographs of a uniplanar external fixator.

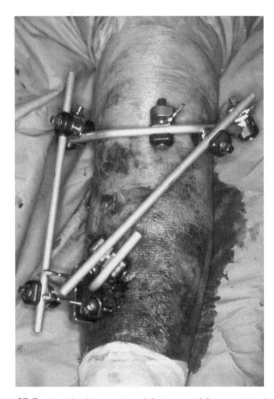

Figure 27-7 A multiplanar external fixator used for a proximal tibial diaphyseal fracture.

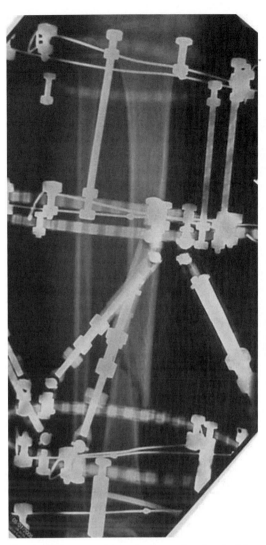
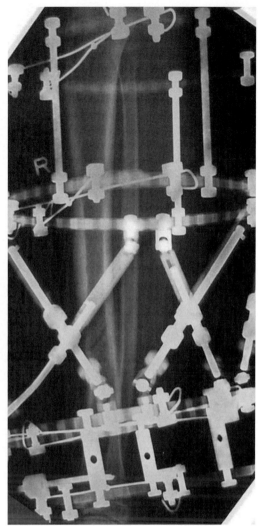

Figure 27-8 A-P and lateral radiographs of a tibial fracture treated with a fine wire ring external fixator.

■ This shows a considerable variation in the duration of external fixation and the delay between removal of the external fixator and intramedullary nailing.

■ Overall, the pin tract sepsis rate is similar to other studies (Table 27-7), although the infection rate is higher than for primary intramedullary nailing.

■ Studies of the technique have suggested it is safer if intramedullary nailing is not undertaken in the presence of discharging pin sites, and a primary exchange can be undertaken if there is no evidence of pin tract sepsis.

TABLE 27-6 RESULTS OF UNIPLANAR AND MULTIPLANAR EXTERNAL FIXATION IN TIBIAL DIAPHYSEAL FRACTURES

Result/Complication	Uniplanar		Multiplanar	
	Range	Average	Range	Average
Open fractures (%)	8.2–100	95.8	76–100	93.1
Union (wk)	20–31.3	25.1	24.7–42.9	30.7
Nonunion (%)	6.2–14	9.4	6.6–41.4	18.6
Infection (%)	0–11.4	5.4	3–26	9.7
Malunion (%)	0–38.6	24.5	3–50	27.9
Refracture (%)	0–4	2.4	3–12.1	2.9
Joint stiffness (%)	10.6–50	31.7	4–50	22.3

TABLE 27-7 RESULTS OF EXTERNAL FIXATION IN GUSTILO IIIB TIBIAL DIAPHYSEAL FRACTURES

Result/Complication	Range	Average
Union time (wk)	23.8–37.7	34
Nonunion (%)	14.2–60	26.7
Infection (%)	11.1–38	16.1
Malunion (%)	9–50	18.9
Refracture (%)	0–6.6	1
Pin sepsis (%)	21.4–100	32.6

- There is a higher deep infection rate if the delay between external fixator removal and intramedullary nailing is prolonged.
- Given the success of primary intramedullary nailing, the only indication for primary external fixation and secondary nailing is in the severely injured patient where rapid primary surgical management is important.

Plating

- Primary plating of tibial diaphyseal fractures (Fig. 27-9) is now less common than 10 years ago.
- The results from the literature are given in Table 27-9.
- Most articles refer to mixed series of closed and open fractures, which accounts for the wide variation in results.
- Plating can give good results, but it is technically more difficult than intramedullary nailing or external fixation.
- It should be remembered that the papers dealing with the management of open tibial fractures were written prior to the introduction of free flaps and fasciocutaneous flaps.
- Thus the results of Table 27-9 are good, although it is unlikely an open surgical method will be consistently better than a closed method of treatment such as intramedullary nailing.

Nonsurgical Treatment

- There are three basic methods for treating tibial diaphyseal fractures nonoperatively: the long-leg cast, the patellar-tendon-bearing cast designed to permit knee

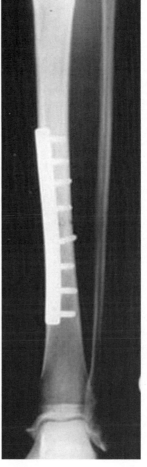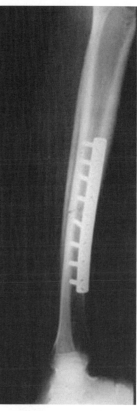

Figure 27-9 A-P and lateral radiographs of a tibial diaphyseal fracture treated with a dynamic compression plate.

movement, and the functional brace designed to allow both knee and hindfoot movement (see Chapter 31).
- The results of all three methods are given in Table 27-10.
  - As with plating, much of the literature concerning nonoperative management was written some time ago.
  - Outcome criteria were somewhat different, and it was often difficult to separate the incidence of delayed union and nonunion.

TABLE 27-8 RESULTS OF PRIMARY EXTERNAL FIXATION AND SECONDARY INTRAMEDULLARY NAILING IN TIBIAL DIAPHYSEAL FRACTURES

Result/Complication	Range	Average
External fixation (wk)	2.4–12	6.1
Delay before nailing (wk)	1.3–31.1	4.2
Pin sepsis (%)	0–100	24.3
Infection (%)	0–66	18.4

TABLE 27-9 RESULTS OF PLATING IN THE MANAGEMENT OF OPEN AND CLOSED TIBIAL DIAPHYSEAL FRACTURES

Result/Complication	Range	Average
Open (%)	0–100	35.9
Union time (wk)	12–42.5	32.1
Nonunion (%)	0–54	9.5
Infection (%)	1–19	4.8
Malunion (%)	2–16.7	7.4
Refracture (%)	0–4.8	2.6
Fixation failure (%)	0–12	3.8

TABLE 27-10 USE OF NONOPERATIVE MANAGEMENT FOR TIBIAL DIAPHYSEAL FRACTURES

Results/Complications	Long-Leg Casts		Patellar-Tendon-Bearing Casts		Functional Braces	
	Range	Average	Range	Average	Range	Average
Open fractures (%)	12–36.3	24.4	0–21	8.4	7.2–31.4	26
Union time (wk)	13.7–19.8	16.5	13.6–26	17.3	15.5–18.7	18
Malunion (%)	9.1–50	15.7	4.4–40	26.4	8.6–40	16.3
Delayed and nonunion (%)	6–24.1	20.4	9.6–27-2	12.3	7.2–32	19.5
Joint stiffness (%)	7–42	26.3	15–43	36.1	26–45	34.6

■ The incidence of nonunion is higher with nonoperative than with operative treatment, however.

■ The incidence of malunion is relatively high as is the incidence of hindfoot stiffness.

■ The problems associated with hindfoot stiffness are often underestimated, but studies have indicated that only 47% of patients managed nonoperatively report a good or excellent result, and only 27% report no problems with running.

■ More recent studies of nonoperative management have tended to concentrate on less severe fractures as surgeons have adopted operative treatment for the more severe fractures.

■ The technique still has a place in the treatment of low-energy fractures in young patients in whom union is rapid and the incidence of hindfoot stiffness is low.

■ Table 27-10 illustrates the problems involved in treating more complex fractures nonoperatively.

■ A number of studies have directly compared intramedullary nailing and nonoperative treatment, and all have favored intramedullary nailing.

■ They have highlighted the improved rates of union and better functional outcome associated with intramedullary nailing.

■ A recent study has suggested that intramedullary nailing is cheaper than nonoperative treatment when complications and time off work is taken into consideration.

■ Table 27-10 also highlights the fact that patellar-tendon-bearing casts and functional braces give the same results as long-leg casts.

■ There is also evidence that tibial diaphyseal malunion is associated with an increased incidence of subtalar stiffness, although it would appear the incidence of knee osteoarthritis after tibial diaphyseal fractures is not influenced by malunion.

Suggested Treatment

The suggested treatment of tibial diaphyseal fractures is shown in Table 27-11.

COMPLICATIONS

■ The incidence of nonunion, infection, and malunion is given in Tables 27-3 to 27-10, and the treatment of

TABLE 27-11 SUGGESTED TREATMENT OF TIBIAL DIAPHYSEAL FRACTURES

Injury	Management
Undisplaced fractures (closed)	Patella-tendon-bearing cast
Displaced fractures (any displacement)	
Closed	Reamed intramedullary nailing
Open	Reamed or unreamed intramedullary nailing
Proximal diaphyseal fractures	
Good alignment	Intramedullary nailing
Poor alignment	Locked plating or periarticular external fixation
Distal diaphyseal fractures	
Outwith 4 cm of ankle joint	Intramedullary nailing
Within 4 cm of ankle joint	
Transverse fracture	Reamed intramedullary nailing
Other fractures	Locked plating or periarticular external fixation
Isolated tibial fractures (intact fibula)	
A3.1 transverse (undisplaced)	Patella-tendon-bearing cast
Others	Intramedullary nailing
Multiply injured	Consider damage control surgery (see Fig. 3-4 in Chapter 3)

TABLE 27-12 PRIMARY AND SECONDARY AMPUTATION RATES IN GUSTILO IIIB AND IIIC OPEN TIBIAL DIAPHYSEAL FRACTURES

Gustilo Grade	Primary Amputation (%)		Secondary Amputation (%)	
	Range	Average	Range	Average
IIIb	0–7	5.2	4.7–23.5	11.9
IIIc	22.2–42.8	34.8	42.8–100	60

these complications is dealt with in the appropriate chapters. There are, however, a number of other complications associated with tibial diaphyseal fracture.

Compartment Syndrome

■ Compartment syndrome is an important complication of tibial diaphyseal fractures. Its incidence, detection, and treatment are discussed in Chapter 38.

Reflex Sympathetic Dystrophy

■ It has been estimated that up to 30% of patients with tibial diaphyseal fractures show signs of reflex sympathetic dystrophy (RSD) (see Chapter 41).
■ Most cases are mild.
■ There is no relationship between the type of treatment and the incidence of RSD.
■ In 78% of patients, the condition resolves within 6 months, but in the remaining 22% there is an association between the severity of the condition and failure of the patient to return to work.

Amputation

■ The indications and techniques of amputation are discussed in Chapter 37.
■ With improved surgical technique the rate of amputation should have decreased, but with increasing numbers of elderly patients being treated there is still a significant amputation rate for both Gustilo IIIb and IIIc open tibial fractures.

■ The rates of primary and secondary amputations are shown in Table 27-12.

SPECIAL CIRCUMSTANCES

Proximal Diaphyseal Fractures

■ Fractures of the proximal tibial diaphysis occur in 5% to 12% of patients depending on the type of institution.
■ They are usually high-energy injuries with 80% occurring in motor vehicle accidents.
■ Over 50% of the fractures have an OTA (AO) type B or C configuration.
■ They are associated with a higher incidence of vascular injury and compartment syndrome.
■ Treatment is more difficult than with fractures of the middle or distal thirds of the diaphysis.
■ Some low-energy proximal tibial diaphyseal fractures may be treated nonoperatively, but nowadays most fractures are treated surgically.
■ The options are intramedullary nailing, plating using a conventional dynamic compression plate or a LISS plate, or external fixation usually using a semicircular hybrid frame or a ring fixator.
■ The comparative results of four treatment methods, given in Table 27-13, show the results of intramedullary nailing are poor.
■ The major problem is malunion, either excessive anterior angulation or a valgus deformity (Fig. 27-10).
   ■ This can be minimized by a number of techniques.
■ It has been suggested that a lateral starting point may be used to reduce the incidence of malalignment, but it is better either to use a temporary external fixator to reduce and hold the fracture while the nail is inserted or to use blocking screws.
■ These screws can be used to correct anterior angulation and valgus malalignment. Figure 27-11 shows a diagrammatic representation of their use.
■ The literature suggests the malunion rate associated with the use of blocking screws is about 9%.
■ Plate fixation is associated with a relatively high infection rate, although the use of the LISS plate (Fig. 27-12) with a minimally invasive approach reduces the rate of infection, possibly at the expense of increased malunion.
■ The results of external fixation (see Fig. 27-7) are good, although the incidence of nonunion is higher than for the other techniques.

TABLE 27-13 RESULTS OF TREATING PROXIMAL TIBIAL DIAPHYSEAL FRACTURES

Results/Complications	Conventional Plate (%)		LISS Plate[a] (%)		IM Nail (%)		External Fixation (%)	
	Range	Average	Range	Average	Range	Average	Range	Average
Open fractures	0–33	12.5	0–3.7	3.6	0–11.1	2.5	0–14.3	3
Nonunion	0–20	2.5	3–4.5	3.6	0–18.7	3	0–12.8	7.9
Malunion	0–40	8.7	9.2–11.6	10.8	0–68.7	20.1	0–42.8	4
Implant failure	0	0	0	0	0–2.5	7.5	0	0

[a]The LISS plate results are taken from series treating both plateau fractures and proximal diaphyseal fractures.

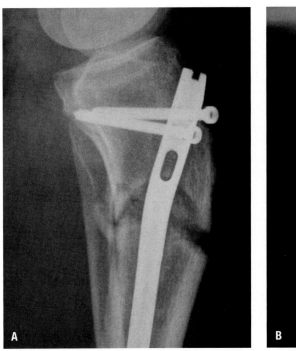

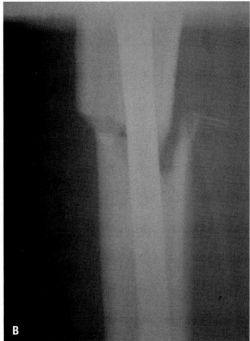

Figure 27-10   Nailing of proximal fractures may be complicated by excessive anterior angulation (**A**) or valgus deformity (**B**).

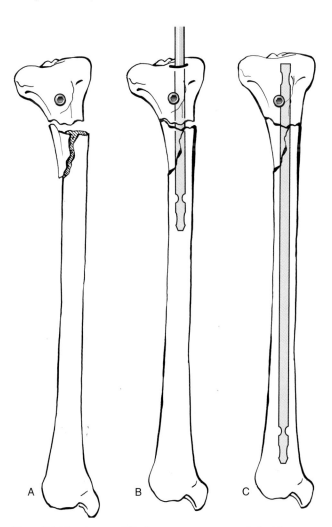

Figure 27-11   The use of blocking screws in proximal tibial fractures.

■ There is no evidence that one type of fixator is superior to another, and most surgeons use a semicircular or circular proximal bar with fine wires or half pins and a conventional diaphyseal construction.

■ Table 27-13 indicates that for proximal tibial diaphyseal fractures, subcutaneous minimally invasive plating or external fixation gives the best results.

Distal Tibial Fractures

■ Most distal tibial diaphyseal fractures can be treated by intramedullary nailing, and nailing is straightforward up to within 4 cm of the ankle joint.

■ Distal to this point nailing is more difficult, particularly if the fracture is oblique or comminuted.

■ Modern intramedullary nails allow the use of very distal cross screws, but it is important to insert two distal cross screws to prevent malalignment.

■ Any associated intra-articular extensions should be stabilized with interfragmentary screws prior to nailing.

■ If the fracture is considered unnailable, either plates or external fixation can be used as described for the treatment of extra-articular tibial plafond fractures.

Isolated Tibial Fractures

■ Until comparatively recently there was considerable debate whether an intact fibula conferred a better or worse prognosis for a tibial diaphyseal fracture.

■ These fractures occur in younger patients.

■ They are usually low-energy injuries with a predominantly OTA (AO) type A fracture morphology (Fig. 27-13).

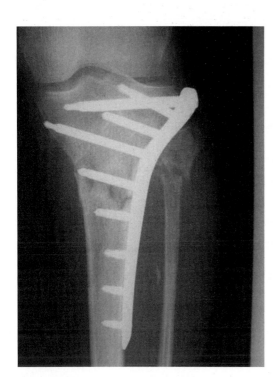
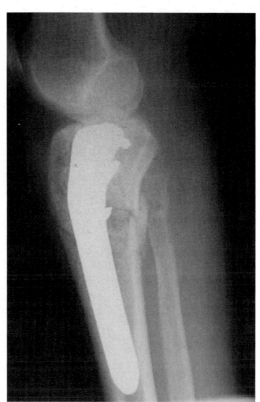

Figure 27-12   A-P and lateral radiographs of a LISS plate used to treat a proximal tibial diaphyseal fracture.

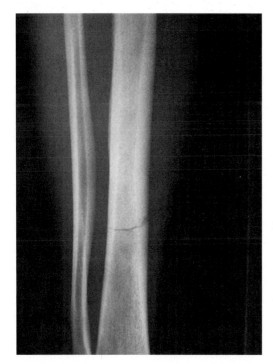
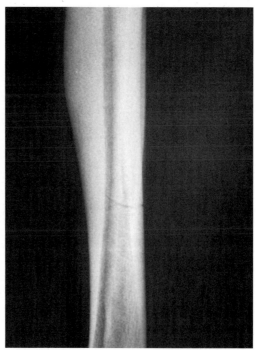

Figure 27-13   A-P and lateral radiographs of an A3.1 isolated tibial fracture.

TABLE 27-14 RESULTS OF TREATING ISOLATED TIBIAL DIAPHYSEAL FRACTURES

Result/Complication	Nonoperative (%)		Reamed IM Nailing (%)		External Fixation (%)	
	Range	Average	Range	Average	Range	Average
Nonunion	0–8.7	3.1	0	0	0	0
Varus deformity	26.4–59.9	32	0	0	0–50	17.6
Refracture	13.7	13.7	0	0	0–33.3	11.8

- Table 27-14 gives the results for nonoperative management, reamed intramedullary nailing, and external fixation.
  - There are very few studies of the operative management of these fractures, but Table 27-14 shows that although the nonunion rate is low, the use of nonoperative management is associated with a very high rate of varus malalignment and a high incidence of refracture.
- It has been shown the only isolated tibial fracture that maintains its position in a cast is the A3.1 transverse fracture.
- All other fracture types tend to displace and should be managed operatively using a reamed intramedullary nail.

Isolated Fibular Fractures

- Most "isolated fibular fractures" are either type C ankle fractures (see Chapter 29) or avulsion fractures of the proximal fibula associated with a knee ligamentous injury (see Chapter 26).
- True isolated fibular fractures are very rare.
- They are usually caused by a fall or a direct blow.
- Treatment is symptomatic with supportive strapping or a below-knee walking cast or brace used.
- Nonunions are extremely rare and best treated by plating and grafting if symptomatic.
- Proximal fibular fractures may cause damage to the superficial peroneal nerve.

Combined Ipsilateral Femoral and Tibial Fractures (Floating Knee)

The management of this condition is detailed in Chapter 23.

Open Fractures

The management of open fractures of the tibia is discussed in Chapter 4.

Bifocal Fractures

- About 4% of tibial diaphyseal fractures are associated with fractures of the plateau, plafond, or ankle, although the combination of diaphyseal and plafond fractures is very rare.
- Most bifocal fractures involve the plateau or ankle.

- The combination of diaphyseal and plateau fractures is best treated by either subcutaneous minimally invasive plating using the LISS system or an external fixator applied as for a proximal tibial diaphyseal fracture (see Fig. 27-7).
- Ankle fractures associated with diaphyseal fractures are treated conventionally using intrafragmentary screws and plates.
- It is important to check if there is an associated posterior malleolar fragment, which may be displaced with the passage of an intramedullary nail.
  - If there is, it should be fixed by intrafragmentary screws prior to nailing.

SUGGESTED READING

Court-Brown CM. Fractures of the tibial and fibula. In: Bucholz RW, Heckman JD, eds. Rockwood and Green's fractures in adults, 5th ed. Philadelphia: Lippincott Williams and Wilkins, 2001:1939–2000.

Court-Brown CM, Christie J, McQueen MM. Closed intramedullary tibial nailing. Its use in closed and type 1 open fractures. J Bone Joint Surg (Br) 1990;72:605–611.

Court-Brown CM, McQueen MM, Quaba AA, et al. Locked intramedullary nailing of open tibial fractures. J Bone Joint Surg (Br) 1991;73:959–964.

Court-Brown CM, Will E, Christie J, et al. Reamed or unreamed nailing for closed tibial fractures. J Bone Joint Surg (Br) 1996; 78:580–583.

Gaebler C, Berger U, Schandelmaier P, et al. Rates and odds ratios for complications in closed and open tibial fractures treated with unreamed, small diameter nails: a multicenter analysis of 467 cases. J Orthop Trauma 2001:15:415–423.

Keating JF, O'Brien PJ, Blachut PA. Interlocking intramedullary nailing of open fractures of the tibia. A prospective, randomised comparison of reamed and unreamed nails. J Bone Joint Surg (Am) 1997;79:334–341.

Müller ME, Nazarian S, Koch P, et al. The comprehensive classification of fractures of long bones. Berlin: Springer-Verlag, 1990.

Riemer BL, DiChristina DG, Cooper A, et al. Nonreamed nailing of tibial diaphyseal fractures in blunt polytrauma patients. J Orthop Trauma 1995;9:66–75.

Sarmiento AA, Gersten LM, Sobol PA, et al. Treated shaft fractures treated with functional braces. Experience with 780 fractures. J Bone Joint Surg (Br) 1989;71:602–609.

Schandelmaier P, Krettek C, Rudolf J, et al. Superior results of tibial rodding versus external fixation in grade 3b fractures. Clin Orthop 1997;342:164–172.

Tornetta P, Bergman M, Watnik N, et al. Treatment of grade-IIIb open tibial fractures. A prospective randomised comparison of external fixation and non-reamed locked nailing. J Bone Joint Surg (Br) 1994;75:13–19.

28 TIBIAL PLAFOND FRACTURES

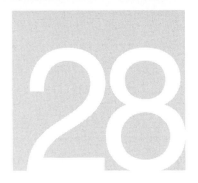

Fractures of the tibial plafond, or pilon fractures, are relatively uncommon. They are frequently high-energy injuries associated with other musculoskeletal damage. They are notoriously difficult to treat, and a high complication rate is associated with all forms of management. The traditional treatment method was plating using AO techniques, but in recent years there has been a shift toward external fixation, often combined with minimal internal fixation. Results have improved somewhat but they remain problematic, and the outcome is poor in many cases. A list of some of the current controversies in the treatment of tibial plafond fractures is given in Box 28-1.

SURGICAL ANATOMY

Tibial plafond fractures are caused by axial loading of the ankle joint. The distal tibia consists of five surfaces: the inferior, anterior, posterior, lateral, and medial (Fig. 28-1). The inferior surface is articular, concave anteroposteriorly, and slightly convex transversely. The inferior surface is wider laterally than medially. The posterior border is lower than the anterior border and in continuity with the posterior surface of the medial malleolus. The lateral articular surface of the ankle joint is formed by the distal fibula.

The dome of the talus is trapezoidal, with the anterior surface broader than the posterior surface. The medial and lateral talar articular facets are contiguous with the distal

tibial articular facets (see Fig. 28-1). The base of the dome of the talus is denser than the distal tibia, and thus talar dome fractures rarely occur in association with tibial plafond fractures. The ligaments, tendons, and neurovascular structures around the ankle joint are illustrated in Figure 29-2. Because plafond fractures are caused by axial loading, rather than rotation, injury to these structures is unusual.

CLASSIFICATION

The original classification of intra-articular plafond fractures was that of Ruëdi and Allgöwer (1979). They divided plafond fractures into three types based on the degree of comminution and displacement. Type 1 injuries are cleavage fractures

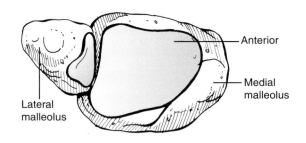
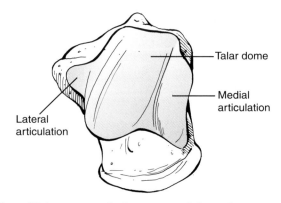

Figure 28-1 Anatomy of inferior aspect of tibia and superior aspect of talus.

BOX 28-1 CURRENT CONTROVERSIES IN THE MANAGEMENT OF TIBIAL PLAFOND FRACTURES

Type A fractures: plating or external fixation?
Type C fractures: Is external fixation better than plating?
What type of external fixator should be used?
Is secondary plating better than primary plating?
Is there a role for intramedullary nailing?
Is compartment syndrome a problem?
What is the incidence of complications?

---

of the distal tibia without significant displacement. Type 2 fractures are displaced but without significant intra-articular or metaphyseal comminution. The type 3 fractures show metaphyseal and/or intra-articular comminution. The Ruëdi-Allgöwer classification has the merit of being brief and easy to remember, but it does not describe the extra-articular or partial articular plafond fractures.

The Ruëdi-Allgöwer classification was extended to the OTA (AO) classification (Fig. 28-2). Type A fractures are extra-articular with A1 fractures having a simple metaphyseal configuration. A2 fractures have a metaphyseal wedge, and A3 fractures are comminuted metaphyseal fractures. In A1 fractures, the suffix .1 to .3 describes the direction of the fracture with .1 spiral, .2 oblique, and .3 transverse. In A2 fractures, .1 refers to posterolateral impaction, .2 to the presence of an anteromedial wedge, and .3 to the fact that the fracture line extends into the diaphysis. In A3 fractures, .1 refers to the presence of three intermediate fragments, .2 to more than three intermediate fragments, and .3 to a fracture extending into the diaphysis.

Type B fractures are partial articular fractures with B1 fractures, split fractures; B2 fractures, split depression; and B3, multifragmentary depression fractures. The suffix .1 to .3 refers to the same characteristics in all three groups. Frontal fractures are .1, sagittal fractures are .2, and metaphyseal multifragmentary fractures are .3.

The type C fractures are those originally described by Ruëdi and Allgöwer. C1 fractures have a simple intra-articular metaphyseal configuration with .1 describing fractures without impaction, .2 fractures with impaction, and .3 fractures extending into the diaphysis. C2 fractures have a simple articular morphology with metaphyseal fragmentation, with .1 referring to impacted fractures, .2 to unimpacted fractures, and .3 to diaphyseal involvement. C3 fractures are the Ruëdi III fractures with extensive articular and metaphyseal damage. The suffix .1 refers to the fact that the comminution is epiphyseal in location. In .2 fractures, it is epiphysiometaphyseal, and in .3 fractures. the comminution extends into the diaphysis.

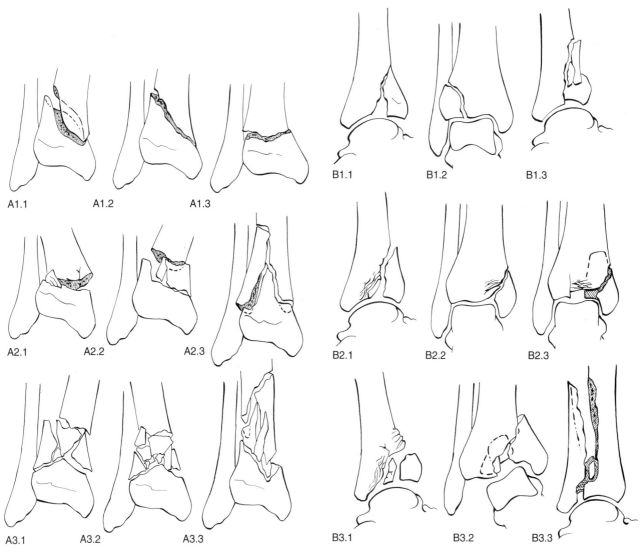

Figure 28-2 The OTA (AO) classification of tibial plafond fractures. *(continued)*

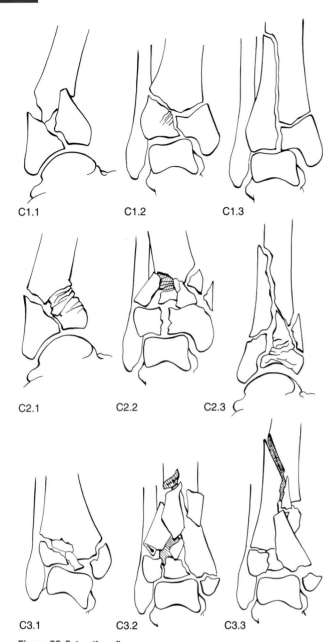

C1.1   C1.2   C1.3

C2.1   C2.2   C2.3

C3.1   C3.2   C3.3

Figure 28-2 *(continued)*

TABLE 28-1 EPIDEMIOLOGY OF TIBIAL PLAFOND FRACTURES	
Proportion of all fractures	0.7%
Average age	39.1 y
Men/women	57%/43%
Distribution	Type D
Incidence	$7.9/10^5/y$
Open fractures	16.6%
Most common causes	
Fall from height	28.5%
Fall	26.2%
Motor vehicle accident	16.6%
Sport	11.9%
OTA (AO) classification	
Type A	40.5%
Type B	30.9%
Type C	28.6%
Most common subgroups	
A1.3	19.0%
B1.1	14.3%
C1.3	11.9%

of posterior malleolar fractures associated with tibial diaphyseal fractures. The most common intra-articular fractures are the C1.3 and C2.3 fractures with a diaphyseal extension. Multifragmentary C3 fractures account for 11.6% of plafond fractures.

Table 28-2 shows that younger patients are injured in falls from a height and sports injuries. Older patients tend to be injured in simple falls and have type A or B fractures. Patients injured in motor vehicle accidents tend to be younger vehicle drivers or older pedestrians.

Associated Injuries

The most common associated injuries are in the ipsilateral leg involving other fractures in the tibia or hindfoot. About 15% of patients have other fractures of the tibia, and 9% have fractures of the axial skeleton. The literature suggests that in level 1 trauma centers up to 8% of plafond fractures are bilateral.

EPIDEMIOLOGY

The epidemiology of tibial plafond fractures is shown in Table 28-1. They have a type D (see Chapter 1) distribution with a unimodal distribution affecting young men and a bimodal female distribution. Open fractures are common with a high incidence of Gustilo type III fractures. There is also a high incidence of associated injuries, with the large European and U.S. level 1 trauma centers reporting up to 55% of patients with associated injuries. The most common subgroups are the A1.3 and B1.1 fractures. The A1.3 subgroup contains a combination of young adults with physeal fractures and elderly patients with transverse insufficiency fractures. The B1.1 group is mainly composed

TABLE 28-2 EPIDEMIOLOGY OF TIBIAL PLAFOND FRACTURES ACCORDING TO THE MODE OF INJURY					
			OTA (AO) Type (%)		
Cause	Age (y)	Open	A	B	C
Fall from height	27.3	25.0	33.3	25.0	41.7
Fall	46.6	9.1	45.4	27.3	27.3
Motor vehicle accident	46.3	42.8	28.6	28.6	42.9
Sport	32.5	0	20.0	60.0	20.0

DIAGNOSIS

History and Physical Examination

- A careful clinical history must be obtained.
- Most patients are young and relatively fit, but the mode of injury may draw attention to the presence of other injuries.
- Patients who have high-energy injuries should be examined according to ATLS principles.
- Neurovascular examination is important.
- Vascular injuries are unusual, but the incidence of compartment syndrome is higher than was previously thought so its signs should be looked for.
- Compartment monitoring is advocated in high-energy injuries.
- Neural damage is also rare but may be associated with later treatment, particularly if fine wires are used around the ankle.
  - The absence of neural damage prior to treatment should be documented.
- Open fractures are relatively common, and the soft tissues should be carefully examined for contamination and associated injuries.
- Degloving in the elderly should always be considered.

- In high-energy fractures there may be considerable soft tissue swelling, and the presence of epidermal blistering or more serious hemorrhagic blistering should be noted.

Radiologic Examination

- Anteroposterior and lateral radiographs are sufficient to diagnose most plafond fractures (Fig. 28-3).
- The extent of articular comminution is often difficult to determine using plain radiographs, and CT scanning is helpful (see Fig. 28-3).
- Anteroposterior and lateral radiographs of the hindfoot, tibia, and knee should be obtained.
- Angiography or Doppler studies are rarely required.

TREATMENT

- There has been considerable debate over the timing of definitive treatment of tibial plafond fractures.
- The presence of significant soft tissue injury associated with high-energy plafond fractures has understandably caused surgeons to be reluctant to operate until the state of the soft tissues has improved.

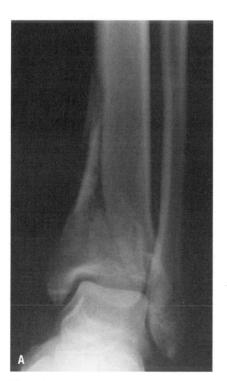
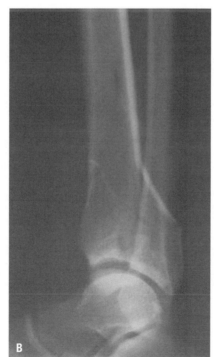
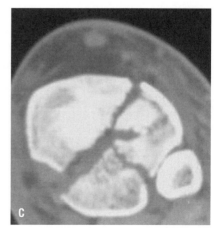

Figure 28-3 (A,B) A-P and lateral radiographs of a C1.3 tibial plafond fracture. (C) A CT scan shows the extent of the intra-articular damage.

■ Unfortunately this is difficult to assess, and inevitably the timing of treatment is a judgment between the state of the soft tissues and the increased difficulty of late surgery.

■ The traditional method of management of type C fractures has been plating through two incisions, one over the distal fibula and the second lateral to the crest of the tibia (Fig. 28-4).

  ■ The fibula was reduced and plated to assist with stability and reduction of the tibial plafond.

  ■ After reduction of fibula plating, a second plate was applied to the tibia.

■ The complications associated with this technique were considerable, and in recent years surgeons have moved toward external fixation, usually combined with minimal internal fixation techniques.

■ Minimally invasive plating using smaller incisions, indirect reduction techniques, and fluoroscopy has also become more popular.

■ External fixation may be used as definitive management or may be applied for a short period to allow the state of the soft tissues to improve.

■ Definitive secondary plating can then be undertaken.

Nonsurgical Treatment

■ The results of nonoperative treatment of displaced intra-articular plafond fractures are poor, and the technique has not been in widespread use for over 30 years.

■ Comparative studies have shown only 54% good and excellent results, with only 32% adequate fracture reduction achieved.

■ Nonoperative treatment should be confined to undisplaced plafond fractures. These are usually type A insufficiency fractures, although occasionally other fracture configurations present without displacement.

■ Treatment involves the use of a below-knee cast or brace and non-weight-bearing mobilization for 10 to 12 weeks.

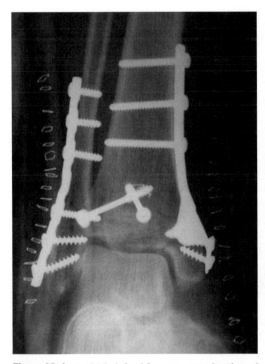 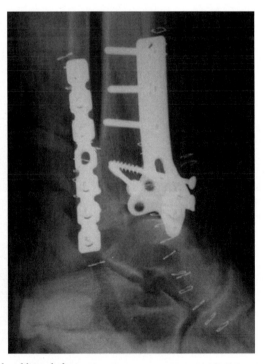

Figure 28-4   A tibial plafond fracture treated with medial and lateral plates.

TABLE 28-3 RESULTS OF THE USE OF TRADITIONAL OPEN PLATING, MINIMALLY INVASIVE PLATING, AND PRIMARY TRANSARTICULAR EXTERNAL FIXATION WITH DELAYED PLATING

Result/Complication	Open Plating +/– Grafting (%)		Minimally Invasive Plating +/– Grafting (%)		Delayed Plating +/– Grafting (%)	
	Range	Average	Range	Average	Range	Average
Excellent/good	25–85.2	59.8	?	?	77–81	79.7
Open	0–52.9	22.6	10–46.4	31.2	28.6–75	43
Skin slough	3–33.3	13.2	0–25	14.6	0–17	5.3
Infection	5.9–33.3	12.1	0–25	14.6	0–12.5	5.2
Nonunion	0–16.6	7.5	?	?	0–4.8	0.9
Malunion	0–13.3	7.5	0–10	4.2	0–4.8	1.7
Moderate/severe osteoarthritis	11.7–51.2	26.7	28.6	28.6	0–28	12.1
Arthrodesis	10–26.6	14.4	28.6	28.6	0–10.8	6

Note: The incidence of primary bone grafting varies between the groups.

Surgical Treatment

Plating

■ The results of open plating, minimally invasive plating, and delayed plating are given in Table 28-3.
■ The two major complications of open plating are skin sloughing and infection.
  ■ These relate to the significant soft tissue injury associated with the fracture.
■ Surgical incisions are difficult to close after plating, and infection and skin sloughing are relatively common.
■ The incidence of nonunion in plating is difficult to evaluate because primary bone grafting is frequently used, an essential part of the technique of rigid plating in comminuted fractures.
  ■ On average about 7% of plafond fractures remain ununited after plating.
■ The incidence of osteoarthritis and late ankle arthrodesis varies somewhat between the techniques, but different studies have used different follow-up periods, and obviously the incidence of osteoarthritis tends to increase with time.
■ There have been very few studies of minimally invasive plating of plafond fracture, but early results do not suggest this technique confers much advantage over open plating.
■ In delayed plating, a transarticular frame is used to support the fracture while the condition of the soft tissue improves.
■ Definitive plating is usually undertaken 2 to 3 weeks after the fracture.
■ Overall the fractures treated by this method have been more severe with a higher incidence of open fractures than in the other two plating methods.
■ Bearing this in mind, the results for this technique are very good, with about 80% excellent and good results.

■ The literature suggests about 5% of patients still experience a degree of skin sloughing, but in most studies this is superficial and not as troublesome as the skin sloughing associated with open primary plating.
■ Percutaneous plating techniques have been developed recently using locking plate technology.
  ■ As yet there are few results of this technique, but it seems likely it will be as useful as it is in tibial plateau fractures.
  ■ It is probable that it will prove very useful in type A extra-articular fractures.
■ Surgeons should be aware of the high incidence of compartment syndrome in high-energy plafond fractures if minimally invasive techniques are used.
  ■ Compartment monitoring should be undertaken under these circumstances.

External Fixation

■ Four basic types of external fixation have been used, and the results associated with their use are given in Table 28-4.
■ The original external fixators were transarticular (Fig. 28-5) and relied on "ligamentotaxis" to reduce the plafond fragment.
■ This technique was unsuccessful, and surgeons moved to periarticular joint-sparing external fixation combined with limited internal fixation where necessary (Fig. 28-6).
■ The frames were unilateral, delta shaped or semicircular, and held with half pins (see Fig. 28-6).
  ■ The results of their use are detailed in Table 28-4.
■ The next evolution was to articulated frames with a hinge at the ankle joint to encourage ankle movement.
■ This principle was unsuccessful with distal radial fractures, and Table 28-4 suggests the results associated

TABLE 28-4 COMPARISON OF THE RESULTS OF DIFFERENT TYPES OF EXTERNAL FIXATION IN THE TREATMENT OF PLAFOND FRACTURES

Result/Complication	Unilateral or Semicircular (%)		Articulated (%)		Hybrid (%)		Ring (%)	
	Range	Average	Range	Average	Range	Average	Range	Average
Excellent/good	30–75	57.6	30–40	35	61.7–80.7	64.5	46.2–71.4	61.7
Open	12.5–60	31.7	18.4–41.7	23	21.4–29.7	25.2	23.1–100	46.8
Infection	0–4.5	1.9	0–8.3	1.6	0–8.1	5.2	0	0
Nonunion	4.2–16.6	9.6	2–8.3	3.3	0–21.9	9.2	0–7.7	2.1
Malunion	0–25	12.5	0–8.2	6.6	3.8–8.1	6.5	0–15.4	6.4
Moderate/severe osteoarthritis	10–60	23.1	30	30	0–15	5.4	0–30.8	10.6
Arthrodesis	0–10	2.9	0–2	1.6	0	0	0–7.7	2.1
Septic arthritis	0–5	1	0	0	0.3–1	0.9	0	0
Pin sepsis	0–37.5	13.9	20.4	20.4	11.5–29.4	19.3	38.1–69.2	48.9
Reflex sympathetic dystrophy	0–22.2	4.8	0–2	1.6	0	0	0	0

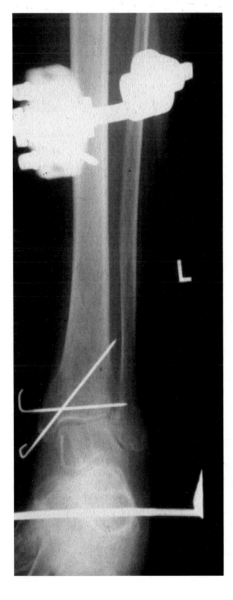
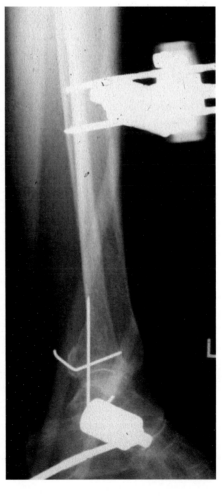

Figure 28-5 A-P and lateral radiographs of transarticular external fixation.

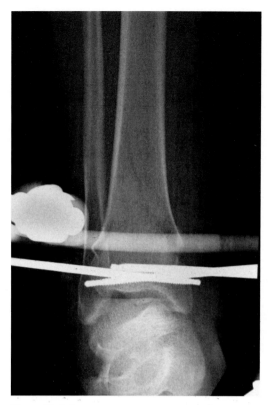
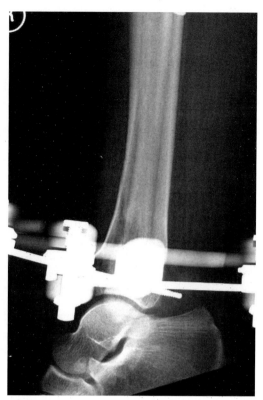

Figure 28-6 A-P and lateral radiographs of periarticular external fixation.

with its use in plafond fractures are no better than when periarticular external fixation is used.

- Hybrid frames with distal fine wires and proximal half pins have been used successfully (Fig. 28-7), although a number of surgeons have favored full ring frames usually using the Ilizarov device.

- Table 28-4 suggests that, as with tibial diaphyseal fractures, the type of external frame has little effect on the final result.

- There are differences in the results shown in Table 28-4, but most of these are due to differences of definition and length of follow-up.

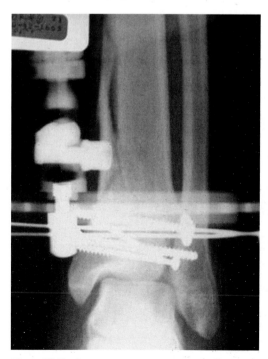
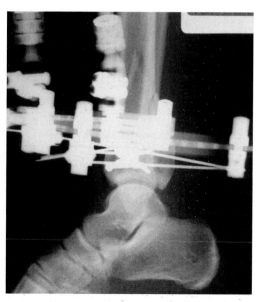

Figure 28-7 A-P and lateral radiographs showing the hybrid fixator used to treat the fracture shown in Figure 28-3.

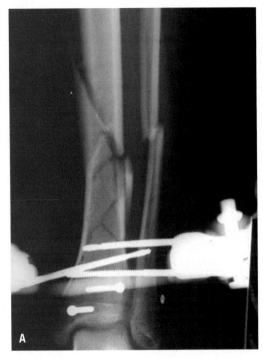
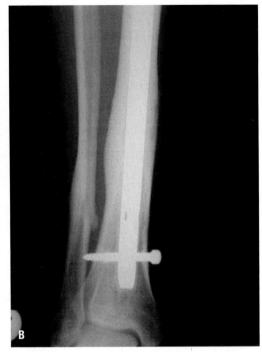

Figure 28-8 (A) A C1.3 plafond fracture treated initially with periarticular external fixation. (B) The metaphysiodi-aphyseal nonunion was treated with a reamed intramedullary nail.

- Overall the results indicate that the increased complexity of articulated frames confers no benefit and that full ring fixators produce similar results to hybrid frames or fixators utilizing half pins.
- One particular problem with external fixation is pin-related neural damage, and an incidence of 7.5% of common peroneal damage has been reported.

Intramedullary Nailing

- There are two indications for intramedullary nailing in the treatment of plafond fractures.
- The change from plating to external fixation increased the incidence of nonunion at the diaphysometaphyseal junction (Fig. 28-8).
  - This had not been a problem with plating because the junctional fracture had been spanned by a plate and often grafted.

- Table 28-4 shows that external fixation is associated with a slightly higher nonunion rate, with most of these between the diaphysis and metaphysis.
  - This nonunion is well treated with a reamed intramedullary nail, provided the metaphyseal fracture has healed and the pin sites are dry prior to nailing (see Fig. 28-8).
- Intramedullary nailing can also be used to treat many displaced type A fractures using the techniques described in Chapters 27 and 33.

Suggested Treatment

- The suggested treatment of tibial plafond fractures is given in Table 28-5.

TABLE 28-5 SUGGESTED TREATMENT OF TIBIAL PLAFOND FRACTURES

Injury	Treatment
Type A extra-articular fractures	Locked plating or periarticular external fixation. Some may be suitable for intramedullary nailing.
Type B partial articular fractures	Interfragmentary screws with neutralization or antiglide plates as required.
Type C complete articular fractures	Primary interfragmentary screw fixation and periarticular external fixation or primary transarticular external fixation and secondary plating.
Multiply injured patients	Consider damage control surgery (see Chapter 3).

COMPLICATIONS

- The treatment of infection, nonunion, and malunion is discussed in the appropriate chapters.
- The incidence of reflex sympathetic dystrophy is probably higher than in the published series used to compile Table 28-4, but it is usually relatively mild and easily treated.
- Reflex sympathetic dystrophy is discussed in more detail in Chapter 41.

Compartment Syndrome

- It is very likely that the incidence of compartment syndrome is higher in plafond fractures than previously thought.
- High-energy fractures of the plafond may be associated with considerable soft tissue damage, but the fascia may still be intact.
- The axial loading implicated in the plafond fracture causes less fascial damage than shearing or rotational injuries.
- The highest incidence that has been reported is 12.5%, but many papers suggest an incidence of over 5%.
- One study reports a 12.5% incidence of late toe clawing, suggestive of missed compartment syndrome.
- With the trend toward either definitive closed management of plafond fractures or primary external fixation and secondary plating, surgeons should be aware of the possibility of compartment syndrome in these high-energy injuries.
- The diagnosis and treatment of compartment syndrome is discussed further in Chapter 38.

Osteoarthritis

- The incidence of moderate and severe osteoarthritis (Fig. 28-9) is listed in Tables 28-3 and 28-4.
- About 85% to 90% of patients who have plafond fractures develop osteoarthritis, although relatively few require ankle arthrodesis.
- The incidence of osteoarthritis correlates with the severity of the fracture and the accuracy of reduction but not with the type of treatment.
- Most articles report limitation of activities because of ankle stiffness, with up to 90% of patients unable to run and 35% to 68% of patients experiencing problems with employment.
- Despite this clear correlation between plafond fractures and social and recreation changes, few patients actually have an ankle arthrodesis (Fig. 28-10) because of osteoarthritis.

SPECIAL SITUATIONS

Combined Tibial Diaphyseal and Plafond Fractures

- The most common combination of fractures is a tibial diaphyseal fracture and a B1.1 posterior malleolar fracture.
- This is best treated by percutaneous anteroposterior interfragmentary screws inserted under fluoroscopic control prior to nailing the tibial diaphyseal fracture.
- More severe plafond/diaphyseal fracture patterns are probably best treated by using external fixation for both fractures.

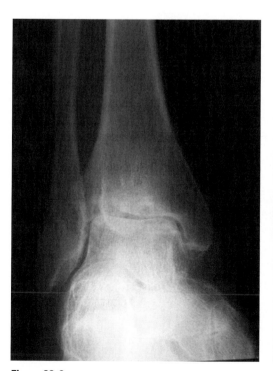
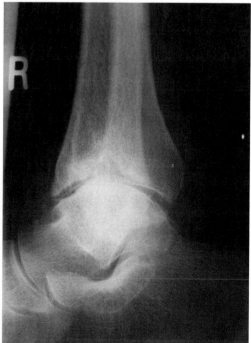

Figure 28-9 A-P and lateral radiographs of ankle osteoarthritis 14 years after a plafond fracture.

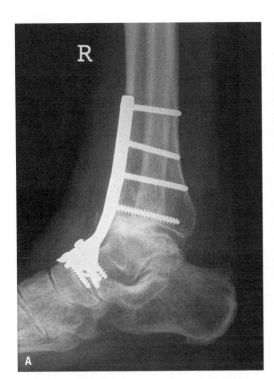
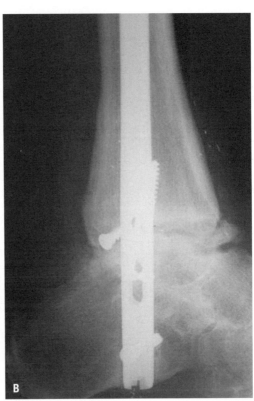

Figure 28-10 Two methods of ankle arthrodesis using a plate (**A**) or a retrograde nail passed proximally through the calcaneus (**B**).

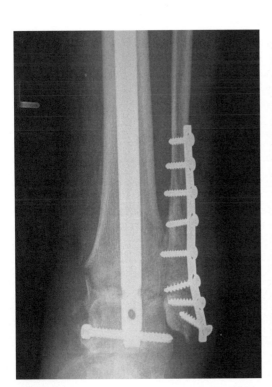
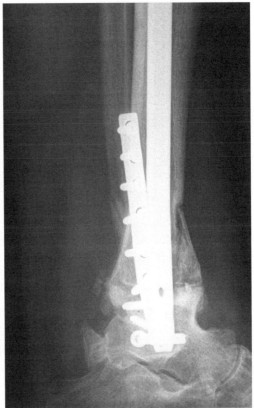

Figure 28-11 A-P and lateral radiographs of a primary arthrodesis using a nail placed into the talus.

Unreconstructable Plafond Fractures

■ Most plafond fractures are reconstructible, and it is certainly worthwhile attempting to reconstruct most C3 fractures.

■ Some are unreconstructable, however, and the difficulty is in choosing the appropriate technique for primary arthrodesis.

■ Clearly there will be a considerable volume of bone loss, and extensive bone grafting is required.

■ Internal fixation techniques are preferred with the options being a long plate spanning the gap between the tibial diaphysis and the talus and midfoot or, preferably, an antegrade intramedullary nail statically locked into the talus and tibia (Fig. 28-11).

■ If the subtalar joint is damaged or very stiff (see Fig. 28-10), a retrograde nail through the calcaneus into the tibia can be used, or alternatively a ring fixator with primary shortening and secondary lengthening may be employed.

SUGGESTED READING

Bartlett CS, Weiner LS. Fractures of the tibial pilon. In: Browner BD, Jupiter JB, Levine AM, et al., eds. Skeletal trauma, 3rd ed. Philadelphia: WB Saunders, 2003:2257–2306.

Blauth M, Bastian L, Krettek C, et al. Surgical options for the treatment of severe tibial pilon fractures: a study of three techniques. J Orthop Trauma 2001;15:153–160.

Helfet DL, Koval K, Pappas J, et al. Intra-articular "pilon" fractures of the tibia. Clin Orthop 1994;298:221–228.

Kim HS, Jahng JS, Kim SS, et al. Treatment of tibial pilon fractures using ring fixators and arthroscopy. Clin Orthop 1997;334:244–250.

Marsh JL. External fixation is the treatment of choice for fractures of the tibial plafond. J Orthop Trauma 1999;13:583–585.

Marsh JL, Saltzman CL. Ankle fractures. In: Bucholz RW, Heckman JD, eds. Rockwood and Green's fractures in adults, 5th ed. Philadelphia: Lippincott Williams and Wilkins, 2001:2001–2090.

Müller ME, Nazarian S, Koch P, et al. The comprehensive classification of fractures of long bones. Berlin: Springer-Verlag, 1990.

Ruëdi T, Allgöwer M. Fractures of the lower end of the tibia into the ankle joint. Injury 1969;1:92–99.

Williams TM, Nepola JV, DeCoster TA, et al. Factors affecting outcome in tibial plafond fractures. Clin Orthop 2004;423:93–98.

ANKLE FRACTURES

Ankle fractures are unusual in that, unlike many other fractures, there has been little debate about the superiority of operative management over nonoperative management for many years. The early studies confirming that displaced ankle fractures should be treated operatively were published in the 1960s and 1970s, and there has been virtually uniform agreement about the principles and techniques of operative treatment of ankle fractures. This consensus has allowed surgeons to concentrate on the treatment of specific types of ankle fracture and to investigate the role of operative management in particular groups of patients. Continuing interest has been expressed about the treatment of ankle fractures, and Box 29-1 lists the areas that remain controversial.

SURGICAL ANATOMY

The ankle joint is formed from the distal fibula, distal tibia, and talus. The joint is saddle shaped and wider laterally than medially in addition to being wider anteriorly than posteriorly (see Fig. 28-1 in Chapter 28). As the ankle dorsiflexes, the fibula rotates externally to accommodate the wider anterior talus. The tibia and fibula are connected by the inferior transverse ligament, which lies posteriorly below the inferior tibiofibular syndesmosis, the inferior tibiofibular syndesmosis itself, and the interosseous membrane. The inferior tibiofibular syndesmosis consists of three main ligaments that may be damaged if a fracture occurs (Fig. 29-1). The anterior and posterior tibiofibular ligaments arise from the anterior and posterior aspects of the distal tibia and insert into the equivalent areas of the distal fibula. Between these ligaments lies the interosseous ligament. The anterior tibiofibular ligament is the weakest in the complex. The interosseous membrane arises above the inferior tibiofibular syndesmosis and then joins the fibula to the tibia throughout its length, finishing distal to the proximal tibiofibular joint.

The tibiofibular complex is attached to the hindfoot medially and laterally by strong ligaments. On the medial side the deltoid ligament is composed of superficial and deep components. The superficial component arises from the medial malleolus and inserts into the navicular, neck of talus, medial border of the sustentaculum tali, and the posteromedial talar tubercle. The deep portion of the deltoid ligament runs between the medial malleolus and the talus. The lateral ligament is composed of

---

BOX 29-1 CURRENT CONTROVERSIES IN THE TREATMENT OF ANKLE FRACTURES

Is surgery required for OTA (AO) B1 fractures?
Should patients with ankle fractures remain non–weight bearing after surgery?
Should metal or bioabsorbable screws be used?
Syndesmotic screws
    In which fractures should they be used?
    How many are required?
    How many cortices should be penetrated?
    How far above the ankle should they be placed?
    Are they needed for type B fractures?
How should ankle fractures in the elderly be treated?
How should ankle fractures in patients with diabetes be treated?
Should ankle sprains be treated surgically?

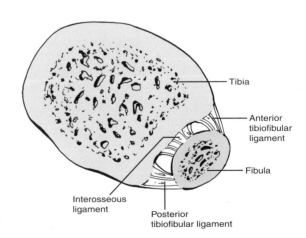

Figure 29-1 The anatomy of the inferior tibiofibular syndesmosis.

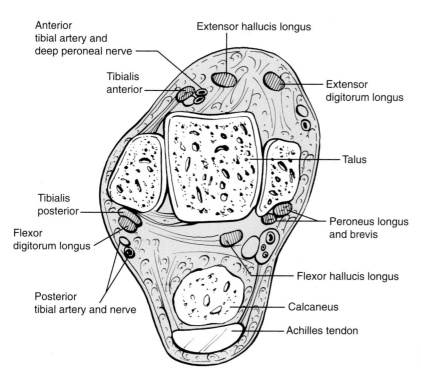

Anterior tibial artery and deep peroneal nerve

Tibialis anterior

Extensor hallucis longus

Extensor digitorum longus

Talus

Tibialis posterior

Flexor digitorum longus

Peroneus longus and brevis

Posterior tibial artery and nerve

Flexor hallucis longus

Calcaneus

Achilles tendon

Figure 29-2   A cross section of the anatomy around the ankle joint.

three main ligaments: the anterior talofibular, calcaneofibular, and posterior talofibular ligaments. The anterior talofibular ligament is the weakest and often injured in ankle sprains. The other two ligaments are much stronger.

The ankle joint is surrounded by tendons and neurovascular structures (Fig. 29-2). The tendons passing across the joint are divided into anterior, medial, lateral, and posterior groups. The anterior tendons are those of tibialis anterior, extensor hallucis longus, extensor digitorum longus, and peroneus tertius. These are restricted by the extensor retinaculum, which also encloses the anterior tibial vessels and the deep peroneal nerve. The terminal branches of the superficial peroneal nerve lie superficial to the extensor retinaculum.

On the medial side, the flexor retinaculum encloses the tendons of tibialis posterior, flexor digitorum longus, and flexor hallucis longus in addition to the posterior tibial artery and accompanying veins and the tibial nerves. The Achilles tendon and plantaris tendon run posteriorly to the ankle joint together with the sural nerve. On the lateral side, the superior peroneal retinaculum encloses the tendons of peroneus longus and peroneus brevis.

CLASSIFICATION

The most common classification in widespread use is the division of ankle fractures into unimalleolar, bimalleolar, or trimalleolar fractures. Clearly this does not describe all ankle fracture types, and in particular it makes no reference to any syndesmotic damage or other soft tissue injury. However it is often used as a quick method of describing infra- or transsyndesmotic fractures.

The two full classifications in use are the Lauge-Hansen (1950) classification and the OTA (AO) classification. The first is a classification based on an analysis of the fracture types as they relate to the position of the foot and the deforming force at the time of fracture. It was particularly useful in the days of nonoperative management, but it is fairly complicated, and the OTA (AO) classification remains in widespread use. This is a morphological classification based on the original Weber (1972) classification. He separated ankle fractures into type A infrasyndesmotic, type B transsyndesmotic, and type C suprasyndesmotic fractures. The OTA (AO) classification has maintained the three basic types but expanded them to include virtually all variants of the ankle fracture (Fig. 29-3).

Type A fractures occur below the level of the inferior tibiofibular syndesmotic ligaments. A1 fractures are unifocal lateral lesions with .1 denoting a lateral ligament rupture, .2 an avulsion fracture of the tip of the lateral malleolus, and .3 an infrasyndesmotic transverse lateral malleolar fracture. In A2 fractures there is an associated medial malleolar fracture, and in A3 fractures there is a posteromedial fracture. In A2 and A3 fractures, the suffixes .1 to .3 represent the same as for A1 fractures.

Type B transsyndesmotic fractures are similarly divided. In B1 fractures, there is a simple oblique/spiral lateral malleolar fracture. The suffix .1 means the anterior tibiofibular ligament is intact. In .2 fractures it is ruptured, or there is an avulsion fracture at the distal anterolateral tibia (Chaput) fracture or an avulsion fracture of the lateral malleolus (Le Fort) fracture. B1.3 fractures are multifragmentary. In B2 fractures, there is a medial lesion, which is a deltoid rupture in B2.1 fractures or a medial malleolar fracture in B2.2 fractures. In B2.3 fractures, there is fragmentation in the lateral malleolus. The B3 group contain fractures that have a

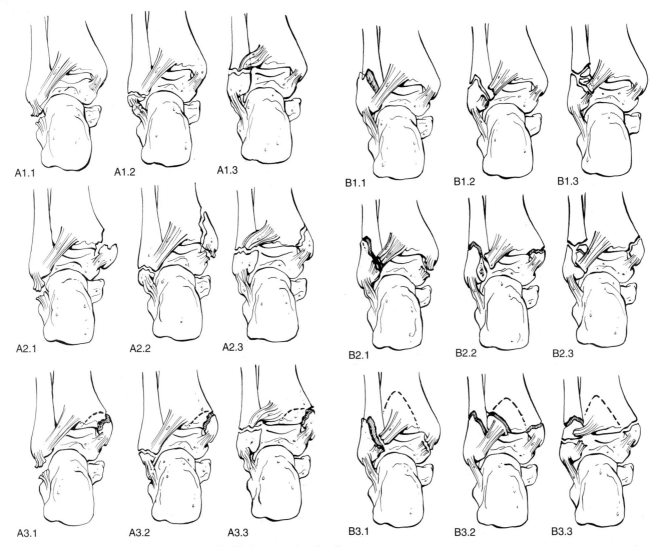

Figure 29-3   The OTA (AO) classification of ankle fractures. *(continued)*

posterior malleolar (Volkmann) fracture, and .1 to .3 refer to the same characteristics seen in the B2 fractures.

In type C fractures, the fibular fractures are suprasyndesmotic. In C1 fractures, there is a simple fibular fracture with damage to at least the anterior tibiofibular ligament. In C2 fractures, the fibular fracture is multifragmentary, and in C3 fractures, it is in the proximal fibula (Maisonneuve fracture). The suffixes .1 to .3 refer to the damage to the medial and posterior malleoli. In .1 fractures there is a deltoid ligament rupture, whereas in .2 fractures there is a medial malleolar fracture, and in .3 fractures there is a posterior malleolar fracture.

PATHOGENESIS

It is important to understand how the different types of ankle fracture occur. This was best described by Lauge-Hansen, who analyzed the effect of different deforming forces on the supinated and pronated foot. He described five different injury patterns, although the effect of dorsiflexion on the pronated foot is to cause a plafond fracture rather than a malleolar fracture. The remaining four injury patterns, illustrated in Figure 29-4, cause malleolar fractures. If the foot is supinated, the deltoid ligament is relaxed and the initial injury is lateral. Conversely, if the foot is pronated, the initial injury is medial.

Injuries to the supinated foot are shown in Figure 29-4A. In supination external rotation injuries, the first stage is damage to the anterior tibiofibular ligaments. Continuing deformation causes a B1 fracture. As the deforming force continues, the posterior tibiofibular ligaments are ruptured or there is a posterior malleolar fracture. The last stage is damage to the medial side causing a B3 fracture. If the supinated foot is adducted, either the lateral ligament ruptures or there is an A1 fracture. Continuing deformation results in an A2 fracture, but the medial fracture is vertical, and associated articular impaction fracture is not uncommon.

Injuries to the pronated foot are shown in Figure 29-4B. If the foot is pronated and an external rotation force is applied, the first injury is a deltoid rupture or an A2.1 fracture. Continuing deformation causes a rupture of the anterior tibiofibular ligament or a fracture of Chaput's tubercle. The

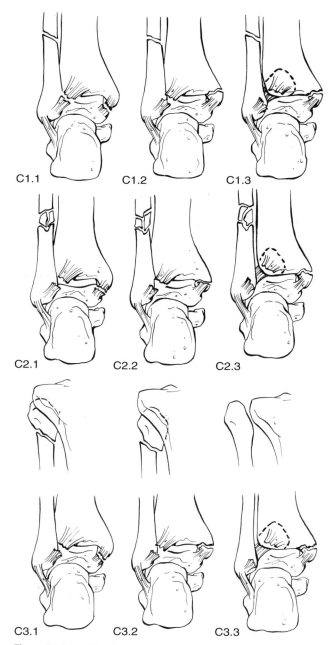

C1.1   C1.2   C1.3

C2.1   C2.2   C2.3

C3.1   C3.2   C3.3

Figure 29-3 *(continued)*

variation in the fracture patterns, but the complete OTA (AO) classification contains all the fracture types that commonly occur.

Interosseous Membrane

There is still debate about the degree of involvement of the interosseous membrane in suprasyndesmotic fractures. There are two different philosophies. A number of surgeons have suggested all suprasyndesmotic fractures are associated with rupture of the interosseous membrane to the level of the fracture even if this is in the proximal fibula. Others believe that in external rotation injuries the fibula rotates on an intact posterior tibiofibular ligament and interosseous membrane, and the fracture occurs at a point of mechanical weakness at the fibular neck. It is interesting to note that suprasyndesmotic fibular fractures do not occur between a point about 12 to 15 cm above the ankle and the fibular neck.

The use of MRI scanning has confirmed an inconstant relationship between the location of the fibular fracture and the extent of interosseous membrane damage. It has also shown that some type B fractures have significant soft tissue injury including interosseous membrane damage. It is likely these fractures have been caused by both external rotation and abduction forces. In type C fractures, abduction forces cause rupture of the interosseous membrane to the level of the fracture, but in pure external rotation injuries, this does not occur and the interosseous membrane is mainly intact, especially if the fracture is at the level of the fibular neck. In injuries caused by both external rotation and abduction forces, the extent of interosseous membrane damage varies.

EPIDEMIOLOGY

The epidemiology of ankle fractures is shown in Table 29-1. They are common fractures affecting men and

next stage is a suprasyndesmotic fibular fracture of the C1 or C3 types. Continuing deformation causes rupture of the posterior tibiofibular ligament or a C1.3 or C3.3 fracture. Abduction of a pronated foot also initially causes deltoid rupture or an A2.1 fracture. The next stage is anterior tibiofibular damage or a Chaput's fracture. The third stage is a multifragmentary C2 fracture with division of the interosseous membrane from the syndesmosis to the level of the fracture. This may be associated with osteochondral impaction. A typical fracture dislocation may then occur (Fig. 29-5).

Figure 29-4 summarizes the fractures associated with external rotation or abduction forces. Many patients present with fractures that have involved both abduction and external rotation forces, however. Thus there may be some

TABLE 29-1 EPIDEMIOLOGY OF ANKLE FRACTURES

Proportion of all fractures	9.0%
Average age	45.9 y
Incidence	100.8/10^5/y
Men/women	47%/53%
Distribution	Type A
Open fractures	1.7%
Most common causes	
Fall	37.5%
Inversion	31.5%
Sport	10.2%
OTA (AO) classification	
Type A	29.7%
Type B	62.5%
Type C	7.8%
Most common subgroups	
B1.1	24.8%
A1.3	12.1%
A1.2	10.6%
B1.3	8.8%

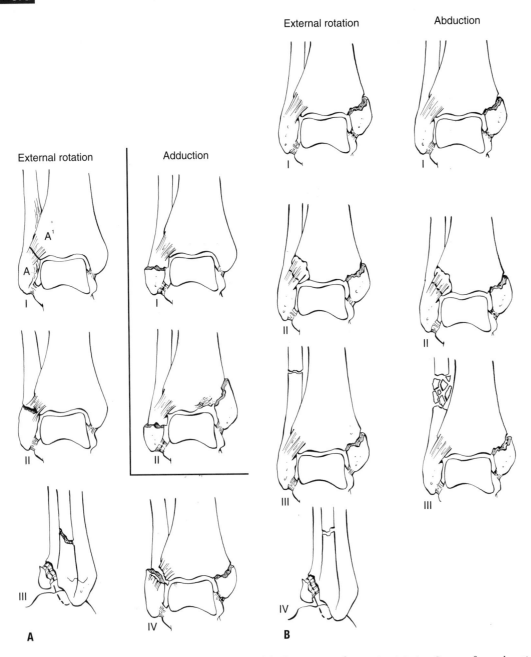

Figure 29-4   (A) The patterns of supination injuries. (B) The patterns of pronation injuries. See text for explanation.

TABLE 29-2 EPIDEMIOLOGY OF THE DIFFERENT CAUSES OF ANKLE FRACTURE

Cause	%	Open (%)	Age (y)	OTA (AO) Type (%)		
				A	B	C
Fall	37.5	0	45	24.2	67.8	7.9
Inversion	31.5	2.5	45.2	32.7	64.3	3
Sport	10.2	3.6		23.6	54.5	21.8
Fall down stairs	7.8	0	43	26.2	69	4.8
Fall from height	4.5	0	35	50	37.5	12.5

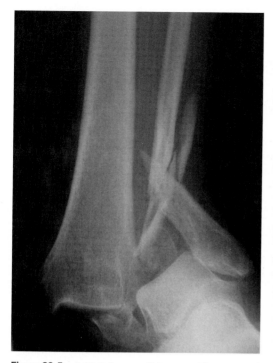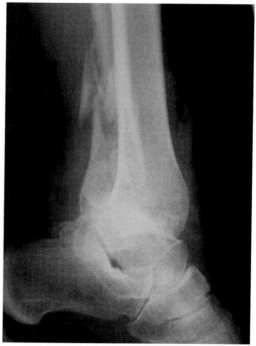

Figure 29-5   A C2.3 fracture dislocation. This is caused by an abduction force applied to a pronated foot.

women equally. They have a type A distribution (see Chapter 1). Open fractures are rare, and most patients present with isolated fractures as a result of low-energy injuries. Type B fractures are by far the most common, with suprasyndesmotic type C fractures relatively unusual. Analysis of OTA (AO) type A and B fractures shows that 70% are isolated lateral malleolar fractures, 6.3% are isolated medial malleolar fractures, 16% are bimalleolar, and 7.5% are trimalleolar fractures.

Table 29-2 shows an analysis of the mode of injury. Inversion injuries and falls are the most common cause of ankle fractures in older patients, with most patients having type B fractures. Type C fractures occur most often after falls from a height or sports injuries. High-energy ankle fractures are comparatively uncommon, with only 4.2% occurring in motor vehicle accidents. There is a significant difference between the epidemiology of isolated lateral malleolar and medial malleolar fractures. Lateral malleolar fractures tend to occur in older patients following low-energy injuries, and medial malleolar fractures occur in younger patients following high-energy injuries.

Associated Injuries

Most ankle fractures are isolated injuries with only about 5% of patients having other musculoskeletal injuries. About 2% of patients with tibial diaphyseal fractures have associated ankle fractures, and indeed most associated fractures are in the ipsilateral lower limb. About 50% of associated fractures are in the ipsilateral foot, mainly affecting the talus and metatarsals. The fall may cause an associated distal radial or proximal humeral fracture, and these should always be checked. Medial malleolar fractures

rarely may cause damage to, or even transect, the tibialis posterior tendon.

DIAGNOSIS

History and Physical Examination

- Most patients present with isolated ankle fractures after low-energy injuries.
- The ankle is painful, swollen, and deformed if a dislocation or subluxation is present.
- Patients who sustain ankle fractures as a result of high-energy trauma must be examined according to ATLS principles because they may well have other injuries.
- Careful examination of the ipsilateral lower limb is important, with particular attention paid to examination of the foot and the proximal fibula to see if there is an associated suprasyndesmotic fracture.
- Open injuries are rare, but, if present, are almost always medial in location and associated with a lateral dislocation.
- Neurovascular damage is also rare and again associated with a fracture-dislocation.
- All fracture-dislocations should be reduced as an emergency to restore the vascular supply to the foot and to take the tension off the skin on the medial side of the joint.
  - Failure to do this has been associated with a 12% incidence of skin necrosis.

Radiologic Examination

- Many patients present with a painful ankle after a fall, but most of them have ankle sprains.

BOX 29-2 OTTAWA RULES FOR ANKLE RADIOLOGY

1. Pain in any malleolar zone and numbers 2, 3, or 4
2. Bone tenderness at posterior edge or lip of lateral malleolus
3. Bone tenderness at posterior edge or lip of medial malleolus
4. Inability to bear weight both immediately and in the emergency department

■ The Ottawa rules (Box 29-2) were introduced to identify which patients with ankle pain should have X-rays.

■ The use of the Ottawa rules is associated with a sensitivity of 98%, with the likelihood of a negative test assessed at about 1 in 100.

■ Anteroposterior and lateral radiographs are usually adequate to diagnose an ankle fracture (Fig. 29-6).

■ A mortise view may be used to identify a syndesmotic injury, although it can usually be inferred from the morphology of the fracture.

  ■ In the mortise view, an anteroposterior radiograph is taken with the leg internally rotated by 15 to 20 degrees.

■ Oblique radiographs may occasionally be used, but they rarely give extra information.

■ Stress views may be used to identify ligamentous damage, and MRI scans may help delineate articular damage and syndesmotic damage but are rarely indicated in the acute situation.

TREATMENT

■ It has been accepted for many years that operative treatment using interfragmentary screws and plates is the preferred treatment method for displaced ankle fractures.

■ There is still debate about the management of B1 fractures where the deltoid ligament is intact because the prognosis for these fractures is good when managed nonoperatively.

■ Controversy about the management of other displaced ankle fractures relates to the technique of fracture fixation rather than to its requirement.

Nonsurgical Treatment

Undisplaced Fractures

■ Many ankle fractures are undisplaced or minimally displaced on presentation and merely require nonoperative management.

  ■ This is particularly true of A1.2 and A1.3 fractures, which comprise 23% of all ankle fractures (see Table 29-1).

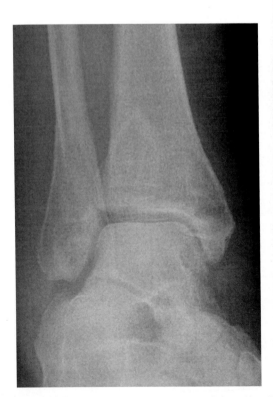 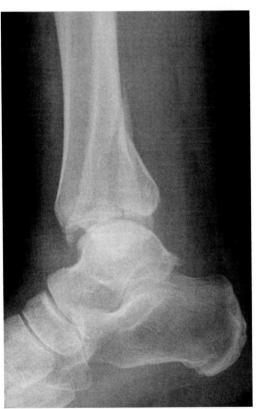

Figure 29-6   A B3.1 fracture subluxation of the ankle. The talus has displaced posteriorly.

TABLE 29-3 COMPARISON OF THE RESULTS OF NONOPERATIVE AND OPERATIVE MANAGEMENT USING AO PRINCIPLES OF RIGID FIXATION

| | OTA (AO) Type (%) | | | | | |
| | A | | B | | C | |
Result	Range	Mean	Range	Mean	Range	Mean
Nonoperative treatment						
Adequate reduction						
Hindfoot dysfunction		0		23.1		20
Osteoarthritis		0		0		20
Inadequate reduction						
Hindfoot dysfunction		50		63.6		68.8
Osteoarthritis		100		90.1		100
Excellent/good	71.4–75	72.9	35–62	53.5	22.7–78.7	29.3
Operative treatment						
Excellent/good	78.2–82.4	81.4	75.6–86.6	80.8	61.8–85.3	72.1

■ It is rarely true of the A2.1 medial malleolar fracture, and early studies detailed poor results with the use of casts in these fractures.

■ Undisplaced fractures should be treated by the application of a weight-bearing cast or brace maintained for 6 weeks.

■ Physical therapy is frequently required after its removal.

■ If a type C fracture (usually a C1.1 or C3.1 fracture) is treated nonoperatively, careful follow-up is required to check that the position is maintained and the syndesmosis does not widen secondarily.

■ This is unusual, but late displacement requires operative treatment.

Displaced Fractures

■ Table 29-3 gives an analysis of the results of nonoperative management compared with operative management using rigid fixation in displaced ankle fractures. These studies were undertaken in the 1960s and 1970s in Germany, Switzerland, and Scandinavia.

   ■ They illustrate the importance of accurate reduction and fixation in displaced fractures but also vindicate the continued use of cast management in undisplaced fractures.

■ Accurate reduction is more difficult to obtain in more complex fractures.

■ In the simpler type A fractures, nonoperative management is almost invariably adequate.

■ Osteoarthritis and hindfoot dysfunction are directly related to the quality of reduction.

Lateral Malleolar Fractures

Intact Deltoid Ligament

■ The fracture in which debate is still ongoing about the role of surgery is the B1 fracture with the intact deltoid ligament (Fig. 29-7).

■ This is often known as the Lauge-Hansen supination-eversion stage II fracture in the literature.

■ The OTA (AO) classification (see Fig. 29-3) indicates that B1.1 fractures have an intact anterior tibiofibular ligament, whereas it is ruptured in B1.2 and B1.3 fractures.

   ■ The state of the ligament is usually unknown, and the important radiologic findings are a spiral or oblique lateral malleolar fracture without talar shift.

■ The argument for surgery is that even 2 mm of fibular displacement is associated with a degree of talar rotation and therefore tibio-talar incongruency.

■ No clinical evidence indicates that operative management gives better results (Table 29-4).

■ Long-term studies of patients with B1 fractures have not shown an increase in ankle osteoarthritis in patients with up to 3 mm of lateral malleolar displacement, and the number of good and excellent results remains about 90% at 25 to 30 years after the fractures.

■ These fractures are best treated by a weight-bearing cast or brace for a 6-week period.

■ Elastic strapping or a supportive shoe also gives good results.

Ruptured Deltoid Ligament

■ If a lateral malleolar fracture is associated with a deltoid ligament rupture (B2.1 fracture), the situation is very different.

■ The patient usually presents with talar shift on the initial anteroposterior or mortise view (Fig. 29-8).

■ Biomechanical studies have indicated that if the talar shift persists, the normal tibio-talar loading is altered considerably.

■ The ankle mortise must be reduced accurately and fibular fixation undertaken.

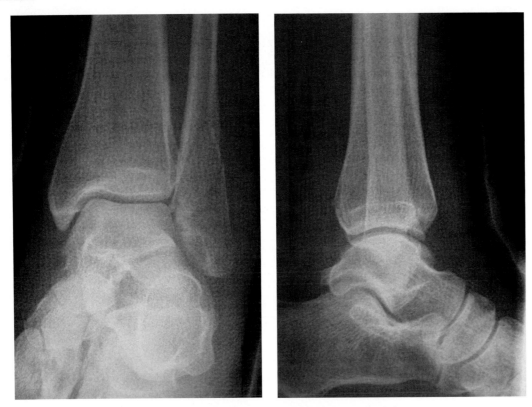

Figure 29-7 A B1.1 fracture. The deltoid ligament is intact and there is no talar shift.

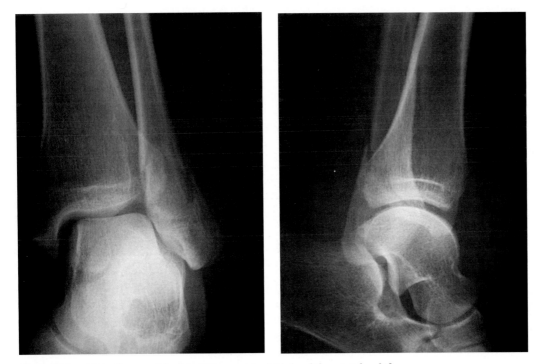

Figure 29-8 A B2.1 fracture. The deltoid ligament is divided and there is talar shift.

TABLE 29-4 RESULTS OF OPERATIVE AND NONOPERATIVE TREATMENT OF B1 FRACTURES

Result/Complication	Operative		Nonoperative	
	Range	Average	Range	Average
Excellent/good (%)	82.8–97.2	94.4	88.2–100	96.9
Severe osteoarthritis (%)	2.6–2.9	2.8	0–7.2	3.8
Return to work (wk)	13–13.5	13.3	6–12.3	8.2

Surgical Treatment

Internal Fixation

- Several techniques are in use for the treatment of lateral malleolar fractures.
- Cerclage wires or staples used to be popular but cannot be recommended now.
- The most common technique involves the use of an interfragmentary screw and a neutralization plate (Fig. 29-9A).
- Alternative techniques utilize two or preferably three interfragmentary screws without a plate (Fig. 29-9B) or the use of a dorsally placed antiglide plate (Fig. 29-9C).
- No evidence in the literature indicates one method is superior to another, although lag screw fixation and the use of a dorsal antiglide plate are associated with a significantly reduced requirement for hardware removal.
- Some evidence indicates that dorsal plating gives better results in osteopenic bone, but essentially the results of all three methods are similar.
- Intramedullary nailing has been used for fibular fractures (Fig. 29-9D).
  - The literature suggests that this method gives similar results to plating and screw fixation, although with an increasingly elderly population, intramedullary nailing may well become more popular.
- There is some debate about the requirement for deltoid ligament repair in a B2.1 fracture, but studies have shown no benefit from deltoid ligament repair, and there are no differences in long-term outcome or ankle stability.
- Should talar shift persist after internal fixation of the fibular in B2.1 fractures, it is often suggested the deltoid ligament may have become trapped in the medial side of the ankle joint.
  - This is extremely rare, and the reason for a persistent talar shift is almost invariably inadequate reduction of the fibula prior to fixation.

Medial Malleolar Fracture

- Isolated A2.1 medial malleolar fractures tend to occur in younger adults following high-energy trauma.
- They are therefore usually displaced and require operative treatment.
- The conventional method of treatment is with two partially threaded 3.5-mm cancellous screws (Fig. 29-10).
- Alternatively, K-wires and a figure-eight tension band can be used for smaller fragments or if there is comminution (Fig. 29-11).

Metallic or Absorbable Screws

- There has been considerable interest in the use of bioabsorbable screws and pins to fix malleolar fragments.
- The implants are made from polyglycolide, polylactide, or glycolide-lactide copolymer.
- The literature is mixed regarding the success of these implants because some patients present with osteolysis related to the screws or pins.
  - In a 9-year study, 1,223 patients with malleolar fractures were treated with absorbable pins and screws.
  - Seventy-four (6.1%) patients had an inflammatory foreign body reaction, and ten of these patients developed late, moderate, or severe ankle osteoarthritis without joint incongruency.
  - Thus there was a severe complication rate of 0.8%.
- Overall the results indicate that, at the moment, metallic implants should be used, although with improving technology bioabsorbable implants may become more popular in the future.

Bimalleolar Fractures

- It was recognized many years ago that displaced bimalleolar fractures should be treated by fixation of both medial and lateral malleoli.
  - Fixation of just the medial malleolus resulted in fracture malposition and severe osteoarthritic change in about 45% of patients.
- The classical B2.2 or B2.3 bimalleolar fractures are treated by internal fixation using the methods already outlined for the lateral and medial malleoli.
- The A2.2 bimalleolar fracture (Fig. 29-12) is caused by adduction of the supinated foot and differs from the B2.2 and B2.3 fractures in several ways.
  - They tend to occur in younger patients after high-energy injury. The medial malleolar fracture line is vertical, and 40% to 45% of these fractures have articular impaction that may require elevation and grafting at the time of surgery.
- The medial malleolus can be fixed by intrafragmentary screws placed at 90 degrees to the axis of the tibia, but an antiglide plate is recommended to prevent proximal migration of the malleolus (see Fig. 29-12).

Trimalleolar Fractures

- As with bimalleolar fractures, the treatment of the B3.2 and B3.3 trimalleolar fractures is operative using the techniques already detailed.

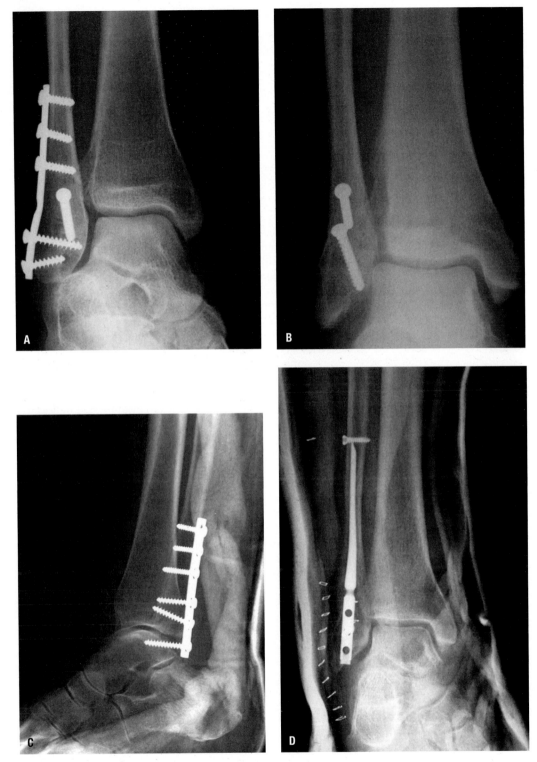

Figure 29-9 Techniques of lateral malleolar fixation. (**A**) Interfragmentary screw and neutralization plate. (**B**) Interfragmentary screws. (**C**) Dorsal antiglide plate. (**D**) Fibular nail.

- The debate concerns the treatment of the posterior malleolar fragment.
  - This is attached to the lateral malleolus by the relatively strong posterior tibiofibular ligament, and when the lateral malleolus is reduced and fixed, a small posterior malleolar fragment tends to reduce, giving a stable congruous ankle.
- If the posterior malleolar fragment is large and displaced, posterior subluxation of the ankle can occur (Fig. 29-13).

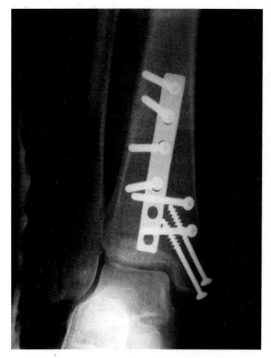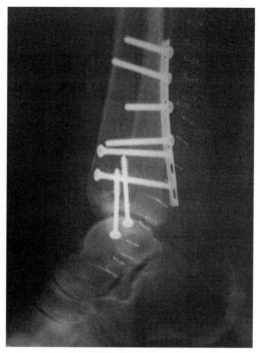

Figure 29-10   An A3.1 fracture with a large posteromedial fragment. A dorsal antiglide plate has been used to prevent posterior ankle dislocation.

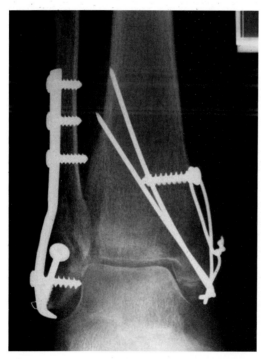

Figure 29-11   The use of K-wires and tension band wiring. This is useful for small medial malleolar fragments.

■ Thus it has been suggested that fragments comprising between 20% and 33% of the ankle joint should be fixed.

■ Most authorities quote 25% as the critical size, but there is little evidence this figure is meaningful.

■ Some experts suggest that functional results may be better after accurate reduction of posterior malleolar fragments that comprise more than 10% of the ankle joint.

■ Treatment should be aimed at achieving anatomical reduction and avoiding posterior subluxation of the ankle joint.

■ Usually fragments comprising less than about 25% of the ankle fixation of the lateral malleolus achieve this (Fig. 29-14).

■ If the ankle is not congruous, the posterior malleolus should be fixed.

   ■ This can be undertaken using two partially threaded 3.5-mm screws (see Fig. 29-10).

   ■ In elderly patients with osteopenic bone, a posterior antiglide plate should be used (see Fig. 29-10) to prevent upward migration of the posterior fragment.

Fracture-Dislocations

■ These are the most serious types of ankle fracture.

■ In older patients they are usually associated with B3.2 or B3.3 trimalleolar fractures, but the classic Dupuytren's fracture-dislocation is a C2 fracture associated with an abduction force.

■ The treatment of fracture-dislocations is the same as for fractures, although emergency reduction is required to minimize the incidence of medial skin necrosis.

■ Both types of dislocations are associated with posttraumatic osteoarthritis, although it is more commonly seen in B3 trimalleolar fractures because the patients are older.

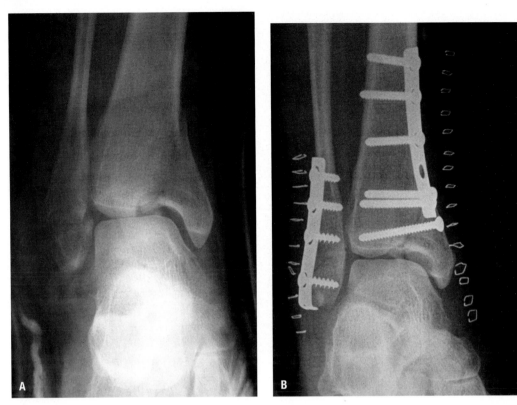

Figure 29-12 An A2.2 adduction fracture. (**A**) The vertical medial fracture line. (**B**) An antiglide plate has been used.

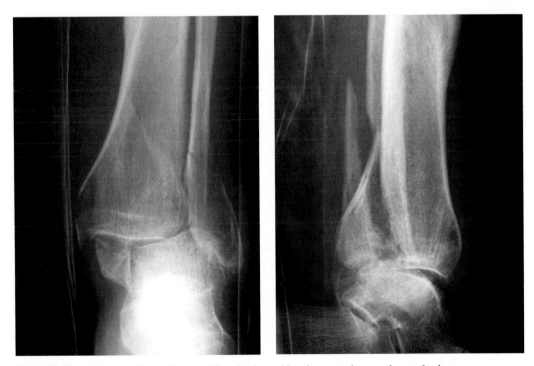

Figure 29-13 A B3.3 trimalleolar fracture. The talus has subluxed posteriorly secondary to displacement of the posterior malleolus.

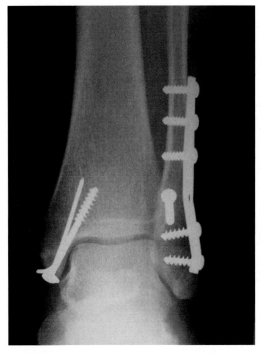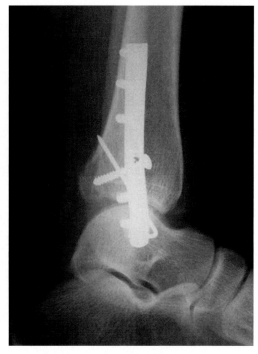

Figure 29-14 A B3.3 fracture with a small posterior malleolar fragment. This has reduced successfully after medial and lateral fixation.

Suprasyndesmotic Fractures

- The treatment of suprasyndesmotic fractures is essentially similar to that of other ankle fractures.
- In low suprasyndesmotic external rotation or abduction fractures, a plate is used to fix the fibula with supplementary screw fixation of an associated medial malleolar fracture.
- The debate concerns the use of syndesmosis screws (Fig. 29-15) placed between the fibula and the tibia to reduce and hold the syndesmosis in accurate alignment.
- In external rotation fractures, a fibular plate, supplemented by the intact interosseous membrane and posterior tibiofibular ligament, will usually restore stability.
- In abduction fractures, there is increased tibiofibular instability, but a fibular plate combined with medial malleolar fixation may well restore stability, although in C2.1 fractures associated with ligamentous instability, the mortise remains unstable and a syndesmotic screw is required.
- In C3 Maisonneuve fractures, the fibular neck should not be internally fixed, and a syndesmotic screw should be used to restore stability.
- It may be difficult to predict the degree of syndesmotic stability after internal fixation of a type C fracture, and therefore all type C fractures must be assessed using a fluoroscope after fixation.
- If external rotation or abduction causes the syndesmosis to open, a syndesmotic screw should be inserted.
- This may also occur in some B2.1 fractures associated with significant soft tissue injury.
- There has been considerable debate about syndesmotic screws, particularly concerning whether one or two screws should be used, whether they should penetrate three or four cortices, and where exactly they should be placed in relation to the ankle joint.
- Little evidence indicates that these arguments matter very much, however, and it is sensible to place one screw through three or four cortices between 2.5 and 4 cm above the ankle joint (see Fig. 29-15).

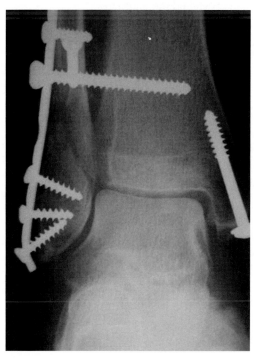

Figure 29-15 A syndesmosis screw placed through a lateral neutralization plate.

TABLE 29-5 SUGGESTED TREATMENT OF ANKLE FRACTURES

Injury	Treatment
Undisplaced fractures	Cast or brace
Displaced fractures	
Lateral malleolus	Interfragmentary screws or plate
	IM nail in osteopenic bone
Medial malleolus	
Large fragment	Cancellous screws
Small fragment	K-wires and tension band
A2.2 fracture	Interfragmentary screws and antiglide plate
Bimalleolar fracture	As above
Trimalleolar fracture	As above
Posterior malleolus	
<25%, congruous	No treatment
>25%, incongruous	Interfragmentary screws +/− antiglide plate
Suprasyndesmotic fractures	
C1.1 or C2.1	Fibula plate; syndesmosis screw if unstable
Other C1 and C2	Lateral and medial fixation using above techniques
C3	Syndesmosis screw

- In an osteopenic bone, all four cortices should be engaged.
- There has also been debate about the optimal position of the foot during syndesmotic screw insertion.
  - There was concern that if the syndesmotic screw was placed with the foot in dorsiflexion, the syndesmosis might be abnormally tightened.
- Biomechanical testing does not indicate this is the case, and the syndesmotic screw can be inserted with the foot in plantarflexion or dorsiflexion.
- The screw should not be lagged.

Postoperative Mobilization

- There has been controversy about the optimal method of managing ankle fractures after fixation.
- Surgeons are concerned that early weight bearing might disrupt their fixation, and they often prescribe 6 weeks of non-weight-bearing mobilization in a cast.
- A considerable number of studies have been undertaken to compare primary cast management, primary mobilization and later cast management, and functional bracing, but no differences have been shown among these three methods of management.
- Similarly, no difference has ever been shown between non-weight-bearing and weight-bearing mobilization in a cast or brace.
- Thus a cast or brace can be used after ankle fixation, and weight bearing should be encouraged.

Suggested Treatment

- The suggested treatment of ankle fractures is shown in Table 29-5.

COMPLICATIONS

- The main complications of the operative treatment of ankle fractures are listed in Table 29-6.
- The incidences of different complications vary among centers, but complications are relatively unusual after ankle fixation.
- In the overall population, the incidence of malunion and implant loosening is unknown but clearly relates to surgical technique.
- The most common complication is wound breakdown or superficial sepsis.
  - This is more common in the elderly, in patients with comorbidities such as alcoholism, schizophrenia, drug addiction, and diabetes, and in patients with more severe fracture types.
- Skin problems are clearly reduced by early surgery and have been shown to increase considerably if surgery is delayed by 24 hours.
  - They are also high in patients with open fractures and where there is skin damage prior to surgery.
- Osteomyelitis is rare and associated with the same factors as skin breakdown. The treatment of osteomyelitis is described in Chapter 40.
- Aseptic nonunions are also rare but more commonly affect the medial (Fig. 29-16) rather than the lateral or posterior malleoli, probably because medial malleolar fractures tend to be high-energy injuries.
  - Treatment is by bone grafting.
- Posttraumatic osteoarthritis is associated with more severe fracture types, and most of the cases analyzed in Table 29-6 were the result of trimalleolar fractures or fracture dislocations.
  - Osteoarthritis can also follow malreduced simpler fracture patterns, particularly if there is persistent talar shift after surgery.

TABLE 29-6 COMPLICATIONS OF ANKLE FRACTURE IN PATIENTS OF ALL AGES AND IN OLDER PATIENTS

Complication	All Patients		Age >60 y	
	Range (%)	Average (%)	Range (%)	Average (%)
Osteomyelitis	0–4.9	1.8	1–3	1.7
Superficial sepsis	2.8–10.3	4.6	5–9	3.7
Nonunion	0–1.7	0.3	0–2.6	0.9
Severe osteoarthritis	0–30.8	1.5	?	?
Malunion	?	?	5–12	5.4

- The onset of posttraumatic osteoarthritis of the ankle tends to be slow unless there is significant talar shift.
- Postoperative malunion can be treated by osteotomy and either fibular lengthening if the fibula is short or fibular derotation if there is a persistent external rotation deformity.
- The reported results of fibular osteotomy are good.
- Severe symptomatic posttraumatic osteoarthritis is treated by arthrodesis.
- Implant loosening is relatively common in osteopenic or osteomalacic bone.
  - This complication may well be reduced by the use of locking plates and intramedullary rods (see Fig. 29-9).
- The incidence of compartment syndrome is very low after ankle fracture.
- The other significant complication is that of pain related to the presence of a lateral malleolar plate.
  - This is estimated to occur in about 30% of patients and not infrequently results in plate removal.
  - The incidence of implant-related pain is less if a dorsal antiglide plate is used.

SPECIAL CIRCUMSTANCES

Fractures in the Elderly

- There has been debate whether elderly patients should be treated surgically in view of the problems of screw fixation in osteopenic bone.

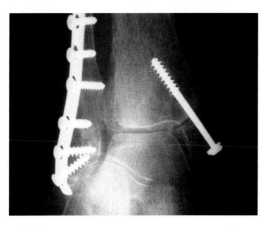

Figure 29-16 A medial malleolar nonunion 15 months after fixation.

- Nonoperative management is associated with all of the complications that caused surgeons to abandon its use in younger patients, however.
- The literature indicates that in patients of at least 60 years of age treated with intrafragmentary screws and plates, the results are very similar to those obtained in younger patients (see Table 29-6).
- Patients with ankle fractures should not be treated differently because of age.

Fractures in Diabetics

- Ankle fractures in diabetics are particularly difficult to treat.
- The complications of both nonoperative and operative treatment are considerable, particularly if the patient has a neuropathic arthropathy.
  - Nonoperative treatment has been shown to be associated with up to 70% malunion and 50% skin breakdown inside a cast.
  - The results of operative management are equally poor, with osteomyelitis averaging 20% and amputation about 10%.
- In open fractures, the results are worse, with about 36% osteomyelitis and 42% below-knee amputations reported.
- The treatment of displaced ankle fractures in young diabetics should be the same as for nondiabetic patients, but in older patients with reduced mobility, nonoperative management can be considered.

Lateral Ligament Injuries

- Injuries to the lateral ligamentous complex in the ankle are common.
- The diagnosis is usually made clinically, with pain usually felt on palpation over the anterior talofibular ligament.
- Arthrography and MRI scans can be used to diagnose lateral ligament damage.
- Treatment is usually nonoperative, although some surgeons advocate ligamentous repair.
- Prospective studies comparing surgical repair, cast management, and the use of an elastic bandage have shown no advantage to any treatment method.
- The patient should be warned that recovery may take 3 to 6 months if there is severe ligamentous damage, but surgery does not improve the prognosis.

Ankle Dislocation

■ Ankle dislocations without an associated fracture are extremely rare and the subject of sporadic case reports.

■ It is said to be caused by extreme plantar flexion and may be associated with a fracture of the posterior process of the talus or with dislocation of the peroneal tendons.

■ Treatment is by closed reduction.

Distal Tibiofibular Dislocation

■ There is a rare fracture dislocation of the ankle where the distal fibula becomes trapped behind the tibia and is irreducible by closed means.

■ Very occasionally the fibula is intact, but usually there is a distal fibular fracture and standard fixation techniques are used.

■ Associated medial malleolar fractures have been reported.

■ If the fibula is intact, a closed manipulation may be attempted, but this is usually unsuccessful and open reduction is required.

SUGGESTED READING

Boden SD, Labropoulos PA, McCowin P, et al. Mechanical consideration of the syndesmosis screw. J Bone Joint Surg (Am) 1989; 71:1548–1555.

Cimino W, Ichtertz D, Slabaugh P. Early mobilization of ankle fractures after open reduction and internal fixation. Clin Orthop 1991;267:152–156.

Court-Brown CM, McBirnie J, Wilson G. Adult ankle fractures: an increasing problem? Acta Orthop Scand 1998;69:43–47.

Harper MC, Hardin G. Posterior malleolar fractures of the ankle associated with external rotation-abduction injuries. Results with and without internal fixation. J Bone Joint Surg (Am) 1988; 70:1348–1356.

Kristensen KD, Hansen T. Closed treatment of ankle fractures. Stage II supination-eversion fractures followed for 20 years. Acta Orthop Scand 1985;56:107–109.

Lauge-Hansen N. Fractures of the ankle: II. Combined experimental-surgical and experimental-roentgenologic investigations. Arch Surg 1950;60:957–985.

Marsh JL, Saltzman CL. Ankle fractures. In: Buchholz RW, Heckman JD, eds. Rockwood and Green's fractures in adults, 5th ed. Philadelphia: Lippincott Williams and Wilkins, 2001:2001–2090.

Müller ME, Nazarian S, Koch P, et al. The comprehensive classification of fractures of long bones. Berlin: Springer-Verlag, 1990.

Pankovich AM. Maisonneuve fracture of the fibula. J Bone Joint Surg (Am) 1976;58:337–342.

Weber BG. Die verletzungen des oberen sprunggelenkes. Bern: Hans Huber, 1966.

FOOT FRACTURES AND DISLOCATIONS

Orthopaedic surgeons commonly encounter foot fractures, and in recent years there has been an increased awareness of their importance and a renewed interest in surgical treatment. This is particularly true of the calcaneus. The use of CT and MRI scans has highlighted the severity of many foot fractures, showing that even apparently simple avulsion fractures may be associated with significant joint damage that may lead to late pain. Despite their relative frequency, remarkably little is known about the epidemiology of foot fractures. This chapter examines the epidemiology of foot fractures in general and the epidemiology, diagnosis, and treatment of individual bones in the foot. Box 30-1 lists a number of the controversies about the management of foot fractures.

EPIDEMIOLOGY

The epidemiology of foot fractures is shown in Table 30-1. There is an approximately equal gender distribution. Predictably, fractures of the metatarsus and phalanges fractures are most commonly seen, although calcaneal fractures

BOX 30-1 CURRENT CONTROVERSIES IN FOOT FRACTURES

How should talar body fractures be treated?
How successful is their treatment?
What are the long-term effects of lateral process fractures of the talus?
Is nonoperative or operative treatment preferable for intra-articular calcaneal fractures?
How should calcaneal fractures be fixed?
Is bone graft required for calcaneal fractures?
How should extra-articular calcaneal fractures be managed?
How common are midfoot fractures?
How should they be treated?
How should Lisfranc fracture-dislocations be treated?
How common are stress fractures of the metatarsus?
How should Jones fractures be treated?

TABLE 30-1 EPIDEMIOLOGY OF FOOT FRACTURES

Proportion of all fractures	12.3%
Average age	39.9 y
Men/women	55%/45%
Incidence	137.1/10⁵/y
Fracture type	
Talus	2.3%
Calcaneus	10.0%
Midfoot	3.7%
Metatarsal	55.0%
Sesamoids	0.1%
Phalanges	28.9%

account for 10% of all foot fractures. Fractures of the midfoot and talus are less common, and fractures of the sesamoids are very rare. Fractures may be associated with dislocations of the hindfoot, midfoot, or the tarsometatarsal joints in particular.

FRACTURES OF THE TALUS

Talar fractures are relatively uncommon but usually severe and associated with considerable morbidity. Their treatment has always challenged orthopaedic surgeons. Initial interest in talar fractures followed the Second World War when aviators' astralagus was described. The classification of talar neck and body fractures was compiled in the 1970s, and there has been little change in classification or management since then. Recent years have seen a renewed interest in the lateral process fracture, mainly because of the popularity of snowboarding!

SURGICAL ANATOMY

The talus is unusual for a number of reasons. Two thirds of its surface is covered with articular cartilage, there are no

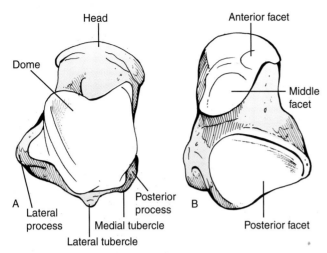

Figure 30-1   The anatomy of the talus. Superior aspect (**A**) and inferior aspect (**B**).

tendons or muscles that originate from or insert into it, and the blood supply is relatively poor, so avascular necrosis is a significant problem after fracture.

The body of the talus is covered superiorly by the trochlear articular cartilage, which is wider anteriorly than posteriorly (Fig. 30-1). The superior articular surface extends medially and laterally to articulate with the medial and lateral malleoli. On the inferior surface of the talar body are three articular facets that articulate with the calcaneus. The body has a wedge-shaped lateral process. Its inferior surface articulates with the lateral aspect of the posterior facet of the calcaneus, and its superolateral surface forms an articulation with the distal fibula. The posterior process is composed of medial and lateral tubercles

that are separated by a groove for the tendon of flexor hallucis longus. An os trigonum or secondary ossification center may be present posteriorly and be confused with a posterior process fracture. The neck extends anteroinferiorly from the body. It deviates 15 to 20 degrees medially in adults. It joins the body to the head of the talus, which articulates with the navicular bone in the midfoot.

The blood supply to the talus comes from three main arteries and their branches. The main blood supply is from the posterior tibial artery, which gives off a branch to the tarsal canal running between the posterior and middle facets. This supplies most of the body. The head and neck are supplied by the dorsalis pedis artery and the artery of the tarsal sinus, a branch of the perforating peroneal artery. The posterior part of the talus is supplied by branches of the posterior tibial artery that enter through the posterior process.

CLASSIFICATION

Two principal classifications cover virtually all talar fractures. These are the Hawkins (1970) classification of talar neck fractures, which was later modified by Canale and Kelly (1978), and the Sneppen (1977) classification of talar body fractures. Hawkins separated talar neck fractures into three types (Fig. 30-2). Type I fractures are undisplaced fractures that exit inferiorly between the middle and posterior facets. Type II fractures are similar, but there is subluxation or dislocation of the subtalar joint, and in type III fractures the body of the talus is dislocated from both subtalar and ankle joints. Canale and Kelly added a type IV fracture, where the talar head is dislocated from the navicular. Hawkins had included these fractures in his type III group.

Sneppen divided talar body fractures into six basic types (Fig. 30-3): Type A fractures are osteochondral fractures.

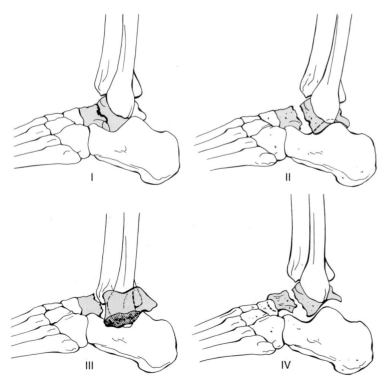

Figure 30-2   The Hawkins (1970) classification of talar neck fractures. Type IV was added by Canale and Kelly (1978). See text for explanation.

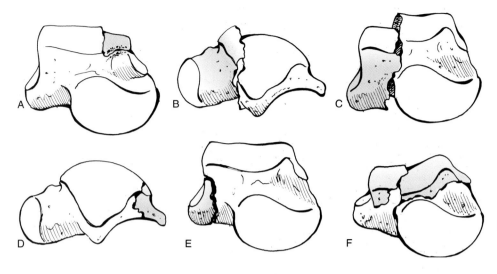

Figure 30-3 The Sneppen (1977) classification of talar body fractures. See text for explanation.

Type B fractures are sagittal shear fractures, and type C fractures are coronal shear fractures. Type D fractures contain the posterior process fractures with the lateral process fractures designated type E. Type F fractures are crush fractures. The classification does not include all variants of talar shear fractures. Boyd and Knight (1942) described the comparatively unusual transverse shear fracture and also pointed out that the sheared fragments could displace and become dislocated from the ankle and subtalar joints in the same way as a type III talar neck fracture.

EPIDEMIOLOGY

The basic epidemiology of talar fractures is shown in Table 30-2. Their rarity means that no talar head fractures were seen during the year analyzed in Chapter 1. Comparative data from a U.S. level 1 trauma center shows a very similar distribution of fractures with 62% talar body fractures, 34% talar neck fractures, and 4% head fractures. The average age of patients with talar fractures is low. The incidence of open fractures varies with the type of institution, but a range of 10.5% to 23.5% is quoted in the literature.

TABLE 30-2 EPIDEMIOLOGY OF TALAR FRACTURES

Proportion of all fractures	0.3%
Proportion of foot fractures	2.3%
Average age	30.5 y
Men/women	82%/18%
Incidence	$3.2/10^5$/y
Distribution	Type C
Open fractures	11.8%
Most common causes	
Falls from height	58.8%
Direct blow	11.8%
Fracture type	
Body	70.6%
Neck	29.4%

Associated Injuries

Talar fractures tend to be high-energy injuries with a very high incidence of associated musculoskeletal injuries. In this series, 17 patients with talar fractures had 31 other musculoskeletal injuries. Analysis showed that 41.1% of patients had calcaneal fractures, 35.3% had metatarsal fractures, and 23.5% had spinal fractures. The literature also records an association between talar body fractures and ankle fractures.

DIAGNOSIS

History and Physical Examination

- Traditionally, most talar fractures have been thought to follow high-energy injuries, and this is true of most neck and body fractures. There is an increasing awareness that lateral process fractures may be caused by sports such as snowboarding, however, and a careful history may reveal the possibility of significant axial loading of the hindfoot in an apparently low-energy injury.
- The clinical presentation is with a swollen painful hindfoot.
- There may be considerable deformity if there is an associated subtalar or ankle dislocation.
- Careful assessment of local swelling, deformity, and the state of the soft tissues must be made with any open wounds carefully examined.
- If there is an associated dislocation, the vascularity of the overlying skin and the foot must be carefully assessed.
- In low-energy injuries, the lateral process should be carefully palpated.

Radiologic Examination

- Talar fractures are complex, but they can usually be diagnosed by anteroposterior and lateral radiographs (Fig. 30-4).

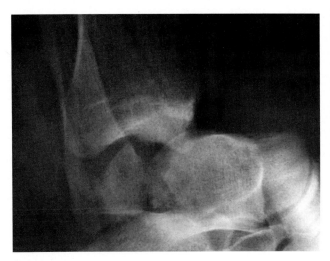
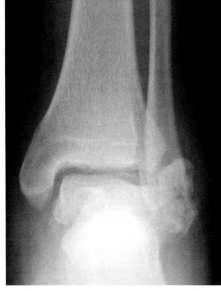

Figure 30-4 A displaced talar body fracture.

- CT scans are useful to delineate the exact fracture pattern and to determine the ease of reconstruction.
  - They are particularly useful in fractures of the talar body where the direction of the shear fracture and the degree of talar dome damage can be assessed.
  - They are also indicated if a lateral process fracture is suspected but radiographs are negative because conventional radiographs may fail to detect as many as 50% of these fractures.
- MRI scans are not required for the primary diagnosis of talar fractures but may well be required for the later detection of avascular necrosis, with serial MRI scans useful for the prediction of recovery of an avascular talar body.
- Careful radiologic assessment of the whole foot, ankle, and distal tibia is important because most associated injuries are in these areas.

TALAR NECK FRACTURES

These were initially described in detail after the Second World War and assumed to occur as a result of hyperdorsiflexion of the foot in flying accidents. Laboratory studies indicate that talar neck fractures are caused by an axial load applied to the plantar aspect of the foot, however.

EPIDEMIOLOGY

The basic epidemiology of talar neck fractures is shown in Table 30-3. They tend to occur in young adults, with men more commonly affected, and have a type C distribution (see Chapter 1). There is a high incidence of open fractures and

associated injuries, most of these in the ipsilateral foot and ankle. All talar neck fractures are caused by high-energy injuries and usually caused by falls from height or motor vehicle accidents. The distribution of the different types of talar neck fractures is taken from the world literature and shows that Hawkins type II fractures are most common.

TREATMENT

Nonsurgical Treatment

- Nonoperative management has always been used for Hawkins type I fractures.
- The treatment protocol is fairly uniform, with 10 to 12 weeks in a non-weight-bearing cast or brace. Surgical management is used if there is secondary fracture displacement.
- No recent series have analyzed nonoperative management of Hawkins type II and III fractures.

TABLE 30-3 EPIDEMIOLOGY OF TALAR NECK FRACTURES	
Proportion of talar fractures	29.4%
Average age	28.4 y
Men/women	60%/40%
Incidence	0.9/10^5/y
Distribution	Type C
Open fractures	20%
Fracture type[a]	
Hawkins I	31%
Hawkins II	43%
Hawkins III	26%

[a]The distribution of talar neck fractures according to the Hawkins classification has been taken from the literature.

TABLE 30-4 RESULTS OF TREATMENT OF TALAR NECK FRACTURES[a]

Result/Complication	Overall (%)		Type I (%)		Type II (%)		Type III[b] (%)	
	Range	Average	Range	Average	Range	Average	Range	Average
Excellent/good	45–96.4	72.7	50–100	87.3	25.6–91.6	45.5	14.2–66.6	60
Open	10–24.7	18.1						
Infection	0–10	3.3						
Avascular necrosis	13–53.2	28.1	0–15.4	3.9	13.6–66.6	25.6	27.2–92.5	69.8
Nonunion	0–6.1	3.9	0–7.7	1.3	0–5.7	2.6	5–13	10.5
Osteoarthritis								
Ankle	30.9–32.9	31.7	15	15	36	36	69	69
Subtalar	36–47.1	45.5	24	24	66	66	63	63

[a]Most type I fractures have been treated nonoperatively, with types II and III fractures treated operatively.
[b]Type IV fractures are included with the type III fractures.

- The older literature suggests an avascular necrosis rate of up to 71%, which is higher than shown in Table 30-4.
- Malunion associated with nonoperative management was problematic and associated with poor results.
- There is now no indication for nonoperative management of Hawkins II or III fractures.

Surgical Treatment

- The standard method of management for Hawkins type II and III fractures is interfragmentary screw fixation using two cannulated screws (Fig. 30-5).
  - Type III and IV fractures should be treated as an emergency because of the associated dislocation.
- The screws can be introduced from anterior to posterior using an anteromedial approach to the distal talus.

- Alternatively, the screws can be inserted percutaneously from posterior to anterior, but reduction is more difficult and malunion more common.
- Table 30-4 summarizes the results of the management of talar neck fractures.
  - The infection rate is low and the major problems are avascular necrosis, osteoarthritis, and nonunion.
  - Avascular necrosis is rare in type I fractures but much more common in types II and III fractures.
  - The nonunion rate also correlates with the severity of the fracture as does the incidence of both ankle and subtalar arthritis.
  - Excellent or good results can be expected after type I injuries but not after type II or type III injuries because of the high incidence of avascular necrosis and osteoarthritis.

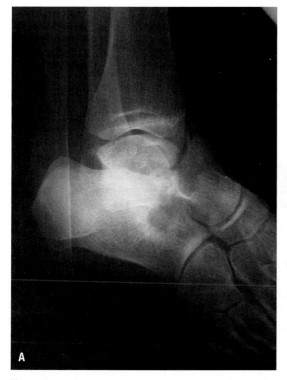
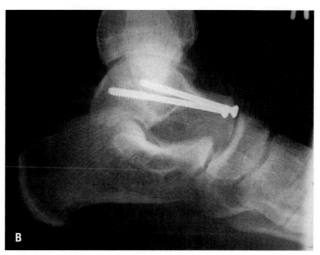

Figure 30-5 (A) A Hawkins II talar neck fracture. (B) This has been fixed with two cancellous screws.

COMPLICATIONS

- Infection is relatively unusual.
- If it cannot be managed according to the principles laid out in Chapter 40, talectomy and subsequent tibiocalcaneal fusion is indicated.
- Treatment of nonunion is discussed in Chapter 39.
- Malunion is relatively unusual if open reduction and internal fixation is used, although if there is comminution of the talar neck, screw fixation can produce a varus deformity that may need to be treated by later osteotomy and bone grafting.

Avascular Necrosis

- This is a radiological diagnosis.
- Initially, there is increased density of the talar body, but as revascularization occurs there is subchondral collapse, secondary osteoarthritic change, and talar dome fragmentation (Fig. 30-6).
- Viability of the talar body is associated with Hawkins sign, that is, subchondral atrophy or rarefaction on routine radiographs.
- This should be seen 6 to 8 weeks after the fracture.
- Treatment of avascular necrosis of the talus depends on the severity of the associated pain, and surgeons are advised to wait and see if the symptoms settle.
  - If operative treatment is required, it is important to identify whether the ankle or subtalar joints are the source of the pain because an appropriate arthrodesis may be beneficial.
  - If there is extensive avascular necrosis, a tibiocalcaneal arthrodesis can be undertaken after resection of the talar body.
  - In the past, a Blair fusion was advocated, with a sliding graft from the anterior distal tibia used to fuse with the calcaneus. Today, however, a retrograde statically locked nail passed from the calcaneus to the tibia, supplemented with bone graft, gives better results.

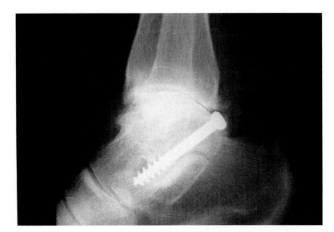

Figure 30-6 Avascular necrosis of the talus and secondary osteoarthritis of the ankle 7 years after a Hawkins II talar neck fracture.

Posttraumatic Osteoarthritis

- Table 30-4 shows that both ankle and subtalar osteoarthritis are relatively common, the incidence correlating with the severity of the fracture.
- Treatment of symptomatic osteoarthritis is by fusion of either or both of the ankle and subtalar joints.
  - If both joints have to be fused, a retrograde intramedullary nail and bone graft can be used (see Fig. 28-10 in Chapter 28).

TALAR BODY FRACTURES

Most shear, compression, and crush fractures of the talar body are caused by axial loading, although fractures of the posterior and lateral processes may occur in twisting injuries, simple falls, or sports injuries.

EPIDEMIOLOGY

The basic epidemiology of talar body fractures is shown in Table 30-5. They are uncommon injuries that usually occur in young men and have a type C distribution (see Chapter 1). Few are open, although this varies according to the type of institution, and up to 18% open talar body fractures have been recorded in level 1 trauma centers. In shear fractures, there is an approximately equal incidence of coronal and sagittal fractures.

TREATMENT

Shear and Crush Fractures

- CT scans should be used to check for displacement of shear fractures.
- If undisplaced (Fig. 30-7), the fracture should be treated nonoperatively with 10 to 12 weeks in a nonweight-bearing cast or brace.

TABLE 30-5 EPIDEMIOLOGY OF TALAR BODY FRACTURES

Proportion of talar fractures	70.6%
Average age	32.1 y
Men/women	92%/8%
Incidence	2.2/10^5/y
Distribution	Type C
Open fractures	8.3%
Fracture type	
Shear/crush	41.6%
Lateral process	25%
Posterior process	25%
Osteochondral	8.3%

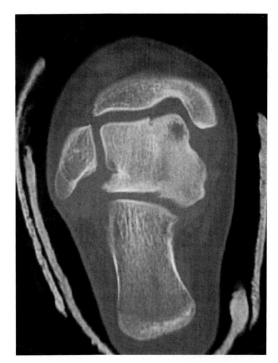

Figure 30-7 A CT scan showing a minimally displaced talar body fracture.

- Displaced fractures should be reduced and fixed with interfragmentary screws.
- Crush fractures should also be reconstructed with interfragmentary screws if possible.
- If it is impossible, primary arthrodesis of the ankle and/or subtalar joints is recommended.
- In severe unreconstructable crush fractures of the talar body, tibiocalcaneal fusion with retrograde intramedullary nailing and grafting should be undertaken.
- If this is done, a careful attempt should be made to preserve the appropriate distance between the calcaneus and distal tibia to ensure optimal foot biomechanics.
- Very little is known about the complications or prognosis of shear or crush fractures of the talar body, but the results documented by Vallier et al. (2003) are interesting.
  - They examined a group of shear and crush talar body fractures and compared the results with a group of very severe talar body fractures that had involvement of the talar neck.
  - The results indicate a high incidence of avascular necrosis, fracture collapse, and ankle and subtalar osteoarthritis (Table 30-6).
  - If symptomatic, treatment is by appropriate ankle and/or subtalar arthrodesis.

Posterior Process Fractures

- Fractures of the posterior process (Fig. 30-8) may involve the whole posterior process or the medial or lateral tubercles.
  - Most are undisplaced or minimally displaced, and nonoperative management is indicated.
  - A below-knee weight-bearing cast or brace should be used for 4 to 6 weeks.

TABLE 30-6 COMPLICATIONS FOLLOWING SHEAR AND CRUSH FRACTURES OF THE TALAR BODY

Complication	Talar Body (%)	Talar Body and Neck (%)
Avascular necrosis	27	55
Fracture collapse	7	36
Osteoarthritis		
Ankle	65	?
Subtalar	35	?

Data from Vallier HA, Nork SE, Benirschke SK, et al. Surgical treatment of talar neck body fractures. J Bone Joint Surg (Am) 2003;85: 1716–1724.

- Nonunion of either the medial or lateral tuberosity may occur, and symptomatic nonunions are best treated by surgical excision.
- Fractures of the whole posterior process are less common.
  - Undisplaced fractures should be treated nonoperatively, but displaced fractures require open reduction and internal fixation with interfragmentary screws.

Lateral Process Fractures

- These fractures (Fig. 30-9) are probably more common than surgeons realize and may be missed when the diagnosis of an ankle sprain is made.
- They are caused by axial loading on an everted foot and may therefore follow a fall, motor vehicle accident, or sports injury.
- Lateral process fractures are particularly important because they may be associated with significant subtalar damage caused by the axial load.
- Late pain after lateral process fractures has been attributed to nonunion but is in fact more commonly caused by subtalar osteoarthritis (see Fig. 30-9).

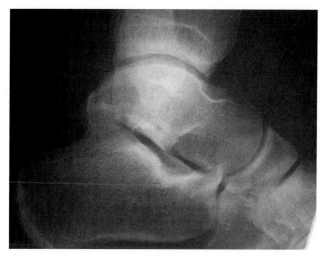

Figure 30-8 A posterior process fracture.

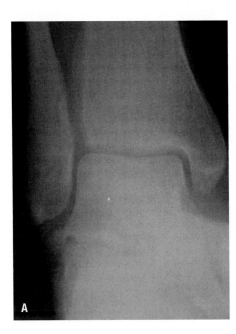

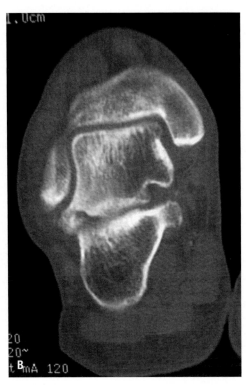

Figure 30-9 A lateral process fracture shown on X-ray (**A**) and CT scan (**B**). Note the subtalar damage on the CT scan.

- Treatment is nonoperative for undisplaced fractures, or if there are small displaced fragments, with 4 to 6 weeks in a weight-bearing cast or brace.
- Larger fragments should be fixed with an interfragmentary screw.
- Late pain should be investigated with a CT or MRI scan.
- If there is symptomatic subtalar osteoarthritis, an arthrodesis is indicated.
- Symptomatic nonunion of small bony fragments should be treated by excision, and larger fragments should be fixed with an interfragmentary screw.

Osteochondral Fractures

The true incidence of osteochondral talar fractures (Fig. 30-10) is difficult to define because a number occur as a result of ankle or plafond injuries.

- The classification of Berndt and Hardy (1959) is shown in Figure 30-11.
    - Stage I lesions consist of subchondral trabecular compression with intact overlying cartilage.
    - Stage II lesions show an incomplete separation of the fragment.
    - Stage III lesions are separate but undisplaced, and in stage IV lesions the fragment has become separate.
    - Some surgeons include subchondral cysts as a IIa lesion, but although these may predispose to fracture there is debate about whether they are traumatic in origin.
- Osteochondral fractures occur anterolaterally and posteromedially on the dome on the talus.
- Stage I lesions are treated nonoperatively with cast or brace immobilization for 6 weeks.

- Early stage II lesions should be similarly treated, but persistently painful lesions should be treated by drilling the subchondral bone.
- Stage III lesions are best treated nonoperatively unless symptoms persist, in which case debridement of the fragment and subchondral drilling should be undertaken.
- Stage IV lesions are usually treated by excision with debridement of the subchondral bone. Larger lesions should be replaced if an accurate reduction can be achieved.

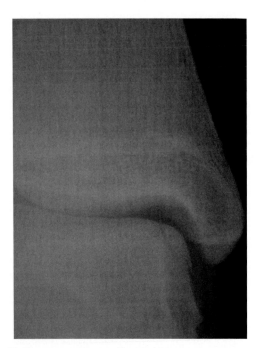

Figure 30-10 A stage III osteochondral fracture.

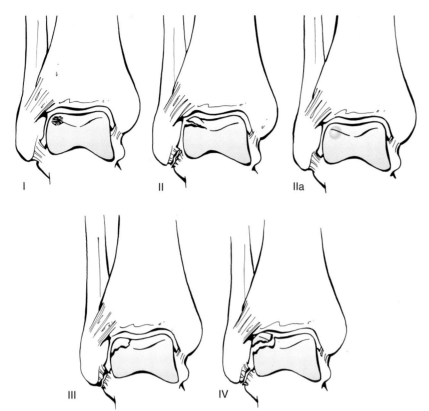

Figure 30-11 The Berndt and Hardy classification of osteochondral talar fractures. See text for explanation.

Talar Head Fractures

- These are very rare.
- They are either shear fractures or impaction fractures.
- Undisplaced shear fractures can be treated nonoperatively with 6 weeks in a cast or brace.
- Displaced shear fractures should be treated by open reduction and internal fixation with interfragmentary screws.
- Impacted fractures are likely to lead to talonavicular osteoarthritis, and if the impaction is severe, a primary talonavicular arthrodesis may be undertaken.
- If the impaction is minor, nonoperative management may be employed with late fusion of a symptomatic talonavicular joint.

Talar Dislocations

Subtalar Dislocation

- Subtalar dislocations (Fig. 30-12) are rare.
- They involve the talocalcaneal and talonavicular joints and may, at times, be associated with a hindfoot fracture, particularly a talar neck fracture.
- About 50% to 65% of subtalar dislocations are associated with other fractures of the foot and ankle.
- Most subtalar dislocations are the result of high-energy injuries such as motor vehicle accidents or falls from a height, but 20% to 25% follow low-energy injuries such as sports injuries.
  - They are caused by rotational forces applied to the hindfoot.

- About 80% of subtalar dislocations are medial, 15% are lateral, and the remainder are either anterior or posterior, although they usually have a component of medial or lateral rotation as well.
- Patients with subtalar dislocation present with deformity of the hindfoot.
  - There is tenting of the skin over the prominent talar head, and between 10% and 40% of the injuries are open.
  - The diagnosis is usually obvious, but care must be taken to check for other foot injuries.
  - Standard anteroposterior, lateral, and oblique X-rays of the foot are required.
  - CT scans show osteochondral fractures and the presence of other occult fractures in the foot.
- Treatment is by closed reduction if possible.
- Open wounds must be treated according to the principles discussed in Chapter 4.
- Approximately 10% to 15% of subtalar dislocations are irreducible by closed means and require open reduction.
  - This is usually caused by the head of the talus buttonholing adjacent soft tissues. In lateral subtalar dislocations the tendon of tibialis posterior may prevent reduction.
- An impaction fracture occasionally may lock the talonavicular joint, preventing reduction.
- After reduction the hindfoot should be immobilized in a weight-bearing cast for 4 to 6 weeks.
- The results are generally poor, with only about 25% of patients having excellent or good results.
  - The results are worse in open injuries and in lateral dislocations.

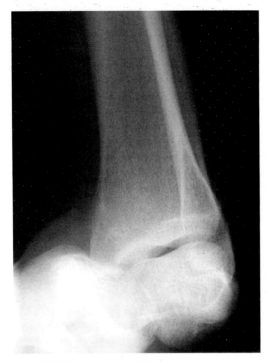

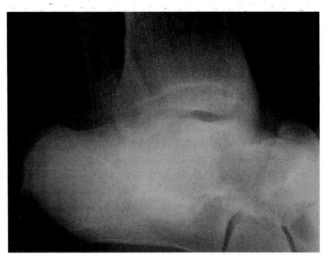

Figure 30-12   A subtalar dislocation.

■ Complications include reflex sympathetic dystrophy, hindfoot stiffness, posttraumatic osteoarthritis, and occasionally avascular necrosis of the talus.

Total Talar Dislocation

■ Total talar dislocation or extrusion of the talus is very rare.

■ The talus can dislocate medially or laterally, and it is caused by continuation of the forces that cause subtalar dislocation.

■ Virtually all of these dislocations are open, and the prognosis is poor.

■ Treatment is by open reduction of the talus with a thorough debridement of all devitalized and contaminated tissues.

■ Casts should be applied and maintained for 6 to 8 weeks.

■ Complications include infection, avascular necrosis, and posttraumatic osteoarthritis, which may necessitate tibiotalar, subtalar, or pantalar arthrodeses.

■ In the largest series reported, Smith et al. (2005) showed that in 27 patients who presented with an extruded talus, 70.4% had associated fractures of the talar neck, body, or lateral process, and 78% had other associated fractures. There was a 7.4% incidence of infection.

Suggested Treatment

■ The suggested treatment of talar fractures is given in Table 30-7.

FRACTURES OF THE CALCANEUS

The calcaneus is the largest bone in the foot. Fractures of the calcaneus are either intra-articular, involving the posterior facet, or extra-articular, usually involving the body or anterior or posterior tuberosities. About 25% to 40% of calcaneal fractures are extra-articular depending on the type of institution. The anatomy of the calcaneus is complex, and fractures can occur in all parts of the bone, although intra-articular fractures have received the most attention.

TABLE 30-7   SUGGESTED TREATMENT OF TALAR FRACTURES

Injury	Treatment
Undisplaced fractures	Cast or brace
Displaced fractures	
Neck	Interfragmentary screws
Body	
Crush/shear	
Reconstructible	Interfragmentary screws
Unreconstructable	Retrograde IM nail and local fusion
Posterior process	Interfragmentary screws
Lateral process	Interfragmentary screws
Osteochondral	See text

SURGICAL ANATOMY

An appreciation of the anatomy of the calcaneus is essential to understand the pathogenesis and treatment of the different fractures. Figure 30-13 shows the lateral, superior, and coronal anatomy of the bone. There are three articular facets-the posterior, middle, and anterior facets all of which articulate with the talus. Intra-articular calcaneal fractures involve the posterior facet. The body of the calcaneus may be fractured without damaging the posterior facet, and both the anterior process and posterior tuberosity can be fractured. The anterior process is attached by the bifurcate ligament to the cuboid and navicular. An anterior process fracture usually involves damage to the calcaneocuboid joint. The posterior tuberosity provides the insertion for the tendo-Achilles, and it may be fractured by direct blow or by a sudden pull of the tendons.

The lateral and medial processes of the posterior tuberosity are the weight-bearing areas of the bone. The medial process gives origin to abductor hallucis, flexor digitorum brevis, and part of abductor digiti minimi, the remainder of abductor digiti minimi arising from the lateral process, which also gives rise to the lateral head of flexor accessorius. The plantar fascia arises from the medial and lateral processes and the intervening posterior tuberosity. There is an oblique ridge on the lateral wall of the calcaneum, which is known as the peroneal trochlea. This gives rise to the inferior peroneal retinaculum, which bridges the tendons of peroneus longus and brevis.

A number of neurovascular structures and tendons run on both sides of the calcaneus. Peroneus longus and brevis tendons pass laterally under the superior and inferior peroneal retinaculae and are at risk in the lateral approach to the bone. The sural nerve runs across the vertical component of the standard extended lateral incision about 3 cm above the tip of the malleolus. It is easily damaged in the

TABLE 30-8 EPIDEMIOLOGY OF CALCANEAL FRACTURES	
Proportion of all fractures	1.2%
Proportion of foot fractures	10.0%
Average age	40.4 y
Men/women	78%/22%
Incidence	13.7/10^5/y
Distribution	Type G
Open fractures	2.7%
Fracture types	
Intra-articular	58.9%
Anterior process	13.7%
Body	6.8%
Posterior tuberosity	2.7%
Medial process	15.1%
Lateral process	2.7%

conventional lateral approach. On the medial side are a number of structures at risk from surgery. The tendons of tibialis posterior, flexor digitorum longus, and flexor hallucis longus all lie under the flexor retinaculum, with the tendon of flexor hallucis longus running under the sustentaculum tali of the calcaneum. The posterior tibial artery branches into the medial and lateral plantar branches under the flexor retinaculum, and the posterior tibial nerve also divides into the medial and lateral plantar nerves at a level just below the arterial bifurcation.

EPIDEMIOLOGY

The basic epidemiology of calcaneal fractures is shown in Table 30-8. They have a different distribution from talar fractures. They are common in younger men but also

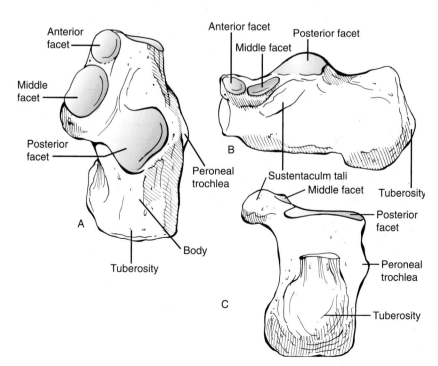

Figure 30-13 The anatomy of the calcaneus showing its superior (**A**), lateral (**B**), and posterior (**C**) aspects.

occur in older men and women, giving them a type G distribution (see Chapter 1). About 60% of calcaneal fractures are intra-articular. The remaining are extra-articular, with fractures of the medial and anterior processes the most common extra-articular fractures.

Intra-Articular Calcaneal Fractures

Intra-articular calcaneal fractures have challenged surgeons for many years, and there is still considerable debate about whether they should be treated operatively or nonoperatively. The early days of fracture fixation involved the use of K-wires, screws, and staples, and results were poor. Both primary and secondary subtalar arthrodeses were used, but again the results did not justify initial optimism. Surgeons returned to nonoperative management, and only in the last 20 to 25 years has there been increased interest in operative management. Better surgical techniques and the introduction of calcaneal plates have improved results, although the debate about the usefulness of surgery continues. The literature is confusing because it is full of retrospective studies employing different surgical techniques and outcome measures.

CLASSIFICATION

To understand any of the classifications, it is important to understand the pathogenesis of intra-articular fractures. This is relatively straightforward and surprisingly constant among fractures, although there are variations in fracture morphology depending on the position of the foot, the magnitude of the deforming force, and the bone quality. Because an axial load is applied to the calcaneus, the primary fracture line is made by the lateral process of the talus being driven downward. The primary calcaneal fracture line runs from anterolateral to posteromedial, dividing the calcaneus into antero-

medial and posterolateral fragments. The position of the primary fracture line may vary from adjacent to the sustentaculum tali on the medial side to relatively close to the lateral wall. As the talus continues to descend, the usually larger posterolateral fragment is secondarily fractured, causing further comminution of the posterior facet, fractures, and bulging of the lateral wall, forward rotation of the posterolateral fragment or fragments, and sometimes calcaneocuboid damage. In a typical fracture, the posterolateral fragment is rotated downward into the body of the calcaneus. If there is a secondary fracture in the axis of the calcaneus, a tongue-type fracture is produced, but if there is a secondary fracture at 90 degrees to the calcaneus, a joint depression fracture occurs (Fig. 30-14A).

The original classification, which still remains in use, is the Essex-Lopresti classification, which simply distinguishes between joint depression and tongue-type fractures (see Fig. 30-14). Many other classifications have been suggested, but it is the Sanders classification that is in widespread use. This is a simple classification based on the position of the primary fracture line and the number of the secondary fragments in the posterior facet (Fig. 30-15). The primary fracture line is defined as having three possible locations, with the number of displaced articular fragments determining the classification number. Thus in type 1 fractures, there may be up to four intra-articular fragments, but they are undisplaced. In type 2 fractures, the primary fracture line creates two fragments, but it is the position of the fracture that determines whether they are 2A, B, or C. In type 3 fractures, there are three displaced intra-articular fragments, and in type 4 fractures, there are four displaced fragments.

EPIDEMIOLOGY

The basic epidemiology of intra-articular calcaneal fractures is shown in Table 30-9. They often occur in middle-aged patients, with men more commonly affected. Open

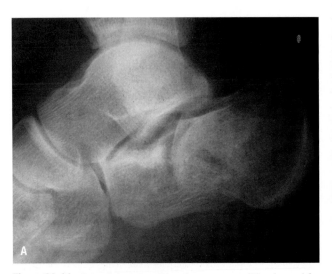
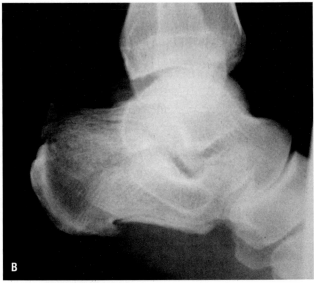

Figure 30-14 Joint depression (**A**) and tongue-type (**B**) calcaneal fractures.

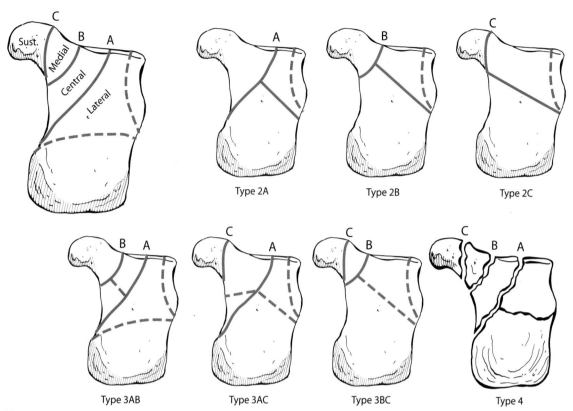

Figure 30-15 The Sanders classification of intra-articular calcaneal fractures. See text for explanation.

fractures are rare but serious when they occur. About 70% of fractures are Sanders type 2 or 3 and potentially reconstructible. About 80% are joint depression fractures.

Analysis of the mode of injury shows that virtually all intra-articular calcaneal fractures follow a fall from a height, motor vehicle accident, or a fall down steps or stairs (Table 30-10). Lower energy fractures occur in older patients. Sanders type 4 fractures occur in motor vehicle accidents or falls from a height.

TABLE 30-9 EPIDEMIOLOGY OF INTRA-ARTICULAR CALCANEAL FRACTURES

Proportion of calcaneal fractures	58.9%
Average age	45.6 y
Men/women	73%/27%
Incidence	8.0/10^5/y
Distribution	Type G
Open fractures	7.0%
Fracture type	
Tongue	18.6%
Joint depression	81.4%
Sanders classification	
Type 1	16.3%
Type 2	46.5%
Type 3	20.9%
Type 4	16.3%

Associated Injuries

The literature indicates that between 7% and 59% of patients with calcaneal fractures have associated musculoskeletal injuries. In the series detailed in Chapter 1 and Table 30-8, the most common associated musculoskeletal injuries involved fractures of the spine, talus, metatarsals, and midfoot, each of which occurred in about 10% of patients. The association with spinal fractures is well known, with other studies showing that up to 30% of patients present with the combination of spinal and calcaneal fractures. These figures come from level 1 trauma centers. About 7% of patients have bilateral fractures.

DIAGNOSIS

History and Physical Examination

- The history is usually straightforward: The patient has usually fallen from a height or been involved in a motor vehicle accident.
- Any associated injuries must be detected, and patients with high-energy injuries should be carefully examined accordingly to ATLS principles.
  - Particular care should be taken to examine for coexisting spinal injuries.
- The calcaneal fracture presents as a very painful swollen hindfoot.
- The incidence of foot compartment syndrome has been estimated as high as 10% and should be looked for.

TABLE 30-10 CAUSES OF INTRA-ARTICULAR CALCANEAL FRACTURES

| | | | Sanders Type (%) | | | |
Cause	Prevalence (%)	Age (y)	1	2	3	4
Fall from height	69.8	42.4	23.3	36.7	23.3	16.7
Motor vehicle accident	13.9	46.2		33.3	16.6	50
Fall on stairs	13.9	57.7		83.3	16.6	

- Neurovascular injury is rare unless the patient has had a crushed foot.
- Careful examination for an open wound is important because open calcaneal fractures are difficult to treat.

Radiologic Examination

- The diagnosis of a displaced intra-articular calcaneal fracture is made by plain radiographs.
- These should include lateral (see Fig. 30-14) and axial views of the hindfoot and an anteroposterior view of the foot to look for involvement of the calcaneocuboid joint.
- Broden's views may be used to visualize the anterior surface of the posterior facet.
    - In these views the foot is in the plantigrade position and the leg internally rotated 30 to 40 degrees.
- Radiographs can be taken with the tube angled 10 to 40 degrees toward the head of the patient.
- Examination of the lateral view of the hindfoot shows two main radiologic landmarks: Bohler's angle and the angle of Gissane (Fig. 30-16).
- Bohler's angle is particularly important because it is flattening of this angle that indicates involvement of the posterior facet.

- CT scans are very useful and should be obtained where possible (Fig. 30-17).
    - They demonstrate the extent of intra-articular damage, the amount of displacement of the intra-articular fragments, the varus angulation of the body of the calcaneus, and the presence of associated calcaneocuboid damage better than standard radiographs.

TREATMENT

- The treatment of intra-articular calcaneal fractures remains contentious, but the literature definitely suggests that operative management gives better results.
- Comparative results of nonoperative management, the use of minimal internal fixation such as K-wires, screws, staples, and other forms of nonrigid fixation, standard plates, and calcaneal plates with a side arm (Fig. 30-18) to control the position of the posterior facet fragments are shown in Table 30-11.
- Analysis indicates that the use of nonrigid fixation gives results similar to those of nonoperative management, and prospective studies comparing nonoperative management with the use of K-wires and bone graft have confirmed this.

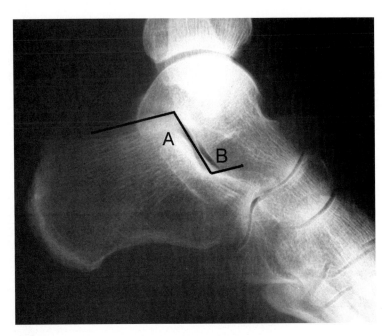

Figure 30-16   The Bohler angle A and the angle of Gissane B. Flattening of the Bohler angle indicates a significant intra-articular fracture (see Fig. 30-14A).

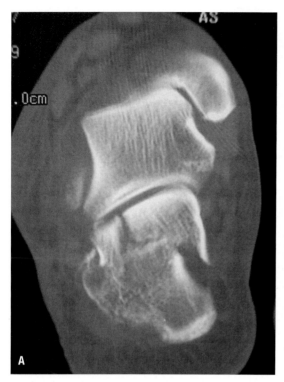
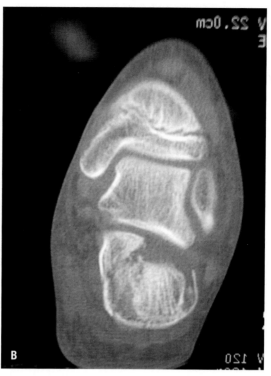

Figure 30-17 CT scans of two calcaneal fractures. (**A**) Type 1 fracture but note the slight varus position of the heel. (**B**) Type 2 fracture in a 15-year-old boy. The posterolateral fragment cannot be seen because it has rotated forward.

■ If operative management is to be undertaken successfully, a lateral plate should be used.

■ The initial plates were standard one-third tubular or reconstruction plates often combined with an interfragmentary screw and bone graft to maintain the reduction of the reduced posterior facet fragments.

■ In the last 10 years, increasing use has been made of calcaneus-specific plates that have a side arm (see Fig. 30-18) or are ovoid in shape to allow rigid fixation of the reduced facet fragments.

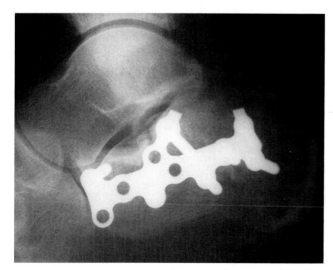

Figure 30-18 A calcaneal plate used to treat a joint depression fracture.

■ Although better results for this type of plate might be expected, Table 30-11 does not confirm this expectation.

▫ As yet there have been many fewer studies using calcaneal plates.

■ Surgery is usually undertaken through a lateral approach curving round the lateral malleolus.

■ The literature does in fact endorse operative management as better than nonoperative management.

■ Most of the recent comparative studies have favored operative management, although different outcome criteria make it difficult to compare them.

■ A recent prospective multicenter study undertaken in Canada also favored operative management, although only in certain groups of patients.

▫ Overall they could not demonstrate an advantage to open reduction and internal fixation, but in younger patients who were not receiving social benefits and who had comminuted fractures that were well reduced, there were clear advantages to open reduction and internal fixation.

■ The literature does not support the use of bone graft if calcaneal plates are used.

■ Some early evidence indicates that the use of calcium phosphate bone cement may facilitate early mobilization.

■ The question arises why there should be a debate about the superiority of open reduction and internal fixation when there is now little doubt that open reduction and internal fixation gives better results than nonoperative management in other severe lower limb intra-articular fractures. A number of factors need to be taken into consideration.

TABLE 30-11 COMPARATIVE RESULTS OF THE TREATMENT OF INTRA-ARTICULAR FRACTURES OF THE CALCANEUS

Result/Complication	Nonoperative Management (%)		K-Wires and Minimal Fixation (%)		Lateral Plate Fixation (%)		Calcaneal Plate Fixation (%)	
	Range	Average	Range	Average	Range	Average	Range	Average
Excellent/good	37–80.9	63.3	50–75.6	59.4	72.7–80	73.4	56–90.2	67.3
Wound complications			0–5.3	3.4	0–33.3	13.6	3–26	13.2
Deep infection			0–2.6	1.7	1–5	1.9	0–39	3.3
Return to work	25–80.9	52.7	26.3–76	62.3	64–84.8	67.8	73.2–94.1	81.2
Subtalar arthrodesis	10.5–15.9	12.6	0–13.1	7.8	2.3–19.2	5.2	0–10.9	7.5

- It seems likely that in most intra-articular calcaneal fractures there is chondral damage, and therefore postoperative pain and subtalar stiffness can be expected despite good radiologic results.
- Many fractures occur in middle-aged men who work as roofers or in other professions where any subtalar dysfunction means their profession is more difficult to pursue.
- The surgery of comminuted intra-articular calcaneal fractures is difficult, and a number of poor results can be expected, particularly in inexperienced hands!
- As with other intra-articular fractures, good evidence indicates that the final results correlate with adequacy of fracture reduction, and even 2 mm of incongruency leads to an increased incidence of subtalar osteoarthritis.
  - This strongly suggests that better results will be obtained in less severe fractures, which is the case in clinical studies.
- It is unlikely that Sanders 4 fractures will fare as well as Sanders 2 or 3 fractures, and primary arthrodesis is suggested for type 4 fractures.

Suggested Treatment

- Table 30-12 outlines the suggested treatment of intra-articular calcaneal fractures.

COMPLICATIONS

- Nonunion is very unusual and virtually always associated with deep infection.

TABLE 30-12 SUGGESTED TREATMENT OF INTRA-ARTICULAR CALCANEAL FRACTURES

Injury	Treatment
Sanders 1 fracture	Nonoperative management
	Non–weight-bearing cast or brace for 6 to 8 weeks
Sanders 2 and 3 fracture	Lateral calcaneal plate
	Bone grafting not required
Sanders 4 fracture	Primary arthrodesis

- An incidence of 1.3% has been reported, but few studies even mention the problem.
- Other problems are more common.

Wound Infection

- Table 30-11 shows that wound complications are relatively common after calcaneal fracture surgery.
- These are more common in diabetics, smokers, and obese patients.
- They also tend to be associated with more severe fractures and with delay between the fracture and surgery.
- An incidence of 50% wound complications has been reported if surgery is delayed by more than 2 weeks.
- Many surgeons believe surgery should be delayed to allow the soft tissues to improve, but no good evidence in the literature supports this belief.

Osteomyelitis

- Osteomyelitis is relatively unusual but more common in open fractures.
- The management of osteomyelitis is discussed in Chapter 40, but calcaneal osteomyelitis is very difficult to treat.
- Debridement with excision of devitalized and infected bone followed by flap cover should be undertaken, but there is a relatively high incidence of below-knee amputation.

Subtalar Stiffness

- Few patients achieve normal subtalar movement after an intra-articular calcaneal fracture, possibly only 3% to 5%.
- On average, 70% to 75% of subtalar motion is regained, but this varies with the severity of the fracture.

Arthrodesis

- Table 30-11 gives the published incidences of subtalar arthrodesis.
- The requirement for subtalar arthrodesis correlates with the severity of injury, with Sanders 4 fractures 5.5 times more likely to require arthrodesis than Sanders 2 fractures.
- Nonoperative treatment is six times more likely to result in arthrodesis than operative treatment, and patients on social support are three times more likely to have a subtalar arthrodesis.

- Calcaneocuboid arthrodesis may be required if there is incongruency of this joint.
- Presumably the factors that determine the likelihood of the requirement for calcaneocuboid arthrodesis are similar to those that determine subtalar arthrodesis, but the literature contains little information.

Compartment Syndrome

- This has been reported to vary between 1% and 10%.
- It should always be considered in intra-articular calcaneal fracture.
- Compartment syndrome is discussed further in Chapter 38.

Nerve Damage

- Sural nerve damage has been reported to occur in about 3% of cases, but the incidence may well be higher.
- It is avoided by identifying and safeguarding the nerve during dissection.
- Damage to the medial and lateral plantar nerves and to calcaneal branches of the tibial nerve can be caused by screw, wire, or drill insertions or by impingement from an exostosis.

Tendon Impingement

- There are two main causes of tendon impingement.
- In nonoperatively managed fractures, the diminution in heel height combined with the displacement of the lateral calcaneal wall means the peroneal tendons may be trapped between the lateral wall and the distal fibula.
  - Treatment is by decompression by lateral wall ostectomy.
- Tendon impingement may occur after plate fixation due to the presence of the plate and screws.
  - This has been reported to occur in as many as 18% of patients.
  - Treatment is by removal of the plate.

Heel Pain

- Heel pain may occur as a result of damage to the heel pad, plantar fasciitis, or the development of calcaneal exostoses.
- It is best treated by the use of orthoses, and the literature suggests about 30% of patients require heel cups, insoles, and other orthotics.

Malunion

- Malunion is particularly common after nonoperative management. The three types are detailed in Table 30-13.

SPECIAL SITUATIONS

Calcaneal Fractures in Adolescents

- The literature suggests about 80% of calcaneal fractures in young adults are intra-articular.
- They are usually Sanders 2 in severity (see Fig. 30-17), and the results of surgical treatment are unquestionably better than in older patients.
- About 75% excellent or good results can be expected, with about 60% return of full subtalar movement.
- Care should be taken to avoid the calcaneal physis when plating the fracture.

Open Fractures

- Open calcaneal fractures are uncommon but associated with significant soft tissue damage.
- Treatment is the same as for closed calcaneal fractures, but the incidence of deep infection is higher.
- The literature quotes the incidence of osteomyelitis as 19% to 31%, but recent studies have suggested an incidence of 8% to 10%.
- The management of open fractures is discussed in detail in Chapter 4.

Primary Arthrodesis

- Most authorities agree that Sanders 2 and 3 fractures should be treated by open reduction and internal fixation, and Sanders 4 fractures are best treated by primary arthrodesis.
- This should be done by restoring the heel height and width as far as possible by open reduction and internal fixation using a lateral calcaneal plate and then undertaking a standard subtalar arthrodesis.
- Analysis of the results has indicated 80% excellent or good results in experienced hands.

Fractures in the Elderly

- It seems likely that the incidence of calcaneal fractures in the elderly will increase and surgeons will be faced with the problems associated with treating osteopenic calcaneal fractures.

TABLE 30-13 TYPES OF CALCANEAL MALUNION AND THEIR TREATMENT

Type	Description	Treatment
I	Large lateral exostosis with or without lateral subtalar osteoarthritis	Lateral exostectomy and peroneal tenolysis
II	Lateral exostosis and subtalar osteoarthritis	Subtalar arthrodesis and lateral exostectomy
III	Subtalar osteoarthritis with varus or valgus angulation	Subtalar arthrodesis, peroneal tenolysis, calcaneal exostectomy and calcaneal osteotomy

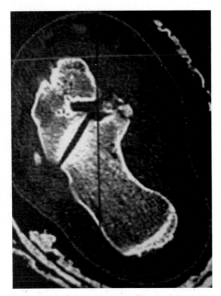

Figure 30-19 A CT scan of a sustentaculum fracture.

■ About 18% of calcaneal fractures occur in patients aged 65 or more, and most are caused by simple falls, falls down stairs, or falls from a low height.

■ The literature suggests that good results can be obtained.

Extra-Articular Calcaneal Fractures

The incidence of the different extra-articular calcaneal fractures is detailed in Table 30-8. In addition to these fractures, surgeons have also described fractures of the sustentaculum tali (Fig. 30-19) and the peroneal trochlea. Both of these are extremely rare.

EPIDEMIOLOGY

The epidemiology of the most common extra-articular calcaneal fractures is given in Table 30-14. This shows an obvious difference between anterior process fractures and fractures of the medial process and body. Anterior process fractures are essentially low-velocity injuries, usually caused by a twisting injury to the hindfoot. Medial process and body fractures tend to be high-energy injuries with most caused by a fall from a height or motor vehicle accidents. The epidemiology of body fractures is similar to that of intra-articular fractures (see Table 30-9). Lateral process and posterior tuberosity fractures are rare, and there is insufficient data to describe their epidemiology.

DIAGNOSIS

History and Physical Examination

■ Patients with extra-articular calcaneal fractures present with a painful swollen hindfoot.

■ There may be other injuries of the foot and ankle, and they should be looked for.

■ There are no reports of compartment syndrome associated with extra-articular fractures, but a careful examination of the foot and ankle should be carried out.

Radiologic Examination

■ Lateral and axial X-rays of the calcaneus diagnose most extra-articular fractures, but the anterior process is notoriously difficult to see on a standard lateral radiograph.

■ An oblique radiograph is indicated if clinical examination suggests the possibility of an anterior process fractures.

■ If in doubt a CT scan will confirm the diagnosis.

TREATMENT

Anterior Process Fractures

■ These fractures (Fig. 30-20) are usually caused by forced inversion with the anterior process avulsed by the bifurcate ligament.

■ They represent an attempt to dislocate or sublux the calcaneocuboid joint, and therefore the joint surfaces may be damaged.

TABLE 30-14 EPIDEMIOLOGY OF THE MOST COMMON EXTRA-ARTICULAR CALCANEAL FRACTURES

	Anterior Process	Medial Process	Body
Average age (y)	36	27.6	41.8
Men/women (%)	60/40	91/9	80/20
Annual incidence	$1.9/10^5$	$2.1/10^5$	$0.9/10^5$
Open (%)	0	0	20
Cause of injury			
Fall from height (%)	40.0	63.6	60
Motor vehicle accident (%)		18.2	20
Twist (%)	40.0		
Fall (%)	10.0	9.1	

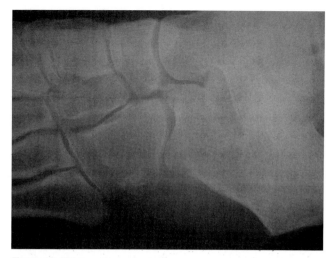

Figure 30-20 An oblique X-ray showing an anterior process fracture.

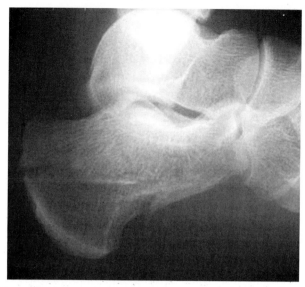

Figure 30-21 A calcaneal body fracture.

- An MRI scan can be used to assess the degree of calcaneocuboid joint damage.
- Treatment is nonoperative unless a large anterior process fragment is displaced, which is extremely rare.
- A weight-bearing cast or brace can be used for 6 to 8 weeks.
- Late pain is not uncommon and often attributed to a nonunion, but it is more likely caused by calcaneocuboid osteoarthritis and should be investigated with an MRI scan.
- If symptomatic arthritis is present, a calcaneocuboid arthrodesis is indicated.

Medial Process Fracture

- These are almost invariably high-energy injuries with the fracture caused by a direct blow.
- Treatment is usually nonoperative, with a weight-bearing cast or brace used to facilitate mobilization.
- Internal fixation can be used if a large medial process fragment is significantly displaced.
- The high-energy nature of this fracture means there is significant local soft tissue damage, and pain can persist for a considerable period.

Calcaneal Body Fractures

- These are usually undisplaced with a fracture that exits on the superior surface of the calcaneus close to but not involving the posterior facet (Fig. 30-21).
- They can be displaced, however.
- Undisplaced fractures are treated nonoperatively with 4 to 6 weeks in a weight-bearing cast or brace, but displaced fractures should be reduced and fixed with a lateral plate.
- It is wise to obtain a CT scan to examine the posterior facet.
  - Even if the facet is intact, there may well be chondral damage, and late subtalar arthrodesis may be required if pain persists.

Lateral Process Fractures

- These are unusual and usually undisplaced.
- Treatment is by the use of a weight-bearing cast or brace for 4 to 6 weeks to facilitate mobilization.
- Nonunion can occur and if symptomatic is treated by excision of the bone fragment.

Tuberosity Fractures

- These are uncommon fractures. They have received attention because they require operative treatment.
- The classic tuberosity fracture is the "parrot beak" fracture, which should be treated by open or closed reduction and screw fixation.
- The variant of this fracture is seen in older patients where a thin shell of the tuberosity fragment is detached (Fig. 30-22).

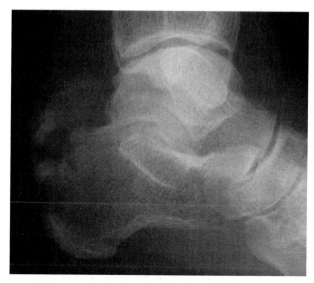

Figure 30-22 A posterior tuberosity fracture.

- The osteopenic nature of the bone means that transosseous sutures may be required.
- Failure to reduce and fix the tuberosity may lead to skin slough and weak plantarflexion.

Calcaneal Dislocations

- Very few cases of dislocation of the subtalar and calcaneocuboid joints, without an associated calcaneal fracture, have been reported.
- These are treated by closed reduction and the use of a walking cast or brace for 6 to 8 weeks.
- Calcaneal fracture-dislocations have also been reported.
  - These occur when the primary calcaneal fracture line is associated with rupture of the calcaneofibular ligament.
  - Under these circumstances, the posterolateral calcaneal fragment moves laterally and the anteromedial fragment and the attached talus move downward so the talus is beside the posterolateral calcaneal fragment.
  - Treatment is by open reduction and internal fixation.

MIDFOOT FRACTURES

Midfoot fractures are relatively unusual. When they occur surgeons should always be aware of the possibility of an associated subluxation or dislocation of either Chopart's or Lisfranc's joints. Minor avulsion fractures of the navicular or cuboid bones may be the only apparent radiological evidence of significant soft tissue or intra-articular damage. Relatively little has been documented about midfoot fractures, but there is an increasing awareness of their importance.

SURGICAL ANATOMY

The bones of the midfoot are the navicular, the cuboid, and the medial, lateral, and intermediate cuneiforms. They are bounded proximally by the distal articular surface's of the talus and calcaneus, forming Chopart's joint. Distally, the cuneiforms and the cuboid form part of Lisfranc's tarsometatarsal joint (Fig. 30-23). The midfoot bones are tightly bound together by interosseous ligaments that also join the midfoot to the hindfoot and forefoot. There is some motion in the midfoot, but most foot motion occurs at the subtalar joint or in the tarsometatarsal joint. Thus successful fusion of the midfoot joints after fracture does not result in major disability. The midfoot and forefoot are divided into medial and lateral columns with the medial two metatarsals and the adjacent midfoot bones forming the medial column, and the lateral three metatarsals and their adjacent midfoot bones forming the lateral column.

Two important ligaments are the bifurcate ligament, which arises from the anterior process of the calcaneus and inserts into the navicular, and the cuboid, although the cuboid component of the ligament is often absent or weak. The spring ligament joins the sustentaculum tali to

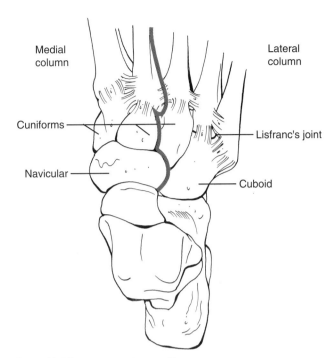

Figure 30-23   Anatomy of the midfoot.

the navicular. The only tendon to insert into the midfoot is tibialis posterior, which inserts into the navicular but sends slips to the sustentaculum tali, all three cuneiforms, the cuboid, and the bases of the second, third, and fourth metatarsals. The flexor hallucis brevis arises from the undersurface of the cuboid and all three cuneiforms.

CLASSIFICATION

The OTA (AO) have produced a classification for midfoot fractures, but it is questionable if such complexity is required for relatively uncommon fractures. Sangeorzan et al. (1989) introduced a classification for navicular fractures that has been adapted to apply to all midfoot bones. Fractures in all three bones are similar and can be characterized using the simple classification shown in Figure 30-24. There are four basic types. Type I fractures are avulsion fractures; type II fractures are shear fractures, which may be coronal (IIA) or sagittal (IIB). Type III fractures are uniarticular impaction fractures, and type IV fractures are biarticular impaction fractures.

EPIDEMIOLOGY

The basic epidemiology of midfoot fractures is shown in Table 30-15. It can be seen that they have a type C distribution (see Chapter 1) occurring in younger patients with an approximately equal gender distribution. There is a relatively high incidence of open fractures, and when open fractures occur they tend to be severe. There is a high incidence of associated injuries.

Cuneiform fractures are rare, with most fractures affecting the navicular or cuboid. Most cuneiform fractures

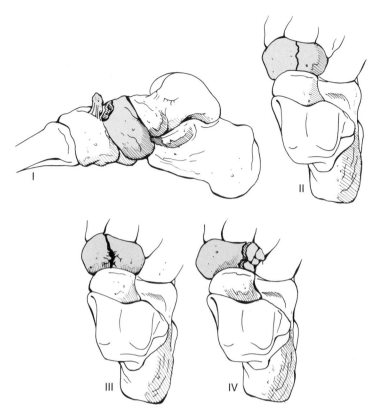

Figure 30-24 Classification of fractures of the midfoot. See text for explanation.

occur in the medial cuneiform. Most fractures are avulsion fractures, although biarticular impaction fractures are not uncommon. The distribution of different fracture types according to the different modes of injury is shown in Table 30-16. Paradoxically, it appears to be younger patients who sustain midfoot fractures from twisting injuries and slightly older patients who are involved in road traffic accidents. Severe type IV biarticular impaction fractures are more common in motor vehicle accidents and falls from a height. Most avulsion fractures are caused by low-energy injuries such as twisting injuries or falls down stairs or steps.

Associated Injuries

There is a very high incidence of associated musculoskeletal injuries with midfoot fractures. About 90% of these injuries are located in the ipsilateral foot or ankle, with the calcaneus and metatarsals most commonly affected. Eleven percent of patients had spinal fractures.

DIAGNOSIS

History and Physical Examination

- As with hindfoot fractures there is a significant incidence of high-energy injuries, and there may well be associated musculoskeletal injuries and injuries to other body systems.
- All patients with high-energy injuries must be examined according to ATLS principles.

TABLE 30-15 EPIDEMIOLOGY OF MIDFOOT FRACTURES

Proportion of all fractures	0.4%
Proportion of foot fractures	3.7%
Average age	36.0 y
Men/women	48%/52%
Incidence	$5.0/10^5/y$
Distribution	Type C
Open fractures	11.1%
Navicular	48.1%
Cuboid	44.4%
Cuneiforms	7.4%
Fracture types	
Avulsion (I)	44.4%
Shear (II)	14.8%
Uniarticular impaction (III)	11.1%
Biarticular impaction (IV)	29.6%

TABLE 30-16 MODES OF INJURY IN MIDFOOT FRACTURES

		Fracture Type (%)			
Cause	Age (y)	I	II	III	IV
Twist	23	66.6	16.6	16.6	
Fall on stairs	33.8	80			20
Fall from height	32.3	28.6	14.3	14.3	42.9
Motor vehicle accident	35.6		20		80

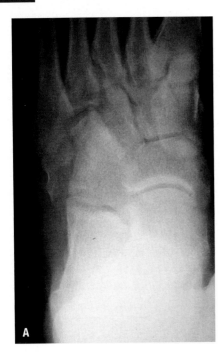
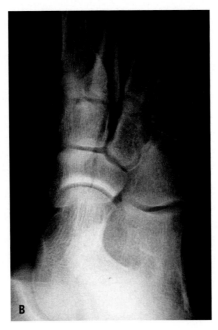

Figure 30-25 Cuboid (**A**) and navicular (**B**) fractures.

- The midfoot fracture presents as a painful, swollen foot.
- The soft tissues must be carefully examined, bearing in mind there is a relatively high incidence of open injuries associated with these fractures.
- It is possible that the foot has been crushed or an automobile tire has passed over it.
  - Under these circumstances, closed or open degloving may be present.
- Neurovascular damage is unusual unless the foot is crushed, but under these circumstances vascular reconstruction is rarely possible and amputation may be required.

Radiologic Examination

- Anteroposterior and lateral radiographs are usually adequate to diagnose midfoot fractures (Fig. 30-25), but in the emergency situation adequate radiographs may not be obtained.
- Oblique views may be helpful to diagnose more subtle avulsion fractures and to delineate the extent of crush fractures.
- A CT scan ideally should be obtained to identify the extent of the fracture and any associated injuries.
- MRI scans are not usually helpful in the acute situation but may be useful secondarily to investigate any chondral damage associated with the fracture.

TREATMENT

- The treatment of midfoot fractures is essentially the same no matter which bone or bones are involved.
- Avulsion fractures rarely need internal fixation, although a displaced avulsed fragment of the navicular tuberosity may require open reduction and internal fixation with an interfragmentary screw.

- Surgeons should be aware of the possibility of an os naviculare or secondary navicular ossification center that may mimic a fracture.
- Undisplaced shear fractures can be treated nonoperatively with a below-knee weight-bearing cast or brace worn for 6 to 8 weeks.
- Displaced shear fractures should be fixed with interfragmentary screws.
- The more difficult decision is how to treat comminuted fractures.
  - The principle to bear in mind is that the length of the medial and lateral columns of the foot must be preserved, which nonoperative management will not achieve in the presence of extensive comminution.
  - If only one articular surface is damaged, nonoperative management may be adequate with late fusion reserved for persistent pain.
  - If the comminution is extensive and the length of medial or lateral column is affected, a primary arthrodesis is indicated with a plate spanning the affected bone.
  - Bone graft will be required.
  - If there is extensive midfoot damage associated with forefoot or hindfoot damage, primary amputation may be required.

Suggested Treatment

- Table 30-17 outlines the treatment of midfoot fractures.

COMPLICATIONS

- The common complications are midfoot osteoarthritis and collapse of the medial or lateral column of the foot.
- Osteoarthritis is treated with appropriate midtarsal arthrodeses, and column collapse by an opening wedge osteotomy, plating, and bone grafting.

TABLE 30-17 SUGGESTED TREATMENT OF MIDFOOT FRACTURES

Fracture	Treatment
Type I (avulsion)	Symptomatic treatment
	Cast or brace if required
	Interfragmentary screw for large displaced navicular tuberosity fragment
Type II (shear)	
Undisplaced	Cast or brace
Displaced	Interfragmentary screw(s)
Type III (uniarticular)	
Minor impaction	Cast or brace. Late arthrodesis if required
Major impaction	Primary arthrodesis
Type IV (biarticular)	Primary arthrodesis. Preservation of column length

■ This is a difficult technique associated with poor results and should be avoided by maintaining the length of the foot by appropriate primary treatment.

■ Severe foot pain secondary to a crush injury and extensive midfoot damage is best treated by amputation with an amputation through the Chopart's joint undertaken if possible.

  ■ If impossible, a below-knee amputation should be performed (see Chapter 37).

MIDFOOT DISLOCATIONS

Calcaneocuboid and talonavicular dislocations are very rare. It is likely that spontaneously reducing subluxations are more common, but their incidence is unknown. They are associated with fractures of the anterior process of the calcaneus and avulsion fractures of the calcaneus, navicular, and cuboid. Dislocations of both the calcaneocuboid and talonavicular joints, have been reported but are very rare. They are caused by high-energy injuries and treated by closed or open reduction followed by the use of a walking cast for 6 to 8 weeks. Instability after reduction is treated by stabilization with K-wires, which can be removed after 6 weeks.

LISFRANC'S DISLOCATION

Dislocation of the tarsometatarsal, or Lisfranc joint (Fig. 30-26), is unusual, and about 20% are missed, resulting in considerable long-term morbidity. The joint consists of the three cuneiform and two cuboid metatarsal articulations (see Fig. 30-23). The stability of the joint is gained from the strong interosseous ligaments and the fact that the second metatarsal articulates with the middle

cuneiform proximal to the articulation of the medial and lateral cuneiforms with the first and third metatarsals. Thus the base of the second metatarsal is recessed into the midfoot, providing stability. As a result, most tarsometatarsal dislocations involve a fracture of the base of the second metatarsal.

Tarsometatarsal ligamentous damage may result from low-energy injuries such as sports injuries or twisting injuries, but dislocation usually follows falls from a height or a motor vehicle accident. The three basic dislocation patterns (Fig. 30-27) are distinguished by the direction of the dislocation and the extent of the ligamentous damage. Type A are total dislocations where there is incongruity of the whole joint. Displacement is uniplanar and can be

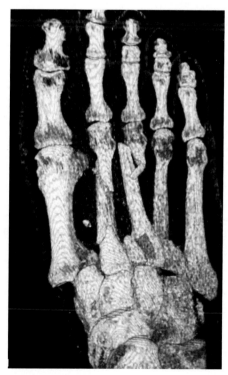

Figure 30-26 A CT scan showing a divergent Lisfranc fracture-dislocation associated with metatarsal fractures.

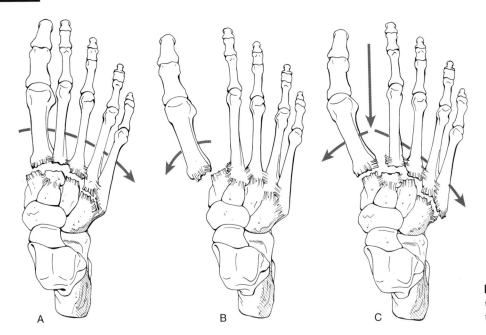

Figure 30-27 Classification of Lisfranc tarsometatarsal fracture-dislocations. See text for explanation.

sagittal, coronal, or both. Type B are partial dislocations, which again can be sagittal, coronal, or both. Medial displacement affects the first metatarsal but may involve adjacent metatarsals as well. Lateral displacement affects one or more of the lateral four metatarsals but not the hallux. Type C dislocations are divergent. Analysis shows that about 37% of Lisfranc dislocations are type A, 54% are type B, and 9% are type C. Between 69% and 85% of Lisfranc dislocations are associated with other fractures in the midfoot or metatarsus (Fig. 30-26).

Diagnosis is usually made from standard anteroposterior and lateral radiographs, but if there is pain in the tarsometatarsal area without an obvious dislocation or fracture, a CT or MRI scan should be obtained to investigate the integrity of the joint because there may be an undisplaced dislocation. Particular attention must be paid to the second metatarsal base to look for fractures and widening of the space between the first and second metatarsals.

Treatment of undisplaced dislocations can be nonoperative with a walking cast or brace applied for 6 to 8 weeks. Most dislocations are displaced, however, and they should be managed by open reduction and internal fixation with interfragmentary screws to hold the reduced joints. K-wires can also be used. Two incisions are usually employed, one over the first web space and the second over the fourth metatarsal. Closed reduction and pinning is difficult and associated with poor results. Primary arthrodesis has not been shown to give better results than open reduction and internal fixation using screws.

The common complications are compartment syndrome, foot pain, posttraumatic osteoarthritis, vascular impairment, and reflex sympathetic dystrophy. The monitoring and treatment of compartment syndrome is discussed in Chapter 38, and reflex sympathetic dystrophy is discussed in Chapter 41. Posttraumatic osteoarthritis occurs in 25% to 35% of patients and is treated by arthrodesis. Missed or neglected Lisfranc dislocations are also treated by arthrodesis of the affected joints.

METATARSAL FRACTURES

These are the most common fractures in the foot. They are usually low-velocity injuries, although they can occur from a variety of different causes. Stress fractures also occur, particularly in military recruits, athletes, or ballet dancers (see Table 6-1 in Chapter 6). Treatment is usually nonoperative and the outcome good, although the Jones fracture of the proximal fifth metatarsal is associated with a high incidence of nonunion. Metatarsal fractures may be isolated or multiple.

SURGICAL ANATOMY

The medial two metatarsals form part of the medial longitudinal arch of the foot, with the lateral three metatarsals forming part of the lateral longitudinal arch. The metatarsals are also arranged in a transverse arch, with the medial side of the transverse arch higher than the lateral side. Metatarsals provide the origins for the dorsal and plantar interossei, and the muscles of the third layer of the foot arise from the inferior surface of the base of each metatarsal. Slips of tibialis posterior insert into the bases of the second, third, and fourth metatarsals. The vascular supply to the area is from branches of the dorsalis pedis artery on the dorsum and branches of the medial and lateral plantar arteries on the sole of the foot. The main nerve supply to the muscles is from the lateral and medial plantar nerves.

CLASSIFICATION

There is no classification in widespread use beyond a description of the position of the fracture. There is an OTA (AO) classification, but it is complex, has no bearing on

TABLE 30-18 EPIDEMIOLOGY OF METATARSAL FRACTURES

Proportion of all fractures	6.8%
Proportion of foot fractures	55.0%
Average age	42.8 y
Men/women	43%/57%
Incidence	75.4/10⁵/y
Distribution	Type A
Open fractures	3.5%
Isolated metatarsal fractures	
Average age	42.1 y
Hallux	1.4%
Second	6.5%
Third	4.8%
Fourth	3.4%
Fifth	74.9%
Multiple metatarsal fractures	
Average age	41.5 y
Two metatarsals	3.9%
Three metatarsals	3.4%
Four metatarsals	1.7%

EPIDEMIOLOGY

The basic epidemiology of metatarsal fractures is shown in Table 30-18. They are more common in women who tend to be older, but overall they have a type A distribution (see Chapter 1). There are very few open fractures or associated injuries. About 75% are isolated fifth metatarsal fractures, with hallux fractures very uncommon. About 9% of metatarsal fractures are multiple. All multiple metatarsal fractures are contiguous. An intact metatarsal between two fractures does not occur. If two metatarsals are fractured, they are commonly the second and third or third and fourth metatarsals. If there are three fractures, it is usually the second, third, and fourth metatarsals that are involved, and virtually all patients who have four metatarsal fractures have fractures involving the second, third, fourth, and fifth metatarsals.

The types of fracture that occur in the different modes of injury are shown in Table 30-19. Twisting injuries overwhelmingly cause fifth metatarsal fractures, which are also common after simple falls, falls down stairs, or sports injuries. High-energy injuries tend to cause multiple fractures or fractures of the medial three metatarsals. Stress fractures account for 2.5% of metatarsal fractures and most commonly affect the second and third metatarsals.

Associated Injuries

There is a low incidence of associated injuries, and very few patients are multiply injured or have open fractures. Most other injuries involve the ipsilateral foot, ankle, or distal tibia.

treatment or outcome, and many surgeons do not use it. The fifth metatarsal is conveniently divided into four zones (Fig. 30-28). Most metatarsal fractures involve the fifth metatarsal, and the fractures in zones 1 and 2, in particular, have different prognoses. In this chapter, metatarsal fractures are categorized by the involved metatarsal(s).

DIAGNOSIS

History and Physical Examination

- The history usually involves a twisting injury or a fall, but if the mode of injury is more severe the surgeon should be aware of the possibility of other injuries to the foot, ankle, and lower tibia and examine the patient accordingly.

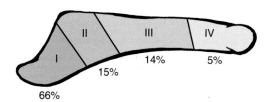

Figure 30-28 The fifth metatarsal zones and prevalence of fracture.

TABLE 30-19 CAUSES OF METATARSAL FRACTURES

		Metatarsal (%)					
Cause	Prevalence (%)	1	2	3	4	5	Multiple
Twist	46.2		1.8	1.8	1.2	92.1	3
Fall	18.3	3.1	4.6	3.1	9.2	73.8	6.1
Fall on stairs	7					88	12
Fall from height	5.1		16.6	16.6		27.7	38.9
Direct blow or crush	10.1	5.5	22.2	11.1	5.5	30.6	25
Sport	7.9	3.6	7.1	3.6		78.6	7.1
Motor vehicle accident	2.8			10	10	60	20
Stress	2.5		44.4	33.3		22.2	

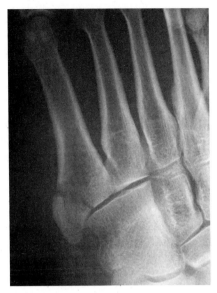

Figure 30-29   A fifth metatarsal base fracture.

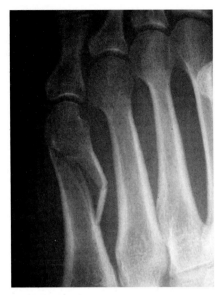

Figure 30-31   A fifth metatarsal shaft fracture.

- The patient usually complains of a painful, swollen forefoot and difficulty walking.
- Neurovascular injuries are very rare unless there has been a severe crush.

Radiologic Examination

- Anteroposterior and lateral radiographs are usually sufficient to diagnose these fractures (Figs. 30-29 to 30-31).
- Care should be taken to examine the Lisfranc joint because metatarsal fractures can be associated with a Lisfranc fracture-dislocation (see Fig. 30-26).
- There is usually no requirement for more sophisticated imaging unless a stress fracture is being considered in which case an MRI scan may be diagnostic.

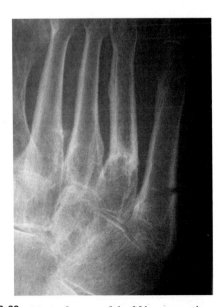

Figure 30-30   A Jones fracture of the fifth metatarsal.

TREATMENT

- Surprisingly, little information is available about the treatment results of metatarsal fractures.
  - The exceptions are fractures of the proximal half of the fifth metatarsal.
- There are no good guidelines about when metatarsal fractures should be internally fixed or studies indicating whether fixation improves gait or not.
- Significantly displaced fractures should be internally fixed, particularly if they are associated with other ipsilateral foot fractures.
  - This is rare, and most isolated metatarsal fractures are treated nonoperatively with good results expected.
- If surgery is required, either K-wires (see Chapter 34) or plates (see Chapter 32) can be used, although most surgeons favor K-wires for the second to fifth metatarsals and reserve plating for the larger hallux metatarsal.

COMPLICATIONS

- The usual complications of metatarsal fractures are late foot pain, malunion, nonunion, and infection if surgery has been undertaken.
- Late foot pain is often difficult to treat and may require the treatment of a malunion or nonunion.
- Orthoses may also be required.
- The management of nonunion, malunion, and infection are discussed in the appropriate chapters.

SPECIAL SITUATIONS

Fifth Metatarsal Fractures

- About 75% of fractures occur in the fifth metatarsal, and they are generally low-energy injuries.

■ The distribution of fifth metatarsal fractures is shown in Figure 30-28.

   ■ About 66% of these fractures occur in zone 1 and are avulsion fractures.

   ■ A further 15% are Jones fractures occurring in zone 2.

   ■ Zone 3 fractures account for about 14% of fifth metatarsal fractures.

■ These may be caused by a simple fall or twist but they also may occur in athletes and present as a stress fracture.

■ Fractures of the neck of the fifth metatarsal are relatively uncommon, accounting for about 5% of fifth metatarsal fractures.

Zone 1 Fractures

■ Avulsion fractures to the proximal fifth metatarsal (see Fig. 30-29) are treated nonoperatively.

■ They are low-energy injuries, and late displacement is extremely rare.

■ Symptomatic nonunion is very uncommon.

■ They should be treated by a supportive strapping or a cast or brace depending on the patient's symptoms.

■ Weight bearing is allowed.

Zone 2 (Jones) Fractures

■ The true Jones fracture (see Fig. 30-30) is not a stress fracture as has been postulated in the literature.

■ It is caused by adduction and axial loading on a plantarflexed foot.

■ It is relatively uncommon, and analysis shows that about 50% are caused by inversion injuries, 15% by simple falls, and 17.5% by sports injuries.

■ The presentation is with a painful forefoot, and radiographs show a transverse fracture in zone 2.

■ The debate is between nonoperative and operative management because of the incidence of nonunion, which has been reported in up to 30% to 35% of patients.

   ■ It is reasonable to employ nonoperative management initially in the form of a walking cast or brace for 6 weeks, but if there is no indication of union at 6 weeks, open reduction and internal fixation should be offered to the patient.

   ■ In athletes, primary open reduction and internal fixation may be selected to reduce the rehabilitation time.

   ■ Surgical treatment is usually with an intramedullary screw or a small plate.

Zone 3 and 4 fractures

■ These may present as stress fractures in athletes or following a twisting injury or fall (see Fig. 30-31).

■ They are treated symptomatically with strapping or a cast or brace depending on the patient's symptoms.

Stress Fractures

■ Stress fractures of the metatarsals (Fig. 30-32) are often referred to as march fractures.

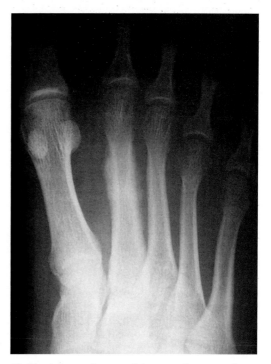

Figure 30-32 A fatigue fracture of the second metatarsal.

■ They are reported as common, but the reports come from specialized centers, and Table 30-19 indicates they are relatively uncommon in the overall population.

■ Patients present with a painful forefoot usually with no history of trauma.

■ There is often a history of unaccustomed exercise such as running or marching.

■ Treatment is symptomatic, and union can be expected.

■ Open reduction and internal fixation should be reserved for nonunions.

■ Stress fractures are discussed further in Chapter 6.

SESAMOID FRACTURES

Table 30-1 shows that fractures of the sesamoid bones are very rare. The sesamoid bones are situated in the tendons of flexor hallucis brevis. They cushion the hallux metatarsal head and help protect flexor hallucis longus, which runs between them. Patients who present with pain in the area of the hallux metatarsal phalangeal joint may have a fractured sesamoid, but the surgeon must be careful not to confuse a fractured sesamoid with a bipartite sesamoid, which occurs in 19% to 31% of the population.

Sesamoid fractures are usually caused by a direct blow to the undersurface of the forefoot, and they are classically seen in dancers and runners, with the latter occasionally presenting with stress fractures of the sesamoid. Diagnosis is often difficult because of the frequency of bipartite sesamoids, but a bone scan or MRI scan may be helpful. Treatment should be nonoperative unless symptoms persist. Treatment alternatives are excision of the sesamoid or bone grafting of the nonunion. The latter should be attempted but sesamoidectomy undertaken if symptoms persist. Sesamoidectomy is not without its complications, however, and hallux deformities and persistent pain have been reported.

PHALANGEAL FRACTURES

Phalangeal fractures are relatively common. It is difficult to estimate their true incidence because many patients do not present to emergency departments or to orthopaedic surgeons. They rarely require operative treatment, and the outcome is generally good, although there are comparatively few good articles detailing the outcome of their treatment.

SURGICAL ANATOMY

Each phalanx of the hallux receives a separate extensor tendon into its base, extensor hallucis longus inserting into the distal phalanx and extensor hallux brevis into the proximal phalanx. On the plantar surface of the hallux, flexor hallucis longus is inserted into the base of the distal phalanx and flexor hallucis brevis, via the two sesamoids, into the base of the proximal phalanx. In the lateral four toes, flexor digitorum brevis inserts into the middle phalanx with flexor digitorum longus inserting into the distal phalanx as in the hand. In the fifth toe, abductor and flexor digiti minimi brevis are inserted into the base of the proximal phalanx.

On the dorsal surface of the lateral four toes, an extensor expansion exists as in the hand formed from extensor digitorum longus, the lumbricals, and the interossei. Tendons of extensor digitorum brevis join the extensor expansions of the second, third, and fourth toes. The tendons of the interossei are inserted directly into the bases of the proximal phalanges as well as into the extensor expansion.

EPIDEMIOLOGY

The basic epidemiology of phalangeal fractures of a foot is shown in Table 30-20. They are quite common, and there

TABLE 30-20 EPIDEMIOLOGY OF PHALANGEAL FRACTURES

Proportion of all fractures	3.6%
Proportion of foot fractures	28.9%
Average age	35.3 y
Men/women	66%/34%
Incidence	39.6/10⁵/y
Distribution	Type C
Open fractures	6.6%
Hallux	19.8%
Average age	33.7 y
Others	80.2%
Average age	37.9 y

TABLE 30-21 CAUSES OF PHALANGEAL FRACTURES

Cause	Average (y)	Prevalence (%)	Hallux (%)	Other Toes (%)
Twist	30.6	7.5	18.7	81.2
Direct blow or crush	36.2	66.5	24.1	75.9
Sport	30.0	13.2	42.9	57.1

is a relatively high incidence of open fractures considering that most are low-energy injuries. Very few have associated injuries. The hallux is affected in about 20% of cases, with most fractures involving a single toe. Table 30-21 shows that most phalangeal fractures are caused by three injury mechanisms twisting injuries, direct blows or crush injuries, and sports injuries with many of the sports injuries actually direct blows or kicks. It is interesting to note that the hallux is more commonly affected in sports injuries.

Associated Injuries

Very few phalangeal fractures are associated with other injuries because most are the result of a kick or direct blow. Most crush injuries to the foot involve the metatarsus or midfoot, and pure crush injuries to the toes are rare, although they can occur.

DIAGNOSIS

History and Physical Examination

- The history is usually straightforward, involving a kick or heavy object dropped on the forefoot.
- There is local pain and swelling.
- The soft tissues must be carefully examined because there is a relatively high incidence of open fractures.

Radiologic Examination

- Anteroposterior and lateral radiographs are usually adequate to diagnose phalangeal fractures (Fig. 30-33).

TREATMENT

- Most phalangeal fractures are relatively minor and either undisplaced or minimally displaced.
- Displaced diaphyseal or intra-articular fractures require reduction and fixation using either interfragmentary screws or, more commonly, K-wires.
- The techniques are discussed in Chapter 34.
- Significantly crushed toes, with an impaired vascular supply, are amputated.
- Nonoperative management is symptomatic.
- Buddy strapping to the adjacent toe may be used.
- Cast or brace management is rarely required.

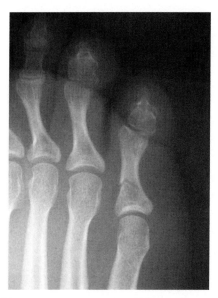

Figure 30-33 A phalangeal fracture of the little toe.

COMPLICATIONS

- There are few complications, although malunion may cause local pain and difficulty wearing shoes.
- Nonunion and infection are unusual, although the latter may occur in diabetic patients or patients with significant peripheral vascular disease.
- The treatment for osteomyelitis is usually amputation.

FOREFOOT DISLOCATIONS

- Pure dislocations of the metatarsophalangeal and interphalangeal joints are relatively unusual.
  - They often follow low-energy injuries such as sports injuries.
- Diagnosis is by standard anteroposterior and lateral radiographs, and treatment is by closed reduction.

- If the dislocation is irreducible, soft tissue interposition is likely and open reduction required.
- If there is instability of the joint after reduction, K-wire fixation is used but rarely required.
- Buddy strapping to the adjacent toe is recommended for stable reduced joints.

SUGGESTED READING

Berndt AL, Hardy M. Transchondral fractures (osteochondritis dissecans) of the talus. J Bone Joint Surg (Am) 1959;41:988–1020.

Berry GK, Stevens, DG, Kreder HJ, et al. Open fractures of the calcaneus: a review of treatment and outcome. J Orthop Trauma 2004: 18;202–206.

Boyd HB, Knight RA. Fractures of the astragalus. South Med J 1942;35:160–167.

Buckley R, Tough S, McCormack R, et al. Operative compared with nonoperative treatment of displaced intra-articular calcaneal fractures: a prospective, randomized, controlled multicenter trial. J Bone Joint Surg (Am) 2002;84:1733–1744.

Canale ST, Kelly FB. Fractures of the neck of the talus: long-term evaluation of seventy-one cases. J Bone Joint Surg (Am) 1978; 60:143–156.

Early JS. Fractures and dislocations of the midfoot and forefoot. In: Bucholz RW, Heckman JD, eds. Rockwood and Green's fractures in adults, 5th ed. Philadelphia: Lippincott Williams and Wilkins, 2001:2181–2245.

Essex-Lopresti P. The mechanism, reduction technique and results in fractures of the os calcis. Br J Surg 1952;39:395–419.

Hawkins LG. Fractures of the lateral process of the talus. J Bone Joint Surg (Am) 1965;47:1170–1175.

Hawkins LG. Fractures of the neck of the talus. J Bone Joint Surg (Am) 1970;52:991–1002.

Rammelt S, Zwipp H. Calcaneus fractures: facts, controversies and recent developments. Injury 2004;35:443–461.

Sanders R. Intra-articular fractures of the calcaneus: present state of the art. J Orthop Trauma 1992;6:252–265.

Sangeorzan B, Benirschke SK, Mosca V, et al. Displaced intra-articular fractures of the tarsal navicular. J Bone Joint Surg (Am) 1989; 71:1504–1510.

Smith CS, Nork SE, Sangeorzan BJ. The extruded talus: results of reimplantation. Washington, DC: American Academy of Orthopaedic Surgeons, 2005.

Sneppen O, Christensen SB, Krogsoe O, et al. Fracture of the body of the talus. Acta Orthop Scand 1977;48:317–324.

Vallier HA, Nork SE, Barei DP, et al. Talar neck fractures: results and outcome. J Bone Joint Surg (Am) 2004;86:1616–1624.

Vallier HA, Nork SE, Benirschke SK, et al. Surgical treatment of talar neck body fractures. J Bone Joint Surg (Am) 2003;85:1716–1724.

NONOPERATIVE MANAGEMENT

Until comparatively recently, nonoperative treatment was the only method of treating fractures and severe soft tissue injuries, but the introduction of anesthesia, antibiotics, improved surgical implants, and better operative techniques has changed the treatment of many fractures. The process of change continues, and probably fewer fractures will be managed nonoperatively in the future as the functional benefits of operative treatment become more apparent to both surgeons and patients. There will always be large numbers of relatively minor fractures in which surgical intervention is unnecessary, however, and nonoperative techniques therefore need to be understood.

Much of the debate about nonoperative or operative management of fractures has centered around the tibial diaphysis, unfortunately, and the arguments for and against surgical treatment of the tibia cannot be extrapolated to other bones. This chapter describes the history of nonoperative management as well as outlines the common methods, and it suggests which methods are appropriate for different fractures should the surgeon select nonoperative management. The indications for nonoperative management are found in the appropriate chapters. If nonoperative management is chosen, Tables 31-1 and 31-2 give recommendations of the optimal methods in upper and lower limb injuries.

TRACTION

Skeletal Traction

Traction was used in many institutions as the principal method of managing femoral diaphyseal fractures until the 1970s, when locked intramedullary nailing became popular. Surgeons also used traction to treat complex tibial diaphyseal fractures they wished to treat nonoperatively but were associated with significant soft tissue damage or comminution. It was also used for the management of pelvic and acetabular fractures.

Most traction methods rely on a splint on which the leg is placed. The proximal end or ring of the splint is placed in the patient's groin, and traction is applied by placing a transosseous pin through the distal femur or proximal tibia. Fixed traction is undertaken when the pin is secured

Fracture Type[a]	Nonoperative Management
Clavicle	Sling and mobilize at 2 wk
Proximal humerus	Sling and mobilize at 2 wk
Humeral diaphysis	Hanging-U slab; brace at 2 to 3 wk
Distal humerus	Long-arm cast
Olecranon	Long-arm cast
Radial head	Sling and mobilize at 2 wk
Radial neck	Sling and mobilize at 2 wk
Forearm diaphysis	
Both bones (undisplaced)	Long-arm cast; forearm cast at 4 wk
Radius only	Forearm cast
Ulna only	Forearm cast
Distal radius and ulna	Forearm cast
Scaphoid	Scaphoid or forearm cast
Other carpal fractures	Forearm cast
Metacarpal fractures	
Undisplaced	Mobilize
Displaced	Burkhalter or James splint; mobilize after 3 wk
Proximal and middle phalangeal fractures	
Undisplaced	Buddy strapping and mobilize
Displaced	Burkhalter, James, or aluminium digit splint; mobilize after 3 wk
Distal phalangeal fractures	Mobilize or mallet splint

[a]See appropriate chapters for suggested management.

to the distal end of the splint by traction cords. In balanced traction the splint is suspended by a pulley system, and a second pulley system is applied to the transosseous pin. Traction with a variable weight then alters the fracture position with countertraction provided with the patient placed in the head-down position by raising the end of the

412

TABLE 31-2 RECOMMENDED NONOPERATIVE TREATMENT METHODS FOR LOWER LIMB FRACTURES IF NONOPERATIVE MANAGEMENT USED

Fracture Type[a]	Management
Pelvis (ring intact)–usually elderly patients	Mobilize full weight bearing as pain permits
Acetabulum (undisplaced)	Non–weight bearing for 4 wk, then full weight bearing
Proximal femur	
Subcapital	Recommended only if anaesthesia considered unsafe
Intertrochanteric	Recommended only if anaesthesia considered unsafe
Femoral diaphysis	Not recommended
Distal femur	
Undisplaced	Hinged knee brace for 6–8 wk
Displaced	Not recommended
Patella	
Undisplaced	Long-leg cast or brace. Mobilize at 4–6 wk
Displaced	Not recommended
Proximal tibia	
Undisplaced	Hinged knee brace for 6–8 wk
Displaced	Not recommended
Tibia diaphysis	Long-leg cast; patellar tendon–bearing cast at 4–6 wk
Distal tibia	Not recommended
Ankle	
Undisplaced	Below-knee cast or brace for 6 wk
Displaced	Not recommended unless significant medical comorbidities (e.g., diabetes). Then as for undisplaced fractures.
Foot	Cast or brace for 6 wk

[a]See appropriate chapters for suggested management.

bed. Once traction is established, the fracture alignment is checked radiologically and pads inserted appropriately to push the femur into the correct alignment. A posterior pad is almost always required under the distal femur because of the posterior sag produced by the effect of gravity.

Many different traction methods have been described. The six basic traction types are shown in Figure 31-1.

- A Thomas splint with a Pearson knee piece (Fig. 31-1A) is a classical traction apparatus employing a splint to support the thigh and a knee splint to support the calf but permit knee flexion.
  - The leg was usually kept straight on the Thomas splint for 4 to 6 weeks to allow healing to start. Then the knee splint was fitted and knee movement allowed.
- A Braun frame and a weight and pulley system (Fig. 31-1B) permits traction in the longitudinal axis of the femur.
  - This is a very simple traction system, and control of the femoral fragments was difficult.
  - Braun frame traction, using skin traction rather than a transosseous pin, is still widely used to rest an injured limb prior to surgery.
- Hamilton-Russell traction (Fig. 31-1C) uses a one-pulley system to provide support for the femur and to apply traction.
  - The mechanical advantage offered by two pulleys at the foot of the bed theoretically meant the longitudinal pull was twice as great as the upward pull, and the resultant traction was at an axis of 30 degrees to the horizontal, approximately in line with the femur.
  - This method of traction does not adequately control femoral fragments, and it was sometimes used after a period of skeletal traction.
- Perkins traction (Fig. 31-1D) is essentially a straight pull along the axis of the femur through a proximal tibial pin but without a splint.
  - The control of femoral alignment was poor.
  - Its purpose was to allow immediate knee flexion, but femoral malunion was common.
  - Perkins advocated the use of a split bed later in the treatment of femoral diaphyseal fractures.
  - In this system the patient sat on a bed with the knee flexed over the mattress.
  - Knee movement was encouraged while ensuring that longitudinal femoral traction was maintained.
- Fisk traction (Fig. 31-1E) consisted of a short Thomas splint and a hinged knee piece.
  - Traction in the axis of the femur was maintained using a proximal tibial transosseous pin, but the patient could flex the hip and knee by pulling on a separate cord attached to the end of the thigh splint.
- In 90-90 traction (Fig. 31-1F), the thigh is pulled upward, and both thigh and knee are at 90 degrees.
  - The advantage of this method is that gravity does not cause a posterior sag of the femoral fragments, a problem associated with all other traction methods.

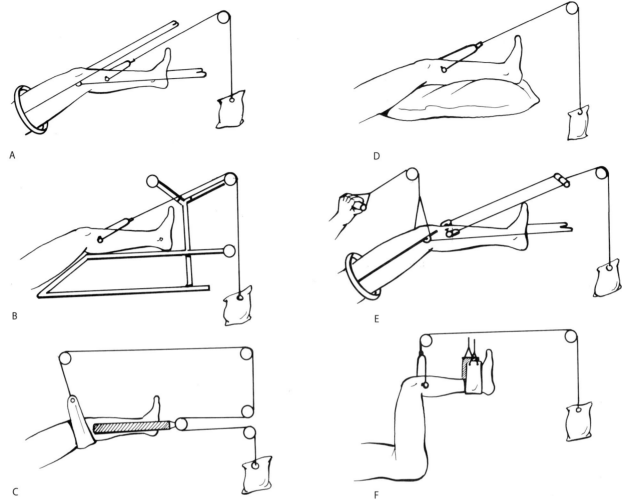

Figure 31-1   Six methods of skeletal traction. See text for explanation.

■ The method was used for proximal femoral diaphyseal fractures where a proximal femoral fragment was flexed by the unopposed action of iliopsoas.

■ This method is still used for pediatric femoral fractures.

Complications

■ The complications associated with skeletal traction are considerable.

■ The major problems are failure to maintain the normal alignment of the femur and significant knee stiffness.

■ Malunion was common, and although surgeons worked hard at preserving knee flexion, a number of studies indicated that flexion of between 90 and 100 degrees was often all that was achieved.

■ The incidence of femoral nonunion is difficult to determine, but refracture was relatively common, suggesting the nonunion incidence was high.

■ Prolonged immobilization in bed was associated with significant medical problems and functional disability.

■ Older patients developed respiratory and urinary complications as well as decubitus ulcers.

■ Younger patients often suffered considerably, with loss of employment and financial hardship.

■ Psychological problems associated with prolonged bed rest were not unusual.

■ Tibial traction is potentially very dangerous and should not be used.

■ It is very easy to distract a tibial diaphyseal fracture with excessive traction and thereby raise the intracompartmental pressure within the leg.

    ■ This may cause compartment syndrome or cause further devascularization of already traumatized muscles, producing muscle tethering and contracture.

Spinal Traction

Unlike skeletal traction, spinal traction remains popular and in widespread use for the management of cervical fractures and dislocations. Traction is commonly used to reduce a fracture or dislocation, thereby decompressing the neural elements and providing a degree of cervical stability. Today traction is rarely used for definitive management, and it is usually changed to a halo-body cast or vest, or the surgeon may opt for later surgical stabilization (see Chapter 18).

There are two principal types of cervical traction: cranial tongs, of which the best known is probably the Gardner Wells tongs, and halo traction.

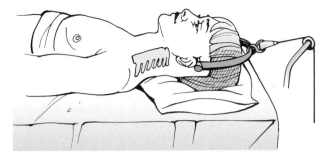

Figure 31-2 The use of cranial tongs to apply cranial traction.

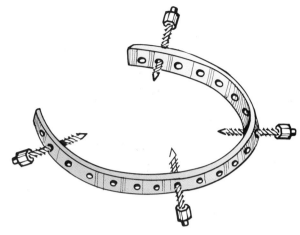

Figure 31-3 A diagram of a halo ring.

Cranial Tongs

■ Cranial tongs consist of a hemicircular frame with two spring-loaded angulated pins (Fig. 31-2) that are placed into the outer table of the skull at points about 1 cm posterior to the external auditory meatus and 1 cm superior to the pinna of each ear.

  ■ Because this is below the widest diameter of the skull, the upward pin angulation means that traction can be applied.

■ Each spring-loaded pin is applied with an insertion torque of 6 to 8 inch pounds.

■ Once the tongs are in position, a simple pulley system can be set up with a weight hanging over the end of the bed or frame (Fig. 31-2).

  ■ Care must be exercised in applying weights in case overdistraction and neural damage occur.

■ The weight required to reduce the spine varies with the position of the fracture, the degree of ligamentous damage, and the size of the patient, but as a rule the surgeon should start with an initial weight of 10 lbs.

  ■ Approximately 5 lb per spinal segment are required to reduce the fracture in most patients, although this is only a guide.

  ■ Thus about a 40-lb load will be needed for a C5-C6 injury, although the exact weight varies and serial imaging is required to check the reduction as the load is increased.

■ A lateral radiograph or fluoroscopic image is then obtained to visualize fracture reduction.

■ The indications for cervical traction are given in Chapter 18.

Halo Ring Traction

■ Closed or open halo rings (Fig. 31-3) are now a popular choice for cervical traction because they can tolerate higher loading than cranial tongs and can also be incorporated into a cast or brace to provide definitive treatment (Fig. 31-4).

■ The halo is attached with four pins, two anterior and two posterior.

■ As with cranial tongs the halo pins must be inserted below the widest diameter of the skull.

  ■ The two anterior pins are placed through stab incisions under local anesthetic about 1 cm above the lateral third of the orbital rim. In this location they are lateral to the supraorbital and supratrochlear nerves.

  ■ The posterior pins are placed about 1 cm above the helix of the ear. To prevent skin necrosis, the posterior pins should not make contact with the ear.

■ Opposing pins should be tightened at the same time to avoid displacement of the ring.

■ Pins should be retightened 24 to 48 hours after the initial application.

■ If a pin becomes loose with time, it can be retightened once to 8 inch-pounds if resistance is met.

Halo-Body Fixation

■ The original halo-body device was a body cast attached to a halo and devised by Perry and Nichol (1959).

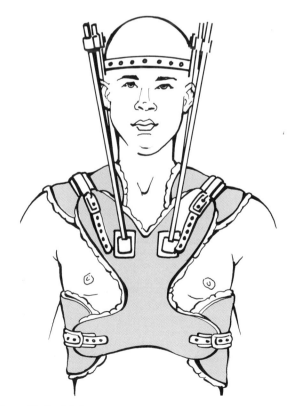

Figure 31-4 A halo vest.

- Halo casts may be useful in patients who are not cooperative or when the appropriate bracing materials are not available, but today halo vests or halo orthoses are in widespread use.
- The vest is usually made of plastic and tightened with buckles or straps.
- It is attached to the halo by two anterior and two posterior rods (see Fig. 31-4).
- The orthosis is worn until union or until the surgeon decides the use of a cervical brace is indicated.

Complications

- As with skeletal traction, a number of complications are associated with cervical spine traction.
- About 10% of patients lose fracture position inside a halo-vest orthosis.
  - It has been estimated that the halo-vest orthosis permits up to 31% of normal cervical spine motion and thus there is always a possibility of loss of reduction.
  - Serial radiographs are essential to check for this.
- Halos are also associated with a number of other complications, some of which are very similar to those associated with external fixation.
  - Pin tract infection has been reported in 6% to 20% of cases, with a high percentage of cases associated with pin loosening. Because the fixation is essentially unicortical, a high incidence of loosening and infection is not surprising.
  - Nerve damage, dural puncture, and skull perforation have all been reported, and when halo-body fixation is used in quadriplegic patients, there is a high incidence of pressure sores, decubitus ulcers, and respiratory complications.
  - Difficulty in swallowing may be associated with overextension of the head and neck.
  - It is obvious that careful follow-up is important if halo-body fixation is used for definitive fracture management.

Thoracolumbar Fractures

- Traction is not used for the definitive management of thoracolumbar fractures, although prolonged bed rest is used.
- This is a well-established method of treating unstable thoracolumbar fractures, although less commonly used today.
- Rotating beds, of which the Stryker bed is the best known, are used.
- These are designed to facilitate skin care, physiotherapy, and personal hygiene.
- Complications associated with the use of these beds are considerable with respiratory complications and decubitus ulcers the particular problems.
- Intensive nursing is required with this method of management.

CASTS

Unlike skeletal traction, the use of casts remains popular for fracture treatment. Indeed, a significant proportion of upper limb injuries and many less severe lower limb injuries

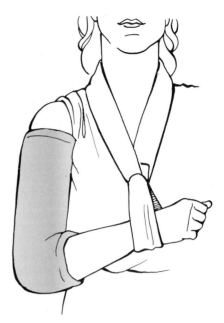

Figure 31-5   A hanging cast.

continue to be treated by the application of casts or slabs despite the rapid expansion of operative fracture surgery. The indications for cast management for most fractures are relative rather than absolute, and nowadays most surgeons reserve the use of casts or braces for less severe fractures, with more severe fractures associated with significant soft tissue damage, comminution, or displacement treated operatively. The decision to treat a patient with a cast obviously may be influenced by the patient's overall health, age, and functional status as much as by the morphology or severity of the fracture. Thus it is difficult to be dogmatic about exact indications for the use of casts.

A number of casts are in common use. In the upper limb, the most common casts used for fracture treatment are the hanging cast, mainly used for humeral diaphyseal fractures (Fig. 31-5); the long-arm cast used for fractures around the elbow and in the forearm (Fig. 31-6); the Colles, or forearm, cast, mainly used for distal radial fractures (Fig. 31-7); the

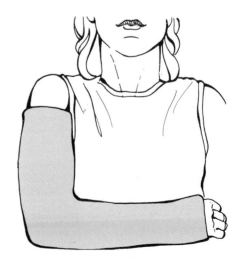

Figure 31-6   A long-arm cast.

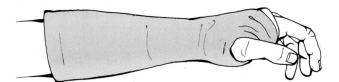

Figure 31-7 A Colles, or forearm, cast.

scaphoid cast used for scaphoid fractures (Fig. 31-8); and the shorter version of the scaphoid cast, the Bruner cast, principally used for fractures and ligamentous damage around the metacarpophalangeal joint of the thumb. A number of plaster slabs or splints used for hand fractures and tendon injuries are detailed in the section dealing with the use of splints.

In the lower limb the most common casts are the long-leg cast used for the initial management of tibial diaphyseal fractures (Fig. 31-9), the patellar tendon–bearing cast used for the definitive management of tibial diaphyseal fractures (Fig. 31-10), and the below-knee cast, most commonly used to treat fractures of the ankle and foot (Fig. 31-11).

Use

Casts are frequently applied to provide a period of pain-free support to fractures that are stable and either undisplaced or minimally displaced. Good examples are seen in many minor distal radial or fibular fractures where reduction is unnecessary and late displacement rare. A supportive cast is all that is required to control pain and facilitate mobilization. Casts may also be used actually to control the position of a fracture that has been reduced by a surgeon. This is clearly more difficult, and the surgeon relies on two principles to achieve success in maintaining the position of unstable diaphyseal fractures in a cast: the principle of three-point fixation, and the hydrostatic effect of the soft tissues between the fractured bone and the rigid external cast.

The principle of three-point fixation is illustrated in Figure 31-12. It relies on the fact that there is a hinge of intact periosteum on the concave side of a diaphyseal fracture. Once the fracture is reduced, the periosteal hinge is tightened, and direct pressure placed on the convex side of the fracture opposite the periosteal hinge supplemented by pressure on the concave side proximally and distally theoretically maintains reduction. The concept is a little naïve, although it will work in low-energy injuries in younger patients. As patients age, however, the periosteum progressively thins and periosteal damage increases, and consequently there may not be a hinge of periosteum across the fracture. In addition, the muscles that span the fracture will tend to cause fracture displacement.

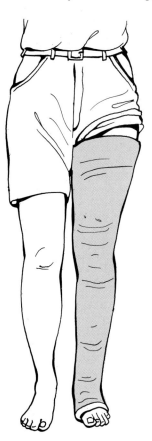

Figure 31-9 A long-leg cast.

Hydrostatic pressure relies on the fact that the soft tissues and the diaphysis are not compressible (Fig. 31-13). Thus when they are encased in a complete cast or brace they essentially become rigid and maintain the position of

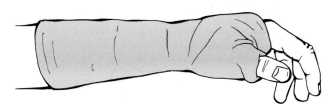

Figure 31-8 A scaphoid cast.

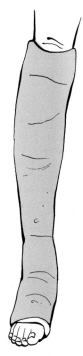

Figure 31-10 A patellar tendon–bearing cast.

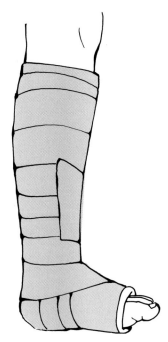

Figure 31-11 A below-knee cast.

the fracture. Again the explanation is a little simplistic and does not take into account active muscle contraction around the fracture.

Application

Casts are applied in a similar manner, no matter which type of cast is used or which material is used to make the cast. Resin-based casts are now more popular than gypsum-based casts because of their light weight and radiolucency. They

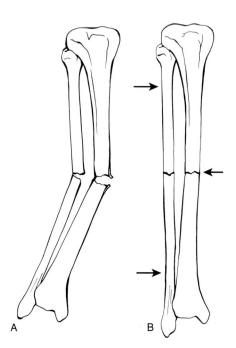

Figure 31-12 Three-point fixation. See text for explanation.

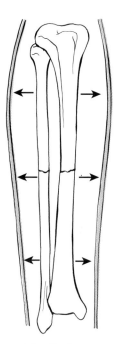

Figure 31-13 The principle of hydrostatic pressure in cast use. See text for explanation.

are not uniformly available throughout the world, however, and the use of gypsum-based casts is still widespread.

- Both types of cast material are frequently used as "slabs," applied soon after injury to give temporary support to an injured limb.
- A full cast is rarely applied immediately after injury because of the potential for the swelling associated with the injury to lead to a compartment syndrome if the limb is encased in a rigid cast.
- Slabs are applied by using a layer of protective stockinette and layers of synthetic wool padding.
- A slab of the appropriate length is then cut and, after soaking, applied to the limb.
- Gypsum-based materials take 36 to 48 hours to completely harden, whereas resin-based casts are hardened fully in 20 to 30 minutes.
- Full casts are applied by wrapping impregnated bandages around the limb after stockinette and synthetic wool have been applied.
- Cast bandages are available in different sizes to cope with different locations.
- If the cast is being used to control the position of a reduced fracture, excessive padding should be avoided because redisplacement of the fracture may occur.
- Cast bandages must be applied carefully, keeping the bandages flat to avoid ridges that may cause soft tissue damage.
- As the cast hardens, the surgeon should manipulate the fracture appropriately.
- Care must be taken not to obstruct joint movement or, if a joint is encased by the cast, it should be placed in the correct position.
- Once the cast is applied, radiographs will confirm if the fracture position is maintained.

- This is rarely a problem if the cast has been used to protect a minor fracture, but if it has been used to stabilize an unstable diaphyseal fracture, it may be necessary to adjust the cast to compensate for residual malalignment.
- Angular malalignment can be corrected by wedging.
  - Radiographs or fluoroscopy are used to identify the fracture site, and the cast is cut circumferentially at the level of the fracture, leaving a hinge of 2 to 3 cm of the cast intact.
  - The location of this intact hinge depends on the direction of the necessary correction.
  - Thus, if the fracture is in valgus, a hinge is placed medially and a varus forcibly applied.
  - The cut in the cast opens as the fracture is reduced and is kept open until further cast material is applied to maintain the reduced position. Fluoroscopic or radiographic control should be used.
- Rotational deformity is often difficult to identify in a cast and may be hard to control.
  - Theoretically, it can be corrected by derotation following a circular cut in the cast opposite the fracture, but this is difficult, and usually it is preferable to remove the cast and start again.
- If cast management is chosen as a definitive method of fracture treatment, surgeons should be aware that control of the position of a displaced diaphyseal fracture is difficult and the fracture position may slip.
  - If this occurs, a decision will need to be made about altering the treatment method.

Types

Upper Limb

Long-Arm Cast
- The classic long-arm cast with the elbow at 90 degrees and the wrist included in the cast (see Fig. 31-6) is less commonly used nowadays because forearm and elbow fractures are often fixed internally.
- It still is used for less severe fractures, although a forearm cast may often be adequate.
- The cast is applied from just below the axilla to just proximal to the metacarpophalangeal joints of the digits, leaving the thumb free.
- The wrist is placed in about 30 degrees of dorsiflexion.
- If the cast is used for an unstable forearm fracture, it is best applied using Chinese finger traps to suspend the forearm to help reduce the fracture.
- If used for a relatively minor elbow injury, this procedure is unnecessary and the cast can be applied with the arm dependent.
- In minor fractures, the wrist may not be included, and a full-arm cylinder may therefore be used.

Hanging Cast or U-Slab
- These casts are routinely used to treat humeral diaphyseal fractures in the acute phase.
- The arm is placed over the lower chest with the elbow at 90 degrees.
- A collar and cuff can be used to maintain the position.
- After applying a layer of stockinette and synthetic wool, a hanging cast can be applied by applying a long-arm cast as shown in Figure 31-5 so the top of the humeral component of the cast is above the humeral fracture.
- Gravity is used to regain humeral length, and the alignment of the fracture can be adjusted by altering the length of the cuff between the neck and the forearm.
  - The shorter the cuff, the more varus is applied to the fracture.
- An alternative is the U-slab, or sugar-tong splint, in which a plaster slab is placed from just below the axilla on the medial side of the arm down and around the elbow and upward to just below the shoulder.
  - The slab is then bandaged to hold it in position and stabilize the fracture.
  - In proximal diaphyseal fractures, the slab can be extended above the shoulder.
  - These casts are often used to maintain humeral reduction with a brace applied after about 2 weeks.

Colles Cast (Forearm Cast)
- The Colles cast is the most popular upper limb cast and is used for the majority of distal radial and ulnar fractures as well as for some carpal injuries.
- The cast extends from below the elbow to just proximal to the metacarpal necks of the digits with the thumb free (see Fig. 31-7).
- The surgeon frequently has to reduce the fracture during cast application, which is achieved by applying traction, slight palmar flexion, and ulnar deviation with the position maintained until the cast hardens.
- The position of extreme palmar flexion should be avoided because it is very painful and may cause medial nerve compression.

Scaphoid Cast
- The scaphoid cast is commonly used to treat scaphoid fractures and pain in the area of the anatomical snuffbox when X-rays do not confirm the presence of a fracture.
- In this cast the wrist is in slight dorsiflexion and the thumb is held in abduction and slight flexion as if a glass was being held between the index finger and thumb (see Fig. 31-8).
- The cast extends from just below the elbow to just proximal to the metacarpal necks of the digits.
- On the thumb the cast extends to just proximal to the interphalangeal joint.
- An extended scaphoid cast may be used for fractures distal to the metacarpophalangeal joint of the thumb, in which case the whole thumb is included.

Bruner Cast
- The Bruner case is a variant of the extended scaphoid cast, which is cut short to release the wrist joint.
- It is particularly useful for the treatment of ligamentous injuries of the thumb metacarpophalangeal joint.

Lower Limb Casts

Below-Knee Cast
- The below-knee cast is the most common cast used for lower limb injuries, including ankle and foot fractures and sprains.

- It is also occasionally used to treat undisplaced lower third tibial diaphyseal fractures.
- The cast is applied from below the level of the fibular neck proximally to the level of the metatarsal heads distally, with the ankle at 90 degrees and the foot in the plantigrade position (see Fig. 31-11).
- The below-knee cast may be applied as the first stage of a long-leg cast used to treat an unstable tibial diaphyseal fracture in the acute phase.
- It can be very difficult to apply a below-knee cast and maintain tibial alignment at the same time.
  - This is best achieved by hanging the leg over the end of a plaster table and maintaining longitudinal traction with the knee and ankle flexed at 90 degrees.
  - Surgeons should be aware of the difficulty in reducing a distal tibial diaphyseal fracture with the foot in the plantigrade position.

Long-Leg Cast
- All other lower limb casts are merely variants of the below-knee cast.
- Surgeons usually apply a long-leg cast to treat unstable tibial diaphyseal fractures in the acute phase, changing to a patellar tendon–bearing cast or brace after a few weeks.
- The long-leg cast is best constructed by applying a below-knee cast and then flexing the knee by about 10 degrees while the thigh extension is applied (see Fig. 31-9).
- Care must be taken not to obstruct hip movement by placing the cast too high in the groin.

Patellar Tendon–Bearing Cast
- The other variant of the below-knee cast is the patellar tendon–bearing cast, usually used to treat tibial diaphyseal fractures after a few weeks in a long-leg cast.
- In this cast the proximal end is extended upward as far as the lower pole of the patellar and molded around the patellar tendon to provide a degree of rotational stability (see Fig. 31-10).
- Care must be taken not to apply pressure over the common peroneal nerve running around the neck of the fibula.

BRACES

Limb Braces

Many different limb braces have been designed, but they fall into three main types used to treat the upper arm, the distal forearm, and the lower leg. Most braces are made of polyethylene or plastic and secured by Velcro or plastic straps or by buckles. Braces tend to be lighter than casts and often used after a short period of cast immobilization once the fracture has become more stable. Other advantages of braces are that they can be tightened as the soft tissue swelling decreases, and they can be removed for personal hygiene and radiological evaluation of the fracture.

- In the upper limb a simple polyethylene or plastic brace is often used to treat humeral diaphyseal fractures after the initial management with a hanging U-slab (Fig. 31-14).

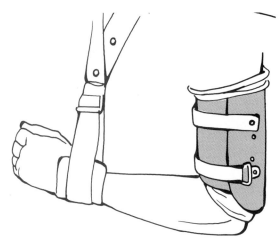

Figure 31-14 An arm brace use to treat humeral diaphyseal fractures.

  - The brace fits around the arm and is wider laterally than medially to support the humerus proximally.
  - It is tightened as required.
- The other brace commonly used in the upper limb is the distal forearm brace, which can be used to treat distal radial fractures (Fig. 31-15).
- Again the braces are light and radiolucent and can be tightened as required.
  - As with humeral braces, they are usually applied after a period of cast immobilization.
- The most popular lower limb brace is the equivalent of the below-knee cast (Fig. 31-16) and used for the same indications.
  - These braces are usually prefabricated and permit early mobilization.
  - They are useful after fracture fixation or to facilitate mobilization after minor fractures or soft tissue injuries of the ankle and foot.
  - The other brace used extensively is the patellar tendon–bearing brace (Fig. 31-17).
  - This is the equivalent of the patellar tendon–bearing cast but allows movement of the ankle.
  - It is fitted with an ankle hinge and a heel cup and thus can be worn inside a shoe.

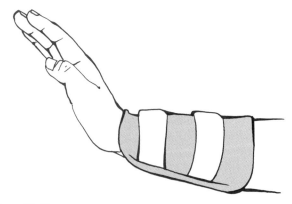

Figure 31-15 A distal forearm brace used to treat distal radial fractures.

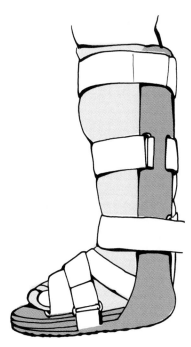

Figure 31-16   A below-knee brace.

■ Occasionally surgeons may make use of a cast brace, a below-knee walking cast attached by medial and lateral hinges to a thigh cast.
　■ This was used to treat femoral diaphyseal fractures after a period of initial traction but is now usually used for protection of the knee after ligament injury.

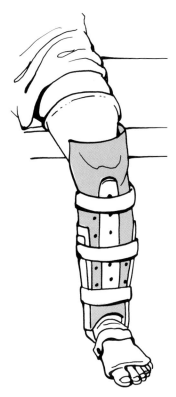

Figure 31-17   A patellar tendon–bearing brace.

BOX 31-1 COMPLICATIONS OF CAST MANAGEMENT

- Malalignment and malunion
- Joint stiffness
- Raised compartment pressure
- Nonunion
- Soft tissue complications

■ Nowadays it is more common to use an off-the-shelf brace made of synthetic material and fitted with integral knee hinges.
　■ This brace is lighter and can be adjusted for tightness.

Complications
The main complications of the use of casts and braces are shown in Box 31-1. Because nonoperative management of fractures was the accepted treatment for so long, there is often a belief it represents an ideal method of management. Although surgeons discuss the complications of operative management, they often ignore the considerable complications of cast management. In addition, there is a scarcity of good information about functional outcome after cast management because many of the papers were written at a time when outcome criteria were less sophisticated.

Malalignment and Malunion
■ The main complications of the use of casts and braces are malunion and joint stiffness.
■ Although advocates of nonoperative management such as Charnley and Sarmiento have highlighted the usefulness of three-point fixation and hydrostatic pressure, nonoperative management usually results in approximate rather than perfect fracture alignment.
■ Operative management became accepted quickly in fractures of the radius and ulna, where malunion was associated with very significant problems.
■ In humeral diaphyseal fractures, where malunion is associated with less functional impact, nonoperative management remains popular.
■ In many fractures, the effects of malunion are underestimated.
　■ Realignment of the normal volar angulation of the distal radius is beneficial, but because remanipulation of the fracture often fails to even restore the neutral position of the distal radius, surgeons merely accepted up to 10 degrees of dorsal angulation despite the fact this was often associated with carpal malalignment and a poor functional outcome.
　■ In nonoperatively treated distal tibial diaphyseal fractures, malunion is common, and studies have shown that many patients experience difficulty in returning to work or normal activities.
　■ Tibial malunion correlates with the incidence of late knee osteoarthritis.

Joint Stiffness
■ Joint stiffness is a major problem associated with the use of casts or braces.

■ It is a combination of a number of problems: capsular contracture, muscle tethering, and possibly raised compartment pressures secondary to the use of a complete cast.

■ Joint stiffness is undoubtedly age related and also depends on the length of time the cast is applied.

■ Thus the incidence of joint stiffness is less in young patients and in patients in whom a cast is used for a short period.

■ No evidence indicates that a forearm cast used to treat a distal radial fracture or a below-knee cast used for an ankle fracture causes stiffness that lasts for more than about 3 months.

■ If casts are used for a prolonged period, however, such as when humeral or tibial diaphyseal fractures are treated, joint stiffness can be a significant, irreversible problem.

■ There is strong implication in the literature dealing with fracture bracing that the use of a brace rather than a cast is associated with less joint stiffness, but little evidence indicates this is actually the case.

■ The three areas in which information exists about joint function either for cast or brace management are the humeral diaphysis, the distal radius, and the tibial diaphysis.

 ■ In none of the studies of these fractures is there evidence that brace management confers improved joint function.

■ Surgeons are in fact frequently using braces to manage less severe fractures, which are associated with a decreased incidence of joint stiffness.

■ Court-Brown (2001) analyzed the use of long-leg casts, patellar tendon–bearing casts, and functional braces in the treatment of tibial diaphyseal fractures, and he showed the incidence of both malunion and joint stiffness was similar in all three types of treatment.

■ If nonoperative management is used, and the problems of joint stiffness minimized, casts or braces should be used for stable fractures associated with little soft tissue damage.

■ In these fractures the duration of cast use is shorter and the incidence of joint stiffness consequently reduced.

Increase in Compartment Pressure

■ The use of complete casts, by preventing the expansion of the soft tissues enclosed within them, can cause an increase in the intracompartmental pressure, which at worse can lead to compartment syndrome.

■ The problem may be lessened by splitting the cast, but high intracompartmental pressures can still occur.

■ The incidence of increased compartment pressure and compartment syndrome associated with cast application is unknown, but the incidence of toe deformities after tibial fracture treatment by a cast has been reported to be about 10%, suggesting compartment problems are relatively common.

Diaphyseal Nonunion

■ It is difficult to compare the incidence of nonunion in cast- or brace-treated fractures with operatively managed fractures because in recent years surgeons have tended to use casts or braces to treat less severe diaphyseal fractures and operative methods for more severe fractures.

■ Nonoperative management of tibial diaphyseal fractures is associated with a higher incidence of nonunion than intramedullary nailing.

■ The requirement for secondary surgery to secure union in a cast- or brace-managed fracture has been reported to be as high as 40% but probably averages 10% to 15%.

Soft Tissue Problems

■ A generation ago surgeons used to refer to "plaster disease," the effect of the use of a circumferential cast on the soft tissues.

■ There was no good definition of plaster disease, but limbs undoubtedly became atrophic, stiff, and dysfunctional after a prolonged period in a cast.

■ It is likely that the syndrome of plaster disease represented a combination of different problems: muscle atrophy, muscle tethering, joint capsular contracture, raised compartment pressure, and possibly reflex sympathetic dystrophy.

 ■ The problem was common and responded only to long-term physiotherapy.

■ One further problem associated with the use of a cast is soft tissue access.

■ This is particularly important in the treatment of open fractures, and cast management should not be used for open fractures or fractures that require fasciotomy.

SPINAL BRACES

Cervical Braces

There are three basic types of cervical braces: soft and hard collars, high cervicothoracic orthoses, and low cervicothoracic orthoses (Fig. 31-18). Within these three types are many different designs, but all have a similar function. Standard cervical collars (Fig. 31-18A) have no place in the treatment of cervical fractures or dislocations, although they are useful for the management of minor soft tissue sprains and whiplash injuries. They allow up to 80% of normal cervical movement and therefore confer little stability to the cervical spine. Their main function is to act as a proprioceptive stimulus to remind patients they should be careful. Rigid collars are useful for emergency neck stabilization, but the most effective way of stabilizing the cervical spine is by strapping the chin and forehead to a rigid spine board.

High cervicothoracic orthoses (Fig. 31-18B) have molded occipitomandibular supports that extend to the upper part of the thorax. Probably the best known example of such a brace is the Philadelphia collar, which is in common use. Studies indicate that it resists 71% of normal cervical flexion and extension, 34% of lateral bending, and 54% of rotation. Other cervical braces show similar results. These types of braces are useful for the management of cervical sprains or to provide temporary immobilization during transport or after surgical stabilization of the cervical spine.

Low cervicothoracic orthoses have the same molded upper support but extend lower down to the lower part of the thorax (Fig. 31-18C). Examples of these braces are the Minerva and SOMI (sternal-occipital-mandibular immobilizer) braces, although there are other designs available.

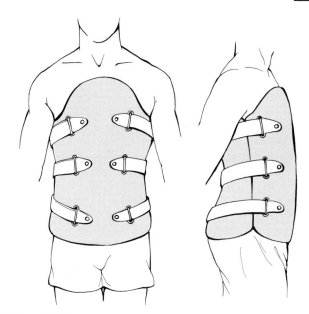

Figure 31-19 A thoraco-lumbar-sacral orthosis.

Thoracic and Lumbar Braces

The goal of thoracolumbar braces is to support the spine by limiting overall trunk motion, decreasing muscular activity, increasing the intra-abdominal pressure, resisting spinal loading, and limiting spinal motion. A number of brace types are available, with the simplest a lumbosacral corset and the most complex an individually modeled thoraco-lumbar-sacral orthosis made from plastic and tightened by buckles or straps (Fig. 31-19). A useful intermediate brace between the lumbosacral corset and the customized orthoses is the Jewett brace (Fig. 31-20). This provides three-point fixation and permits spinal extension but prevents flexion.

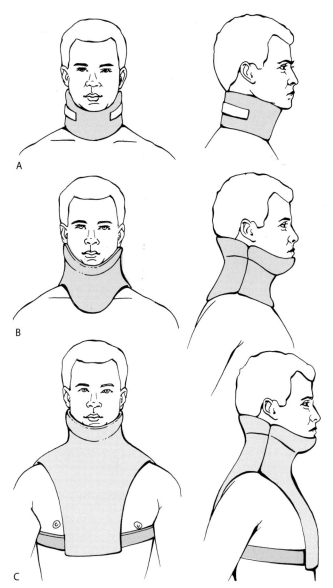

Figure 31-18 Different types of cervical braces. (**A**) A cervical collar. (**B**) A high cervicothoracic orthosis. (**C**) A low cervicothoracic orthosis.

Low cervicothoracic orthoses are better than high cervicothoracic orthoses in resisting cervical rotation and sagittal movement in the mid and lower cervical spine, but similar to high cervicothoracic braces they do not prevent all cervical movement. If any neck brace is used to treat an unstable fracture, the surgeon must be careful to obtain serial radiographs to check that the fracture reduction is maintained until union.

Complications
- The main complication of spinal braces is the same as limb braces, namely loss of reduction of the fracture.
- Even low cervicothoracic orthoses permit neck movement, and thus their use does not guarantee maintenance of the position in unstable fractures.
- A poorly fitted brace may be uncomfortable and cause skin and soft tissue irritation and damage.

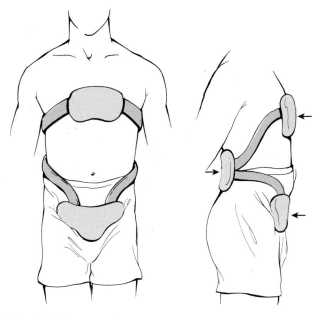

Figure 31-20 A Jewett brace.

Lumbar corsets, like cervical collars, are essentially proprioceptive and serve to remind the patient to take care. They are used in the treatment of low back pain, but their only use in spinal injury is in the management of stable minor fractures or soft tissue injuries. The Jewett brace is useful in the treatment of injuries between T6 and L3, which are unstable in flexion. Studies have shown that it reduces intersegmental motion and flexion at the thoracolumbar junction, whereas lateral bending and axial rotation remain unaffected. It has been shown to be effective in the treatment of one- or two-column fractures, but not in the treatment of three-column fractures. Custom molded thoraco-lumbar-sacral orthoses provide more stability, but maintenance of reduction of unstable thoracolumbar fractures cannot be guaranteed and serial radiographs of the fracture are required if nonoperative management of unstable thoracolumbar fractures is undertaken.

Complications

- The complications of thoracolumbar braces are essentially the same as for cervical braces, namely difficulty in maintaining fracture reduction, patient compliance, and skin problems.

Slings, Bandages, and Support Strapping

- A number of minor injuries, soft tissue sprains, and fractures are treated by support and analgesia with mobilization of the affected area encouraged after a relatively short period.
- Tubular elastic support bandages are frequently used to treat minor soft tissue injuries such as ankle and foot sprains, wrist sprains, or minor ligament damage in other joints.
- A number of upper limb fractures are treated by the use of slings, which may be supplemented by bandaging.
- Fractures of the clavicle, proximal humerus, and radial head and neck are often treated by sling support until the discomfort settles enough to allow joint movement.
- Several different methods of bandaging have been used to treat clavicle fractures in an effort to reduce pain and maintain fracture reduction.
  - The figure-eight bandage is still used.
  - This is placed anteriorly around both shoulders and crossed over at the level of the upper thoracic spine.
  - As it is tightened it extends the shoulders, ideally reducing the fracture.
  - It loosens quickly, unfortunately, and no evidence indicates it is better than a sling.
- For fractures of the clavicle, proximal humerus, and radial head and neck treated nonoperatively, 2 weeks in a sling followed by mobilization is all that is required.
- Another area where strapping is useful is in the management of stable undisplaced fractures of the phalanges of the hand and foot.
- These fractures can be treated by buddy strapping the affected digit to an adjacent digit (Fig. 31-21).
  - Usually two strips of half-inch tape are used, placed around the proximal middle phalanges with protective gauze placed between the fingers.
  - The joints should be left free to allow mobilization.

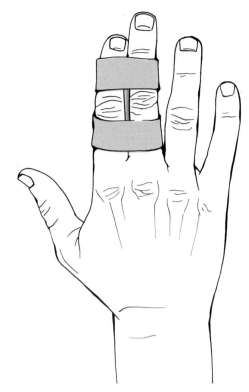

Figure 31-21   Buddy strapping.

- This type of strapping loosens quickly, and the patient, or a companion, must be taught how to replace it.
- The thumb spica elastoplast splint around the thenar eminence and proximal phalanx of the thumb (Fig. 31-22) may also be helpful for sprains or minor tears of the collateral ligaments of the metacarpocarpal phalangeal joint of the thumb.

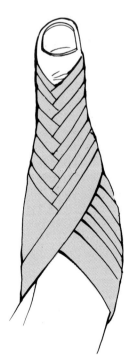

Figure 31-22   A thumb spica.

■ Again the strapping will loosen after a few days and may need to be replaced.

■ Buddy strapping and thumb spicas are not useful for the treatment of unstable fractures and do little more than provide a degree of stabilization for minor injuries.

Splints

Many different splints have been designed, usually for the immobilization of hand injuries, typically fractures of the metacarpals or phalanges or damage to the extensor and flexor tendons of the hand. It is beyond the scope of this book to describe all the different splints designed for use in the hand, and if more information is required, *Green's Operative Hand Surgery* (2005) should be consulted. Many hand injuries can be treated by the use of a few simple splints, however.

■ Many metacarpal fractures require no treatment beyond pain relief and mobilization, but if splintage is required, two separate splints are in popular use.

■ The Burkhalter splint is used for metacarpal and proximal phalangeal fractures (Fig. 31-23).
  ■ The wrist is placed in 40 degrees of extension, and a Colles short-arm cast is applied.
  ■ Once the cast hardens, a dorsal slab is applied with the metacarpophalangeal joints in 70 to 90 degrees of flexion.
  ■ The slab is extended to just proximal to the proximal interphalangeal joints, which are allowed to mobilize.
  ■ Distal extension of the splint allows more distal fractures to be treated with an extension block if necessary.
  ■ This splint relies on the intact dorsal extensor mechanism of the fingers acting as a tension band and thereby maintaining the position of the fracture.

■ An alternative splint or slab is the volar slab with the fingers placed in the James position of 70 to 90 degrees of flexion of the metacarpophalangeal joints and full extension of the proximal interphalangeal joints and distal interphalangeal joints (Fig. 31-24).
  ■ The principle behind this splint is that the collateral ligaments of the metacarpal phalangeal joints and both interphalangeal joints are at full stretch in this position and therefore contractures will not occur.

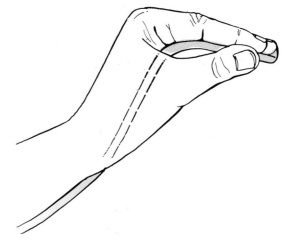

Figure 31-24 A volar slab.

■ This position is useful for the treatment of both metacarpal and phalangeal fractures.

■ The whole hand can be immobilized if a volar slab is used, or one finger can be immobilized by the use of an aluminium-backed foam splint.

■ Aluminium-backed foam splints are very useful in digital injuries.
  ■ They can be applied to the volar or dorsal aspects of the digits to immobilize fractures or joints after dislocation has been reduced.
  ■ They are also useful for resting the fingers after soft tissue injuries, and a volar splint can be particularly used for maintaining extension following a volar plate injury.
  ■ These splints are cut and molded appropriately and held by adhesive strapping (Fig. 31-25).

■ Mallet fingers caused by either avulsion of the extensor tendons from the distal phalanx or by a fracture of the distal phalanx are well treated by the use of a mallet finger splint (Fig. 31-26).
  ■ An appropriately sized splint is applied to the digit with the distal interphalangeal joint in full extension.
  ■ If this method of management is used, the patient should be taught that the distal interphalangeal joint must be kept extended for a period of 6 weeks.

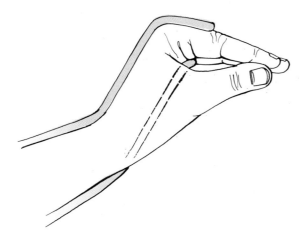

Figure 31-23 A Burkhalter splint.

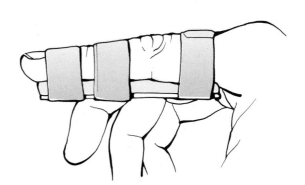

Figure 31-25 An aluminium-backed foam splint.

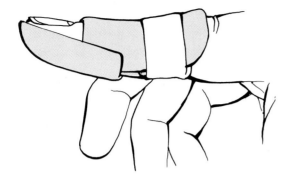

Figure 31-26   A mallet finger splint.

Complications

- As with all methods of nonoperative fracture management, the main complication of the use of splints is failure to maintain the reduced position of the fracture.
- Thus, like casts or braces, splints are frequently used to treat simple fractures, with more complicated fractures treated by operative means.
- Patient compliance and soft tissue abrasion can be a problem.

SUGGESTED READING

Charnley J. Closed treatment of common fractures, 3rd ed. Edinburgh: Churchill Livingstone, 1961.

Court-Brown CM. Fractures of the tibial and fibula. In: Bucholz RW, Heckman JD, eds. Rockwood and Green's fractures in adults, 5th ed. Philadelphia: Lippincott Williams and Wilkins, 2001:1939–2000.

Fjalestad T, Stromsoe K, Salvesen P, et al. Functional results of braced humeral diaphyseal fractures; why do 38% lose external rotation of the shoulder? Arch Orthop Trauma Surg 2000;120:281–285.

Green DP, Hotchkiss RN, Pederson WC, Wolfe SW, eds. Green's operative hand surgery, 5th ed. New York: Churchill Livingstone, 2005.

Kuntscher M, Blazek J, Bruner S, et al. Functional bracing after operative treatment of metacarpal fractures. Unfallchirurg 2002;105:1109–1114.

McQueen MM, Hajducka C, Court-Brown CM. Redisplaced unstable fractures of the distal radius: a prospective randomised comparison of four methods of treatment. J Bone Joint Surg (Br) 1996;78:99–104.

Milner SA, Davis TR, Muir KR, et al. Long-term outcome after tibial shaft fracture: is malunion important? J Bone Joint Surg (Am) 2002;84:971–980.

Sarmiento A. A functional below-the-knee brace for tibial fractures. A report on its use in one hundred thirty-five cases. J Bone Joint Surg (Am) 1970;52:295–311.

Sarmiento A, Gersten LM, Sobol PA, et al. Treated shaft fractures treated with functional braces. Experience with 780 fractures. J Bone Joint Surg (Br) 1989;71:602–609.

Sarmiento A, Horowitch A, Aboulafia A, et al. Functional bracing of comminuted extra-articular fractures of the distal third of the humerus. J Bone Joint Surg (Br) 1990;72:283–287.

Sarmiento A, Latta LL. Functional fracture bracing. Berlin: Springer-Verlag, 1995.

Stern PJ. Fractures of the metacarpals and phalanges. In: Green DP, Hotchkiss RN, Pederson WC, eds. Green's operative hand surgery, 4th ed. New York: Churchill Livingstone, 1999.

Tropiano P, Huang RC, Louis CA, et al. Functional and radiographic outcome of thoracolumbar and lumbar burst fractures managed by closed orthopaedic reduction and casting. Spine 2003;28:2459–2465.

PLATING

The first bone plate was used in 1886 by Hansmann in Hamburg, Germany. He employed the novel concept of inserting percutaneous screws that protruded through the skin like external fixator pins! The acceptance of plate fixation was fairly rapid and popularized by three orthopaedic surgeons in particular. Albin Lambotte in Belgium, William Arbuthnott Lane in England, and William Sherman in the United States not only developed plating systems but also undertook clinical research to improve both plate design and patient management. Lane and Sherman plates dominated fracture treatment for several decades, but it was the work of Robert Bagby in the United States and Robert Danis, professor of theoretical and practical surgery at the University of Brussels, that changed plating techniques and stimulated worldwide interest in the techniques. Danis invented a "coapteur," or compression plate, that facilitated fracture reduction and rigid fixation. His work influenced the AO (Arbeitgemeindschaft für Ostéosynthesfragen) group, which has been responsible for virtually all innovation in plate design and surgical techniques since the 1950s.

FRACTURE COMPRESSION

The basic philosophy of the AO group between the 1950s and mid-1970s was essentially that of Danis. They believed in accurate fracture reduction and rigid fracture fixation. The concept of fracture compression is central to their treatment methods, usually achieved by the use of a lag screw whose simple principle is illustrated in Figure 32-1. After reduction of the fracture, a screw is inserted at right angles to the fracture line. The proximal cortex is overdrilled to allow the screw to slide within the cortex. Tightening of the screw causes compression of the fracture. An alternative to the lag screw is the partially threaded screw, which, when tightened, also causes fracture compression (Fig. 32-1). In long spiral fractures, a number of lag screws can be inserted to secure the fracture. This technique is particularly applicable to external rotation fractures of the lateral malleolus (see Fig. 32-2). If this technique is used, care must be taken to alter the angle of insertion of the screws around the spiral fracture so they are inserted at 90 degrees to the fracture

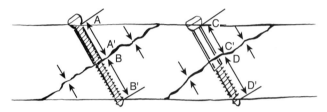

Figure 32-1   A diagram of the use of the lag screw (left) and the partially threaded screw (right). A-A' is overdrilled, and B-B' is drilled and tapped normally. C-C' is not overdrilled, but the screw is partially threaded. D-D' is drilled and tapped normally.

line. In most other fractures, the use of a lag screw may produce compression and temporary stabilization of a fracture, but by themselves lag screws not infrequently provide insufficient mechanical stability. A plate is then required to stabilize the fracture.

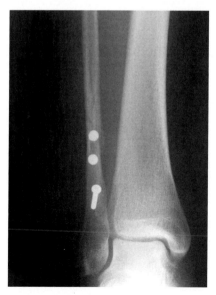

Figure 32-2   The use of three lag screws to fix a lateral malleolar fracture.

PLATE DESIGN

Many different plates have been designed. Plates are produced in different lengths and sizes to fit all bones. They are conventionally defined by the size of the screw they are designed to take and the number of screw holes they contain. Thus a 10-hole 3.5 plate has 10 screw holes and is designed to be used with 3.5-mm screws. Screws in common use vary between 1 mm and 6.5 mm in diameter. In recent years, with better metallurgy and improved operative technique, surgeons have tended to use smaller plates.

Neutralization Plates

All early plates were neutralization plates with round or oval holes (Fig. 32-3). They were designed to hold bone after the fracture had been reduced and fixed with one or more interfragmentary screws. These plates have some disadvantages. Round-hole plates do not allow much variation in screw placement; modern plates are more versatile. In good-quality bone, however, a lag screw and neutralization plate may be all that is required to hold a fracture until union occurs. An example of this is in the fibula where one type of neutralization plate, the one-third tubular plate, is commonly used (see Fig. 32-3). This plate has oval holes to permit some variation in screw placement, but fracture compression is not possible. It is only 1 mm thick and therefore provides less rigid fixation. One-third tubular plates are also commonly used in the forearm, olecranon, and distal ulna.

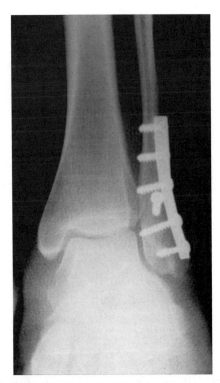

Figure 32-3   The use of a neutralization plate on a lateral malleolar fracture.

Reconstruction Plates

Reconstruction plates (Fig. 32-4) are stainless steel neutralization plates that are available in 3.5 and 4.5 sizes. They are designed to be more easily contoured than dynamic compression plates and therefore are particularly useful in bones with a complex morphology such as those of the pelvis, acetabulum, clavicle, and distal humerus. They are designed with deep notches between the holes to facilitate contouring, but the plates are not as strong as dynamic compression plates, and excessive contouring can weaken them. The screw holes are oval, but their design does not permit compression.

Dynamic Compression Plates

The dynamic compression plate (DCP) was introduced in 1969 (see Fig. 32-4). This plate revolutionized fracture treatment. The screw holes are oval and shaped such that if a screw is placed in the proximal part of the screw hole closest to the fracture and then tightened, the screw head slips distally, resulting in fracture compression if the plate is already secured to the other bone fragment. The lag screw became unnecessary, and compression could be achieved in transverse fractures where inserting a lag screw was impossible (see Fig. 27-9 in Chapter 27). The design of the screw holes allows screws to be angled up to 7 degrees in the transverse plane and up to 25 degrees in the longitudinal plane. The DCP can be used in compression mode or in neutralization mode.

Despite the advanced design of the DCP, it had much the same basic problems associated with neutralization plates. The insertion of any plate requires open surgery and significant soft tissue mobilization. The periosteal circulation is unavoidably damaged, and in diaphyseal fractures this is associated with an increased incidence of infection and nonunion when compared with less invasive techniques such as intramedullary nailing. In an attempt to minimize periosteal damage, the low-contact dynamic compression plate (LC-DCP) was devised.

The LC-DCP is available in a variety of sizes in stainless steel or titanium. The screw holes are the same as in a dynamic compression plate, but the undersurface of the plate is scalloped to reduce the surface area in contact with the periosteum. This alteration of plate design also facilitated plate contouring. Clinical studies have not defined the superiority of the LC-DCP over the DCP, but the LC-DCP design has been retained in more recent plates.

Locking Compression Plates

Locking compression plates (LCP) are the most recent plate to be devised. Early results are very promising, particularly when they are used in osteopenic bone. The design of the screw hole has been changed to permit the screw heads to screw into the plate itself. This gives a more rigid plate/screw construct and has been described as an internal fixator. The principle is that if all the screws are fixed to the plate they will all have to loosen if the plate becomes detached from osteopenic bone.

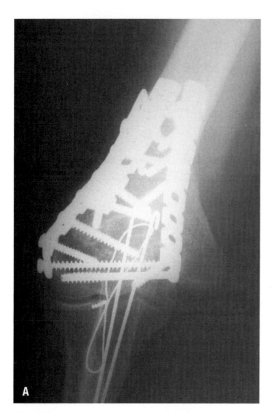
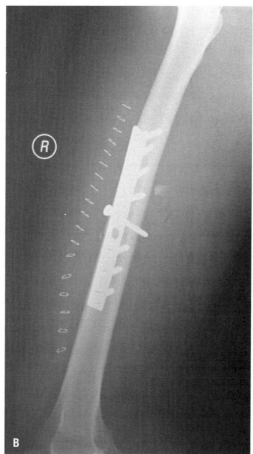

Figure 32-4 (A) The use of reconstruction plates on the distal humerus. The middle plate was used to stabilize a tricortical autograft from the iliac crest. (B) A dynamic compression plate used on a femur. Note the oval screw holes, which permit compression.

There are two variants of the threaded screw hole. In one the screw thread is the only option available on the plate. This is found in a number of location-specific plates for the distal femur, proximal (Fig. 32-5) and distal tibia, and the proximal humerus. These plates can be inserted using both open and minimally invasive techniques. The second screw hole is a combination hole consisting of a DCP and threaded screw hole together (Fig. 32-6). This is available in straight plates but also in T- or L-shaped plates, reconstruction plates, and volar curved plates for the distal radius. The advantage of the combination hole is that either standard or locking screws can be used. If a locking plate is used, there are a number of points of surgical technique (Box 32-1).

Blade Plates

Blade plates are modified plates designed to be used in a few specific locations. The plate is prebent so one end is placed into the metaphyseal area of the bone while the other is secured to the diaphysis in the usual way using bone screws. Blade plates were popularized for use in the proximal and distal femur (see Fig. 24-4 in Chapter 24). Proximal femoral blade plates are supplied with a variety of blade/shaft angles. They are rarely used for fresh fractures nowadays but are still used for valgizing subtrochanteric osteotomies (see Fig. 39-11 in Chapter 39). The distal femoral blade plate has a 95-degree blade plate angle. Its use in fresh fractures has largely been replaced by dynamic condylar screw/plate systems, but the blade plate is still occasionally used.

Blade plates are used in two other locations. Small blade plates for use in metacarpal and phalangeal fractures

---

BOX 32-1 POINTS OF SURGICAL TECHNIQUE IN THE USE OF LOCKING PLATES

- Unicortical screws can be used in good-quality bone, but the use of bicortical screws is advised in osteoporotic bone.
- Plates cannot be placed eccentrically on bone because the locking screws cannot be angled to allow placement.
- Locking screws cannot be used to pull the plate onto bone.
- Screws inserted at more than 10 degrees to the correct vertical axis will not grip the plate and will be mechanically weak.
- The alignment of metaphyseal screws cannot be altered to avoid an adjacent joint. Care must be taken to place the plate correctly so the screws are extra-articular.

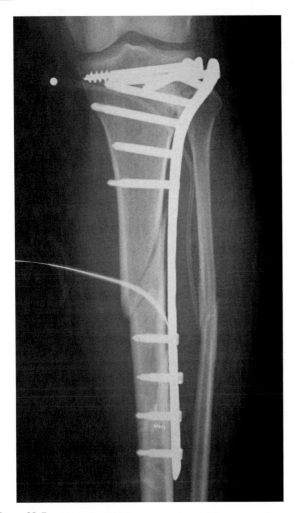

Figure 32-5   A locking (LISS) plate used to stabilize a complex proximal tibial fracture.

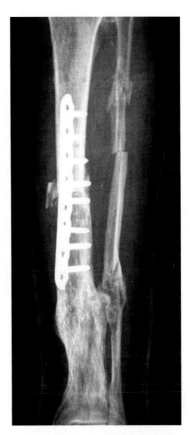

Figure 32-6   A locking compression plate used for a tibial nonunion. The earlier malunion made IM nailing impossible.

(Fig. 32-7) are available, and the recently devised acromioclavicular hook plate is essentially a blade plate in which the blade is placed through the acromioclavicular joint under the acromion and the plate is screwed to the distal clavicle. This plate is mainly used for reduction and fixation of Neer type II distal clavicle fractures (see Fig. 10-8 in Chapter 10).

Location-Specific Plates

In recent years there has been increasing interest in plates designed for specific locations. These are virtually all used to treat metaphyseal or intra-articular fractures or to treat fractures in small irregularly shaped bones such as the calcaneus (Fig. 32-8). Currently location-specific plates exist for the treatment of many fractures including those of the spine (see Fig. 18-15 in Chapter 18), distal clavicle (see Fig. 10-8 in Chapter 10), proximal humerus, distal humerus, proximal ulna, distal radius (see Fig. 16-12 in Chapter 16), metacarpals and phalanges (Fig. 32-7), pelvis, proximal femur (see Fig. 21-13 in Chapter 21), distal femur (see Fig. 24-6 in Chapter 24), proximal tibia (see Fig. 26-11 in Chapter 26), distal tibia (see Fig. 28-4 in Chapter 28), and calcaneus (Fig. 32-8). Most of these plates act as neutralization plates, although newer designs have incorporated the concept of the threaded screw hole

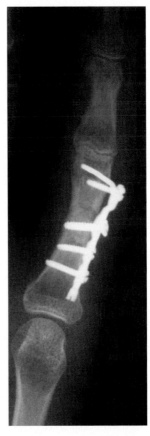

Figure 32-7   A blade plate used to fix a proximal phalangeal fracture.

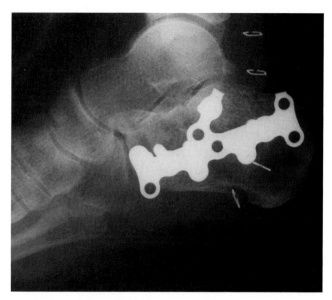

Figure 32-8 A location-specific calcaneal plate.

and may well prove advantageous in the treatment of osteopenic metaphyseal fractures.

PLATE APPLICATION

Plate application is usually straightforward, but the surgeon must consider a number of factors.

Soft Tissue Mobilization

Care must be taken to mobilize the soft tissues from the bone to allow plate application without unnecessary devitalization of the bone ends or any intermediate bone fragments. This is a particular problem in comminuted fractures where multiple attempts at fracture reduction may well cause significant devascularization leading to nonunion or infection.

Fracture Reduction

Care must be taken to reduce the fracture accurately. Plating is the most rigid of the commonly used fracture treatment methods, and if a fracture is plated in distraction or in significant malposition, nonunion may occur. Bone-holding forceps should be used to maintain the reduced position while a lag screw or plate is applied.

Plate Contouring

Plate rigidity means that plates must be contoured to the shape of the bone. Failure to do this may result in fracture malposition and nonunion or malunion. Plate templates and benders are provided within the plating systems to facilitate contouring.

Selection of Plate Type

The different plate types and their application methods are described in this chapter. The surgeon must select an appropriate plate for the fracture being treated.

Number of Screws

In diaphyseal fractures there should be three bicortical screws above and below the fracture. More may be required in complex fractures or in osteopenic bone where fixation is poor. In metaphyseal or intra-articular fractures, the number of metaphyseal screws is dictated by the fracture pattern, but it is generally better to increase the number of screws, particularly in elderly patients.

PLATING TECHNIQUES

Plates can be applied in a number of different ways depending on the fracture location, fracture morphology, and reason for surgery.

Tension Band Plating

One of the most common reasons for applying a plate is to stabilize a diaphyseal fracture in anatomical alignment while it unites. This is commonly done for fractures of the clavicle, humeral diaphysis, forearm diaphyses, and metacarpals, and for periprosthetic femoral fractures. The best examples of tension band plating are seen in eccentrically loaded bones such as the femur where the ground reaction force passes medial to the axis of the bone (Fig. 32-9). With a plate placed on the lateral side of the femur, the fracture will be compressed. If the plate is placed on the medial side of the femur, the fracture

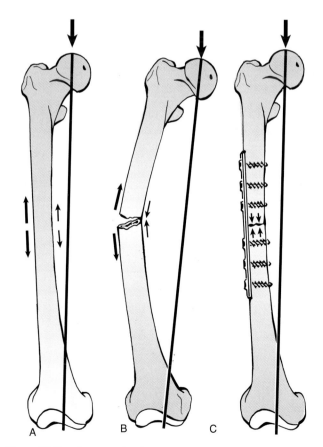

Figure 32-9 The principle of tension band plating. See text for explanation.

will open laterally. For this principle to work, the medial cortex of the bone obviously must be intact.

Buttress or Antiglide Plating

Buttress or antiglide plates are used for the treatment of intra-articular fractures with a shearing component (Fig. 32-10). The intra-articular fracture is reduced and held with interfragmentary screws, but the orientation of the fracture line means there is potential for slippage of the fracture fragments. This can be avoided by using a buttress or antiglide plate. The plate is contoured to fit the metaphyseal area around the fracture and only needs to be screwed to the diaphysis proximal to the distal end of the fracture, although there is no reason why supplementary fixation through the plate should not be used. This technique is particularly useful for volar displaced fractures of the proximal radius (see Fig. 16-14 in Chapter 16), fractures of the proximal tibia and fractures of the posterior (see Fig. 32-10), and medial and lateral malleoli of the ankle (see Figs. 29-12 and 29-9, respectively, in Chapter 29).

Biological or Bridge Plating

One of the criticisms leveled at diaphyseal plating has been the requirement for extensive soft tissue dissection to permit accurate reconstruction of the bone fragments prior to the use of interfragmentary screws and a plate. Obviously the greater the comminution, the more the dissection and the higher the incidence of complications such as infection or nonunion. To counteract this, surgeons apply plates across comminuted areas with minimal dissection at the fracture site (Fig. 32-11). Thus the principle of anatomical reconstruction is abolished, and the technique of bridge plating essentially mimics intramedullary nailing or external fixation with retention of the soft tissues at the fracture site.

This technique is obviously designed for use in comminuted diaphyseal fractures and has therefore been largely superseded by intramedullary nailing. It remains a useful technique in fibular fixation, however. If used, surgeons must be aware of the requirement for a longer plate because only proximal and distal screw fixation can be used.

Wave Plating

One of the difficulties in using a broad 4.5 DCP or LCP to stabilize an atrophic nonunion was there was essentially no room left for the bone graft. Surgeons wishing to use plating had to strip enough soft tissues from around the bone to permit corticocancellous bone grafting. Unfortunately, the more they damaged the soft tissues, the lower the incidence of union. Wave plating refers to the

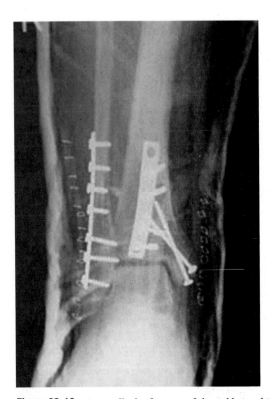
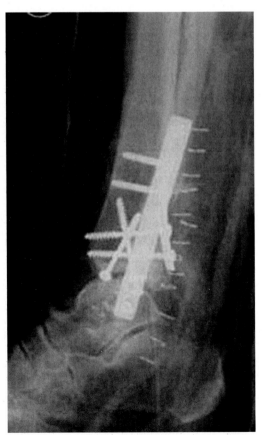

Figure 32-10   A trimalleolar fracture of the ankle in which an antiglide plate has been used to stabilize the posterior malleolus.

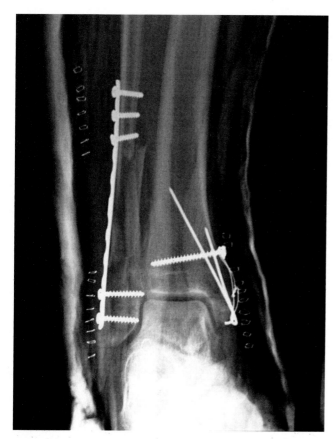

Figure 32-11 A bridge plate used to stabilize a comminuted lateral malleolar fracture. The skin overlying the comminuted area was not incised.

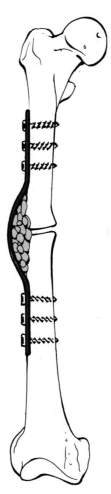

Figure 32-12 A wave plate with underlying bone graft.

use of a contoured 4.5 plate, usually on the femur, which allows bone graft to be placed between the plate and the cortex (Fig. 32-12). This technique may be useful if plating is required as, for example, if there is a nonunion of a periprosthetic femoral fracture, but most lower limb long-bone nonunions are treated by intramedullary nailing.

Subcutaneous Plating

A number of disadvantages are associated with the requirement for long incisions to allow plate application. Not only is there extensive soft tissue stripping as the fracture site is exposed, but the greater the soft tissue dissection, the more difficult it is to reduce the fracture by indirect means such as traction. An alternative is the use of subcutaneous plating. The plate is inserted through a small incision at a point where the subcutaneous tissues are relatively thin, such as the distal femur or proximal tibia.

The fracture is reduced by traction with the intact soft tissue envelope assisting with reduction. The plate is inserted through a small incision using fluoroscopy to position the plate on the bone. A jig is attached to the plate that facilitates insertion of the screws under fluoroscopic control. Subcutaneous plating is not appropriate for all metaphyseal and intra-articular fractures. Intra-articular comminution may require open reduction of the fracture prior to fixation with interfragmentary screws, and not all metaphyseal and spiral diaphyseal fractures are easily

reduced by closed means. The technique is particularly useful for the distal femur and proximal tibia and likely to become more popular.

PLATING OF SPECIFIC FRACTURES

Obviously there are alternative options to treating all fractures, but plating remains a standard treatment method for many fractures. Table 32-1 gives a list of the plates recommended for different locations if plating is chosen as the method of management.

Clavicle Fractures

- Clavicle plating is used both primarily and for the treatment of nonunion (see Chapter 10).
- Middle-third clavicle fractures are usually plated with an appropriately contoured 3.5 reconstruction plate (see Fig. 10-6 in Chapter 10) or a location-specific plate.
- Hook plating is routinely used for Neer II (Robinson 3B1 and 3B2) lateral clavicle fractures (see Fig. 10-8 in Chapter 10).
- Both incisions overlie the clavicle, and care must be taken not to damage the underlying subclavian vein.

TABLE 32-1 DIFFERENT TYPES OF PLATES IN COMMON USE IN DIFFERENT LOCATIONS

Fracture Location	3.5	4.5	Locked[a]	LSP	Other
Clavicle diaphysis	Reconstruction			X	
Clavicle distal	Hook			X	
Proximal humerus	T/L-shaped		X	X	
Humeral diaphysis		DCP/LCP	X	X	
Distal humerus	One-third tubular reconstruction			X	
Proximal ulna	One-third tubular			X	
Proximal radius					1.5 or 2.0 T
Forearm diaphysis	DCP/LCP				
Distal radius	T-shaped		X	X	
Metacarpal/phalanx diaphysis					1.5/2.0 DCP
Metacarpal/phalanx Intra-articular					1.5/2.0 T Blade
Spine				X	
Pelvis	Reconstruction DCP/LCP		X	X	
Acetabulum	Reconstruction			X	
Proximal femur					DHS
Femoral diaphysis		DCP LCP	X		Cable plate
Distal femur			X	X	DCS Blade
Proximal tibia	T/L-shaped	T/L	X	X	
Tibial diaphysis		DCP	X		
Tibial plafond	Cloverleaf One-third tubular		X	X	
Ankle	One-third tubular reconstruction		X		
Calcaneus			X	X	
Metatarsal/phalanx Diaphysis	One-third tubular				1.5/2.0 DCP
Metatarsal/phalanx Intra-articular					1.5/2.0 T Blade

LSP, location-specific plate.
[a]Locked means a locked plate is commonly used.

Proximal Humeral Plating

■ Proximal humeral plating (see Chapter 11) is usually used for translated two-part fractures in younger patients.
■ A 3.5 or 4.5 T-plate is usually used (see Fig. 11-8 in Chapter 11), although modern location-specific locked proximal humeral plates are now available.
■ The plate is applied to the lateral aspect of the proximal humerus using cancellous screws in the humeral head and cortical screws in the proximal diaphysis.
■ An anterior approach is usually used.
■ Care must be taken not to damage the long head of the biceps lying anteriorly over the proximal humerus or the axillary nerve.

Humeral Diaphyseal Plating

■ The humeral diaphysis (see Chapter 12) is usually plated with a 4.5 DCP (see Fig. 12-5 in Chapter 12) or LC-DCP, although increasingly locking plates are used because humeral fractures often occur in osteopenic bone (see Fig. 12-11 in Chapter 12).
■ Plates are inserted through an anterolateral approach or a posterior approach. The latter approach is more useful for distal diaphyseal fractures.
■ Care must be taken not to damage the radial nerve and particularly not to compress it under the plate.

Distal Humeral Plating

■ Distal humeral plating for intra-articular fractures (see Chapter 13) is usually undertaken using a 3.5 one-third tubular plate on the medial distal humeral column and a 3.5 reconstruction plate on the lateral column, although variations may be used depending on the fracture morphology (see Fig. 13-8 in Chapter 13).
■ Location-specific distal humeral plates can also be used.
■ Condylar fractures are occasionally plated using a 3.5 one-third tubular antiglide plate.

- A 2.0 antiglide plate can be used for capitellar fractures (see Fig. 13-7 in Chapter 13).
- In intra-articular fractures, the incision is posterior and an olecranon osteotomy is usually undertaken.
- Care should be taken not to damage the ulnar nerve.

Proximal Ulnar Plating

- Olecranon fractures may be plated with an appropriately contoured 3.5 one-third tubular or reconstruction plate (see Fig. 14-12 in Chapter 14), although location-specific proximal ulnar plates can be used.
- Proximal ulnar diaphyseal fractures are usually plated using a 3.5 reconstruction plate, DCP, or LC-DCP (see Fig. 12-9 in Chapter 12).
- A posterior incision is used.

Proximal Radial Plating

- Displaced radial neck fractures may be plated using a 1.5-mm T-plate (see Fig. 14-9 in Chapter 14) applied to the lateral aspect of the radial head and neck.
- The posterior interosseous nerve is at risk of damage.
- A lateral approach is used.

Radial and Ulnar Diaphyseal Plating

- Fractures of the radial and ulnar diaphyses are treated similarly no matter whether they are isolated fractures, Monteggia or Galeazzi fracture-dislocations, or fractures of both bones of the forearm (see Fig. 15-3 in Chapter 15).
- Plating is usually undertaken with 3.5 DCP or LCP plates.
- Two incisions are usually used.

Distal Radial Plating

Volar Plating

- Volar displaced distal radial fractures are usually plated using a buttress or antiglide technique.
- A neutralization 3.5 T-plate is used with appropriate contouring to restore the normal volar angulation of the distal radius.
- There is increasing interest in volar plating of dorsally angulated distal radial fractures using locked plates (see Fig. 16-12 in Chapter 16).
- Care must be taken to reduce the fracture prior to plating, to contour the plate (see Fig. 16-14 in Chapter 16), and to ensure the screws placed into the distal radial fragment are extra-articular!

Dorsal Plating

- Dorsally displaced distal radial fractures can be treated by distal plating.
- Two types of plate are in common use.
- A neutralization 3.5 T-plate can be used with screws placed into the distal fragment and the distal diaphysis (see Fig. 16-11 in Chapter 16).
- Alternatively, a location-specific distal radius plate can be used.

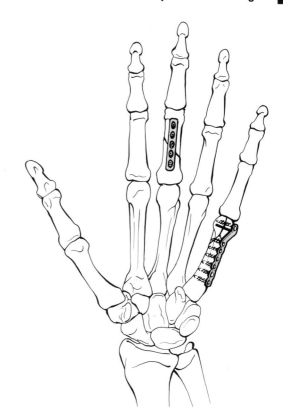

Figure 32-13 Diagram of the use of plates on the metacarpals and phalanges.

- As with volar plating, it is important to check that the volar angulation of the distal radius has been restored after fixation.

Metacarpal and Phalangeal Plating

- Diaphyseal fractures of the metacarpals and phalanges can be plated using 1.5 or 2.0 LC-DCP plates depending on the size of the bone.
- Intra-articular fractures can be plated, although many are treated by K-wires or by intrafragmentary screw fixation.
- If plating is used, 1.5 or 2.0 T-plates or blade plates are useful (Figs. 32-7 and 32-13).

Pelvic and Acetabular Plating

- Plates are commonly used to treat both pelvic and acetabular fractures.
- Most pelvic plates are used to treat posttraumatic pelvic instability usually following a period of external fixation, maintained until the patient is hemodynamically stable.
- The most common plates used are reconstruction plates because the necessary contouring is easily achieved.
- Locking compression plates can also be used.
- Plates are usually applied to stabilize the pubic symphysis in open book or vertical shear type fractures or to stabilize the sacroiliac joints in vertical shear fractures (Fig. 32-14). If the pubic symphysis is being stabilized, the options are to use a 3.5 or 4.5 DCP or LCP

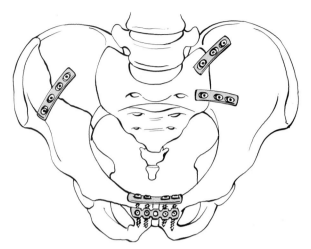

Figure 32-14 Two plates used to stabilize the pubic symphysis. A posterior iliosacral screw has also been used.

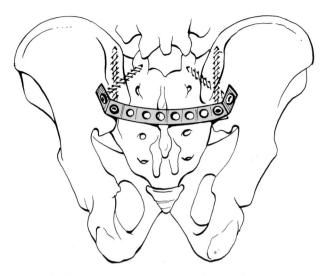

Figure 32-15 A diagram demonstrating the use of a posterior sacroiliac bridge plate.

superiorly over the symphysis or to use a superiorly located 3.5 DCP or LCP supplemented by an anteriorly placed 3.5 reconstruction plate.

- Sacroiliac stability can be achieved by using two anterior 3-hole 3.5 DCPs or the equivalent LCPs.
- If this technique is used, care must be taken not to damage a sacral nerve root.
- Alternatively, a contoured sacroiliac plate can be placed posteriorly.
- This is a bridge plate with screws placed in both iliac wings and not in the sacrum (Fig. 32-15).
- Acetabular plating usually involves applying 3.5 reconstruction plates to the posterior and anterior columns around the acetabulum.
- Anterior column plates tend to be longer than posterior column plates, which are commonly used to stabilize the posterior acetabulum after a posterior fracture-dislocation (Fig. 32-16).

Spinal Plating

- Location-specific plates are used in the cervical spine (see Fig. 18-15 in Chapter 18).
- Thoracolumbar posterior and anterior instrumentation devices are essentially location-specific plates (see Fig. 19-9 in Chapter 19).

Proximal Femoral Plating

- Intertrochanteric or basicervical fractures are usually treated using a location-specific hip screw/plate system (DHS) (see Fig. 21.2-13 in Chapter 21).
- The plate is a neutralization plate.
- A lateral approach is used.

Femoral Diaphyseal Plating

- Femoral diaphyseal plating is rarely used in the acute situation because most femoral fractures are treated by intramedullary nailing, but the technique continues to be useful for the treatment of periprosthetic fractures.

- It may be useful if the intramedullary canal is very narrow or if there is an associated proximal femoral fracture (see Fig. 23-7 in Chapter 23).
- Two main types of plates are used for the femur.
- The standard 4.5 DCP or LCP can be used for acute fractures in normal femora or in periprosthetic fractures (see Fig. 7-6 in Chapter 7).
  - These plates are applied to the lateral aspect of the femur.

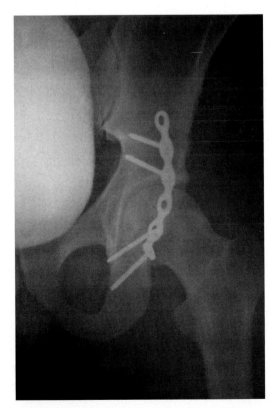

Figure 32-16 A posterior acetabular plate. This is an antiglide plate and has been used to treat the fracture shown in Figure 21.1-3.

■ Medial bone defects should be reconstructed with bone grafts.

■ If the plate is used to treat a periprosthetic fracture around or distal to a hip prosthesis, the screws will have to be angulated to avoid the prosthesis.

■ This is usually straightforward if a conventional cemented prosthesis has been used but may be impossible if a canal filling press-fit prosthesis has been used.

■ Unicortical screws can then be used, but stability is poor.

■ An alternative is to employ a plate designed to be used with both screws and cable loops.

■ The plate either has sculpted areas on the dorsal aspect to allow cable loops to be passed round it and secured with a clamp or it has holes through it.

■ Not infrequently the plate is used with a combination of loops and screws (see Fig. 7-5 in Chapter 7).

■ Care must be taken when passing the loops around the femur to keep the cables close to the bone and not to damage the perforating vessels.

Distal Femoral Plating

■ Distal femoral fractures can be plated using three different techniques, all of which require a lateral approach.

■ They can be treated using a condylar screw/plate system (see Figs. 7-2 and 24-5 in Chapters 7 and 24, respectively), which is very similar to the hip screw/plate systems used for intertrochanteric and basicervical fractures.

■ The difference is that the condylar screw is inserted at 95 degrees to the lateral cortex of the femur after insertion of a guide wire and drilling and reaming of the screw insertion hole.

■ Once the condylar screw is inserted, a side plate is placed over the proximal end of the condylar screw and screwed down to the lateral femur, usually in neutralization mode.

■ Obviously if an intra-articular distal femoral fracture is being treated, the intra-articular fragments must be reduced and fixed with interfragmentary screws prior to the insertion of the condylar screw.

■ If this is required, care must be taken to assess where the condylar screw will be placed, so the interfragmentary screws can be placed appropriately to avoid interference with the passage of the condylar screw.

■ An alternative plating technique involves the use of a 95-degree angled blade plate (see Fig. 24-4 in Chapter 24).

■ This is inserted after accurate reduction of the fracture.

■ The technique is more difficult than that of the condylar screw plate system and now rarely used.

■ The third method of plating distal femoral fractures involves the use of a location-specific distal femoral plate with locking screws (see Fig. 24-6 in Chapter 24).

■ This is designed to be inserted using a minimally invasive technique, and the plate is placed through a small skin incision at the level of the lateral femoral condyle.

■ The fracture is reduced by indirect means, although direct open reduction may be required if there are displaced intra-articular fragments.

■ Fluoroscopy is used to position the plate and to assist with positioning the screws, although the screws are inserted percutaneously using a plate-mounted jig.

■ The plate can also be inserted using a conventional open technique.

Proximal Tibial Plating

■ Lateral tibial plateau fractures are conventionally plated using an L- or T-shaped buttress or antiglide plate placed on the lateral aspect of the proximal tibia (see Fig. 26-7 in Chapter 26).

■ An anterolateral curved incision is usually used.

■ The intra-articular fracture is reduced and fixed with intrafragmentary screws and the plate applied to the lateral aspect of the proximal tibia.

■ An alternative technique involves the use of a location-specific proximal tibial plate inserted percutaneously in much the same manner as the distal femoral plate (see Fig. 26-11 in Chapter 26).

■ The plate is inserted through a small incision over the proximal lateral tibial condyle, and the screws are inserted percutaneously using a fluoroscopic control and a plate-mounted jig.

■ Bicondylar tibial fractures are now commonly treated by external fixation, but the use of two plates remains an option (see Fig. 26-8 in Chapter 26).

■ Surgeons should be aware that the technique necessitates significant soft tissue stripping.

■ Bicondylar fractures should be approached through a longitudinal anterior midline incision and bilateral T- or L-plates used to buttress both condyles.

■ It is usually easiest to reduce and fix the least comminuted condyle to the proximal tibial diaphysis and then fix the more extensively damaged condyle secondarily.

■ Other interfragmentary screws will be required, and both plates may need to be relatively long to achieve adequate distal fixation.

■ Proximal tibial diaphyseal fractures are often difficult to nail, and a location-specific plate may be used (see Fig. 27-12 in Chapter 27).

Tibial Diaphyseal Plating

■ Tibial diaphyseal fractures are rarely plated nowadays because intramedullary nailing is the preferred option.

■ If plating is to be undertaken, the plate is placed on the anteromedial subcutaneous border of the tibia through an incision 1 cm lateral to the subcutaneous border of the tibia.

■ The method of plating will depend on the type of fracture.

■ The relatively common spiral tibial fracture is best treated by reduction and fixation with lag interfragmentary screws. Then a neutralization plate is applied, frequently a DCP or LCP placed in neutralization mode.

■ Transverse tibial fractures should be plated with a DCP or LCP using the compression facility (see Fig. 27-9 in Chapter 27), and comminuted fractures are best treated using a bridge plate technique with minimal dissection of the comminuted area and the use of a longer plate.

■ Fractures associated with wedge or butterfly fragments can be treated by the use of two lagged interfragmentary screws and then stabilized with a DCP or LCP.

Distal Tibial Plating

■ As with proximal tibial fractures, external fixation has become more popular in the management of distal tibial fractures.

■ Plating remains popular mainly for OTA (AO) type B and C distal tibial fractures.

■ In OTA (AO) type B partial articular fractures, interfragmentary screws are used to reconstruct the distal tibia.
  ■ If the bone fragments are relatively small, the use of interfragmentary screws may be adequate, but in more extensive fractures a supplementary neutralization plate is used.
  ■ This is usually a cloverleaf-shape plate placed on the medial aspect of the lower tibia.

■ In type C, complete articular distal tibial fractures, two plates are commonly used.
  ■ The fibula is usually plated first using a one-third tubular plate, although an LCP can be used.
  ■ Once the fibula is out to the length and stabilized, the tibia is reconstructed using interfragmentary screws and a supplementary cloverleaf plate used in neutralization mode (see Fig. 28-4 in Chapter 28).
  ■ The cloverleaf plate is placed on the medial side of the distal tibia.

■ An alternative plating technique is to use a location-specific distal tibial plate that utilizes threaded screws.
  ■ As with modern distal femoral or proximal tibial plates, the plate can be inserted percutaneously and fluoroscopy used to insert the screws.
  ■ Any intra-articular fragments need to be reduced and held with interfragmentary screws prior to plate application.

■ Plating of tibial plafond fractures is a particularly difficult technique, requiring skill and experience.
  ■ Great care must be taken with soft tissue mobilization and fracture reduction.
  ■ The distal tibial articular surface is difficult to visualize adequately, and not infrequently fragments of the articular surface may be displaced by 2 to 3 cm proximally into the distal tibial metaphysis.

Ankle Fractures

■ Fibular plating remains the treatment of choice for most ankle fractures.

■ This may be supplemented by medial and/or posterior malleolar screw fixation in bimalleolar or trimalleolar fractures, but most transsyndesmotic and suprasyndesmotic ankle fractures are treated by fibular plating.

■ External rotation fractures of the fibula are treated by reduction and stabilization with one or more interfragmentary screws followed by the application of a one-third

tubular neutralization plate that needs to be contoured over the flare of the lateral malleolus (see Fig. 29-9 in Chapter 29).

■ If there is significant comminution, a bridge plate technique can be used with screws placed proximal and distal to the fracture site (see Fig. 32-11).

■ Care should be taken not to strip the comminuted fragments from their blood supply.

■ Distal fibular plates can be placed laterally or posteriorly (see Fig. 29-9 in Chapter 29).

■ Medial malleolar antiglide plating is relatively uncommon and usually undertaken in adduction injuries in which there is a vertical fracture line.

■ The relatively large medial malleolar fragment can be reduced and fixed with interfragmentary screws, but it is wise to buttress the fixation with an antiglide plate, which can be a short one-third tubular plate, reconstruction plate, or LCP (see Fig. 29-12 in Chapter 29).

■ The use of posterior malleolar plates is also unusual because most smaller posterior malleolar fragments do not require surgical treatment.

■ An antiglide plate may be used if the posterior malleolar fragment is more than 25% (see Fig. 32-10).
  ■ Posterior malleolar plating is discussed in more detail in Chapter 29.

■ Large posteromedial, or Volkmann, fragments require reduction and fixation.

■ The use of two or three interfragmentary screws may be adequate, but in large fragments it is wise to supplement this fixation with an antiglide plate.

■ There may be a medial malleolar fracture together with the posteromedial fragment.

■ An extended posteromedial incision allows screw fixation of the medial malleolar fragment and antiglide plate fixation of the posteromedial fragment (Fig. 32-10).

Calcaneal Fractures

■ Displaced intra-articular calcaneal fractures are frequently treated by reduction of the fracture followed by the application of a calcaneal plate to the lateral wall of the calcaneus.

■ Prior to the use of specialized calcaneal plates, surgeons used straight plates applied to the lateral wall of the calcaneus, but it was found the posterior facet fragments tended to redisplace inferiorly.

■ Calcaneal plates were developed that had a side arm, which allowed screws to be placed into the reconstructed posterior facet fragment (see Fig. 32-8).

■ The surgeon may choose to use an separate interfragmentary screw to fix the reconstructed articular surface internally or may elect to place the interfragmentary screw through the plate.

■ The plate is a neutralization plate, which is inserted through an extended lateral incision.

■ During insertion care must be taken not to damage the sural nerve or the peroneal tendons.

■ Calcaneal locking plates exist, but as yet no evidence indicates the results associated with their use are better than those of standard locking plates.

Metatarsal Plating

■ Most metatarsal fractures are treated nonoperatively, but if plating is undertaken the surgeon can use a 2.0 LC-DCP plate or a 3.5 one-third tubular plate depending on the size of the bone.

SUGGESTED READING

Chandler RW. Principles of internal fixation. In: Bucholz RW, Heckman JD, eds. Rockwood and Green's fractures in adults, 5th ed. Philadelphia: Lippincott, Williams and Wilkins, 2001.

Cole PA, Zlowodzki M, Kregor PJ. Treatment of proximal tibia fractures using the less invasive stabilization system: Surgical experience and early clinical results in 77 fractures. J Orthop Trauma 2004;18:528–535.

Kregor PJ, ed. Less invasive stabilisation system for the tibia. Injury 2003;34(Suppl 1).

Perren SM. The biomechanics and biology of internal fixation using plates and nails. Orthopedics 1989;12:21–33.

Rüedi TP, Murphy WM. AO principles of fracture management. Stuttgart: Thieme, 2000.

Schatzker J, Sanderson R, Murnaghan JP. The holding power of orthopaedic screws: in vivo. Clin Orthop 1975;108:115–116.

Schütz M, Südkamp NP. Revolution in plate osteosynthesis: new internal fixator systems. J Orthop Sci 2003;8:252–258.

Sommer C, ed. Locking compression plate–LCP—a new AO principle. Injury 2003;34(Suppl 2).

Sommer C, Babst R, Müller M, et al. Locking compression plate loosening and plate breakage: a report of four cases. J Orthop Trauma 2004;18:571–577.

Weight M, Collinge C. Early results of the less invasive stabilization for mechanically unstable fractures of the distal femur (AO/OTA Types A2, A3, C2 and C3). J Orthop Trauma 2004;18:503–508.

33 INTRAMEDULLARY NAILING

Prior to the First World War, intramedullary nailing was confined to the use of bone pegs inserted into long-bone fractures using an open technique. Metal nails were introduced after the First World War by Hey Groves in England but were popularized by Gerhard Küntscher of Germany after the Second World War. He devised locked nails with proximal and distal locking bolts, reconstruction nails, and the closed insertion techniques in use today. The nails in current use have evolved from the early designs of Klemm and Schellman in Germany and Grosse and Kempf in France. Femoral nailing, using locked nails, became popular in the 1970s, and tibial nailing in the 1980s and 1990s. Humeral nailing using flexible unlocked nails has been used sporadically over the last 30 to 40 years, but there has been recent interest in the use of both antegrade and retrograde locked nails for the stabilization of humeral diaphyseal fractures. The results of humeral nailing have not been as convincing as those of femoral or tibial nailing, however, and the procedure is not in widespread use. Nailing of the forearm bones has been undertaken, but plating remains the treatment of choice for these fractures.

NAIL DESIGN

Unlike plates and external fixators, most nails are of a similar design. Flexible, small-diameter unlocked nails or pins are rarely used in adults, although they remain popular in the treatment of long-bone fractures in children. All locked nails have a similar design. The main mechanical difference relates to whether they are solid or hollow; the former is stiffer than the latter. The main controversy in intramedullary nailing recently has concerned the use of reaming to facilitate nail insertion.

REAMING

The original intramedullary nails were unlocked, and most were inserted using reaming to enlarge the diameter of the intramedullary canal, thereby allowing the introduction of wider, stronger nails. Stability depended on the area of contact between the nail and the endosteal surface of the intramedullary canal, and reaming increased fracture stability. Reamed nailing remained popular until the 1990s when animal experiments suggested reaming has a deleterious effect on the endosteal blood supply. Other work showed that reaming has a beneficial effect on periosteal blood flow and periosteal new bone formation. Subsequent clinical trials in patients with both closed and open femoral (see Table 23-4 in Chapter 23) and tibial diaphyseal fractures (see Tables 27-3 to 27-5 in Chapter 27) have indicated that reaming does have a positive effect on bone union, but the effect is in inverse proportion to the degree of soft tissue injury associated with the fracture. In less severe closed tibial fractures (see Table 27-3 in Chapter 27), it has been shown that unreamed nailing is associated with an increase in nonunion compared with reamed nailing, whereas in severe open fractures the benefits from reaming are much less (see Tables 27-4 and 27-5 in Chapter 27). The role of exchange reamed nailing in the treatment of nonunion is discussed in Chapter 39.

Intramedullary nailing is currently the preferred method of treating virtually all femoral diaphyseal fractures and most tibial diaphyseal fractures. To undertake intramedullary nailing successfully, all the correct equipment must be available. This includes a full set of nail sizes, reaming equipment, nail extraction equipment, a specialized nailing table, and fluoroscopy.

FEMORAL NAILING

Femoral nailing can be undertaken through an antegrade (Fig. 33-1) or retrograde (Fig. 33-2) approach. Antegrade nailing, through the piriformis fossa or tip of the greater trochanter, is regarded as the gold standard and the more common procedure. Retrograde nailing through the intercondylar notch is becoming more popular. Surgeons should be familiar with both techniques.

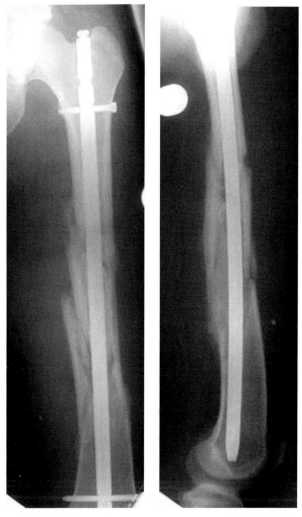

Figure 33-1 A-P and lateral X-rays of a type C femoral diaphyseal fracture treated with an antegrade statically locked nail.

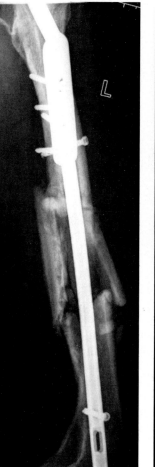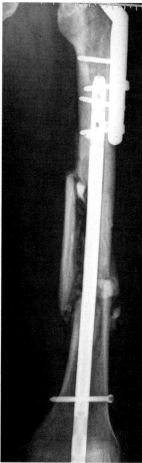

Figure 33-2 A-P and lateral X-rays of a retrograde nail used to treat a type C femoral fracture associated with a proximal femoral fracture.

ANTEGRADE NAILING

Surgical Technique

■ Position the patient.
  ■ Supine or lateral positions can be used.
  ■ The supine position is most commonly used (Fig. 33-3).
    ■ The leg is slightly adducted.
    ■ The position gives good access for fluoroscopy.
    ■ There is easy access for distal cross screw insertion.
  ■ The lateral position gives easier access to the greater trochanter.
    ■ It is easier to reduce a proximal femoral fracture with a flexed proximal fragment.
    ■ It is useful if there is a hip flexion contracture.
    ■ There is less easy access for fluoroscopy and distal cross screw insertion.
■ Reduce the fracture.
  ■ This can be done on a fracture table, with a femoral distractor or by manual traction.

  ■ If a fracture table is used, the setup is shown in Figure 33-3.
  ■ Traction can be applied with a distal femoral or proximal tibial transfixion pin or by using a traction boot.
  ■ A fracture distractor is a uniplanar external fixator specifically designed for the indirect reduction of diaphyseal fractures.
  ■ If a femoral distractor is used, the pins should be placed so as not to interfere with nail insertion.
  ■ Manual traction can be used, but it is difficult to maintain for a prolonged period, and rotational malalignment is a problem.
  ■ Check the reduction before nailing. Do not nail an irreducible fracture.
■ Make the incision.
  ■ The incision starts at the greater trochanter and extends proximally for 10 to 15 cm.
    ■ If minimally invasive techniques are used, a small incision is made about 10 cm proximal to the greater trochanter.
    ■ Both fascia and muscle are incised.
■ Choose the starting point.

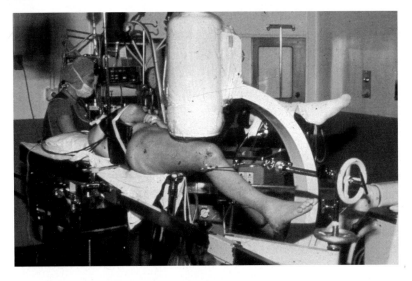

Figure 33-3 The setup for antegrade femoral nailing using a nailing table.

- Selection of the correct starting point is important.
  - Palpate the greater trochanter and piriformis fossa medial to it.
  - Use a bone awl or drill to penetrate the proximal femur in the piriformis fossa, under fluoroscopic control.
  - Insert a hand reamer through the proximal femoral metaphysis.
  - Avoid too medial or too lateral a starting point.
    - If too medial, there may be a femoral neck fracture.
    - If too lateral, medial femoral comminution may occur.
- Pass an olive-tipped guide wire down the intramedullary canal.
  - It should be centrally located in the distal femur.
- Ream the intramedullary canal (omit if unreamed nail is used).

- Reduce the fracture while reaming.
  - Undertake reaming in 0.5-mm increments.
  - Ream the intramedullary canal to 1 to 1.5 mm more than the proposed nail diameter.
  - A 12-mm nail is commonly used, unless the intramedullary canal is wide.
  - Do not force reamers down the intramedullary canal.
  - Assess correct nail length.
- Insert nail.
  - Make sure fracture is reduced as nail is inserted.
- Insert locking screws.
  - Use jig for proximal locking screws.
  - Freehand technique is usually used for distal screws (see Box 33-1 and Fig. 33-4).
  - One proximal and one distal screw are sufficient, unless fracture is very proximal or distal or bone is osteopenic.

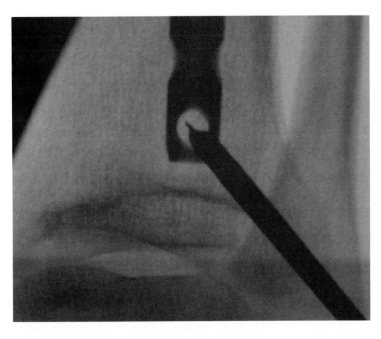

Figure 33-4 The freehand technique for distal cross screw insertion. It is important to visualize the screw hole as a full circle and seek the center of the circle with an awl or drill bit.

1. Align fluoroscope so distal screw hole is full circle. Do not start if distal screw hole is an ellipse.
2. Place metal awl, pointed pin, or drill bit on skin so tip is in middle of circle (see Fig. 33-4).
3. Make skin incision: 1 cm in tibia and humerus, 2 cm in femur.
4. Place awl, pin, or drill on bone so it is central in distal screw hole.
5. Use alignment of C-arm to determine direction of drill.
6. Drill through both cortices and locking hole in nail.
7. Measure screw length.
8. Insert screw.

■ The results of antegrade femoral nailing are given in Tables 23-4, 23-7, and 23-8 in Chapter 23.

Cross Screw Insertion

The insertion of proximal and distal cross screws is similar in all long bones, no matter which bone is being nailed or which direction the screws are going. Proximal cross screws are easy to insert using the jig supplied with the nailing system. Because the nails tend to deform as they are passed down the medullary canal, distal targeting jigs are much less successful. Usually a freehand technique is employed (see Box 33-1).

Dynamic locking refers to the placement of a proximal or distal cross screw only. This allows fracture site compression but should only be used for stable fracture configurations. Thus it is essentially confined to transverse or short oblique configurations. If there is any doubt about the inherent stability of the fracture, a static lock should be used with cross screws placed proximally and distally. This will stabilize all fracture configurations. In most fractures only one proximal and distal cross screw is required, but two or more can be used if the fracture is very proximal or distal or the bone is osteopenic.

Complications

■ A number of complications are associated with antegrade femoral nailing (Table 33-1).

TABLE 33-1 COMPLICATIONS ASSOCIATED WITH ANTEGRADE FEMORAL NAILING

Complication	Range (%)	Average (%)
Femoral neck fractures	0–2.5	1
Femoral comminution	0–5	3
External rotation deformity	0–55	10
Neurological damage	0–6	1
Heterotopic ossification	60–68	65
Nail breakage	0–3	1
Avascular necrosis	Rare	<1

■ With the exception of heterotopic ossification, complications are rare.

Femoral Neck Fracture

■ The most serious complication of femoral nailing is damage to the femoral neck and head.
■ Two types of femoral neck fracture are associated with femoral nailing.
■ If the nail entry point is too medial or posterior and the intramedullary canal is narrow, an iatrogenic femoral neck fracture can occur.
  ▪ It is often difficult to know if these fractures were present prior to nailing. If there is any doubt about the presence of a femoral neck fracture prior to nailing, a preoperative CT or MRI scan should be obtained.
  ▪ In periarticular fractures the intramedullary nail can be left and three proximal femoral screws placed into the femoral neck and head behind the intramedullary nail (see Fig. 23-7 in chapter 23).
  ▪ If the fracture in extra-capsular it is best treated with a long reconstruction nail with a screw placed in the femoral neck (see Fig. 23-7 in Chapter 23).
  ▪ The prognosis is good.
■ A second type of insufficiency femoral neck fracture occurs after nailing in older patients and presents up to 3 months after surgery.
  ▪ They have been estimated to occur in 2.3% of patients and are more common if the fracture is in the proximal third and the bone is osteopenic.

Avascular Necrosis

■ Avascular necrosis of the femoral head has been reported after intramedullary nailing of femoral diaphyseal fractures in adolescents.
■ The condition is probably caused by injury to the medial circumflex artery near the piriformis fossa, which interferes with the vasculature of the femoral head.
■ The incidence of the condition is unknown but is probably low, although the effects are devastating.

Proximal Femoral Comminution

▪ If the starting point is too lateral, the nail may be passed medially and damage the medial femoral cortex.
▪ If the diaphyseal fracture is in the proximal third, this may result in fracture propagation and increased comminution.
▪ This is not usually a problem if a statically locked nail is then used, unless the comminution involves the lesser trochanter, in which case a reconstruction nail should be used to stabilize the fracture.
▪ Proximal femoral comminution is less common if more flexible slotted intramedullary nails are used, but if the surgeon uses a solid stiffer nail, particular care must be taken in selecting the entry point in the proximal femur.

Heterotopic Ossification

▪ Heterotopic ossification in the hip abductors after femoral nailing has been reported in up to 68% of cases.
▪ The most common symptom is proximal femoral discomfort.

■ About 75% of patients present with either no heterotopic ossification or with a focus of less than 2 cm in length, and severe heterotopic ossification is rare.
■ Reamed nailing causes a higher incidence of heterotopic ossification than unreamed nailing.
■ Despite its relatively high incidence, heterotopic ossification rarely requires treatment, although large ossific deposits may require excision.

External Rotation Deformity

■ It is relatively easy to externally rotate the femur during intramedullary nailing, particularly if a fracture table is not used and the surgeon relies on the assistant to maintain alignment.
■ The incidence of external rotation deformity may be high, but the studies investigating the incidence have used fluoroscopy to determine the incidence, and clinically very few patients are left with an external rotation deformity that requires surgical treatment.
■ Surgeons should be aware of the problem and ensure proper rotational alignment prior to nailing.

Neurological Damage

■ Neurological damage is infrequent, but damage to the common peroneal, pudendal, and sciatic nerves has been reported.
■ Common peroneal nerve damage usually follows excessive traction but may be caused by the inappropriate insertion of a proximal tibial traction pin.
■ Pudendal nerve damage is the most common neurological problem associated with nailing, and again it is caused by traction, with the pudendal neuropraxia caused by the position of the traction post in the groin.
  ▪ The incidence of pudendal neuropraxia has been estimated at approximately 3%.
  ▪ It presents with numbness of the penis and scrotum and erectile dysfunction in men and genitoperoneal dysesthesia in women.
  ▪ The condition is self-limiting but worrying for the patients, who should be reassured the dysesthesia will resolve.
■ Nerve damage is discussed further in Chapter 41.

Nail and Cross Screw Breakage

■ The incidence of broken nails has been reported to be as high as 3.3%, but with modern nails the incidence is probably nearer 1%.
■ Nail breakage is usually associated with nonunion, which should be looked for if nail breakage occurs.
■ Broken cannulated nails are usually easy to remove by taking out the proximal segment and then using a long hook to remove the distal segment.
■ Removing the distal end of a solid nail is more difficult, and the nonunion site may have to be opened.
■ Broken cross screws are encountered relatively frequently, particularly if the fracture is comminuted or distracted slightly during nailing.
■ Occasionally they may break before the fracture is stable and the reduction may be lost, requiring renailing.
■ Usually the broken screw is a problem only if the nail needs to be removed.

■ Screws usually break with a section of the distal part of the screw still contained within the nail, and attempted nail extraction without screw removal will cause cortical damage.
  ▪ The proximal part of the screw is easy to remove.
  ▪ The distal part is best removed by inserting a thin blunt pin such as a Steinmann pin into the proximal screw hole and tapping out the distal part of the screw, which can then be removed through a separate incision.

Other Complications

■ Vascular damage is rare, but an arteriovenous fistula of the femoral vessels has been reported as has knee damage from a nail or piece of bone being hammered into the knee during nail insertion.

RETROGRADE NAILING

Retrograde femoral nailing has become popular in the last 10 years. The early retrograde nails were inserted through the medial femoral condyle, but now locking nails are inserted through the intercondylar notch of the distal femur (see Fig. 33-2). Obviously all femoral diaphyseal fractures can theoretically be treated by antegrade nailing, but retrograde nailing has a number of relative indications, which are listed in Box 33-2. The technique may be particularly useful in the multiply injured patient because it allows a femoral fracture to be nailed while chest, abdominal, or cranial surgery is undertaken. It also useful in morbidly obese patients and in those patients who present with a floating knee, a combination of femoral and tibial diaphyseal fractures (see Chapter 23). Other indications are less common.

Surgical Technique

■ Position the patient.
  ▪ The patient is positioned supine on a radiolucent table with the knee flexed to 40 degrees (Fig. 33-5).
■ Reduce the fracture.
  ▪ This is done by manual traction.
    ▪ Check the reduction before nailing. Do not nail an irreducible fracture.
■ Make the incision.
  ▪ A 2- to 3-cm vertical skin incision is made in or medial to the midline.
    ▪ Dissection is medial to the patellar tendon.
    ▪ Palpate the intercondylar notch.

BOX 33-2 INDICATIONS FOR RETROGRADE FEMORAL NAILING

■ Obesity
■ Pregnancy
■ Ipsilateral femoral and tibial fractures (floating knee)
■ Ipsilateral acetabular or pelvic fracture
■ Ipsilateral proximal and diaphyseal fractures
■ Distal diaphyseal or supracondylar fracture
■ Multiple injuries

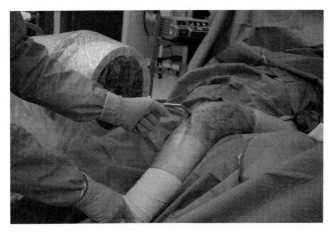

Figure 33-5 The setup for retrograde femoral nailing.

- Choose the starting point.
  - Use the fluoroscope to visualize the entry point 1 cm anterior to the femoral attachment of the posterior cruciate ligament.
    - Use a bone awl or drill to make the starting point (see Fig. 33-5).
    - Use a hand reamer to broach the distal femoral metaphysis.
- Pass an olive-tipped guide wire up the intramedullary canal.
  - It should be centrally located in the proximal femur.
- Ream the intramedullary canal (omit if unreamed nail is used).
  - Reduce the fracture while reaming.
    - Undertake reaming in 0.5-mm increments.
    - Ream the intramedullary canal to 1 to 1.5 mm more than the proposed nail diameter.
    - A 12-mm nail is commonly used, unless the intramedullary canal is wide.
    - Do not force reamers up the intramedullary canal.
    - Assess correct nail length.
- Insert nail.
  - Make sure fracture is reduced as nail is inserted.
- Insert locking screws.
  - Use a jig for distal locking screws.
  - Freehand technique is usually used for proximal screws.
    - The technique is similar to that for distal cross insertion in antegrade nailing (see Box 33-1).
    - Proximal locking screws are more easily lost in soft tissues. Tie suture around neck of screw prior to insertion.
    - One proximal and one distal screw are sufficient, unless fracture is very proximal or distal or bone is osteopenic.
  - The results of retrograde femoral nailing are given in Table 23-6 in Chapter 23.

Complications

- The relatively recent popularity of retrograde nailing means that little has been published about the complications of the technique.

- There will be cases of increased fracture comminution, neurovascular damage, and broken hardware as in antegrade nailing.
- Septic arthritis and heterotopic ossification in the knee have been reported, but the main concern relates to knee pain and stiffness.
- It has been reported that up to 30% of patients may complain of knee pain, but the pain is usually mild, and similar knee pain has been reported after an antegrade femoral nailing.

RECONSTRUCTION NAILS

Reconstruction, or third-generation, nails are interlocking nails in which the proximal lock is gained by placing a specifically designed hip screw or two cancellous screws through the nail into the femoral neck and head (Fig. 33-6). Distal locking is achieved by percutaneously inserted screws as in standard femoral nailing. Reconstruction nails are generally available in two lengths. Short reconstruction nails are known as proximal femoral nails and used for the treatment of intertrochanteric fractures (see Fig. 21.2-14 in Chapter 21), particularly those with an unstable fracture morphology such as the reverse obliquity fracture. Their

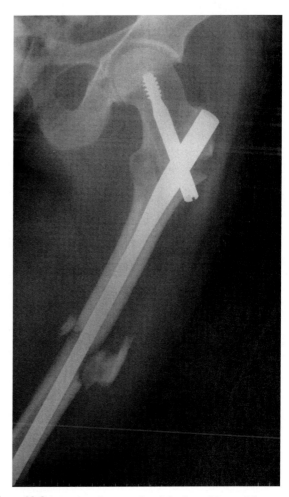

Figure 33-6 Combined proximal and diaphyseal femoral fractures treated with a long reconstruction nail.

use is discussed in Chapter 21. Long reconstruction nails extend the whole length of the femur and have been used increasingly for a number of indications, which are listed in Box 33-3.

Both nail types are inserted in the same way as antegrade femoral nails. Reconstruction nails are stiffer than conventional femoral nails, and insertion through the greater trochanter is ill advised, particularly if there is a subtrochanteric fracture or metastasis. Reaming is undertaken in the usual way, but the proximal 12 to 15 cm of the femur may need to be reamed to about 17 mm to accommodate the increased diameter of the nail. Proximal screws are inserted with a jig, as are distal screws in shorter reconstruction nails. In the longer reconstruction nails, distal screws are inserted freehand.

TIBIAL NAILING

Intramedullary nailing has become a popular technique for treating open and closed tibial diaphyseal fractures. Nails are used with and without reaming. The results associated with both techniques are given in Tables 27-2 to 27-4 in Chapter 27.

Tibial nailing (Fig. 33-7) is easier than femoral nailing. Virtually all tibial fractures reduce with straight traction, which can be maintained on a traction table (Fig. 33-8), by the use of a femoral distractor, or by manual traction.

SURGICAL TECHNIQUE

■ Position the patient.
  ■ The patient is positioned supine with the knee flexed to 90 degrees.
    ■ Either a fracture table (see Fig. 33-8) or conventional table can be used.
■ Reduce the fracture.
  ■ This is best done on a fracture table but can be done on a conventional table with a femoral distractor or by manual traction.
    ■ If a fracture table is used, the setup is shown in Fig. 33-8.
    ■ Traction can be applied with a calcaneal transfixion pin or, more commonly, by using a traction boot.

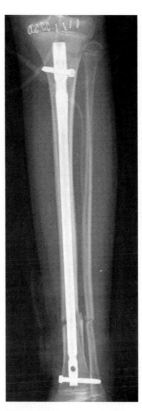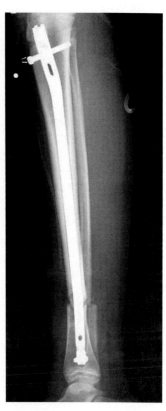

Figure 33-7 A statically locked tibial nail used to treat the open fracture shown in Figures 4.1 and 4.2 in Chapter 4.

    ■ A femoral distractor may be useful for proximal diaphyseal fractures.
    ■ If a femoral distractor is used, the pins should be placed so as not to interfere with nail insertion.
    ■ Manual traction can be used, but it is difficult to maintain for a prolonged period, and rotational malalignment is a problem.
  ■ Check the reduction before nailing. Do not nail an irreducible fracture.
■ Make the incision.
  ■ A vertical or transverse incision can be used.
  ■ A vertical incision is made from the tibial tuberosity to the patella.
  ■ A transverse incision is made halfway between the tibial tuberosity and the joint line.
    ■ It should be 3 cm in length.
    ■ It is in Langer's lines and heals better than a vertical incision.
■ Choose the starting point.
  ■ The starting point is just above the tibial tuberosity.
    ■ If a stiffer solid nail is used, the starting point is higher.
    ■ Avoid damage to the anterior horns of the menisci if a solid nail is used.
    ■ A bone awl is used to make the starting point.
    ■ Use a curved hand reamer to broach the proximal tibial metaphysis.
■ Pass an olive-tipped guide wire down the intramedullary canal.
  ■ It should be centrally located in the distal tibia.

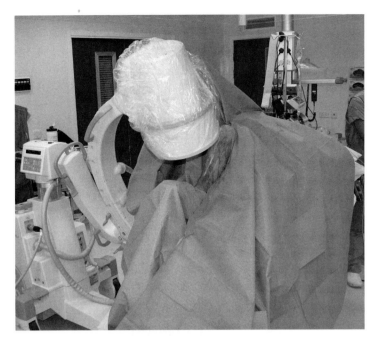

Figure 33-8 The setup for tibial nailing.

■ Ream the intramedullary canal (omit if unreamed nail is used).
  ■ Reduce the fracture while reaming.
    ■ Undertake reaming in 0.5-mm increments.
    ■ Ream the intramedullary canal to 1 to 1.5 mm more than the proposed nail diameter.
    ■ An 11-mm nail is commonly used, unless the intramedullary canal is wide.
    ■ Do not force reamers down the intramedullary canal.
    ■ Assess correct nail length.
■ Insert nail.
  ■ Make sure fracture is reduced as nail is inserted.
■ Insert locking screws.
  ■ Use jig for proximal locking screws.
  ■ Freehand technique is usually used for distal screws (Box 33-1 and Fig. 33-4).
  ■ One proximal and one distal screw are sufficient, unless fracture is very proximal or distal or bone is osteopenic.
■ The results of tibial nailing are given in Tables 27-3 to 27-5 in Chapter 27.

COMPLICATIONS

■ Table 33-2 lists the complications associated with tibial nailing.

Knee Pain

■ This is the most common complication, occurring in 55% to 70% of patients.
■ It is more common in younger, more active, patients, but there does not seem to be any association between pain and the surgical approach.
■ Nail insertion through or medial to the patellar tendon results in the same incidence of pain.

■ Knee pain can affect 33% of people at rest, and 90% of patients complain of some discomfort on squatting.
■ About 80% of patients either have no pain or only mild pain.
  ■ The rest complain of more significant discomfort.
■ The cause is unknown, but pain is often relieved by nail removal.
■ It may be caused by coincidental articular, meniscal, or ligamentous injury, but in the absence of other obvious injury the pain is probably caused by scarring of the gliding tissues in front of the knee.

Neurological Damage

■ The incidence of neurological damage associated with nailing varies considerably as does the incidence of neurological damage caused by the fracture itself.
■ Damage to the common peroneal nerve as well as to the superficial and deep peroneal nerves has been reported, as has damage to the saphenous and sural nerves during cross screw insertion.

TABLE 33-2 COMPLICATIONS ASSOCIATED WITH TIBIAL NAILING

Complication	Range (%)	Average (%)
Knee pain	55–70	60
Neurological damage	2–30	5
Vascular damage	Very rare	<1
Nail breakage	0–6	1
Screw breakage		
Reamed nails	0–3	3
Unreamed nails	10–52	25
Thermal necrosis	Rare	<1

■ Neurological damage associated with intramedullary nailing should be rare if the correct surgical technique is followed.

Vascular Damage

■ Vascular damage is very rare, but damage to the popliteal artery can be caused during the insertion of proximal anteroposterior cross screws.

■ Damage to the medial inferior genicular artery has also been reported, as has distal cross screw occlusion of the posterior tibial and peroneal arteries.

Hardware Breakage

■ Nail and cross screw breakage depends on the diameter of the nail and cross screws, the type of metal used, and whether the fracture unites.

■ Most nail breakages are associated with an untreated nonunion.

■ In general, thinner unreamed nails have a higher incidence of breakage as do the smaller diameter locking screws associated with their use.

■ Broken nails are treated by removal and renailing.

■ Broken cross screws are rarely problematic but can be difficult to remove.

■ Screw removal is described in the section on femoral nailing.

Thermal Necrosis

■ Heat-induced thermal necrosis of the bone and overlying soft tissue has been reported.

■ This is a serious complication that may well lead to infection and the need for extensive reconstructive surgery.

■ It is rare and best avoided by the use of sharp reamers and good reaming technique.

■ Reaming should never be forced, and if the reamer fails to progress it should be withdrawn, the flutes cleaned, and the process restarted.

Bone Damage

■ As with femoral nailing, tibial nailing may cause propagation of undisplaced fracture lines.

■ This is rarely a problem if static locking is used.

■ A problem specific to tibial nailing is the displacement of an occult posterior malleolar fragment during nailing.

■ About 2% of patients have ipsilateral ankle and tibial diaphyseal fractures. This complication can be avoided if the ankle fracture is fixed with interfragmentary screws prior to intramedullary nailing.

HUMERAL NAILING

Humeral nailing (see Fig. 12-6 in Chapter 12) is usually straightforward, but surgeons should be aware that the distal humerus flattens anteroposteriorly, and therefore the intramedullary canal of the humerus is relatively shorter than those of the femur and tibia. A number of humeral

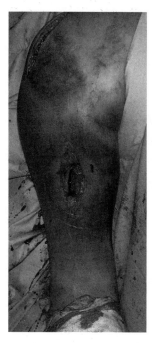

Figure 33-9   The use of the sitting position for antegrade humeral nailing. The fracture was a Gustilo II open fracture.

fractures are in the distal third of the bone, and the relatively short canal makes these fractures difficult to treat by intramedullary nailing. Humeral intramedullary nails can be inserted using both antegrade (Fig. 33-9) and retrograde techniques. The results of both techniques are given in Table 12-4 in Chapter 12.

Surgeons must remember that unlike the femur and tibia, a major nerve, the radial nerve, passes around the middiaphysis of the humerus. Trapping of the radial nerve within the diaphysis can occur in some distal diaphyseal fractures. This is referred to as the Holstein-Lewis lesion (see Fig. 12-10 in Chapter 12). If the patient presents with a radial nerve palsy or the fracture cannot be reduced prior to nailing, the surgeon should never undertake closed nailing in case the radial nerve is trapped.

ANTEGRADE NAILING

SURGICAL TECHNIQUE

■ Position the patient.
  ■ The patient is positioned supine on a radiolucent table and rotated by 30 degrees with the shoulder supported by a pillow.
  ■ Alternatively, the patient can be sitting at 30 to 45 degrees (see Fig. 33-9).

■ Reduce the fracture.
  ■ This is done by manual traction.
    ■ Check the reduction before nailing. Do not nail an irreducible fracture.

■ Make the incision.
  ■ A 4-cm incision is made laterally from the acromion.
    ■ The deltoid is split.

- The rotator cuff is incised.
- Choose the starting point.
    - The starting point is the lateral aspect of the humeral head.
        - Use a narrow bone awl or drill to make the starting point.
        - Use a hand reamer to broach the proximal humeral metaphysis.
- Pass a guide wire down the intramedullary canal.
    - It should be centrally located in the distal humerus.
- Ream the intramedullary canal (omit if unreamed nail is used).
    - Reduce the fracture while reaming.
        - Reaming is undertaken in 0.5-mm increments.
        - The intramedullary canal should be reamed to 1 mm more than the proposed nail diameter.
        - A 9- or 10-mm nail is commonly used, unless the intramedullary canal is wide.
        - Do not force reamers down the intramedullary canal.
        - Assess correct nail length.
- Insert nail.
    - Make sure fracture is reduced as nail is inserted.
- Insert locking screws.
    - Use jig for proximal locking screws.
    - Freehand technique is usually used for distal screws.
        - The technique is similar to that for distal cross insertion in antegrade femoral or tibial nailing (see Box 33-1).
    - One proximal and one distal screw are sufficient, unless fracture is very proximal or distal or bone is osteopenic.
- The results of antegrade humeral nailing are given in Table 12-4 in Chapter 12.

COMPLICATIONS

- The main complications of antegrade humeral nailing are listed in Table 33-3.

Shoulder Dysfunction

- The principal complication of antegrade humeral nailing is rotator cuff damage.

- The effect of this is age related, and it is likely that younger patients, with good muscle quality, will not have significant problems.
- Because the average age of patients with humeral diaphyseal fracture is about 55 years (see Table 12-1 in Chapter 12), rotator cuff damage from the advancing nail can be expected in many patients.
- Shoulder dysfunction has been estimated to occur in up to 100% of patients, although the incidence obviously depends on the surgeon's definition of what constitutes shoulder dysfunction.
- Significant rotator cuff damage occurs in about 70% of patients treated by antegrade humeral nailing.
- Shoulder pain and stiffness obviously can also follow failure to bury the nail within the proximal humerus, and direct impingement of the proximal nail on the acromion can occur.

Neurological Damage

- Neurological damage may be associated with the humeral fracture (see Chapter 12).
- Antegrade nailing may also cause damage to the radial nerve as a result of reaming and the insertion of the nail, the axillary nerve as a result of proximal cross screw insertion, and the radial, musculocutaneous, and median nerves following distal cross screw insertion.
- It is difficult to separate the incidence of radial nerve damage from that associated with the fracture, but radial nerve damage from nailing probably occurs in about 3% of cases.
- Nerve damage secondary to cross screw insertion can be minimized by good surgical technique.
- Drills and cross screws should not be inserted through stab incisions.
- A tissue guard should be used when drilling or inserting cross screws.

Vascular Damage

- Vascular damage is very rare, but brachial artery damage can occur following the insertion of distal cross screws.
- The incidence of vascular damage is minimized by good surgical technique.

Other Complications

- Increased fracture comminution occurs in about 10% of antegrade humeral nailing.
- Heterotopic ossification in the deltoid has been reported.

RETROGRADE NAILING

In an effort to avoid the rotator cuff problems associated with antegrade nailing, some surgeons favor retrograde humeral nailing with the nail passed proximally from just above the olecranon fossa.

TABLE 33-3 COMPLICATIONS ASSOCIATED WITH ANTEGRADE HUMERAL NAILING

Complication	Range (%)	Average (%)
Shoulder dysfunction	0–100	70
Radial nerve palsy	0–5	3
Other neurological damage	Rare	<1
Vascular damage	Rare	<1

SURGICAL TECHNIQUE

- Position the patient.
  - The patient is placed in the prone position with the arm abducted and a support under the cubital fossa to allow elbow flexion.
- Reduce the fracture.
  - This is done by manual traction.
    - Check the reduction before nailing. Do not nail an irreducible fracture.
- Make the incision.
  - A 7- to 8-cm posterior longitudinal incision is made in the midline.
    - The triceps is split to expose the distal diaphysis and the olecranon fossa.
- Choose the starting point.
  - The starting point is just above the olecranon fossa.
    - Use a drill to make the starting point.
    - Do not use an osteotome.
    - Use bone nibblers carefully to enlarge starting point.
    - Take care not to fracture the distal humerus between the starting point and the fracture.
- Pass a guide wire up the intramedullary canal.
  - It should be centrally located in the proximal humerus.
- Ream the intramedullary canal (omit if unreamed nail is used).
  - Reduce the fracture while reaming.
    - Undertake reaming in 0.5-mm increments.
    - Ream the intramedullary canal to 1 mm more than the proposed nail diameter.
    - A 9- or 10-mm nail is commonly used, unless the intramedullary canal is wide.
    - Do not force reamers up the intramedullary canal.
    - Assess correct nail length.
- Insert nail.
  - Make sure fracture is reduced as nail is inserted.
- Insert locking screws.
  - Use jig for distal locking screws.
  - Freehand technique is usually used for proximal screws.
    - The technique is similar to that for distal cross insertion in antegrade femoral or tibial nailing (see Box 33-1).
  - One proximal and one distal screw are sufficient, unless fracture is very proximal or distal or bone is osteopenic.

- The results of retrograde humeral nailing are given in Table 12-4 in Chapter 12.

COMPLICATIONS

- The main complications of retrograde humeral nailing are shown in Table 33-4.
- The principal complication of retrograde humeral nailing is elbow dysfunction, which may take the form of pain or elbow stiffness.
  - This occurs in up to 13% of patients.
- Comminution of the distal humerus may also occur, particularly if the fracture is in the distal diaphysis.
  - This is said to occur in 4% to 7% of fractures, but minor comminution is probably very much more common.
- There is no theoretical reason why the incidence of radial nerve palsy should differ between antegrade and retrograde humeral nailing. The axillary nerve is at risk from the insertion of anteroposterior proximal cross screws.

FOREARM NAILING

Forearm nailing using unlocked nails has been in use for over 60 years, although the results associated with their use were poor with high incidences of nonunion, malunion, and poor forearm function. The excellent results associated with forearm plating have ensured that the use of more modern locked forearm nails is sporadic and confined to specific indications such as failed forearm plating, segmental fractures, and fractures in pathological bone (see Fig. 15-6 in Chapter 15). Even these indications are relative!

- Ulnar nails are inserted through the proximal ulna using a short longitudinal incision and manual traction to reduce the fracture.
- Radial nails are inserted through a short longitudinal incision overlying the radial styloid.
- The main complication of forearm nailing is difficulty in achieving a satisfactory reduction, particularly in terms of radial or ulnar rotation.
- Increased fracture comminution is possible as is neurological or vascular damage associated with cross screw insertion.
- The posterior interosseous nerve is particularly at risk.
- It is impossible to assess incidences of these complications because forearm nailing is not widely practiced.

NAIL REMOVAL

Nail removal is usually undertaken at the request of the patient or in an attempt to relieve proximal thigh or knee pain. It is straightforward, provided the proximal end of the nail can be located. In the femur the high incidence of heterotopic ossification means the surgeon may have to excise

TABLE 33-4 COMPLICATIONS ASSOCIATED WITH RETROGRADE HUMERAL NAILING

Complication	Range (%)	Average (%)
Elbow dysfunction	3–13	5
Entry portal comminution	4–7	5
Radial nerve palsy	0–5	3
Other neurological damage	Rare	<1
Vascular damage	Rare	<1

bone from the abductor musculature to locate the nail. This is not a problem in the tibia, but tibial nails are often buried in the bone and may be difficult to locate. If there is an anteroposterior screw present, it can be partially withdrawn and may then act as a guide to the position of the proximal end of the nail. Once the end of the nail is located, it should be cleared of soft tissue and bone, the appropriate extractor inserted, and the nail removed. All cross screws obviously should be removed prior to nail extraction. Very occasionally the proximal end of a tibial nail cannot be located because bone has grown into it. Under these circumstances the nail should probably be left because the dissection required to remove the nail is considerable. The patient should be warned preoperatively about this possibility.

SUGGESTED READING

Court-Brown CM. Fractures of the tibia and fibula. In: Bucholz RW, Heckman JD, eds. Rockwood and Green's fractures in adults, 5th ed. Philadelphia: Lippincott Williams & Wilkins, 2001.

Court-Brown CM. Femoral diaphyseal fractures. In: Browner BD, Jupiter JB, Levine AM, et al., eds. Skeletal trauma, 3rd ed. Philadelphia: WB Saunders, 2003.

Court-Brown CM. Reamed intramedullary tibial nailing: an overview and analysis of 1106 cases. J Orthop Trauma 2004;18:96–101.

Farragos AF, Schemitsch EH, McKee MD. Complications of intramedullary nailing for fractures of the humeral shaft: A review. J Orthop Trauma 1999;13:258–267.

Franklin JL, Winquist RA, Benirschke SK, et al. Broken intramedullary nails. J Bone Joint Surg (Br) 1998;70:1463–1471.

Grosse A, Christie J, Taglang G, et al. Open adult femoral shaft fracture treated by early intramedullary nailing. J Bone Joint Surg (Br) 1993;75:562–565.

Hupel TM, Weinberg JA, Aksenov SA, et al. Effect of unreamed, limited reamed, and standard reamed intramedullary nailing on cortical bone porosity and new bone formation. J Orthop Trauma 2001;15:18–27.

Ingman AM, Waters DA. Locked intramedullary nailing of humeral shaft fractures. J Bone Joint Surg (Br) 1994;76:23–29.

Küntscher G, Maatz R. Technik der Marknagelung. Leipzig: Thieme, 1945.

McKee MD, Waddell JP. Intramedullary nailing of femoral fractures in morbidly obese patients. J Trauma 1994;36:208–210.

Patton JT, Cook RE, Adams CI, et al. Late fracture of the hip after reamed intramedullary nailing of the femur. J Bone Joint Surg (Br) 2000;82:967–971.

Rommens PM, Verbruggen J, Broos PL. Retrograde locked nailing of humeral shaft fractures. J Bone Joint Surg (Br) 1995;77:84–89.

Schemitsch EH, Bhandari M. Fractures of the humeral shaft. In: Browner BD, Jupiter JB, Levine AM, et al., eds. Skeletal trauma, 3rd ed. Philadelphia: WB Saunders, 2003.

Trafton PG. Tibial shaft fractures. In: Browner BD, Jupiter JB, Levine AM, et al., eds. Skeletal trauma, 3rd ed. Philadelphia: WB Saunders, 2003.

34 OTHER INTERNAL FIXATION TECHNIQUES

Many fractures are treated by methods other than casting or bracing, plating, intramedullary nailing, or external fixation. The size of the bone or the fractured bone fragments or the location of the fracture within the bone may suggest the use of a number of different fracture treatment methods. These are usually screws, threaded or plain pointed metal wires usually known as Kirschner wires (K-wires), tension band wiring, or cerclage wire or loops. Obviously these techniques can be used in virtually any location in the body, but in this chapter the common indications are described.

KIRSCHNER WIRES

Niehaus is credited with the first use of closed reduction and pin fixation of fracture fragments under radiological control in 1904, and the technique is still in widespread use. Threaded or unthreaded pointed wires are available in a range of sizes. The commonly used wires have diameters of between 1.1 and 2.5 mm. In the imperial system the most commonly used wires have diameters of 0.32, 0.45, and 0.62 inches. They can be used in many different locations, but there are a number of areas in which their use is popular, and these are described here.

Temporary Fracture Fixation

K-wires are widely used for temporary fracture fixation prior to the introduction of a bone screw or a plate. Temporary K-wires are mainly used in the reconstruction of metaphyseal or intra-articular fractures. The intra-articular surface is reconstructed using bone-holding forceps to maintain the reduction. One or more K-wires are then placed across the reconstructed bone to maintain its position. Interfragmentary screws can then be used to provide definitive fracture fixation. The technique is straightforward, but care must be taken to assess the position of the screws prior to inserting the K-wires because it can be relatively easy to place them so they obstruct the subsequent passage of the screws. Usually the K-wires are removed after screw fixation, but they can be cut short and left in situ if the surgeon feels this will provide appropriate

supplementary fracture fixation. Many modern plates have holes specifically to facilitate temporary K-wire fixation.

Definitive Fracture Fixation

K-wires are used for definitive management in a number of different locations. The choice for the surgeon is whether to leave the proximal end of the K-wire out of the skin to aid with later removal or to place the end of the wire subcutaneously and thereby make removal somewhat more difficult. There is no real answer to this, and both methods are acceptable. Obviously leaving the proximal end of the K-wire out of the skin is associated with an increased incidence of superficial infection. However, as with external fixator pins, osteomyelitis is very rare and the infection usually remains superficial. Unlike external fixator pins, most K-wires are inserted for a relatively short period and complications are few, although if they are inserted adjacent to a joint, skin and soft tissue tethering can be a nuisance.

K-wires should be inserted through both cortices no matter where they are used. Even if they are used as part of a tension band, they will function better if placed through two cortices. Unicortical wires usually loosen fairly quickly. Surgeons must be particularly careful when using K-wires in cortical fractures of small bones such as the metacarpals or phalanges because the K-wire can distract the fracture during insertion and thereby cause a nonunion. It is important to reduce these fractures and hold the reduction firmly prior to the insertion of K-wires across both cortices.

UPPER LIMB
Proximal Humerus

- The concept of using percutaneous K-wire fixation to treat fractures of the proximal humerus (see Fig. 11-7 in Chapter 11) is attractive, but in reality the procedure is more difficult than it looks, and overall the results are poor (see Table 11-4 in Chapter 11).
- The proximal humerus is reduced by closed means with the patient anesthetized in the beach chair position.
- A fluoroscope is used to check that the fracture is reduced, and three or four K-wires are inserted.

■ The technique is not recommended in older osteoporotic patients because the pins frequently loosen and migrate, resulting in loss of fracture position.

■ Because proximal humeral fractures are relatively uncommon in younger patients, the indications for this technique are limited, but it is useful in the management of Salter-Harris II physeal fractures of the proximal humerus where union is rapid and the bone quality is good.

Distal Radius

■ There are four circumstances in which K-wires are commonly used in the distal radius.

■ In Kapandji intrafocal pinning (Fig. 34-1A), one or more K-wires are placed into the distal radial fracture to assist with fracture reduction and to splint the fracture.

■ The initial pin is introduced radially between the first and second extensor compartments parallel to the fracture line.

■ A second pin is introduced into the fracture between the third and fourth extensor compartments, again parallel to the fracture.

■ Both pins are then directed obliquely at about 45 degrees to the long axis of the radius and driven through the distal radial cortex. This helps restore the normal volar tilt and radial length.

■ Kapanjii pinning was initially described for the treatment of unstable extra-articular fractures in younger patients, and it is more effective in fractures that do not have volar comminution or where the bone is not osteoporotic.

■ Because most distal radial fractures actually occur in osteoporotic bone, its scope is probably limited, but it is widely used.

■ Results of this technique are given in Table 16-6 in Chapter 16.

■ K-wire fixation can also be used to treat distal radial fractures by passing two or more K-wires into the reduced fracture.

■ The fracture is reduced by longitudinal traction and palmar translation and probably best stabilized by crossing the K-wires over the fracture site as shown in Figure 34-1B.

■ Both pins are placed dorsally, one starting at the radial styloid and the second between the third and fifth extensor compartments on the ulnar aspect of the distal radius.

■ Surgeons also use one or two K-wires to fix radial styloid fractures.

■ These are passed from the tip of the radial styloid across the fracture through the distal radial cortex (Fig. 34-1C).

■ As with the Kapandji technique, the use of crossed K-wires works better in younger bone, and K-wires, even when supplemented by a cast, cannot be guaranteed to maintain fracture reduction in osteoporotic bone.

■ K-wires may also be used to provide supplementary fixation following the application of a trans-articular external fixator (Fig. 34-2; see also Fig. 16-8 in Chapter 16).

■ After the application of the trans-articular external fixator (see Chapters 16 and 35), K-wires are placed percutaneously to help reduce and maintain the position of the fracture fragments.

■ The results of the technique are given in Table 16-5 in Chapter 16.

■ The exact number and position of the K-wires depends on the morphology of the fracture and the extent of the comminution.

Carpal Injuries

■ The use of K-wires in the carpus is usually reserved for carpal dislocations, which may be associated with a fracture.

■ There are uncommon carpal conditions such as capitate-hamate diastasis when K-wires might be used, but the common indication for the use of K-wires in the carpus is to treat acute perilunate instability, which presents either as a scapholunate dissociation or as a perilunate dislocation that may be associated with fractures of the scaphoid, capitate, triquetrium, or distal radius (see Chapter 17).

■ The treatment of scapholunate dissociation involves closed or open reduction of the carpus and triangular

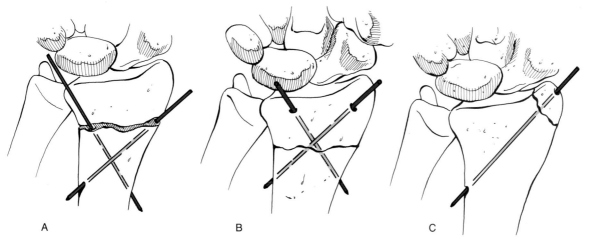

A   B   C

Figure 34-1 Three common methods of using K-wires in the treatment of distal radial fractures. See text for explanation.

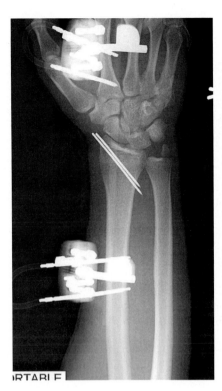

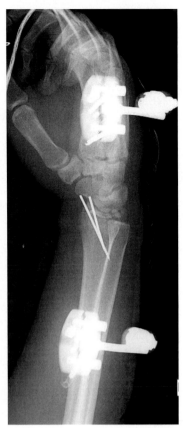

IRTABLE

Figure 34-2 The use of periarticular external fixation with K-wires to treat a fracture-dislocation of the radio-carpal joint.

fixation of the capitolunate, scapholunate, and scaphocapitate joints (Fig. 34-3).

■ The exact orientation of the K-wires is determined at the time of surgery, and other configurations may be used (see Fig. 17.1-12 in Chapter 17).

■ Treatment of the different variants of perilunate dislocation is similar.

■ The lunate must be reduced by open or closed means.

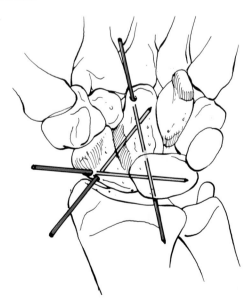

Figure 34-3 The treatment of scapholunate dissociation using K-wires.

■ In perilunate dislocation without an associated fracture, the K-wire insertion pattern is the same as for a scapholunate dissociation (see Fig. 34-3).

■ If there is an associated fracture, it is best treated by scaphoid screw fixation, although two K-wires can be used.

■ Because the carpal K-wires have been used to treat ligamentous instability, they should be left in position for 8 to 10 weeks.

■ See Chapter 17 for more information about carpal injuries.

Carpometacarpal Fracture-Dislocations

■ Some injuries result in carpometacarpal dislocations or in comminuted fractures of the bases of the metacarpals associated with dislocation of one or more carpometacarpal joints.

■ If an isolated carpometacarpal dislocation occurs, it tends to be at the base of the more mobile little finger.

■ The general principle of management with K-wires is similar no matter which joints are involved.

■ Reduction of the comminuted fracture of the base of the metacarpal is best achieved closed by direct traction and ligamentotaxis.

■ Open reduction is often very difficult because of the degree of comminution.

■ Once the fracture is reduced, the fluoroscope is used to assist in the insertion of a K-wire through the intact proximal shaft of the metacarpal into the adjacent carpal bone.

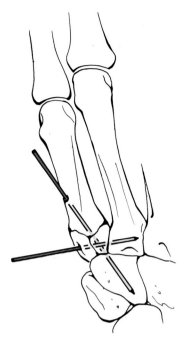

Figure 34-4 Treatment of carpometacarpal fracture-dislocations using K-wires. See text for explanation.

- A second K-wire is used to stabilize the proximal metacarpal bone fragments (Fig. 34-4).
- If there are multiple fracture-dislocations, each carpometacarpal joint needs to be similarly treated.

Metacarpal and Phalangeal Fractures

- The treatment of displaced metacarpal and phalangeal fractures is commonly undertaken with K-wires, although a number of the older methods of management involving K-wires and interosseous or cerclage wires have now been replaced by the use of interfragmentary screws.
- There are many published methods describing the management of metacarpal and phalangeal fractures with K-wires.

Bennett's Fracture

- The management of the Bennett's fracture-dislocation of the thumb metacarpal with K-wires (see Fig. 17.2-8 in Chapter 17) is very similar to the management of the other carpometacarpal fracture-dislocations, but it merits individual discussion because it is common.
- Reduction of the fracture is undertaken by traction with manual pressure applied to the base of the metacarpal.
- Two K-wires should be used, one placed through the radial aspect of the base of the thumb metacarpal proximally into the adjacent carpus and the second placed between the thumb metacarpal and the metacarpal of the index finger.
- It is the same configuration as shown in Figure 34-4.

Rolando's Fracture

- This three-part intra-articular fracture (see Fig. 17.2-9 in Chapter 17) can be treated in a similar way to the Bennett's fracture.
- Again, reduction of the fracture is achieved by traction, and the reduced position of the intra-articular fragments at the base of the thumb metacarpal is maintained by the use of a K-wire in the manner shown in Figure 34-4.
- A second K-wire can be placed from the base of the thumb metacarpal into the adjacent carpus.

Metacarpal Diaphyseal Fractures

- There are a number of techniques described using K-wires in the treatment of metacarpal diaphyseal fractures.
  - The most common of these are shown in Figure 34-5.

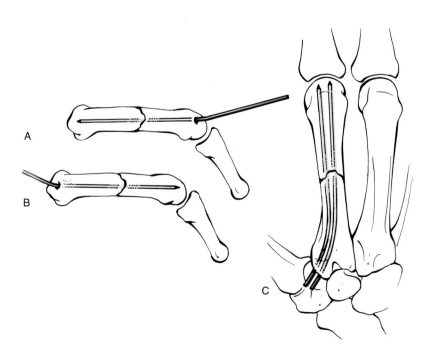

Figure 34-5 Three methods for fixing metacarpal diaphyseal fractures with longitudinal K-wires. See text for explanation.

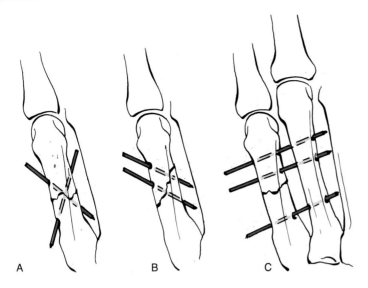

A   B   C

Figure 34-6 Three methods for fixing metacarpal diaphyseal fractures with crossed or parallel K-wires. See text for explanation.

■ Metacarpal fractures can be treated by intramedullary K-wire insertion with the K-wires introduced proximally or distally.
  ■ If a distal insertion is used, the metacarpophalangeal joint is flexed and the wire inserted through the dorsum of the head or neck of the metacarpal (Fig. 34-5A).
  ■ The same principle applies if the wires are placed proximally in the metacarpal.
  ■ To avoid damage to the carpometacarpal joint, one or two thin flexible wires may be used with a dorsal entry point (Fig. 34-5B).
  ■ If the fifth metacarpal diaphysis is fractured, two or more flexible wires can be passed from proximal to distal through the base of the fifth metacarpal (Fig. 34-5C).
■ Alternative fixation methods include the use of crossed K-wires for transverse fractures (Fig. 34-6A).
  ■ These are relatively difficult to insert and need to be passed obliquely across the fracture, being careful not to damage the extensor tendons or the digital nerves.
  ■ The fracture must be held in a reduced position as the K-wires are passed across it.
  ■ The K-wires tend to distract the fracture, and if the fracture is held in distraction, the incidence of nonunion is high.
  ■ Two or more parallel K-wires can be used to immobilize an oblique or spiral metacarpal fracture, but again, fracture distraction may occur if the reduction position is not held firmly prior to pin insertion (Fig. 34-6B).
■ Transverse fractures of the fifth metacarpal diaphysis are relatively common and well treated by the use of K-wires.
  ■ Access is clearly easier than in the other metacarpals, and the best method of K-wire fixation utilizes two parallel K-wires passed through the fifth metacarpal diaphysis distal to the fracture into the diaphysis of the fourth metacarpal.
  ■ Two distal K-wires are used to minimize the risk of rotation of the distal fragment.

■ A single K-wire is passed in a similar fashion proximal to the fracture. These metacarpal pins should be removed after 3 or 4 weeks (Fig. 34-6C).

Metacarpal Neck Fractures
■ The most common metacarpal neck fracture occurs in the fifth metacarpal and is known as a boxer's fracture.
■ If operative treatment is required, this is best treated using the method shown in Figure 34-7, which is similar to the treatment of fifth metacarpal diaphyseal fractures.
■ Two K-wires should be passed through the neck and head of the fifth metacarpal into the fourth metacarpal (see Fig. 17.2-4 in Chapter 17).
■ One K-wire is passed in a similar fashion proximal to the fracture.

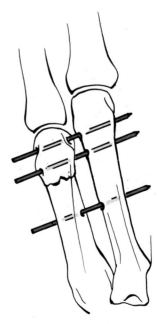

Figure 34-7 Parallel K-wires used to treat a boxer's fracture of the fifth metacarpal neck.

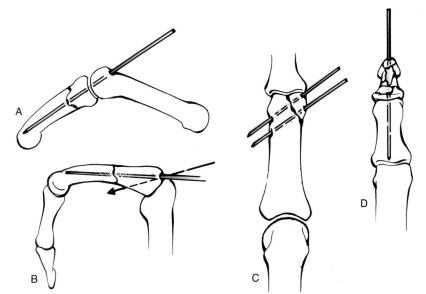

Figure 34-8 Four methods of fixing phalangeal fractures with K-wires. See text for explanation.

- Two distal K-wires are used because of the mobility of the fifth metacarpal head.
- The K-wires should be left in position for 3 to 4 weeks. Intramedullary fixation can also be used utilizing the technique shown in Figure 34-5A.

Phalangeal Fractures

- The treatment of phalangeal fractures with K-wires is not dissimilar to that of metacarpal fractures.
- Proximal phalangeal fractures can be treated by intramedullary fixation, but the proximity of the fracture to the metacarpophalangeal joint means the K-wire is placed through the head of the metacarpal with the metacarpophalangeal joint in flexion.
  - The reduced position of the fracture is checked by fluoroscopy and the K-wire passed distally into the proximal phalanx (Fig. 34-8A).
  - Intramedullary techniques can also be used for more distal phalangeal fractures by passing one or more flexible K-wires distally from the interphalangeal joint (Fig. 34-8B).
  - Crossed wires may be used as shown in Figure 34-6A, but as with metacarpal fractures care must be taken not to distract the fracture during wire insertion.
  - Parallel K-wires can also be used for spiral and oblique fractures in the same manner as for metacarpal fractures (see Fig. 34-6B).
  - Intra-articular fractures of the inter-phalangeal joints can be treated using K-wires in the same way as demonstrated in Figure 34-8C, but the technique is very difficult because the fragments are usually very small.
- Distal phalangeal K-wires can be used to stabilize a crush fracture or to treat a mallet finger.
  - These are either inserted through the tip of the distal phalanx in a retrograde manner into the proximal part of the distal phalanx if the damage is not too severe, or, if there is significant damage to the distal phalanx, the K-wire can be inserted across

the distal interphalangeal joint into the middle phalanx (Fig. 34-8D).
  - Mallet fingers can also be treated with a transarticular K-wire to maintain extension of the distal interphalangeal joint.

LOWER LIMB

Ankle Fractures

- Two K-wires can be used to stabilize the medial malleolus in ankle fractures in elderly patients with osteoporotic bone.
- The K-wires can be inserted percutaneously, although an open reduction is usually required.
- They may be augmented with a tension band (see Fig. 29-11 in Chapter 29).
- If this technique is used, it must be remembered that the fixation is not rigid and the supplementary below-knee walking cast is required.

Fracture-Dislocations of the Foot

- As with carpal or carpometacarpal fracture-dislocations, K-wires are useful in the management of dislocations or fracture-dislocations of the foot.
- They can be used in all dislocations with the number and configuration of the K-wires determined by the nature of the injury.
- Their use has been described in calcaneal fracture-dislocations, subtalar dislocations, and midfoot fracture-dislocations as well as in severe crush injuries. The joints need to be realigned by open or closed means, and the indication for the use of K-wires is usually persistent subluxation or instability of the involved joint.
- Usually the ankle and subtalar joints are stable after reduction, although even a minor associated fracture may alter this.

- Joints such as the talonavicular joint and the calcaneocuboid joint have no inherent stability and rely on their capsules and ligaments to provide stability.
  - Thus the requirement for K-wire fixation of these joints is relatively common.
- Because the wires are being used because of significant soft tissue trauma, they should be kept in position for 8 to 12 weeks depending on the surgeon's assessment of the degree of damage.

Lisfranc Fracture-Dislocation

- The Lisfranc fracture-dislocation is commonly stabilized with K-wires after reduction.
- It is tempting to reduce the tarsometatarsal joints by closed reduction, but the reduction is often imperfect, and open reduction is recommended.
- Several K-wires are required to stabilize the joints, and as with other fracture-dislocations they should be left in position for 8 to 12 weeks to allow the soft tissues to heal (Fig. 34-9).

Metatarsal Fractures

- The use of K-wires for the treatment of metatarsal fractures is similar to their use in metacarpal fractures, although the central three metatarsals are usually treated

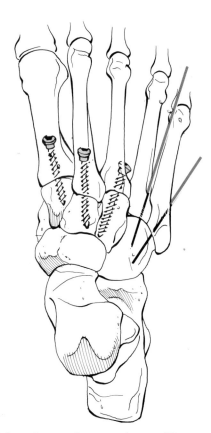

Figure 34-9   A diagram illustrating the use of K-wires and screws in a Lisfranc fracture-dislocation.

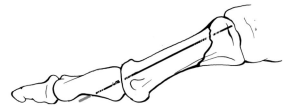

Figure 34-10   A longitudinal K-wire used for a metatarsal fracture. See text for explanation.

by intramedullary K-wiring with the wires either inserted distally and passed proximally using a closed technique under fluoroscopic control or inserted using an open technique.
- If this is done the wires can be driven distally through the fracture site, the fracture reduced, and the wire driven proximally into the proximal fracture fragment.
- In both techniques the K-wire will penetrate the proximal phalanx of the toe (Fig. 34-10).
  - This is required if good metatarsal reduction is to be achieved.
- If the K-wire is placed under the proximal phalanx, dorsiflexion of the metatarsophalangeal joint causes metatarsal malunion.
  - The K-wire is removed in 3 to 4 weeks.
- These techniques are applicable to both metaphyseal and metatarsal neck fractures.
- Hallux metatarsal fractures can be treated by K-wires, although screw and plate fixation is more commonly used today.
  - If K-wires are used, the techniques are the same as those described for metacarpal fractures.
- Fifth metatarsal diaphyseal fractures can be treated with proximally inserted intramedullary K-wires using the same technique shown in Figure 34-5C for metacarpal fractures.

Phalangeal Fractures

- K-wiring of phalangeal fractures in the foot is essentially restricted to the treatment of crushed toes.
- If there is extensive soft tissue and bone damage, K-wires can be used to straighten the toes while the fracture unites.
- The wires are placed through the distal phalanx and passed across the interphalangeal joints into the proximal phalanges or, if they are damaged, into the metacarpal heads (Fig. 34-8D).

TENSION BAND WIRING

- The tension band principle is used in the management of a number of fractures.
  - All curved tubular structures under axial load have a compression and a tension side.

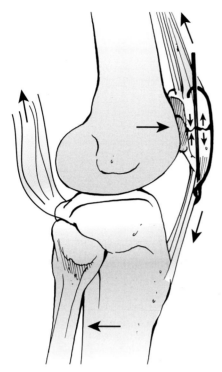

Figure 34-11   The principle of tension band wiring. See text for details.

■ This is illustrated with reference to the patella in Figure 34-11.

■ An eccentric force on the concave side of the bone increases the differential between the compression and tension sides.

■ In the patella this force differential is produced by hamstring muscle action.

■ A tension band placed on the tension side tends to neutralize the forces on each side of the bone, and the stronger the tension band, the more the forces are neutralized.

■ If the tension band is sufficiently strong, the tension forces can be converted to compression forces.

■ The action of the quadriceps converts the tension force on the concave side to a compressive force, and

knee movement therefore compresses the fracture and facilitates union (see Fig. 25-6 in Chapter 25).

■ The principle of tension banding is used for patellar, olecranon, and proximal humeral fractures (Fig. 34-12).

  ■ The same arrangement of two K-wires and a figure-eight wire loop can also be used for both medial (see Fig. 29-11 in Chapter 29) and lateral malleoli and in the distal clavicle (Fig. 34-13), although because there is no muscle action in these locations, it is strictly not a tension band but merely a method of fixing a fracture in the distal part of a long bone.

■ The technique is simple and varies little in different locations.

  ■ Two parallel K-wires are placed across the reduced fracture and a wire loop fixed distal to the fracture by placing it through the bone as in the olecranon, over both ends of the K-wires as in the patella, or over a screw as in the proximal humerus (see Fig. 34-12).

  ■ The figure-of-eight is tightened, and the ends of the K-wires cut and turned.

  ■ Motion is then permitted.

  ■ Figure 34-12 shows that the technique applied to the proximal humerus is slightly different in that K-wires are not used if a greater tuberosity fracture is treated.

■ The principle can be used for surgical neck fractures of the proximal humerus.

  ■ Two intramedullary pins or rods can be placed down the humerus and a tension band system used.

  ■ If this is done the pins need to be removed after union and the surgeon must be aware of the potential problem of rotator cuff damage.

  ■ It is not unusual to have to remove all tension band injuries because in the locations they are used they are subcutaneous and may well cause later problems.

K-Wire Migration

■ Surgeons should be aware of the potential problems of K-wire migration.

■ Usually K-wires merely back out and cause superficial infection.

■ They can migrate for considerable distances, however (see Fig. 34-13).

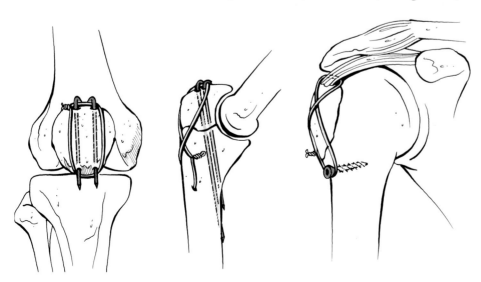

Figure 34-12   The use of tension band wiring in the patella, olecranon, and proximal humerus.

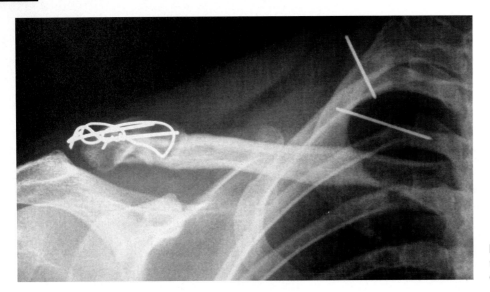

Figure 34-13   K-wire migration from tension band wiring used for a distal clavicular fracture.

- They have been known to enter the great vessels and pleural cavities.

Cerclage Wires

- Cerclage wires have been used since the middle of the 19th century. They are still occasionally used to stabilize diaphyseal bone fragments (Fig. 34-14), although the

requirement for this is now much less following the introduction of locked intramedullary nails.
- Cerclage wires and loops are still widely used for other indications.
  - They may be used to treat proximal femoral periprosthetic fractures in which the femoral prosthesis remains well secured (see Fig. 7-5 in Chapter 7).
  - They can also be used to stabilize the proximal femur if there is a calcar fracture during the insertion of a hemiarthroplasty prosthesis, as occasionally happens.
  - The other indication for cerclage wires is in the management of stellate patellar fractures.
  - Although K-wires and tension banding are commonly used to treat patellar fractures, a circumferential wire may be required to reconstruct the patella if there is significant comminution (Fig. 34-15A; see also Fig. 25-4 in Chapter 25).

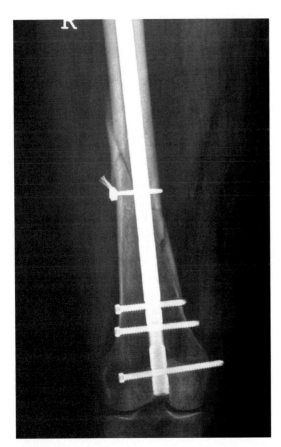

Figure 34-14   A cerclage wire loop used to facilitate reduction in a long spiral fracture of the femur.

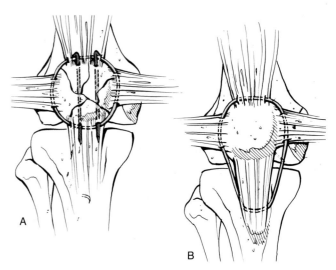

Figure 34-15   The use of wire loops around the patella. These may be used for stellate patellar fractures (**A**) or to maintain the position of the patella (**B**).

- A wire loop may also be used to protect the repair of a patellar tendon or if the distal pole of the patellar has to be excised and the soft tissues reconstructed (see Fig. 25-8 in Chapter 25).
  - Under these circumstances, a wire is placed around the superior surface of the patella and either through a transosseous hole just below the tibial tuberosity or around a screw in the same location (Fig. 34-15B).
  - Care should be taken not to lower the patella while tensioning the wire.
  - The use of a circumferential wire under these circumstances permits early knee flexion while protecting the patellar tendon repair.
  - The wire should be removed after about 12 weeks to facilitate joint movement.

SCREW FIXATION

Bone screws were used throughout the 20th century, but the AO group have been responsible for most of the innovations in screw technology. Their screws were designed for use with plates, although they can be used on their own. Many different screws have been manufactured.

Recently surgeons have designed screws that are not part of a plating system and are used for interfragmentary fixation with the screws buried in the bone. The best examples of these types of screws are the Herbert screw (Fig. 34-16A), which utilizes two threaded areas of different pitch to promote fracture compression, and the Acutrak screws (Fig. 34-16B; see also Fig. 17.1-4 in Chapter 17), which are tapered screws with a variable pitch. Both were originally designed for scaphoid fixation, although they are now used in other locations. Many of the indications for K-wire fixation have now been replaced by the use of interfragmentary screws.

The principle of the use of interfragmentary or lag screws was described in Chapter 32 (see Fig. 32-1), and although they are not used very often for diaphyseal fractures they continue to be used in metaphyseal fractures and in the small bones of the hand and feet. Cortical and cancellous bone screws are commonly available between 1.0 mm and 6.5 mm in diameter and in varying lengths. Cannulated screws can be used to increase precision in screw placement, although the basic principles of screw

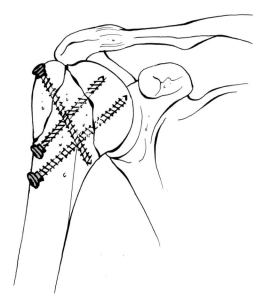

Figure 34-17   The use of interfragmentary screws in the proximal humerus.

insertion are the same. In recent years the use of tapered screws or screws with two different pitches has extended the indications for screw fixation in metaphyseal fractures and in fractures of the small bones of the hand and foot. Screw fixation can be used to treat virtually any fracture, but the more common indications are described.

Proximal Humerus

- Interfragmentary screw fixation of proximal humeral fractures is becoming more popular, with isolated greater tuberosity fractures often treated by screw fixation (Fig. 34-17).
- It is possible to reduce some valgus-impacted proximal humeral fractures by introducing a blunt probe percutaneously and reducing the fracture under fluoroscopic control.
- Once the humeral head is reduced, the greater tuberosity can be placed under it and temporary K-wires used to maintain alignment.

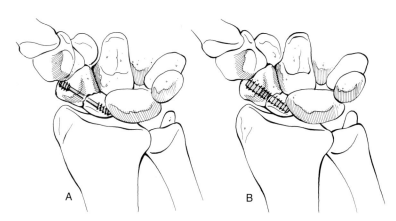

A   B

Figure 34-16   Examples of two headless compression screws. The Herbert screw (**A**) and the Acutrak screw (**B**).

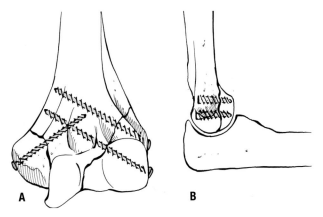

Figure 34-18   The use of screws in the distal humerus. These are mainly used for epicondylar or condylar fractures (**A**) or for capitellar fractures (**B**).

■ Several 3.5-mm interfragmentary screws can then be used to fix the fracture (Fig. 34-17; see also Fig. 11-14 in Chapter 11).

■ The results of this technique in the treatment of three- and four-part proximal humeral fractures are given in Tables 11-6 and 11-7 in Chapter 11.

Distal Humerus

■ Screw fixation can be used to fix isolated lateral or medial epicondylar or condylar fractures or capitellar fractures.

■ Epicondylar fractures can usually be fixed with one interfragmentary 3.5-mm cancellous screw with condylar fractures similarly fixed, although two screws may be required (Fig. 34-18A).

■ Capitellar fractures are more difficult to treat because they involve a shear fracture of the anterior capitellum.
  ■ These fractures can be fixed with interfragmentary screws either placed posteriorly or anteriorly.
  ■ If a posterior approach is used, it should be remembered that the capitellar fragment may only consist of a shell of cancellous bone and good fixation is sometimes difficult to achieve.
  ■ If the anterior approach is selected, the screws must be placed through the articular surface and therefore must be countersunk if a conventional screw is used.
  ■ The alternative method is to use a headless tapered screw (Fig. 34-18B; see also Fig. 13-4 in Chapter 13).
  ■ The results of screw fixation of capitellar fractures are given in Table 13-3 in Chapter 13.

Proximal Radius

■ Interfragmentary screw fixation is often used to treat radial head fractures (see Fig. 14-5 in Chapter 14). One or two 2.0- or 2.7-mm screws can be used.

■ Alternatively, headless tapered screws or screws with two different screw pitches may be used.

■ The results of this treatment method are given in Table 14-5 in Chapter 14.

Distal Radius

■ The only common indication for screw fixation of distal radial fractures is in partial articular fractures, of which the radial styloid fracture is the most common.

■ One or two 3.5-mm interfragmentary cancellous screws should be used.

Scaphoid

■ Screw fixation of the scaphoid is usually undertaken to treat scaphoid nonunion, but increasingly surgeons are using the technique for primary fracture fixation.

■ Because of the proximity of the different intercarpal joints, it is important not to have a prominent screw head, and headless screws are used (see Fig. 34-16B; see also Fig. 17.1-4 in Chapter 17).

■ These screws can either be inserted open or using a closed technique under fluoroscopic control.

■ The results of screw fixation of scaphoid fractures are given in Table 17.1-5 in Chapter 17.

Metacarpal and Phalangeal Fractures

■ Indications for the use of interfragmentary screws in the metacarpals and phalanges are shown in Figure 34-19.

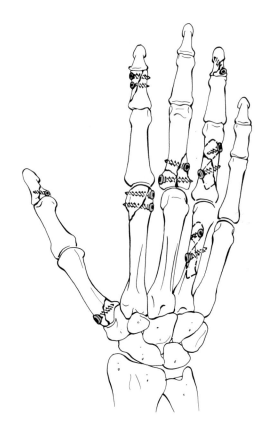

Figure 34-19   A diagram illustrating the use of screws in the metacarpals and phalanges.

- Interfragmentary screws essentially are useful for fixing intra-articular metacarpal or phalangeal fractures or spiral or oblique diaphyseal fractures.
- Transverse diaphyseal fractures should be treated by alternative means.
- The treatment of metacarpal and phalangeal fractures is discussed in Chapter 17.

Proximal Femoral Fractures

- The nails or pegs used to fix subcapital fractures were made initially of metal, ivory, or bone, and often two nails or pegs were used.
  - In 1917 Smith-Petersen published the results of the use of a single triflanged nail that was hammered into the femoral neck and head.
  - Cannulated versions soon became available, and the single hip nail became a popular implant.
  - Multiple pinning of femoral neck fractures was introduced in the 1930s, and a number of surgeons refined this technique with the Deyerle instrumentation becoming very popular.
  - Since then, multiple pin or nail fixation has become the method of choice for subcapital fractures, and currently most surgeons use three hip screws or pins to treat femoral neck fractures (see Fig. 21.2-6 in Chapter 21).
- The use of more implants does not confer any additional biomechanical or clinical advantage.
- The technique is undertaken under fluoroscopic control, and a hip fracture table should be used.
  - The patient is placed on the table with the affected leg under traction and in slight internal rotation.
  - A padded post placed in the groin provides countertraction.
  - The contralateral leg is supported in flexion and abduction by a padded splint under the calf.
  - This facilitates access for the fluoroscope.
  - It is essential that good anteroposterior and lateral images of the proximal femur are obtained prior to the commencement of surgery.
- Hip pinning can be undertaken percutaneously, but there is no great advantage and it is usually easier to make a 3- to 5-cm lateral incision opposite the lesser tuberosity.
- Biomechanical and clinical studies have shown that three screws should be placed inferiorly, anteriorly, and posteriorly in the femoral neck to buttress the three adjacent cortices.
- The results of screw fixation of proximal femoral fractures are given in Tables 21.2-6 to 21.2-8 in Chapter 21.

Proximal Tibia

- Interfragmentary screw fixation is used commonly to treat undisplaced or minimally displaced shear fractures of the lateral tibial condyle.
- Two or three screws are inserted percutaneously under fluoroscopic control to close the lateral condylar fracture.

- If there is a depression fracture of the lateral tibial condyle, plate fixation is often used, but recent work has indicated that if the depressed fragment is elevated and the reduced position maintained by calcium phosphate bone cement, percutaneous screws are often adequate to maintain the reduction until union (see Fig. 26-9 in Chapter 26).
- Surgeons should be aware that most such fractures occur in osteoporotic bone, and screw loosening may still be a problem.
- Interfragmentary screws are often used in conjunction with other treatment methods for more complex proximal tibial fractures (see Figs. 26-10 and 26-11 in Chapter 26).

Distal Tibia

- Pilon fractures are rarely treated solely by screw fixation, although frequently interfragmentary screws may be used to supplement plate fixation (see Fig. 28-4 in Chapter 28).
- Screw fixation may be used for type B partial articular pilon fractures where there is an anterior split fracture of the distal tibia.

Ankle

- Screw fixation of the ankle is undertaken for five main indications (Fig. 34-20).
- Long spiral fractures of the lateral malleolus can be fixed with two or three 3.5-mm interfragmentary screws (Fig. 34-20A; see also Fig. 29-9B in Chapter 29).
- Medial malleolar fractures are usually fixed by two 3.5-mm screws (see Fig. 29-10A in Chapter 29).
- Because most medial malleolar fractures are avulsion fractures caused by external rotation or abduction forces, two diagonal 3.5-mm cancellous screws placed upward from the tip of the malleolus are commonly used (Fig. 34-20A).
- In adduction injuries, the medial malleolus is sheared off and the fracture line is consequently vertical.
  - Under these circumstances two transverse screws can be used (Fig. 34-20B), although an antiglide plate should be used if the medial fragment is large (see Fig. 29-12 in Chapter 29).
- Small posterior malleolar fractures can be fixed with one or two 3.5-mm cortical screws inserted anteriorly into the posterior fragment (Fig. 34-20D), and if there is a large Tillaux-Chaput anterior fragment, this is usually fixed with one 3.5-mm cancellous screw (Fig. 34-20A).
- Occasionally there may be an anterior fibular fracture at the insertion of the anterior tibiofibular syndesmosis or a larger posterolateral fragment at the tibial origin of the posterior tibiofibular syndesmosis.
- Both of these can be fixed with interfragmentary 3.5-mm screws (Fig. 34-20C and D).

Syndesmosis Screws
- In type C ankle fractures associated with a tibiofibular diastasis, one or two syndesmosis screws may be inserted (see Fig. 29-15 in Chapter 29).

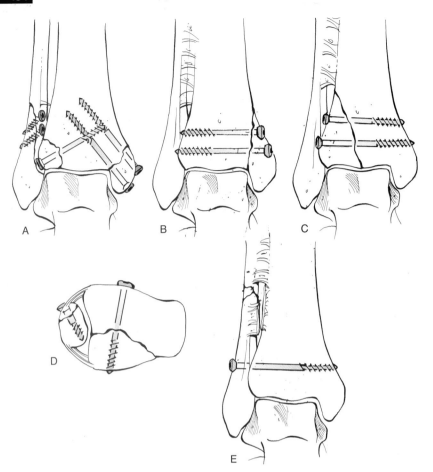

Figure 34-20 The main indications for screw fixation of the ankle. See text for explanation.

- There is debate about whether one or two screws should be used and whether the screws should penetrate the medial cortex of the tibia, but this is probably academic. No evidence indicates that one syndesmosis screw regime is better than another.
- One or two screws should be inserted through the distal fibula into the distal tibia (Fig. 34-20E).
- Surgeons should remember that the fibula lies postero-lateral to the tibia and angle the diastasis screw upward during insertion.
- The screws should not be lag screws because closure of the syndesmosis may compromise ankle function.

Talus

- Of all the bones in the foot, the talus is the one most commonly treated with screw fixation.
- Because of its size, relative inaccessibility, and large articular surface area, the use of plate fixation is impossible and screw fixation is used for most displaced talar fractures.
- Screw fixation is used for fractures of the talar neck, body, and head.
- The fractures of the talar body that may be fixed with screws are fractures of the lateral process, posterior process, and large osteochondral fractures affecting the dome of the talus.

Talar Neck Fractures

- Talar neck fractures are usually treated by two 3.5-mm cancellous screws inserted along the axis of the talus after reduction (Fig. 34-21A; see also Fig. 30-5 in Chapter 30).
- The screws can be inserted from anterior to posterior or from posterior to anterior.
  - The advantage of anterior to posterior screws is that the surgeon will usually have undertaken an anterior approach to reduce the fracture and the positioning of the screws is straightforward, with one screw placed on each side of the talar head.
- The lateral screw can be placed extra-articularly on the superior aspect of the neck of the talus, but the medial screw needs to be countersunk into the superior part of the articular surface.
- If the screws are placed from posterior to anterior, articular damage is avoided, but screw placement is more difficult and requires separate posterior incisions.

Talar Body Fractures

- Crush fractures of the talar body are comminuted inter-articular fractures and require accurate reconstruction and fixation.

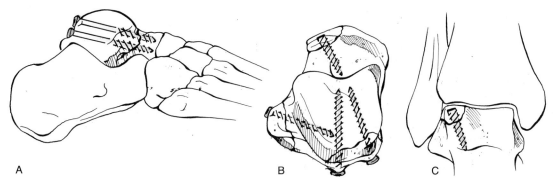

Figure 34-21 The use of screw fixation in the talus. See text for explanation.

- The exact method of reconstruction depends on the morphology of the fracture, but usually 3.5-mm cancellous screws are used (Fig. 34-22).
- Visualization of these fractures is often difficult, and a medial or lateral malleolar osteotomy may be required to achieve adequate reduction and fixation.

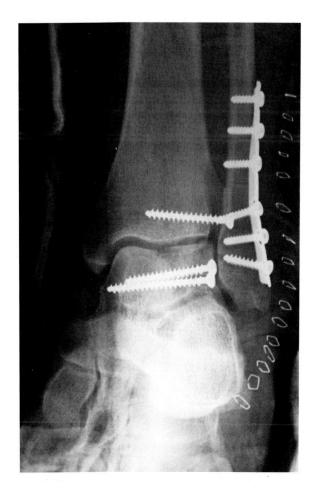

Figure 34-22 A comminuted crush fracture of the talus treated with interfragmentary screws. Note the articular damage. A lateral malleolar osteotomy was used to improve exposure.

- Fractures of the lateral and posterior process of the talus may be fixed by screw fixation depending on their size (Fig. 34-21B).
- Again, 3.5-mm cancellous screws are used.
- Osteochondral talar dome fractures rarely require fixation, but fractures that have a relatively large bony component may be treated by the use of headless screws (Fig. 34-21C).
- Talar head fractures are unusual, but if they are displaced they require screw fixation (Fig. 34-21B).

Calcaneus

- Screw fixation in the calcaneus may be used to supplement plate fixation, particularly if the calcaneal fracture has involved the calcaneocuboid joint.
- The only other indication for screw fixation in the calcaneus is if a posterior tuberosity fracture occurs as a result of avulsion by the tendo-Achilles.
  - This is usually fixed by one 4.5-mm or two 3.5-mm cancellous screws.

Other Foot Fractures and Dislocations

- Screw fixation may be used for isolated fractures of the tarsus with fractures of the navicular most commonly treated by this method.
- Screw fixation may also be used for Lisfranc tarsometatarsal fracture-dislocations in the same way as K-wires are used (see Fig. 34-9).
- Interfragmentary screws are rarely used for metatarsal fracture treatment, although they are occasionally used for spiral or oblique fractures of the hallux metatarsal.
- They are used to treat nonunions of the Jones fracture of the proximal diaphysis of the fifth metatarsal.

SUTURE ANCHORS

- Suture anchors are used increasingly in orthopaedic trauma surgery for the stabilization of soft tissues.
- They are therefore particularly useful in the treatment of a rotator cuff avulsion associated with glenohumeral

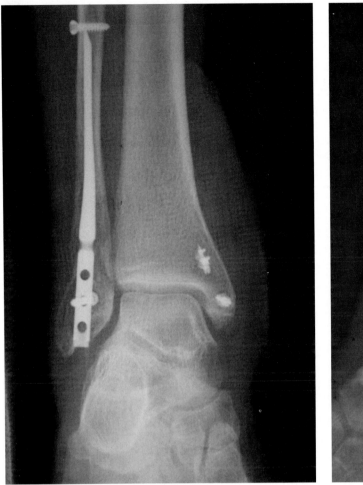
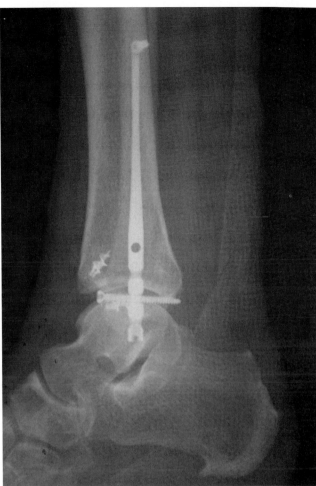

Figure 34-23   The use of suture anchors to reconstruct the medial soft tissues in an ankle fracture-dislocation.

dislocation in the elderly or for treating patellar tendon avulsions from the inferior pole of the patellar.

- They can be used to treat any soft tissue avulsions (Fig. 34-23), but they are not usually used for the treatment of fractures.

SUGGESTED READING

Chandler RW. Principles of internal fixation. In: Bucholz RW, Heckman JD, eds. Rockwood and Green's fractures in adults, 5th ed. Philadelphia: Lippincott Williams & Wilkins, 2001.

Fang RH, Chang TL. Watch out for the K-wire: painful experiences in two cases. Br J Plast Surg 2002;55:698–699.

Fitzgerald JA, Southgate GW. Cerclage wiring in the management of comminuted fractures of the femoral shaft. Injury 1987;18: 111–116.

Galanakis I, Aligizakis A, Katonis P, et al. Treatment of closed unstable metacarpal fractures using percutaneous transverse fixation with Kirschner wires. J Trauma 2003;55:509–513.

Hargreaves DG, Drew SJ, Eckersley R. Kirschner wire pin tract infection rates: a randomised controlled trial between percutaneous and buried wires. J Hand Surg (Br) 2004;29:374–376.

Horton TC, Hatton M, Davis TR. A prospective randomized controlled study of fixation of long oblique and spiral shaft fractures of the proximal phalanx: closed reduction and percutaneous Kirschner wiring versus open reduction and lag screw fixation. J Hand Surg (Br) 2003;28:5–9.

Karlsson MK, Hasserius R, Besjakov J, et al. Comparison of tension-band and figure-of-eight wiring techniques for treatment of olecranon fractures. J Shoulder Elbow Surg 2002;11:377–382.

Lee CA, Birkedal JP, Dickerson EA, et al. Stabilization of Lisfranc joint injuries: a biomechanical study. Foot Ankle Int 2004;25:365–370.

EXTERNAL FIXATION

The first use of an external device to control the position of bone fragments was by Malgaigne in 1843 in Paris. He designed a metal claw to facilitate reduction and immobilization of patellar fractures. About the same time Cucel and Rigaud in Strasbourg used two wood screws and a leather thong to immobilize an olecranon fracture. Following these early devices there was considerable interest in external fixation, and by the beginning of the 20th century a number of surgeons had not only advocated external fixation but recorded their results. Two of the main proponents of the technique were Clayton Parkhill of Denver, Colorado, and Albin Lambotte of Antwerp, Belgium. Both of these surgeons used unilateral frames. Multiplanar external frames became popular in the 1930s and 1940s following the work of Roger Anderson in Seattle, Washington, and Raoul Hoffmann in Geneva, Switzerland.

The first circular frame was designed by Hempel and Block in 1923. This fixator utilized tensioned fine wires. It was the work of Gavril Ilizarov in Russia after the Second World War, however, that created the current interest in circular frames. He was faced with a considerable number of wounded ex-servicemen and a crippled economy. He utilized simple components to construct rigid external fixator frames. His main contributions to fracture management were the promotion of distraction osteogenesis and the manufacture of a rigid frame that permitted the transportation of bone segments. His techniques have become very useful in the reconstruction of posttraumatic deformity and in the treatment of osteomyelitis (see Chapter 40).

EXTERNAL FIXATOR DESIGN

External fixators can be used to construct many different configurations, and many different designs have been devised. The three basic designs of external fixators are uniplanar frames, multiplanar frames, and circular frames. There has been considerable debate about the rigidity with which frames should be applied, with some surgeons preferring rigid frames and others less rigid designs to encourage callus formation. Much biomechanical work has been done, but no clinical evidence indicates one fixator or frame type is better than another.

Uniplanar Frames

The main role of uniplanar frames (Fig. 35-1) is in the treatment of diaphyseal fractures, although in recent years unilateral frames have been devised that allow limb lengthening and bone transport. A relatively large number of unilateral devices are available, but they are basically similar and rely on the use of four or six half pins placed into the diaphysis above and below a fracture. Pins are secured to a bar or to one or two rods. Unilateral frames are usually applied to the

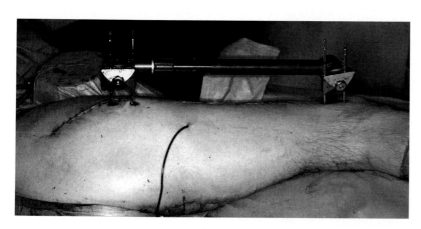

Figure 35-1 A uniplanar external fixator.

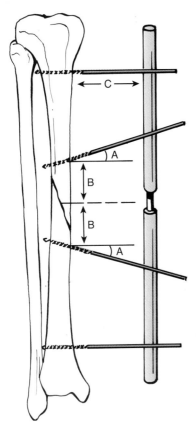

Figure 35-2 Diagram of the factors involved in frame stiffness. Pin angle (**A**), pin distance (**B**), and pin length (**C**). See text for explanation.

lateral aspect of the humerus, femur, or tibia or to the anteromedial border of the tibia.

Biomechanical testing has shown that uniplanar frames are as stiff as bilateral frames. The stiffness of unilateral frames can be altered by a number of simple adjustments (Fig. 35-2). Most unilateral frames use two half pins above and below the fracture (Figs. 35-1 and 35-2). Increased fracture stiffness can be achieved by reducing the pin length (Fig. 35-2C), the pin angle (Fig. 35-2A), and the distance between the inner pins and the fracture

(Fig. 35-2B). It is also achieved by increasing the distance between the outer pins and the fracture and, in the tibia, by applying the fixator in a lateral rather than an anteromedial location. The addition of a third half pin on each side of the fracture does not increase fracture stiffness.

Unilateral fixators are generally not used for metaphyseal or intra-articular fractures. The main exception to this is in the treatment of distal radial fractures where unilateral frames can be applied in transarticular (joint spanning) or periarticular (joint sparing) modes. In transarticular external fixation, pins are placed proximal and distal to a joint and its associated fracture (Fig. 35-3). The pins are inserted in a similar manner as for a diaphyseal fracture with the same biomechanical criteria applying. Periarticular distal radial external fixation (Fig. 35-4) is strictly speaking not unilateral, in that the pins placed into the distal radial fragment are not in the same plane as the fixator bar, but effectively the construct works as a uniplanar device. Uniplanar frames can be used to span other joints, but in practical terms the only other intra-articular or periarticular fractures treated by unilateral frames are those of the hand phalanges (Fig. 35-5).

Multiplanar Frames

With the acceptance of intramedullary nailing as the optimal method of managing lower limb diaphyseal fractures, the use of multiplanar frames has become more popular in the management of metaphyseal fractures, particularly those of the proximal and distal tibia (Fig. 35-6). They can also be used to stabilize pelvic fractures (Fig. 35-7).

As with uniplanar frames the stiffness of multiplanar frames can be increased, although there is no indication from clinical studies as to the optimal fixator design or configuration. To increase fracture stiffness, the fixator bars should be increased in number and the pin length reduced by placing the bars as close to the limb as possible in the same way as shown in Figure 35-2 for uniplanar frames. Fracture stiffness is also increased by placing a bar transversely between the longitudinal bars running on each side of the limb. In constructing any complex frame the surgeon should be aware of the need for soft tissue access, particularly in open fractures.

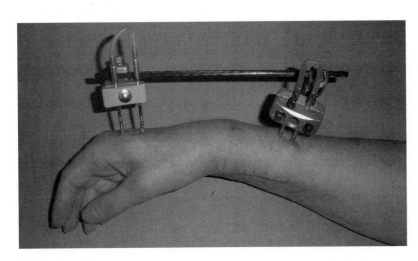

Figure 35-3 A transarticular (joint spanning) external fixator.

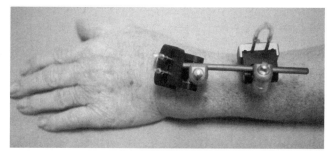

Figure 35-4 A periarticular (joint sparing) external fixator.

Multiplanar fixators can be used in periarticular mode or transarticular mode. Periarticular fixators are applied with half pins or tensioned wires in the metaphysis, and today it is usual to use a triangular system connecting a circular or semicircular metaphyseal bar to half pins in the diaphysis (see Fig. 35-6). This type of frame is used fairly commonly for tibial plateau and pilon fractures and infrequently in other locations. Transarticular multiplanar frames tend to be used if the surgeon either considers the metaphyseal or intra-articular fracture unreconstructable and proposes a later arthrodesis or if it is decided to delay definitive reconstruction because of significant soft tissue damage and swelling. This usually applies to type C pilon fractures (see Table 28-4 in Chapter 28), and under these circumstances a frame may be constructed to cross the ankle and subtalar joints. Occasionally the surgeon may

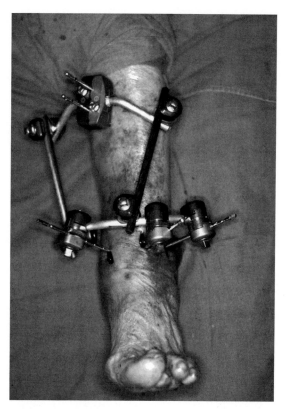

Figure 35-6 A triangular external fixator used to treat a plafond fracture.

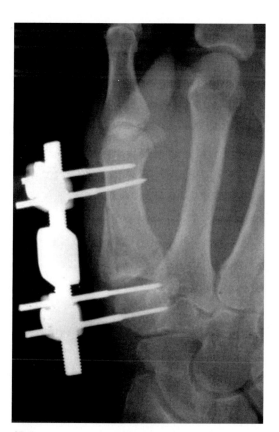

Figure 35-5 A unilateral external fixator use to treat an intra-articular metacarpal fracture using ligamentotaxis.

elect to use a transarticular frame to try to reduce a complex intra-articular fracture by relying on the intact soft tissues adjacent to the fracture to pull the fracture fragments into the reduced position. This is referred to as ligamentotaxis. Unfortunately, in the severity of fracture in which ligamentotaxis is usually used, the complex nature of the fracture means the bone fragments are not all connected to soft tissues and reduction is usually imperfect. The technique is most commonly used in intra-articular fractures of the distal radius.

Circular Frames

In recent years there has been considerable interest in the use of circular frames, mainly for posttraumatic reconstruction. The fact that bone segments can be easily transported and the frames can be hinged to correct deformity has meant that a range of problems such as infection, nonunion, and malunion can be treated successfully. This type of frame is assembled using circular rings placed around the limbs. Each ring is secured to two, or sometimes three, tensioned fine wires placed through the limb. The rings are then connected using threaded rods (Fig. 35-8). Obviously many different configurations can be constructed, but the biomechanical properties are similar to those illustrated in Figure 35-2. Each ring/fine wire assembly can be thought of as equivalent to the half-pin/pin clamp assembly of a unilateral frame (see Fig. 35-1), and the same basic biomechanical principles apply. To increase the stiffness of the frame, the inner ring/wire assemblies should be

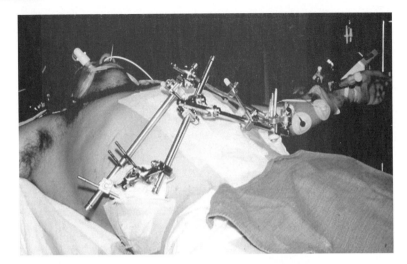

Figure 35-7 A pelvic external fixator.

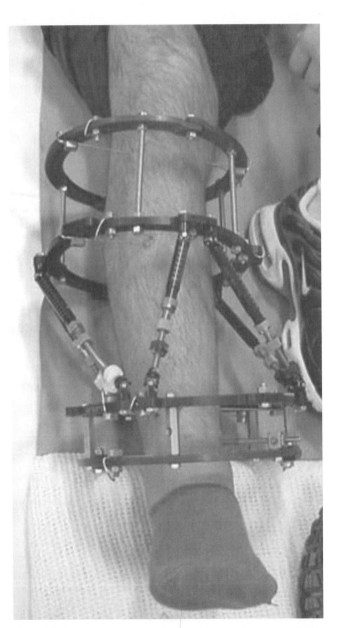

Figure 35-8 A circular frame using fine wires used to treat a tibial fracture.

close to the fracture with the outer ring/wire assemblies as distant as possible. Given the constraints imposed by the use of fixed ring/wire assemblies, stiffness can not be altered by changing the pin length.

Fine wire fixation does not require circular rings, and surgeons may use semicircular or 270-degree rings to secure the wires. There has been increasing interest recently in the use of hybrid frames, which use tensioned fine wires in the metaphysis and half pins in the diaphysis (Fig. 35-9). The advantages of these are obvious because the prolonged use of a full ring fixator for metaphyseal fractures is associated with significant muscle penetration and joint stiffness. This type of hybrid frame is particularly useful for tibial plateau and pilon fractures.

EXTERNAL FIXATOR PINS

There are two basic pin designs, the half pin and the transfixion fine wire. Half pins are available in different sizes depending on the size of the frame to be applied, but most are between 2 mm and 6 mm in diameter. Some are self-tapping and some are conical in design. A recent innovation has been to cover the threaded portion of the pin with hydroxyapatite in an attempt to minimize pin loosening.

Half Pins

Half-pin insertion is straightforward, but the surgeon should follow a few basic rules because adherence to good surgical technique minimizes the later complications of loosening and infection (Box 35-1).

Fine Wires

In contrast to half pins, fine wires may be inserted percutaneously, but if they are inserted in areas where underlying structures such as nerves and blood vessels are at risk, the same insertion technique as for half pins should be used (see Box 35-1). As fine wires are unthreaded, the risks of twisting the underlying soft tissues are less, although soft tissue transfixion is clearly a possibility. It is important to have a good knowledge of the local anatomy

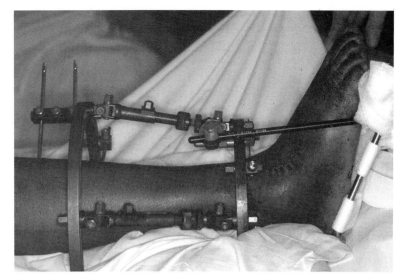

Figure 35-9 A hybrid frame used to treat the plafond fracture shown in Figure 28-3.

when inserting both half pins and fine wires, but with fine wires it is particularly important to understand the anatomy of the area distal to the bone where the fine wires emerge from the skin. An alternative to standard fine wires is the use of an olive wire with a small bulb placed on the wire. This is useful for reducing fracture fragments. If an olive is to be used, the half-pin technique of insertion should be employed (see Box 35-1). Postoperatively, the treatment of the pin tracts is similar to that of half pins. A local pressure dressing can be applied around each percutaneously inserted wire after cleansing. Where a skin incision has been made, the treatment is the same as for half pins.

Pin Loosening and Infection

If care is taken during pin insertion, loosening is unusual. The most common cause of loosening is poor insertion technique. If pins loosen, they become infected, and the treatment of a loose infected pin is removal and repositioning. If there is clinical or radiological evidence of bone involvement, the infected pin track should be curetted and cleaned. If the infection is confined to the adjacent soft tissues, local debridement and cleansing is adequate.

BOX 35-1 RULES FOR HALF-PIN INSERTION

1. Do not insert percutaneously through stab incisions. There is significant risk of nerve, tendon, or vessel damage.
2. Use 1- to 1.5-cm incision for each half pin. The incision will need to be longer if two half pins are inserted close together as in the distal radius or pelvis.
3. Incise subcutaneous tissues down to bone and protect them.
4. Predrill cortical bone.
5. Insert half pins by hand because power insertion may cause bone necrosis, resulting in a ring sequestrum, pin loosening, and sepsis.
6. Penetrate both cortices.
7. Release skin if tented on pins.
8. Do not suture pin incisions.
9. Apply antiseptic dressings.

COMMON FIXATOR APPLICATIONS

- Surgeons can apply fixators in many locations and it is impossible to describe them all.
- There are a few basic frames in use and, if necessary, these frame designs can be modified to permit treatment of many different fractures.

Distal Radius

- Two types of distal radial frame are in common use.
- The periarticular frame is used for extra-articular and undisplaced intra-articular distal radial fractures (see Fig. 35-4).
- The transarticular frame (see Fig. 35-3) is used for complex intra-articular fractures. The principle of ligamentotaxis is used to reduce the fracture, although fracture reduction is often facilitated and maintained by the use of supplementary K-wires (see Figure 16-8 in Chapter 16).

Periarticular Distal Radial Fixation

- Periarticular or joint sparing external fixation of the distal radius consists of placing two half pins into the distal radial fragment and two further half pins into the distal radial diaphysis (see Fig. 35-4).
- The distal two pins are placed under fluoroscopic control.
- The entry points are defined by palpating Gerdy's tubercle or on the dorsum of the distal radius.
- Two 1-cm parallel longitudinal incisions are made on each side of Gerdy's tubercle.
- Blunt dissection is then used to expose the radius on each side of the tubercle and the adjacent extensor pollicis longus tendon.
- The wrist is rotated into the lateral position, and a fluoroscope used to position the first distal half pin.
- The pin is placed on the posterior cortex and angled to be parallel with the distal radial articular surface.
- It is then inserted, without predrilling, just under the subchondral bone parallel to the distal radial joint surface to penetrate the anterior cortex (Fig. 35-10).
- A second pin is then inserted parallel to the first about 1 cm apart. Volar angulation of the distal fragment is

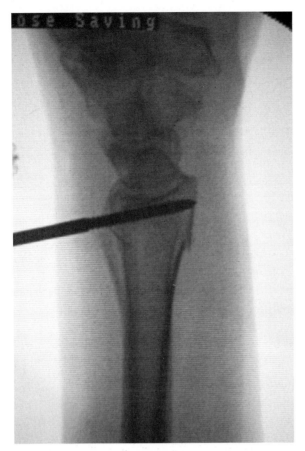

Figure 35-10 The insertion of a distal pin in a periarticular distal radial frame. See text for surgical technique.

simply achieved by angulating the pins under fluoroscopic control.

- Two radial diaphyseal pins are inserted through a 2-cm incision placed anteriorly over the distal radial diaphysis about 7.5 to 8 cm proximal to the fracture.
- Care should be taken to avoid damage to the superficial branch of the radial nerve.
- The frame can then be assembled (see Fig. 35-4).
- The results of the use of periarticular distal radial external fixation are given in Table 16-5 in Chapter 16.

Transarticular Distal Radial Fixation

- A transarticular or joint spanning frame is applied using the same technique for the proximal pins as described for the periarticular frames.
- Two pins are placed in the distal radial diaphysis.
- A similar technique is used to place two parallel half pins in the second metacarpal diaphysis.
- A dorsoradial incision is made over the metacarpal and the bone exposed on the radial side of the extensor tendon.
- Two predrilled parallel half pins are inserted and the frame is then assembled (see Fig. 35-3).
- Although longitudinal traction is required to facilitate distal radial reduction, excessive traction should be avoided because it is associated with an increased incidence of reflex sympathetic dystrophy (see Chapter 41).

- The results of the use of transarticular distal radial external fixation are given in Tables 16-5 and 16-7 in Chapter 16.

Pelvic External Fixation

- A number of pelvic frame configurations have been advocated, but nowadays external fixation is rarely used to treat pelvic fractures. Internal fixation is preferred.
- A pelvic frame is applied in the acute situation to stabilize an unstable pelvis and minimize hemorrhage, so a simple frame configuration is essential.
- The surgeon should be aware that in a multiply injured patient a laparotomy may well be needed, and the frame should not obstruct this operation.
- The most practical frame to assemble is with two 5-mm half pins placed into each anterior iliac crest just behind each anterior superior iliac spine.
- It can be difficult to angle the half pins correctly to ensure that the threaded portions lie between the inner and outer tables of the ileum.
- A 5-cm skin incision should be used and the iliac crest exposed by sharp dissection.
- The surgeon can then palpate the inner and outer tables and place two pins appropriately.
- The bilateral pins should be connected by rods placed over the lower abdomen (see Fig. 35-7).
- They should be angled upward to allow for abdominal distension, and if a laparotomy is required they should also be angled downward to facilitate access.

Femoral External Fixation

- External fixation of the femur is very rarely indicated as the definitive method of management, but it is used as a temporary treatment method under a number of circumstances.
  - Military surgeons may externally fix the femur prior to evacuating casualties to second-line hospitals.
  - In civilian practice surgeons may use external fixation in the multiply injured patient in whom damage control surgery is indicated (see Chapter 3).
  - Under these circumstances a temporary femoral diaphyseal fixator may be used.
  - Occasionally a temporary transarticular knee-spanning external frame may be applied if there is significant damage to the lower femur.
- If a femoral diaphyseal fixator is to be used, it is placed laterally and usually consists of four half pins inserted through the vastus lateralis into the femur.
  - Although speed of application may be vital, it is important to insert the femoral half pins correctly because the surgeon will probably wish to change the fixation to an intramedullary nail within a few days.
  - Poorly inserted pins increase the incidence of sepsis and may actually prevent appropriate secondary surgery.

Tibial External Fixation

- Diaphyseal external fixation should be undertaken with a uniplanar frame.
  - There is no indication for more complex frames if the fracture is diaphyseal.

- If the fracture involves both the metaphysis and diaphysis, a multiplanar or hybrid frame may be required.
- The application of a unilateral tibial diaphyseal frame is straightforward.
- The fracture is reduced and four pins inserted (see Fig. 35-1).
- The pins should be placed in the subcutaneous anteromedial border of the tibia because there is no muscle penetration and therefore ankle and subtalar movement is facilitated.
- A laterally placed frame provides greater fracture stability, but there is no clinical indication this is important, and the associated muscle penetration may cause hindfoot stiffness.
- The results of the use of external fixation in tibial diaphyseal fractures are given in Tables 27-6 and 27-7 in Chapter 27.

Proximal Tibial External Fixation

- The design of frames used to stabilize tibial plateau and pilon fractures is very similar.
- Two basic methods are employed.
  - The metaphysis can be stabilized by three half pins assembled around a semicircular bar or by two tensioned fine wires on a ring.
- Care must be taken not to damage the common peroneal nerve.
  - This is most likely to occur with the insertion of a fine wire.
- The other major structure to avoid is the patellar tendon to facilitate knee movement.
- No matter whether proximal half pins or wires are used, the diaphyseal fixation should be with two or three half pins inserted into the anteromedial border of the tibia.
- If a full ring frame is used, muscle penetration will obviously occur, and because hybrid frames provide excellent fracture stability their use is preferred.
- The results of the use of external fixation in proximal tibial fractures are given in Table 26-9 in Chapter 26.

Distal Tibial External Fixation

- The same basic frame is used for pilon fractures as for plateau fractures.
- The distal metaphysis is stabilized with three half pins (see Fig. 35-6) or two tensioned fine wires placed as shown in Figure 35-9.
- More care is required with pin and wire placement because of the number of tendons, nerves, and vessels in the area.
- If a transarticular frame is used for severe pilon fractures, the distal pins are placed in the hindfoot.
- The results of the use of external fixation in distal tibial fractures are given in Table 28-4 in Chapter 28.

COMPLICATIONS

There are three principal complications of external fixation: pin tract sepsis, malunion, and patient compliance. Diaphyseal external fixators have also been associated with a higher incidence of nonunion than internal fixation methods, but this may well reflect the severity of fractures treated with external fixation and the fact that fracture malposition is more common with external fixation. Comparative studies of open tibial diaphyseal fractures treated with external fixation and intramedullary nailing have indicated a higher incidence of nonunion with external fixation (see Tables 27-4 to 27-7 in Chapter 27).

Most of the complications arise in the treatment of diaphyseal fractures because of the length of time the fixator needs to be in position. Metaphyseal fractures unite more quickly than diaphyseal fractures, and the problems are consequently less. In distal radial fractures where the fixator is retained for only 6 weeks, the major problem is superficial pin sepsis, which is usually easily treated. In tibial metaphyseal fractures, a frame is usually retained for 10 to 12 weeks, and again the complications are relatively minor with pin sepsis the most important.

In diaphyseal fractures, the external frame may need to be in position for up to 6 months or even longer, depending on the severity of the fracture. It is often tempting to remove the frame early after the soft tissue problems have resolved and apply a cast. This is associated with a high incidence of malunion, however, if the frame is removed before the fracture has begun to unite. Malunion also follows a poor initial reduction, and surgeons should remember that most uniplanar frames are not very forgiving and require perfect reduction before the frame is applied.

The incidence of pin sepsis varies, but most authorities quote between 20% and 50%. Its treatment has been detailed already. Usually it is not serious and can be treated fairly easily. Occasionally pins need to be repositioned, however, and even more occasionally osteomyelitis can occur. It can be a particular problem if a surgeon wishes to change from primary external fixation to secondary intramedullary nailing because it is ill advisable to nail a long bone in the presence of a discharging pin tract. Under these circumstances the pin tract sepsis should be treated and allowed to resolve before nailing is undertaken.

Patient compliance varies with the length of time the frame is worn. This is a particular problem with ring fixators used for reconstructive work because the frame may be worn for a very prolonged period. Psychological counseling may even be required in some cases. In selecting an external fixator, the surgeon must assess whether the patient will cope with a prolonged period of external fixation. Many elderly patients find it very difficult to look after the frame, and they may require prolonged hospitalization or rehabilitation merely because they have been treated with an external fixation device.

SUGGESTED READING

Behrens F. General theory and principles of external fixation. Clin Orthop 1989;241:15–23.

Behrens F, Searls K. External fixation of the tibia. Basic concepts and prospective evaluation. J Bone Joint Surg (Br) 1986;68:246–254.

Calhoun JH, Li F, Ledbetter BR, et al. Biomechanics of the Ilizarov fixator for fracture fixation. Clin Orthop 1992;280:15–22.

Court-Brown CM. The effect of external fixation on bone healing and bone blood supply. An experimental study. Clin Orthop 1985;210:278–289.

Ertel, W, Keel M, Eid K, et al. Control of severe hemorrhage using C-clamp and pelvic packing in multiply injured patients with pelvic disruption. J Orthop Trauma 2001;15:468–474.

Hildebrand F, Giannoudis P, Krettek C, et al. Damage control: extremities. Injury 2004;35:678–689.

Huiskes R, Chao EY. Guidelines for external fixator frame rigidity and stresses. J Orthop Res 1986;4:68–75.

Hutson JJ, Zych GA. Treatment of comminuted intraarticular distal femur fractures with limited internal and external tensioned wire fixation. J Orthop Trauma 2000;14:405–413.

Ilizarov G. The tension stress effect on the genesis and growth of tissues: I. The influence of stability of fixation and soft tissue preservation. Clin Orthop 1989;238:249–281.

Kershaw CJ, Cunningham JL, Kenwright J. Tibial external fixation, weight bearing, and fracture movement. Clin Orthop 1993;293:28–36.

Matthews LS, Green CA, Goldstein SA. The thermal effects of skeletal fixation pin insertion in bone. J Bone Joint Surg (Am) 1984;66:1077–1083.

McQueen MM. Redisplaced unstable fractures of the distal radius. A randomised, prospective study of bridging versus non-bridging external fixation. J Bone Joint Surg (Br) 1998;80:665–669.

Paley D, Maar DC. Ilizarov bone transport treatment for tibial defects. J Orthop Trauma 2000;14:76–85.

Saleh M, Royston S. Management of nonunion of fractures by distraction with correction of angulation and shortening. J Bone Joint Surg (Br) 1996;78:105–109.

Tornetta P, Weiner L, Bergman M, et al. Pilon fractures: treatment with combined internal and external fixation. J Orthop Trauma 1993;7:489–496.

ARTHROPLASTY

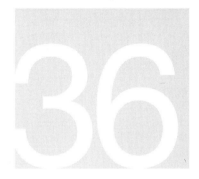

The use of arthroplasty to treat acute fractures used to be confined to the hip, but in recent years increased interest has been expressed in the use of primary knee, shoulder, elbow, and radial head arthroplasties. As the numbers of fractures in elderly osteoporotic patients increases, arthroplasty will assume greater importance in fracture management. This chapter concentrates on the surgical aspects of the use of hip, knee, shoulder, elbow, and proximal radial arthroplasty in the treatment of acute fractures.

HIP ARTHROPLASTY

Hemiarthroplasty

The first hip arthroplasties were either excision or interpositional arthroplasties and used to treat degenerative or infected joints. Gluck in Germany and Hey-Groves in England both used ivory proximal femoral prostheses to treat osteoarthritis, and the Judet brothers in Paris invented an acrylic hemiarthroplasty, which had a stem that was placed down the femoral neck into the trochanteric region of the proximal femur. This device stimulated further research, and it was soon found that improved fixation was gained by placing the stem of the proximal femoral prosthesis down the femoral canal. In 1943 Austin Moore and Harold Bohlmann, in the United States, described the use of a metal prosthesis to replace the upper end of the femur in a patient with a giant cell tumor. Moore then devised his classic hemiarthroplasty prosthesis shown in Figure 36-1. The Moore hemiarthroplasty is a press-fit uncemented prosthesis that is still in widespread use and undoubtedly the most durable of all the prostheses devised in the 20th century. The Thomson hemiarthroplasty prosthesis was also developed in the 1950s. This had a narrower solid stem that facilitated the use of bone cement, and the cemented Thomson prosthesis is still in use. Later hemiarthroplasty prostheses have followed the basic designs of Moore and Thomson, although today a number of press-fit modular hemiarthroplasty prostheses are available.

Surgical Technique

- There are several approaches through which hip prostheses can be inserted.
- They must be inserted either posterior or anterior to the greater trochanter.
- The patient is usually placed in the lateral position.
- The two most popular approaches are the posterolateral, or Southern, approach and the anterolateral, or Hardinge, approach.
- There are a number of variations of these approaches.
- The insertion of cemented hemiarthroplasties is described here. Uncemented prostheses are used, but these should be reserved for the very elderly and infirm.

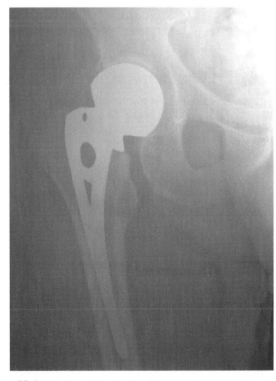

Figure 36-1 A Moore's hemiarthroplasty.

Posterolateral Approach

- In the posterolateral approach, the hip is entered behind the proximal femur.
- The patient is placed in the lateral position.
- A skin incision is made from about 15 cm below the greater trochanter to the greater trochanter, then about 10 cm toward the posterior inferior iliac spine.
- The fascia lata and gluteus maximus are divided and retracted.
- The sciatic nerve is protected.
- The external rotators are divided.
- A capsulotomy is undertaken and the cervical neck and head are exposed.
- The femoral head is removed and its diameter assessed.
- The neck is trimmed to fit the flange of the prosthesis and the femoral canal is reamed.
- A box chisel or gouge is used to remove bone from the greater trochanter.
- The size of the femoral stem is assessed and the correct size of implant is selected.
- A cement plug is inserted into the intramedullary canal.
- Cement pressurization techniques are used.
- The implant is inserted and the hip reduced, and the wound is closed in layers.

Anterolateral Approach

- In the anterolateral approach, the hip joint is approached down the front of the trochanters and femoral neck.
- The patient is placed in the lateral position.
- A 20-cm incision is made parallel to the femur and centered on the greater trochanter.
- The iliotibial tract is incised, and the tensor fascia lata is retracted anteriorly and gluteus maximus posteriorly.
- The vastus lateralis is incised longitudinally and left in continuity with the gluteus medius, which is incised for about 3 to 4 cm.
- The tissues are mobilized from the front of the proximal femur.
- The leg is externally rotated and flexed to expose the hip joint.
- The femoral head is removed and its diameter assessed.
- The neck is trimmed to fit the flange of the prosthesis, and the femoral canal is reamed.
- A box chisel or gouge is employed to remove bone from the greater trochanter.
- The size of femoral stem is assessed and the correct size of implant selected.
- A cement plug is inserted into the intramedullary canal.
- Pressurization techniques are used.
- The implant is inserted and the hip reduced, and the wound is closed in layers.

Complications

- The main intraoperative complications associated with the use of a hemiarthroplasty prosthesis are periprosthetic fractures and prosthesis malalignment.
- If the prosthesis is too large, there is a risk of periprosthetic fracture of the acetabulum or the proximal femur (see Figs. 7-7 and 7-4, respectively, in Chapter 7).

- The most common periprosthetic fractures are actually minor longitudinal fractures of the calcar caused by using too large a prosthesis.
  - If a minor calcar crack occurs, it may not need any treatment if the crack is small and prosthesis is stable, but if there is concern that the fracture might propagate distally, it should be treated by the use of one or two cerclage wires or loops.
  - If a more serious periprosthetic fracture occurs, the surgeon may have to use a cemented long-stem prosthesis to stabilize the hip joint.
- Implant malposition usually occurs because of failure to follow correct surgical techniques.
  Surgeons should remember that most of the patients receiving hip prostheses after fracture are frail, elderly, and osteoporotic.
  - It is relatively easy to penetrate the lateral or posterior femoral cortices if the prosthesis is inserted incorrectly.
  - Attention to correct surgical technique will prevent this.
- Care must be taken not to damage the sciatic nerve in the posterior approach and the superior gluteal nerve in the lateral approach.
- The most common late complication of the use of a hemiarthroplasty is hip pain.
  - This is more common in uncemented prostheses and younger patients.
  - It may result from the use of too small an uncemented prosthesis.
  - In active patients it may be caused by the articulation of the metal head in a normal acetabulum.
- Full details of the results and complications of hemiarthroplasty are given in Tables 21.2-8 to 21.2-10 in Chapter 21.

Bipolar Arthroplasty

The bipolar arthroplasty was popularized by Bateman in the 1970s as an alternative to the traditional Moore or Thomson hemiarthroplasty. These prostheses consist of the femoral component of a total hip arthroplasty with a hemiarthroplasty head placed on the conventional arthroplasty head (Fig. 36-2). Theoretically, the two heads facilitate hip movement, but little evidence indicates this is the case, and recent studies have not indicated any particular advantage over standard hemiarthroplasty prostheses (see Table 21.2-9 in Chapter 21).

Bipolar prostheses are inserted through the same approaches as hemiarthroplasty prostheses, and the basic surgical technique is very similar. The main differences between the two types of implant are the fact that the femoral stems of bipolar prostheses are usually the same stems used for total hip replacement. They can be inserted as an uncemented press-fit prosthesis or with bone cement. The head that articulates with the acetabulum is applied over a smaller femoral head, which is often 28 or 32 mm in size. The results of bipolar arthroplasty are given in Table 21.2-9 in Chapter 21.

Radiological studies have shown that bipolar prostheses rarely function as a total hip replacement with movement

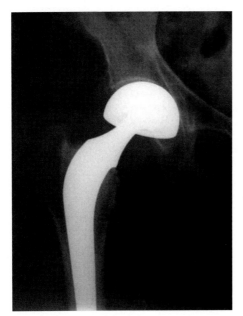

Figure 36-2   A bipolar arthroplasty.

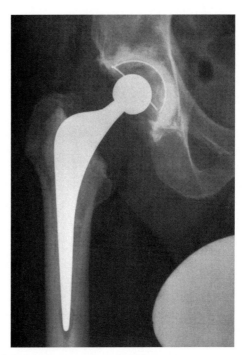

Figure 36-3   A total hip arthroplasty.

between the two heads. They usually function as a hemiarthroplasty with movement at the interface between the acetabulum and the larger head. Any benefit from their use derives mainly from the fact that they are usually cemented, and the results of cemented hemiarthroplasties are better than those of uncemented devices (see Table 21.2-10 in Chapter 21).

Complications
- The perioperative complications of bipolar prostheses are the same as those for hemiarthroplasty and dealt with similarly.

Hip Replacement

Total hip replacement followed the early work of Moore and Thomson. Charnley is correctly regarded as the father of hip arthroplasty, but recognition of the work of McKee of Norwich, England, in 1950 is important. He visited Thomson in New York, adopted the Thomson stem, and then designed a chrome cobalt socket that was secured with acrylic cement. It was McKee's design that was first used in the United States.

Total hip replacement is increasingly being used to treat displaced subcapital fractures, particularly in younger and fitter patients (Fig. 36-3). The surgical approaches are the same as those for hemiarthroplasty or bipolar arthroplasties, and the technique of inserting the stem is similar to that for a bipolar prosthesis. The acetabulum is inserted after appropriate reaming and size assessment. Cemented or uncemented acetabular prostheses may be used.

Complications
- The perioperative complications of total hip replacement are the same as for hemiarthroplasty or bipolar arthroplasty.

- In addition to the problems of periprosthetic fractures and malalignment of the femoral stem, it is also possible to malalign the acetabular prosthesis, and care must be taken to set the prosthesis in the correct degree of anteversion during insertion.
- Dislocation is a particular problem associated with arthroplasty following proximal femoral fracture.
- It occurs in about 10% of cases (see Table 21.2-8 in Chapter 21), but there is no good evidence it remains a long-term problem or that it varies with the approach.

KNEE REPLACEMENT

As with hip arthroplasty, the earliest knee arthroplasties were excisional or interpositional. Gluck inserted ivory knee replacements in Germany in the late 19th century, but his infection rate was very high and he was heavily criticized. The first metal interpositional knee arthroplasty was devised by Boyd in the United States in 1938, and several similar devices were used up to the 1960s with some success. The first hinged knee replacement was used by Jean and Robert Judet in 1947. Hinged knee replacements became popular, but it did not take long to find out they were associated with a relatively high incidence of patellar instability, prosthetic loosening, and infection. They continued to be used in some European centers up to the 1980s for elective knee arthroplasty, but most surgeons adopted the use of unconstrained condylar prostheses following the work of Freeman in London and Insall in New York. These devices can be used to treat impaction fractures of the proximal tibia, but they are not used for distal femoral fractures.

The use of hinged knee replacements for degenerative or inflammatory arthropathies has now virtually ceased, although they occasionally have a role in revision surgery.

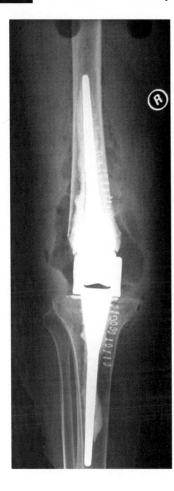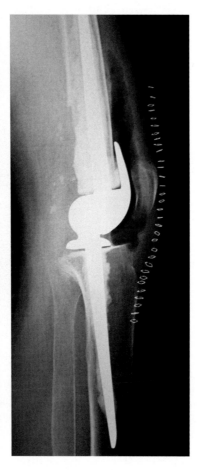

Figure 36-4   A-P and lateral radiographs of a hinged knee arthroplasty used to treat a type C distal femoral fracture in a 91-year-old woman.

The dramatic increase in osteoporotic fractures in the very elderly has caused orthopaedic trauma surgeons to reexamine their use in low supracondylar and intercondylar femoral fractures (Fig. 36-4), and good results have been reported (see Chapter 24).

Surgical Technique

- The patient is placed in the supine position.
- A tourniquet is used.
- A longitudinal anterior midline incision is used. It extends over the lower femur, patella, and upper tibia.
- The fascia, muscles, and retinacular ligaments are incised medial to the patella, which is mobilized laterally.
- Once the femoral condyles have been exposed, the fracture fragments are removed.
- This should be done using sharp dissection to mobilize the cruciate and collateral ligaments from the femoral condyle.
- The knee should be placed in flexion during removal of the fracture fragments.
- This facilitates the surgery and protects the popliteal vessels and nerve.
- The proximal tibia is exposed by excising the meniscal remnants and using an oscillating saw to remove the proximal tibia.
- The arthroplasty is then cemented into position and the femoral and tibial components connected.

Complications

- The use of a hinged knee arthroplasty is relatively straightforward, and complications are few.
- Given the osteoporotic nature of the bone, surgeons may be faced with a more comminuted fracture than they expected from examination of the initial radiographs.
- If this is the case, cerclage wires or loops may be required to stabilize longitudinal cracks in the bone prior to the introduction of the femoral prosthesis.
- Periprosthetic fractures are very unusual.
- The surgeon should guard against prosthesis malposition by carefully orientating the tibial prosthesis into the correct position and then rotating the femoral prosthesis appropriately during insertion.
- The operation must be restricted to the very elderly or infirm.

SHOULDER REPLACEMENT

The earliest arthroplasties of the shoulder were excision arthroplasties, but the results were very poor. The use of a metal hemiarthroplasty in the management of proximal humeral fractures was documented by Charles Neer of New York in 1955, and it is to Neer that the credit must go for introducing and popularizing the use of shoulder hemiarthroplasty in trauma (Fig. 36-5).

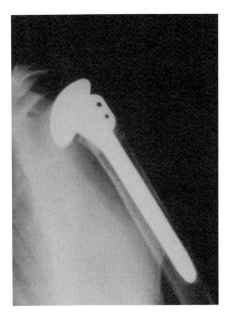

Figure 36-5 A shoulder hemiarthroplasty.

ELBOW ARTHROPLASTY

As with the other joints discussed in this chapter, the early arthroplasties performed on the elbow joint were excision arthroplasties, not infrequently performed to treat tuberculosis. Interpositional arthroplasty utilizing fascia lata tied around the distal humerus after distal humeral excision was also used. The first metal hinged elbow arthroplasty was reported by Dee in 1972, and since then many different elbow prostheses have been devised. As with the knee the original elbow hinge designs gave way to unconstrained prostheses, but hinged devices are usually used for trauma. The Coonrad hinged arthroplasty was developed in the 1970s and has been used extensively for the management of posttraumatic arthritis. Its modification into the Coonrad-Morrey prosthesis has improved the design and provided a prosthesis that has been shown to be useful in the treatment of distal humeral fractures and nonunions in elderly patients (Fig. 36-6).

Surgical Technique

- The patient can be positioned in the supine position with a sandbag under the shoulder and the arm over the chest.
- Alternatively, the patient can be in the lateral position with the arm supported by a U-shaped support, allowing the elbow to flex to 90 degrees.
- A posterior incision is made passing lateral to the medial epicondyle and medial to the tip of the olecranon.
- The ulnar nerve is located on the medial side of the distal humerus running posterior to the medial epicondyle. It is transposed anteriorly.
- An incision is made along the medial aspect of the triceps and extended over the elbow joint onto the medial aspect of the olecranon and down over the medial aspect of the proximal ulnar diaphysis.
- The tissues, including the posterior capsule, are elevated using sharp dissection and displaced laterally.
  - This allows the ulna to be displaced laterally and facilitates access to the distal humerus.
- About 1 cm of the tip of the olecranon is excised with an oscillating saw to facilitate exposure of the distal humerus but, more importantly, to allow the ulnar prosthesis to be passed easily down the ulna later in the operation.
- In a primary bicondylar fracture, the distal humerus can be discarded.
  - If it is preserved, appropriate cuts are made to allow the insertion of the prosthesis, which is cemented into position.
- The soft tissues are then reconstructed and the wound closed.

Surgical Technique

- Shoulder prostheses are inserted through a deltopectoral approach.
- The patient is positioned in the beach chair position.
- The incision starts at the coracoid process and extends inferiorly for about 20 cm in line with the anterior edge of the deltoid muscle.
- The space between the pectoralis major and deltoid is exposed and opened.
- The cephalic vein is retracted laterally with the deltoid.
- The clavipectoral fascia is incised and the upper half of the pectoralis major insertion is mobilized to facilitate exposure.
- The rotator cuff interval is identified and opened.
- The greater and lesser tuberosities are identified and the humeral head removed.
- The stem size of the implant is assessed and selected.
- The prosthesis is cemented into position, making sure the degree of retroversion and the alignment with the glenoid are correct.
- The tuberosities are reduced and attached with wire or heavy suture.
- The wound is closed in layers.
- It is important to position the prosthesis and the tuberosities accurately (see Chapter 11). The results of shoulder hemiarthroplasty are given in Table 11-8 in Chapter 11.

Complications

- The main complications of shoulder hemiarthroplasty are tuberosity malposition and failure to align the head of the prosthesis with the glenoid (see Chapter 11).

Complications

- There are relatively few complications of elbow arthroplasty if the correct surgical technique is used.
- Periprosthetic fractures are discussed in Chapter 7.

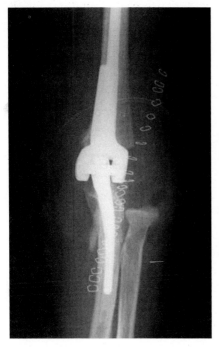
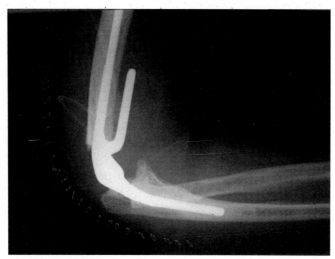

Figure 36-6   A-P and lateral radiographs of a semiconstrained elbow replacement.

■ Elbow stiffness may occur in the elderly, but overall the results are good.

■ The results of elbow arthroplasty in the treatment of distal humeral fractures and nonunions are given in Tables 13-5 and 13-7 in Chapter 13.

PROXIMAL RADIAL ARTHROPLASTY

Kellog Speed reported on the use of a metallic radial head cap in 1941, and Cherry described the use of an acrylic radial head in the management of a radial head fracture in 1953. Credit for popularizing the use of radial head spacers or hemiarthroplasty prostheses must go to Swanson, who described the use of silicone spacers in 1981. Since then surgeons have become concerned about wear debris associated with the use of silicone implants and have returned to the use of metal radial head hemiarthroplasties (Fig. 36-7). The main indications remain the treatment of comminuted radial head fractures, particularly if they are associated with a complex ulnar fracture or a dislocation (see Chapter 14). However, as with other arthroplasties, it is likely they will be used increasingly to treat radial head fractures in elderly patients in the future.

Surgical Technique

■ A 10-cm midlateral incision is made, centered on the elbow joint, and dissection is carried out down to the annular ligament, which is incised.

■ The radial head is removed and the radial neck trimmed back.

■ Care must be taken to avoid damage to the posterior interosseous nerve.

■ The correct size of radial head is selected and the head is inserted.

■ The annular ligament is repaired and the wound closed in layers.

Complications

■ There are few intraoperative complications of the use of radial head prostheses.

■ Dislocation or subluxation may occur if the wrong size of prosthesis is selected and the periarticular soft tissues around the elbow are not balanced properly.

■ This is more likely in complex fracture-dislocations.

■ The results of radial head replacement are given in Table 14-7 in Chapter 14.

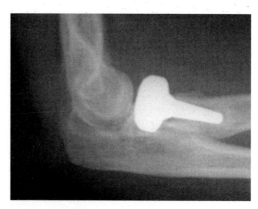

Figure 36-7   A radial head replacement.

SUGGESTED READING

Bell KM, Johnstone AJ, Court-Brown CM. Primary knee arthroplasty for distal femoral fractures in elderly patients. J Bone Joint Surg (Br) 1992;74:400–402.

Boileau P, Walch G, Krishnan SG. Tuberosity osteosynthesis and hemiarthroplasty for four part fractures of the proximal humerus. Tech Shoulder Elbow Surg 2000;1:96–109.

Kamineni S, Morrey BF. Distal humeral fractures treated with non-custom total elbow replacement. J Bone Joint Surg (Am) 2004;86:940–947.

King GJ. Management of comminuted radial head fractures with replacement arthroplasty. Hand Clin 2004;20:429–441.

Lu-yao GL, Keller RB, Littenburg B, et al. Outcomes after displaced fractures of the femoral neck: a meta-analysis of one hundred and six published reports. J Bone Joint Surg (Am) 1994;76:15–25.

Mabry TM, Prpa B, Haidukewych GJ, et al. Long-term results of total hip arthroplasty for femoral neck fracture nonunion. J Bone Joint Surg (Am) 2004;86:2263–2267.

McKee MD, Jupiter JB. Trauma to the adult elbow. In: Browner BD, Jupiter JB, Levine AM, et al., eds. Skeletal trauma, 3rd ed. Philadelphia: WB Saunders, 2003.

Ong BC, Maurer SG, Aharonoff GB, et al. Unipolar versus bipolar hemiarthroplasty: functional outcome after femoral neck fracture at a minimum of thirty-six months follow up. J Orthop Trauma 2002:16;317–322.

Parker MJ, Gurusamy K. Arthroplasties (with and without bone cement) for proximal femoral fractures in adults. Cochrane Database Syst Rev 2004;(2):CD 001706.

Robinson CM, Page RS, Hill RM, et al. Primary hemiarthroplasty for treatment of proximal humeral fractures. J Bone Joint Surg (Am) 2003;85:1215–1223.

Sipila J, Hyvonen P, Partanen J, et al. Early revision after hemiarthroplasty and osteosynthesis of cervical hip fracture: short-term function mortality unchanged in 102 patients. Acta Orthop Scand 2004;75:402–407.

37 AMPUTATIONS

Amputations have been undertaken for several thousand years. Evidence indicates they were performed in Neolithic times, although they may well have been punitive as well as therapeutic. Hippocrates discussed amputations in some detail, but amputation between healthy and diseased tissue was first recommended by Celsus in the first century. The introduction of gunpowder and cannon shot into warfare in the middle of the 14th century greatly increased the number of open fractures and must have resulted in a huge increase in the requirement for amputation. Despite this, little progress was made until the 17th century when a number of surgeons devised flaps to cover amputation stumps. Amputation at this time was crude, to say the least. Surgeons relied on speed and dexterity. The introduction of anesthesia in the 19th century improved matters, but the amputation rate and mortality associated with open fractures remained high. At this time the amputation rates following major limb surgery in large European city hospitals varied between 25% and 63%.

By the time of the Second World War, improved orthopaedic and plastic surgery techniques were available, but so were better weapons, and the amputation rate during the Second World War was 5.3% compared with 2% to 3% in the First World War. The incidence of amputations decreased during the Korean and Vietnam conflicts, but it has only been comparatively recently that the amputation rate has markedly abated. The decline has followed the introduction of better triage and improved orthopaedic techniques, but the major reason has been the introduction of free flaps and the improvement in local flaps in the last 20 years.

CLASSIFICATION

A number of classifications of the severely injured extremity have been proposed. These include the Mangled Extremity Syndrome Index (MESI), the Predictive Salvage Index (PSI), the Mangled Extremity Severity Score (MESS), the Limb Salvage Index (LSI), and the NISSSA, a modification of the MESS system based on nerve injury, ischemia, soft tissue contamination, skeletal injury, shock, and age. It is beyond the scope of this chapter to discuss all of these systems in detail, but they have been critically examined by Bonanni and colleagues (1993), who were sceptical about their usefulness. Dirschl and Dahners (1996) have also examined these systems in detail.

The most popular system said to be predictive of the requirement for amputation is the Mangled Extremity Severity Score (MESS) (Table 37-1). It is relatively simple to apply both pre- or perioperatively, unlike some of the other classifications that can only be applied retrospectively. The initial studies indicated that a score of 7 predicted amputation with 100% accuracy. Later studies suggested a sensitivity of 22% and a specificity of 53%. Most studies have suggested that the MESS score, and the other scoring systems, should be used as an aid to predict the requirement for amputation, rather than the sole predictor.

TABLE 37-1 MANGLED EXTREMITY SEVERITY SCORE (MESS)

Injury	Score
Skeletal/soft tissue injury	
Low energy (stab, simple fracture, low-velocity gunshot wound)	1
Medium energy (open or multiple fractures, dislocation)	2
High-energy (close-range shotgun, high-velocity gunshot, crush)	3
Very high energy (preceding criteria plus gross contamination, soft tissue avulsion)	4
Limb ischemia (score doubled for ischemia >6 hr)	
Pulse reduced or absent but perfusion normal	1
Pulseless, paresthesias, diminished capillary refill	2
Cool, paralyzed, insensate, numb	3
Shock	
Systolic blood pressure always >90 mm Hg	0
Hypotensive transiently	1
Persistent hypotension	2
Age	
<30 y	0
30–50 y	1
>50 y	2

GOALS

The overall aim of an amputation performed for trauma is to excise the damaged area but preserve maximal function while obtaining good soft tissue cover. Care must be taken to assess which type of amputation will give the best long-term function for the patient. In severely injured patients, this may well take second place to saving the patient's life, but in most patients, consideration of outcome should be more than just short-term fracture treatment. Plastic surgery techniques may be used to lengthen stumps or to cover exposed bone, allowing a joint to be preserved. This is particularly true of tibial fractures where a below-knee amputation should be performed if at all possible because their functional results are much better than that of above-knee amputations.

UPPER LIMB AMPUTATIONS

- With the exception of digital amputations, upper limb amputations are uncommon.
- Most amputations are undertaken because of severe open injury, and Table 4-2 in Chapter 4 highlights the relatively low incidence of Gustilo type III fractures in the upper limb.
- The requirement for digital amputation is still considerable, although in many countries improved industrial and workplace legislation has reduced the need for this operation.

Digital Amputation

- The common reasons for digital amputation are trauma, infection, Dupytren's contracture, and neoplasia, but it has been estimated that about 90% of digital amputations follow trauma.
- The aims of digital amputation are listed in Box 37-1.
  - All are important, but the maintenance of maximal function is the surgical priority.
- The surgeon may have to decide between amputation and reimplantation of the digits.
- Single digits are rarely reimplanted because studies have shown that reimplanted digits rarely have normal sensation and function and often merely interfere with hand function.
- If possible the thumb should be reimplanted because its function is unique and makes up about 50% of the use of the hand.

BOX 37-1 AIMS OF DIGITAL AMPUTATION

- Maintain maximal function.
- Ensure that the digital stump does not interfere with hand use.
- Achieve good soft tissue closure without tension.
- Minimize stump tenderness.
- Strive for the best cosmesis possible.

BOX 37-2 PRINCIPLES OF DIGITAL AMPUTATION

- Conserve length if possible. Soft tissue cover takes priority over length.
- Amputate through adjacent joint if residual phalanx <1 cm in length.
- If the amputation is through the PIPJ or DIPJ, trim the phalangeal condyles.
- Do not suture flexor and extensor tendons over stump.
- Cut digital nerves as proximal as possible and cauterize.
- Ensure that flaps site scar dorsal to midaxial line of finger.
- Do not suture flaps under tension.

- If there are multiple traumatic digital amputations, the surgeon should aim at retaining at least two fingers.
- If reimplantation is to be successful, the digit should not have been crushed or significantly contaminated.
- The reimplantation operation should be undertaken expeditiously, and the severed digit should be stored in a plastic bag cooled in ice during transport.

Distal Phalangeal Amputation

- Traumatic amputations of the tip of the finger through the distal phalanx are common.
  - They may be treated using split skin grafting or various flaps, but often the surgeon may elect to shorten the distal phalanx and suture the soft tissues.
- There are a number of principles the surgeon should follow if a digital amputation is performed (Box 37-2).
- It is important to plan the soft tissue flaps so the resulting scar is dorsal to the midaxial line of the finger.
- The scar should not be placed over the anterior aspect of the pulp because it is used for gripping.
- Where possible, a long volar flap (Fig. 37-1A) or volar and dorsal flaps should be used (see Fig. 37-1B).
  - If the latter technique is used, the volar flap should be longer than the dorsal flap to ensure the resulting scar is placed appropriately.
  - A dorsal flap should not be used because the sutures are then placed on the pulp of the finger and the nail bed is moved distally and anteriorly, forming a hooked nail.
- It is unwise to leave a small piece of the distal phalanx behind in an effort to spare the distal interphalangeal joint.
  - If the phalangeal remnant is less than about 1 cm in length, it tends to flex and restrict digital function.
- Under these circumstances, amputation through the distal interphalangeal joint is recommended.
- If this is done, the distal end of the middle phalanx should be trimmed to resemble the normal distal phalangeal tuft.
  - This is done by removing the lateral condyles of the phalanx.
- The flexor and extensor tendons should not be sutured over the end of the bone because both extensor and flexor tendons arise from a common muscle origin, and suturing the tendons together interferes with function in the other digits.

A   B   C

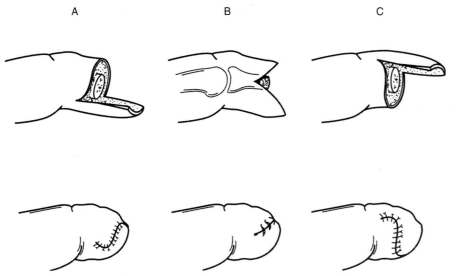

Figure 37-1   Skin flaps used in digital amputation. See text for explanation.

■ The nerves should be sectioned as far proximally as possible and then cauterized.
  ■ This reduces the incidence of neuroma formation at the level of the amputation.
■ The accompanying vessels are cauterized to avoid hemorrhage, and the skin is sutured without tension.

Middle Phalangeal Amputations

■ The principles that govern amputation through the middle phalanx are essentially the same as for distal phalangeal amputations (see Box 37-2), although there are some differences.
■ A dorsal flap can be used to cover the amputation stump if the suture line is placed proximal to the reconstructed pulp (Fig. 37-1C).
■ The location of the amputation with reference to the insertion of flexor digitorum superficialis determines the function of the finger.
  ■ If the amputation is distal to the insertion of flexor digitorum superficialis, the finger will be able to grasp.
  ■ If amputation is proximal to the insertion, function is markedly impaired. It is better to amputate through the proximal interphalangeal joint with trimming of the condyles, as described for distal phalangeal amputations.

Proximal Phalangeal Amputation

■ As with distal and middle phalangeal amputations, the principles in Box 37-2 apply to proximal phalangeal fractures.
■ Length should be preserved, but soft tissue cover and function are more important.
■ If the amputation level is distal and the proximal phalangeal stump is relatively long, finger function is reasonable.
■ Intrinsic function allows for flexion to about 45 degrees, and the stump helps maintain objects in the palm of the hand.
■ If the stump is short or the amputation level is through the metacarpophalangeal joint, there is a cosmetic deformity, and the gap left by removal of either the long or index fingers allows objects to drop from the hand.

■ Under these circumstances a ray amputation should be performed.

Ray Amputation

■ Ray amputations should be considered if an amputation is necessary at the metacarpophalangeal joint or slightly distal to it.
■ In the index and little fingers, the operation is straightforward and consists of a racquet incision placed around the middle of the proximal phalanx and extending proximally dorsolaterally and dorsomedially over the hand (Fig. 37-2).
■ The base of the metacarpal is cut obliquely. Cosmesis and hand function are good.
■ Ray amputation of the middle and ring fingers is more difficult.
  ■ It can be done by removal of the finger through a racquet incision around the proximal phalanx, which continues dorsally over the metacarpal.

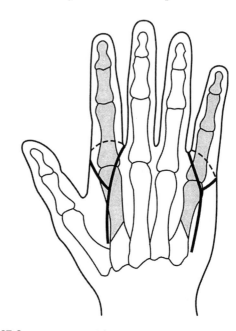

Figure 37-2   Incisions used for ray amputation.

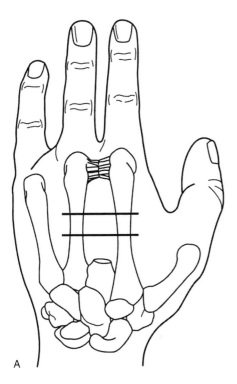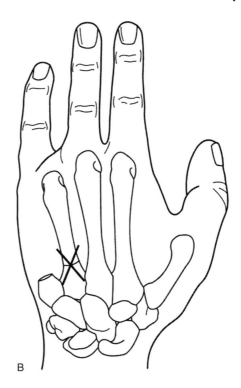

Figure 37-3 Reconstruction techniques in ray amputation.

- The metacarpal is then cut near the base, and a subperiosteal dissection is carried out to free the metacarpal.
- The nerves and vessels are cut and cauterized as distally as possible, and the space between the adjacent fingers is closed by suturing the transverse ligaments and holding the metacarpals together with K-wires while the soft tissues heal (Fig. 37-3A).
- The little or index fingers can be transposed onto the osteotomized proximal metacarpals of the ring and long fingers. The osteotomy should be held with K-wires or a plate (Fig. 37-3B).

Multiple Digital Amputations
- Where a number of digits have been severely injured, the general principle is save as much viable tissue as possible at the time of the initial surgical procedure.
- Later procedures will aim at preserving as much length as possible and providing good soft tissue cover.
- The surgical procedures undertaken depend on the severity and location of the injury, but possible procedures involve finger transposition, implantation of the hallux to the thumb, and lengthening of the thumb.
    - As a minimum it is important to try and restore thumb and index finger function, but ideally two fingers should be reconstructed in addition to the thumb.

Complications of Digital Amputation
- A number of inevitable complications are associated with digital amputation.
- There may well be restriction of function and cosmetic problems, but there are other complications (Box 37-3).

- Ray amputations tend to alter hand function considerably, but cosmesis tends not to be such a problem.

Other Upper Limb Amputations
- Other upper limb amputations are very rarely undertaken. The general principles are the same no matter what level of amputation is performed.
- Once the hand is removed, the main objective of upper limb amputation is to preserve as much limb length as possible so a prosthesis can be fitted.

BOX 37-3 COMPLICATIONS OF DIGITAL AND RAY AMPUTATIONS

Digital Amputation
Hand dysfunction
Pain
Digital neuromas
Cosmesis
Finger tip injuries
    30% to 50% cold intolerance
    30% dysesthesia

Ray Amputation
20% loss of power grip, key pinch, and supination strength
50% loss of pronation strength
Index ray amputation
    Hyperesthesia
    Carpal tunnel syndrome following flexor tendon migration

- If necessary, plastic surgery techniques can be used to preserve or create limb length.
- Free flaps used to create limb length are associated with a higher incidence of skin breakdown and ulceration than flaps fashioned from local tissue.
- The conventional amputation levels are transcarpal, disarticulation through the wrist, below elbow, disarticulation through the elbow, above elbow, shoulder disarticulation, and four-quarter amputation.
  - The last two amputations are so rarely required in the management of trauma that they are not described in this chapter.

Transcarpal Amputation

- If possible a transcarpal amputation is preferred to a wrist disarticulation because radiocarpal function is preserved and the arm is therefore more useful.
  - It is also easier to fit a prosthesis.
- Because transcarpal amputations are undertaken because of very severe injury to the hand, it is difficult to be precise about surgical technique.
- The objectives are essentially the same as for digital amputation, namely presentation of length and function with good soft tissue cover supplemented by flap cover if it helps preserve the radiocarpal joint.

Wrist Disarticulation

- If the radiocarpal joint cannot be preserved, a wrist disarticulation is performed.
  - This confers certain advantages over any amputation performed through the forearm because the radial styloid flare improves prosthetic fitting and use.
  - The other major advantage is that full pronation and supination are maintained.
- The operation is best performed using dorsal and volar flaps with the volar flap longer than the dorsal flap to ensure the scar is on the dorsum of the wrist (Fig. 37-4A).
- The distal radioulnar joint must be protected to preserve rotation.

Forearm Amputation

- If a forearm amputation is undertaken, the surgeon should attempt to preserve length. Essentially the longer the forearm stump, the better the degree of rotation.
- In trauma work the flaps are dictated by the local damage to the soft tissues of the forearm, but ideally equal anterior and posterior flaps should be used (see Fig. 37-4B).
- As with all amputations, the level of bone transection is proximal to the level of soft tissue dissection to allow the soft tissues to be closed without tension.

Elbow Disarticulation

- The advantage of elbow disarticulation over an above-elbow amputation is that the prosthesis can be fitted better over the humeral condyles.
- Flap cover depends on local damage, but equal anterior and posterior flaps (see Fig. 37-4C) are a good way of closing the soft tissues over the stump.

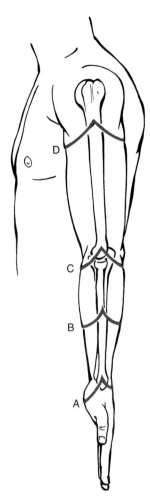

Figure 37-4   Amputation levels in the arm. See text for explanation.

Above-Elbow Amputation

- As with below-elbow amputation, the surgeon should strive to preserve length where possible.
  - Split thickness skin grafting or free flap cover can be used where necessary.
- It is important to try to preserve the proximal humerus and therefore the shape of the shoulder, and ideally the bone cut should be below the level of axilla.
- More proximal amputations function as a shoulder disarticulation with no shoulder mobility.
- Flap cover depends on available tissue but as with other upper limb amputations, equal anterior and posterior flaps can be used (see Fig. 37-4D).

Lower Limb Amputations

- Amputations of the lower limb are much more commonly performed than amputations of the upper limb.
  - They are usually performed because of severe injury to the leg that has frequently been caused by road traffic accidents, falls from a height, or work-related injuries.
- Today most amputations follow Gustilo type IIIb or IIIc fractures, and the incidence of amputation following a closed or Gustilo type I, II, or IIIa fracture should be extremely low.

BOX 37-4 ABSOLUTE AND RELATIVE INDICATIONS FOR AMPUTATION

Absolute Indications
Avulsed lower extremity
Unreconstructable bone damage
Severe soft tissue destruction
Warm ischemia time >6 hr

Relative Indications
Age
Gustilo IIIb or IIIc fracture in a multiply injured patient
Severe damage to ipsilateral foot
Femoral or posterior tibial nerve transaction
Major soft tissue loss
Uncontrollable hemorrhage (coagulopathy)
Poor prefracture function
Prefracture medical comorbidities
Soft tissue infection
Osteomyelitis

■ With improved orthopaedic surgery, plastic surgery and vascular surgery many limbs can be salvaged, but it is questionable whether limb salvage is always in the patient's best interest.

■ A modern lightweight below-knee prosthesis may allow a patient to return to virtually normal function 6 weeks after a Gustilo type IIIb or IIIc fracture, but the sequential reconstructive pathway of bone resection, bone transport, and grafting may take several years and still result in a dysfunctional leg.

■ The few absolute indications for amputation are straightforward. A number of relative indications need to be considered (Box 37-4), but they must be interpreted carefully.

■ Age by itself is not an indication for amputation, but increasing age does increase the relevance of the other indications.

   ■ In older patients, circumferential degloving or uncontrollable hemorrhage because of a coagulopathy in a multiply injured patient may well be an indication for amputation, whereas they would not be in a younger patient.

■ It must be emphasized that the indications in Box 37-4 are relative, and frequently more than one will need to be present to suggest that amputation is the best course of action.

   ■ A Gustilo IIIb fracture in an elderly patient with preexisting peripheral vascular disease or diabetes mellitus who mobilizes poorly might well benefit from amputation rather than a prolonged limb reconstruction program.

■ If amputation is thought to be the best course of action, it should be performed early.

■ Once a program of reconstruction has been started, it is difficult for both patient and surgeon to make the decision to amputate.

   ■ Failure to do so ensures a lengthy, costly program of multiple hospital admissions and operations, which may prove physically, psychologically, and financially expensive for the patient.

■ As has already been pointed out, the predictive scoring systems are not adequate to allow an accurate prediction of the need for amputation. The decision has to be made by the surgeon in consultation with the patient and an experienced colleague.

■ A review of the literature is interesting in that it tends to point to amputation having a similar functional outcome when compared to limb reconstruction.

■ Most of the studies are retrospective, and it is very difficult to compare the severity of injury among different studies.

■ Good evidence indicates that amputations are associated with a reduced hospitalization time, fewer surgical procedures, and less hospitalization costs.

■ Few studies take into account the long-term cost of prostheses, and if this is done it is probable that amputation is actually as expensive as limb reconstruction.

   ■ Financial considerations should be secondary to patient function, and it is interesting to note that patients with amputations seem to do as well as patients in whom limb reconstruction is undertaken.

■ A prospective analysis of 569 patients with severe leg trauma carried out by the LEAP study group in the United States has shown that soft tissue injury is the most important determinant of amputation. The 2-year outcomes from amputations were equivalent to those of patients who had had limb reconstruction.

   ■ This suggests that although limbs capable of being reconstructed should be, amputation is a reasonable alternative in those limbs in which reconstruction is going to be very difficult and prolonged.

Level of Amputation

■ As with the upper limb, it is important to conserve as much length as possible in lower limb amputation.

   ■ Examination of the metabolic cost of walking with a lower limb amputation shows that the higher the amputation, the lower the velocity of walking and the greater the energy required.

   ■ Below-knee amputees expend approximately 25% more energy in walking on the level than able-bodied people.

■ It has also been shown that the average velocity of patients with a below-knee amputation is 87% of normal compared with 63% of normal if the patient has an above-knee amputation.

   ■ Above-knee amputees inevitably adjust their lifestyle to cope with the greater metabolic demands placed on them, but functionally they are very restricted compared with below-knee amputees.

■ It is therefore very important that surgeons strive to obtain a below-knee amputation even if it means using plastic surgery techniques to gain length.

■ It is also important that surgeons do not convert a below-knee amputation to an above-knee amputation without good cause.

Toe Amputations

■ Toe amputations are very similar to finger amputations.

■ The maintenance of length is less important than obtaining good soft tissue cover.

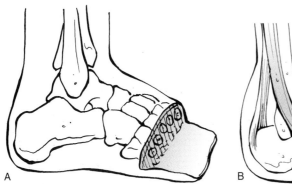 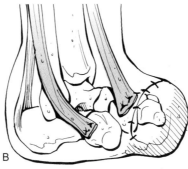 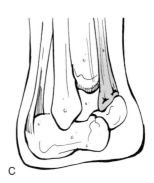

A   B   C

Figure 37-5   Three types of foot amputation. (**A**) Transmetatarsal amputation. (**B**) Tarsometatarsal amputation. (**C**) Midtarsal amputation. See text for explanation.

- Flap cover is dictated by the location and quality of the remaining soft tissues, but ideally a long plantar flap or plantar and dorsal flaps should be used (Fig. 37-1A and B).
- If two flaps are used, the plantar flap should be longer than the dorsal flap to ensure that the scar is away from the weight-bearing surface.
- A long dorsal flap should not be used because the scar will tend to bear weight and a hooked toenail may occur.
- It is easiest to amputate the smaller toes through an interphalangeal joint, but if possible length should be conserved in the hallux, although not at the expense of soft tissue cover.
- The functional impairment of losing the hallux is relatively mild and consists of a mild decrease in walking stability during the terminal stance phase of gait.
- When amputating the second toe, it is advisable to try and retain length of the proximal phalanx because it helps minimize the drift of the hallux toward the third toe.
- If the fifth toe is amputated, it is better to cut the metatarsal neck obliquely to preserve the shape of the foot.

Midfoot Amputations

- Midfoot amputations are rarely performed for trauma but are very useful.
  - They allow weight bearing without a prosthesis, although shoe modification is usually required.
- The stump is usually comfortable, and good long-term function is the rule, provided the correct surgical technique is used.
- It is important to preserve as much midfoot length as possible, provided there is good soft tissue cover.
- All midfoot amputations tend to be associated with an equinus deformity, and the shorter the midfoot stump the more the tendency to equinus.
- There are three types of midfoot amputation: the transmetatarsal amputation, the tarsometatarsal amputation through Lisfranc's joint, and the midtarsal amputation through Chopart's joint (Fig. 37-5).
- The problem with all these amputations is that the hindfoot tends to go into equinus because of the unopposed action of gastrocnemius and soleus.
- To compensate, it is advisable to suture the tendon of tibialis anterior into the dorsal surface of the remaining hindfoot.

- The tendon of peroneus brevis should be sutured to the lateral aspect of the remaining hindfoot.
- It is also advisable to undertake a tendo-Achilles lengthening, and the combination of this and the muscle transfers tends to maintain the plantargrade position of the hindfoot.
  - Ideally, a long plantar flap should be used, sutured over the end of the stump to keep the scar away from the weight-bearing surface.

Ankle Disarticulation

- Ankle disarticulation, or Syme's amputation, was initially popularized because it provided an end-bearing stump, although the leg was slightly short.
  - It became less popular as prostheses improved, although a good prosthesis can be fitted over a Syme's amputation.
- Most surgeons would probably now treat a severe injury of the hindfoot with a below-knee amputation, although there are some advantages to Syme's amputation.
- Early weight bearing is allowed and patients require little, if any, gait retraining.
- The amputation is probably used most commonly for the treatment of diabetic and vascular foot problems, but is still useful for the management of severe hindfoot trauma.
- The operative technique is straightforward, and the skin flaps and bone cuts are illustrated in Fig. 37-6.
- It is important that the heel pad be in good condition to allow weight bearing on the stump.
- The calcaneus and talus are resected as are the lateral and medial malleoli.
- Care must be taken not to damage the posterior tibial artery because it supplies the heel skin.
- The suture line is situated anterior and proximal to the weight-bearing area.

Below-Knee Amputation

- Below-knee amputations are the most common amputations that most orthopaedic surgeons have to perform.
- There are two commonly used methods of undertaking a below-knee amputation. The first is the use of a long posterior myocutaneous flap (Fig. 37-7A), and the second involves the use of two equal anterior and posterior flaps (Fig. 37-7B).

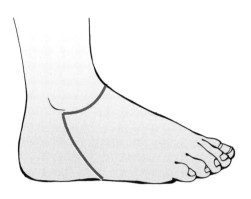
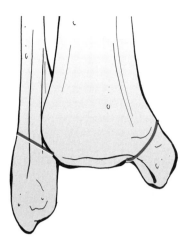

Figure 37-6 The skin flaps and areas of bone resection in a Syme's amputation.

- A variant of the latter technique is the use of two skew flaps, which are anteromedial and posterolateral fasciocutaneous flaps.
- In traumatic situations it is often impossible to use a long posterior myocutaneous flap because the soft tissues are severely damaged, and frequently the surgeon has to use whatever soft tissue is available.
- The tibia should be cut about 12 to 15 cm distal to the knee joint with the fibula cut 1 to 1.5 cm shorter.
- Modern prosthetic fitting allows for a shorter tibial stump, and the tibia can be cut as proximal as just below the tibial tuberosity.
  - Under these circumstances, the fibula should be excised to narrow the amputation stump. The anterior aspect of the distal tibia should be beveled at about 45 to 60 degrees to minimize pressure on the overlying soft tissues.

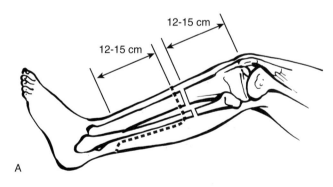
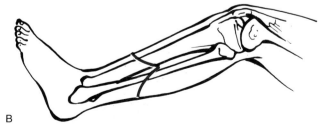

Figure 37-7 Two types of below-knee amputation. (**A**) This technique uses a long posterior myocutaneous flap. (**B**) Two equal anterior and posterior flaps are used.

- If a long posterior myocutaneous flap is used, the gastrocnemius should be sutured to the front of the tibia. The skin must not be closed under tension.
- Where possible, the surgeon should preserve the length of a below-knee amputation stump. A number of techniques allow a patient to have a below-knee amputation rather than an above-knee amputation.
- Good results have been reported with the use of microvascular free flaps, although the surgery is complex and time consuming and some patients are troubled with skin breakdown.
- A second option is to use the skin of the sole of the foot to cover the amputation stump if the skin of the sole of the foot is intact.
  - Ideally, the skin should be transferred with an intact neurovascular supply to maintain the stump.
  - If this is not possible, the skin can be transferred, using microvascular techniques, as a free flap. The advantage of this technique is that length is preserved and the patient has tough heel skin on the amputation stump.
- A third alternative is to use a turn-up flap (Fig. 37-8). If there is extensive damage to the proximal tibia and fibula such that an amputation is required, the distal tibia can be turned upward using a long posterior myocutaneous flap.
  - This unusual technique may be helpful in preserving limb length.

Knee Disarticulation

- Today it is possible to fit a below-knee prosthesis to a below-knee amputation stump where the tibia has been cut just below the tibial tuberosity.
  - Thus undertaking a knee disarticulation over a below-knee amputation has no advantages.
- A knee disarticulation does confer some advantages over an above-knee amputation.
  - The stump is end bearing and requires less energy to walk than with an above-knee prosthesis.
  - The skin flaps are essentially those of the below-knee amputation with a long posterior myocutaneous flap or anterior and posterior skin flaps used.

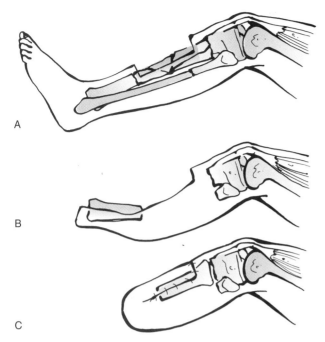

Figure 37-8   Diagram of a turn-up flap. See text for details.

Above-Knee Amputation

- Ideally an above-knee amputation should be undertaken using a medial, adductor-based myocutaneous flap (Fig. 37-9).
- This allows the adductors to be passed around the distal femur and sutured to the bone.
- Thus the thigh does not drift into abduction as it tends to with the conventional above-knee amputation using anterior and posterior flaps and cutting the muscles around the end of the amputated femur.
- This results in an "adductor lurch" gait pattern associated with high-energy consumption.
- In trauma cases the distal soft tissues of the thigh may well be damaged, and it is not always possible to use an adductor-based myocutaneous flap.

Hip Disarticulation

- Hip disarticulation is very rarely required in trauma cases. The main indications are severe damage to the groin with massive injury to the vessels or nerves or a severe crush injury to the thigh resulting in thigh muscle necrosis.
- Ideally, a racquet incision is used and the gluteal muscles with the overlying buttock skin are preserved to close the disarticulation defect.
- In severe trauma this may not be possible, and the skin flaps are based on whichever local muscles are preserved.

COMPLICATIONS

- Because traumatic amputations often do not permit the use of the ideal flap, patients do complain of stump pain and difficulty in fitting and wearing prostheses.

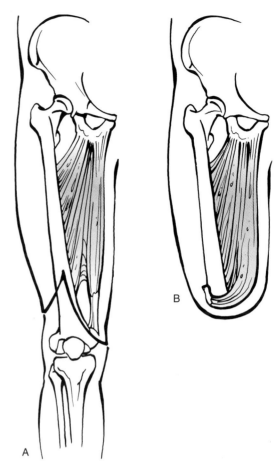

Figure 37-9   Above-knee amputation. See text for details.

- Modern prosthetic management has improved markedly, however, and usually traumatic amputees can be accommodated successfully.
- Phantom pain is a common problem with all amputations.
- There may be a wide spectrum of symptoms from the sensation of feeling the absent limb through to burning dysesthesia. Patients who do not experience phantom pain soon after amputation tend not to experience it later.
- The symptoms usually settle down about 3 to 6 months after amputation, but in those in which phantom pain persists, medication is rarely useful.
- The other main complication associated with amputations is the development of neuromas.
- The best treatment is prevention, and the cut nerve ends should be buried deep in the soft tissues away from the pressure areas and the scar.
- If symptoms from a neuroma occur, excision can be carried out.

SUGGESTED READING

Bonanni F, Rhodes M, Lucke JF. The futility of predictive scoring of mangled lower extremities. J Trauma 1993;34:99–104.
Bosse MJ, MacKenzie EJ, Kellam JF, et al. An analysis of outcomes of reconstruction or amputation after leg-threatening injuries. N Engl J Med 2002;347:1924–1931.

Bowker JH, San Giovanni TP, Pinzur MS. North American experience with knee disarticulation with use of a posterior myofasciocutaneous flap. Healing rate and functional results in seventy-seven patients. J Bone Joint Surg (Am) 2000;82:1571–1574.

Dirschl DR, Dahners LE. The mangled extremity: when should it be amputated? J Am Acad Othop Surg 1998;12:460–463.

Fairhurst MJ. The function of below-knee amputee versus the patient with salvaged grade III tibial fracture. Clin Orthop 1994;301: 227–232.

Gottschalk FA. Traumatic amputations. In: Bucholz RW, Heckman JD, eds. Rockwood and Green's fractures in adults, 5th ed. Philadelphia: Lippincott Williams & Wilkins, 2001.

Johansen K, Daines M, Howey T, et al. Objective criteria accurately predict amputation following lower extremity trauma. J Trauma 1990;30:568–572.

Lange RH. Limb reconstruction versus amputation decision making in massive lower extremity trauma. Clin Orthop 1989;243:92–99.

Louis DS, Jebson PJL, Graham TJ. Amputations. In: Green DP, Hotchkiss RN, Peterson WC, eds. Green's operative hand surgery, 4th ed. New York: Churchill Livingstone, 1999.

MacKenzie EJ, Bosse MJ, Castillo RC, et al. Functional outcomes following trauma-related lower-extremity amputation. J Bone Joint Surg (Am) 2004;86:1636–1645.

McCarthy ML, MacKenzie EJ, Edwin D, et al. Psychological distress associated with severe lower-limb injury. J Bone Joint Surg (Am) 2003;85:1689–1697.

Pinzur MS. Amputations in trauma. In: Browner BD, Jupiter JB, Levine AM, et al., eds. Skeletal trauma, 3rd ed. Philadelphia: WB Saunders, 2003.

Pinzur MS, Angelats JK, Light TR, et al. Functional outcome following traumatic upper limb amputation and prosthetic limb fitting. J Hand Surg (Am) 1994;19:836–839.

Pozo JL, Powell B, Andrews BG, et al. The timing of amputation for lower limb trauma. J Bone Joint Surg (Br) 1990;72:288–292.

Swiontkowski MF, MacKenzie EJ, Bosse MJ, et al. Factors influencing the decision to amputate or reconstruct after high-energy lower extremity trauma. J Trauma 2002;52:641–649.

Woo SH, Kim JS, Seul JH. Immediate toe-to-hand transfer in acute hand injuries: overall results, compared with results for elective cases. Plast Reconstr Surg 2004;113:882–892.

ACUTE COMPARTMENT SYNDROME

Acute compartment syndrome occurs when pressure rises within a confined space in the body, resulting in a critical reduction of the blood flow to the tissues contained within the space. Without urgent decompression, tissue ischemia, necrosis, and functional impairment occur. The acute compartment syndrome should be differentiated from other related conditions (Table 38-1). The current controversies associated with acute compartment syndrome are detailed in Box 38-1.

SURGICAL ANATOMY

Leg

The four leg compartments and their contents are listed in Table 38-2, along with the signs of acute compartment syndrome in each compartment. Their relationship to each other and the other structures in the leg can be seen in Figure 27-1 in Chapter 27.

Foot

There are four main compartments in the foot, medial, central, lateral, and interosseous. These can be subdivided into two central compartments, a separate adductor hallucis compartment and four separate compartments for the interosseous muscles, making a total of nine compartments (Table 38-3). The deep central or calcaneal compartment communicates with the deep posterior compartment of the leg. The barrier between the superficial central and calcaneal compartments is thought to become incompetent at a pressure of 10 mm Hg. In practice, therefore, it is probably sufficient, especially in forefoot injuries, to decompress the interosseous, medial, lateral, and central compartments, usually through dorsal incisions (Fig. 38-1). In hindfoot injuries, the calcaneal, medial, and superficial central compartments can be decompressed through a medial incision from behind the heel extending distally. The clinical diagnosis of acute compartment syndrome should be suspected in the presence of severe swelling, but differentiating the affected compartments is extremely difficult.

Thigh

The thigh contains the three main compartments listed in Table 38-4 and illustrated in Figure 23-1 in Chapter 23.

TABLE 38-1 DEFINITIONS OF CONDITIONS ASSOCIATED WITH ACUTE COMPARTMENT SYNDROME

Condition	Definition
Acute compartment syndrome	Raised ICP to a level requiring decompression to prevent muscle necrosis
Volkmann's ischemic contracture	The end stage of acute compartment syndrome with muscle necrosis and contracture
Exertional compartment syndrome	Raised ICP during exercise causing ischemic muscle pain; resolves with rest
Crush syndrome	Systemic effects of muscle necrosis caused by prolonged compression of a muscle group or groups

ICP, intracompartmental pressure.

BOX 38-1 CURRENT CONTROVERSIES ASSOCIATED WITH ACUTE COMPARTMENT SYNDROME

The role of monitoring versus clinical diagnosis of acute compartment syndrome
The pressure threshold for decompression
Double-incision versus single-incision fasciotomy in the leg
Techniques of closure: gradual closure versus split skin grafting
The role of fasciotomy when muscle necrosis is inevitable

TABLE 38-2 COMPARTMENTS OF THE LEG, THEIR CONTENTS, AND THE CLINICAL SIGNS OF ACUTE COMPARTMENT SYNDROME

Compartment	Contents	Signs
Anterior	Tibialis anterior Extensor digitorum longus Extensor hallucis longus Peroneus tertius Anterior tibial nerve and vessels	Pain, passive flexion ankle/toes Numbness, first web space Weakness, ankle/toe flexion
Lateral	Peroneus longus Peroneus brevis Superficial peroneal nerve	Pain, passive foot inversion Numbness, dorsum of foot Weakness, eversion
Superficial posterior	Gastrocnemius Soleus Plantaris Sural nerve	Pain, passive ankle extension Numbness, dorsolateral foot Weakness, plantar flexion
Deep posterior	Tibialis posterior Flexor digitorum longus Flexor hallucis longus Posterior tibial nerve	Pain, passive ankle/toe extension/ foot eversion Numbness, sole of foot Weakness, toe/ankle flexion, foot inversion

TABLE 38-3 COMPARTMENTS OF THE FOOT AND THEIR CONTENTS

Compartment	Contents
Medial	Intrinsic muscles of the great toe
Lateral	Flexor digiti minimi Abductor digiti minimi
Central	
Superficial	Flexor digitorum brevis
Deep (calcaneal)	Quadratus plantae
Adductor hallucis	Adductor hallucis
Interosseous × 4	Interosseous muscles Digital nerves

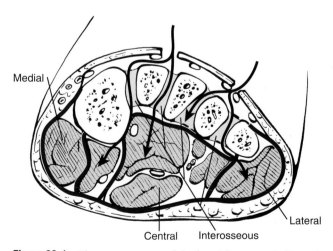

Figure 38-1 The compartments of the foot. The arrows indicate the fasciotomies required for adequate decompression.

Forearm

The forearm contains three compartments: volar, dorsal, and "the mobile wad" (see Fig. 15-1 in Chapter 15). The compartments are listed in Table 38-5 along with their contents and the clinical signs of acute compartment syndrome. It has been suggested that the volar compartment of the forearm contains three spaces, the superficial volar, deep volar, and pronator quadratus spaces, but in practice it is not usually necessary to distinguish among these at fasciotomy. Volar compartment syndrome can cause characteristic wrist and finger flexor spasm.

Hand

It is generally considered that the hand has ten muscle compartments: one thenar, one hypothenar, one adductor pollicis, four dorsal interosseous, and three volar interosseous compartments (Fig. 38-2). Their contents are listed in Table 38-6. As in the foot, differentiation clinically among the affected compartments is extremely difficult. There may be stretch pain involving the intrinsic muscles and intrinsic paralysis. The volar interosseous compartments lie on the volar aspect of the metacarpals, but it is unlikely these are functionally separate from the dorsal interosseous compartments because the tissue barrier between the two cannot withstand pressures of more than 15 mm Hg.

Arm

The compartments of the arm, their contents, and clinical signs of acute compartment syndrome are detailed in Table 38-7. The anatomy of the arm is shown in Figure 12-1 in Chapter 12.

TABLE 38-4 COMPARTMENTS OF THE THIGH, THEIR CONTENTS, AND SIGNS OF ACUTE COMPARTMENT SYNDROME

Compartment	Contents	Signs
Anterior	Quadriceps muscles Sartorius Femoral nerve	Pain, passive knee flexion Numbness, medial leg/foot Weakness, knee extension
Posterior	Hamstring muscles Sciatic nerve	Pain, passive knee extension Sensory changes rare Weakness, knee flexion
Adductor	Adductor muscles Obturator nerve	Pain, passive hip abduction Sensory changes rare Weakness, hip adduction

TABLE 38-5 COMPARTMENTS OF THE FOREARM, THEIR CONTENTS, AND THE SIGNS OF ACUTE COMPARTMENT SYNDROME

Compartment	Contents	Signs
Volar	Flexor carpi radialis longus and brevis Flexor digitorum superficialis and profundus Pronator teres Pronator quadratus Median nerve Ulnar nerve	Pain, passive wrist/finger extension Numbness, median/ulnar distribution Weakness, wrist/finger flexion Weakness, median/ulnar motor function in hand
Dorsal	Extensor digitorum Extensor pollicis longus Abductor pollicis longus Extensor carpi ulnaris	Pain, passive wrist/finger flexion Weakness, wrist/finger flexion
Mobile wad	Brachioradialis Extensor carpi radialis brevis and longus Superficial branch radial nerve	Pain, passive wrist flexion/elbow extension Weakness, wrist extension/elbow flexion

TABLE 38-6 COMPARTMENTS OF THE HAND AND THEIR CONTENTS

Compartment	Contents
Thenar	Abductor pollicis brevis Flexor pollicis brevis Opponens pollicis
Hypothenar	Abductor digiti minimi Flexor digiti minimi Opponens digiti minimi
Dorsal interosseous × 4	Dorsal interossei
Volar interossei × 3	Volar interossei
Adductor pollicis	Adductor pollicis

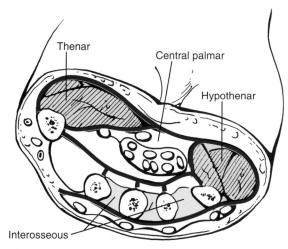

Figure 38-2   The compartments of the hand.

TABLE 38-8 EPIDEMIOLOGY OF ACUTE COMPARTMENT SYNDROME

Average age	32 y
Men/women	90%/10%
Distribution	Type B
Incidence	$3.1/10^5/y$
Causes	
Motor vehicle accident	21.4%
Sport	20.1%
Crush	9.8%
Fall	9.2%
Underlying conditions	
Tibial fracture	36%
Soft tissue injury	23.2%
Distal radius fracture	9.8%
Crush syndrome	7.9%
Forearm fracture	7.9%

EPIDEMIOLOGY

Knowledge of the epidemiology of acute compartment syndrome is important to define the patient at risk of developing the condition and therefore allow prompt diagnosis and treatment, which is the key to a successful outcome. The epidemiology of all cases of acute compartment syndrome is shown in Table 38-8.

The most common reason for the development of acute compartment syndrome is a fracture in around 70% of cases. The most common fracture implicated is the tibial diaphyseal fracture. The epidemiology of acute compartment syndrome associated with tibial fracture is detailed in Table 38-9.

About 30% of all cases of acute compartment syndrome occur in the absence of fracture with over 20% following soft tissue injury (see Table 38.8). These patients tend to be older and have more medical comorbidities than those with a fracture. The epidemiology of this group is detailed in Table 38-10.

The second most common fracture complicated by acute compartment syndrome is the fracture of the distal radius. The demographics of the patients with distal radius

fractures complicated by acute compartment syndrome are very different from the general population sustaining distal radius fractures who are usually middle aged to elderly women with an average age of 55 years. The epidemiology of acute compartment syndrome complicating distal radius fracture is shown in Table 38-11. Other less common causes of acute compartment syndrome are listed in Box 38-2.

It is now recognized that from adolescence, younger patients are at more risk of compartment syndrome. In tibial diaphyseal fracture, the prevalence of acute compartment syndrome is three times higher in the under-35-year-old age group, and in distal radial fractures, the prevalence is 35 times less in the older age group. Male gender is also a risk factor.

High-energy injury is generally believed to increase the risks of developing an acute compartment syndrome. However, in a study of tibial diaphyseal fractures complicated by acute compartment syndrome, the proportion of high- and low-energy injuries showed a slight preponderance of low-energy injuries. In the same population were an equal number of high-energy and low-energy injuries in tibial diaphyseal fractures uncomplicated by acute compartment syndrome. This suggests that acute compartment syndrome

TABLE 38-7 COMPARTMENTS OF THE ARM, THEIR CONTENTS, AND CLINICAL SIGNS OF ACUTE COMPARTMENT SYNDROME

Compartment	Contents	Signs
Anterior	Biceps	Pain, passive elbow extension
	Brachialis	Numbness, median/ulnar distribution
	Coracobrachialis	Weakness, elbow flexion
	Median nerve	Weakness, median/ulnar motor function
	Ulnar nerve	
	Musculocutaneous nerve	
	Radial nerve (distal third)	
Posterior	Triceps	Pain, passive elbow flexion
	Radial nerve	Numbness, ulnar/radial distribution
	Ulnar nerve (distally)	Weakness, elbow extension
		Weakness, radial/ulnar motor function

TABLE 38-9 EPIDEMIOLOGY OF ACUTE COMPARTMENT SYNDROME COMPLICATING TIBIAL DIAPHYSEAL FRACTURE

Average age	30 y
Men/women	93%/7%
Distribution	Type B
Prevalence	
Closed fractures	4.3%–7%
Open fractures	3.3%–9.1%
Incidence	
Men	$6.9/10^5/y$
Women	$0.2/10^5/y$
Compartment involved	
Anterior	100%
Lateral	40.7%
Deep posterior	40%
Superficial posterior	30.5%

TABLE 38-10 EPIDEMIOLOGY OF ACUTE COMPARTMENT SYNDROME BECAUSE OF SOFT TISSUE INJURY[a]

Age	36 y
Men/women	84%/16%
Distribution	Type G
Incidence	
Men	$3.7/10^5/y$
Women	$0.3/10^5/y$
Compartments involved	
Lower leg	53%
Forearm	24%
Thigh	15%
Foot	5%
Hand	2%

[a]Excludes patients with crush syndrome.

TABLE 38-11 EPIDEMIOLOGY OF ACUTE COMPARTMENT SYNDROME COMPLICATING DISTAL RADIUS FRACTURES

Average age	26 y
Men/women	94%/6%
Distribution	Type B
Incidence	
Men	$1.9/10^5/y$
Women	$0.05/10^5/y$
Prevalence	0.25%
Compartments involved	
Volar forearm	87.5%
Volar forearm/hand	6.25%
Hand	6.25%

BOX 38-2 UNDERLYING CAUSES OF ACUTE COMPARTMENT SYNDROME

Conditions increasing the volume of compartment contents
Fracture
Soft tissue injury
Crush syndrome (including use of the lithotomy position)
Revascularization
Exercise
Fluid infusion (including arthroscopy)
Arterial puncture
Ruptured ganglia/cysts
Osteotomy
Snake bite

Nephrotic syndrome
Leukemic infiltration
Viral myositis
Acute hematogenous osteomyelitis

Conditions reducing compartment volume
Burns
Repair of muscle hernia

Medical comorbidity
Diabetes
Hypothyroidism
Bleeding diathesis/ anticoagulants

BOX 38-3 RISK FACTORS FOR THE DEVELOPMENT OF ACUTE COMPARTMENT SYNDROME

- Youth
- Male gender
- Tibial fracture
- High-energy forearm fracture
- High-energy femoral diaphyseal fracture
- Bleeding diathesis/anticoagulants

may be more prevalent after low-energy injury in diaphyseal fractures, possibly because in low-energy injury the compartment boundaries are less likely to be disrupted, and an "autodecompression" effect is avoided. It is important to note that open tibial diaphyseal fractures remain at risk of acute compartment syndrome, which occurs in around 3%, but less severe open fractures are at more risk, possibly also because of the lack of disruption of the compartment boundaries.

However, metaphyseal fractures (e.g., distal radius fractures) associated with high-energy injury are more likely to be complicated by acute compartment syndrome, possibly because the energy of the injury is directed at the bone ends, leaving the compartments relatively intact. There is also a preponderance of young men sustaining these types of injury.

The likely explanation for the preponderance of young men with acute compartment syndrome is that they have relatively large muscle volumes, although their compartment size does not change after growth is complete. Thus young men may have less space for swelling of the muscle after injury. The older person presumably has smaller hypotrophic muscles, allowing more space for swelling. Hypertension may also have a protective effect in the older patient. The possible risk factors for the development of acute compartment syndrome are shown in Box 38-3.

PATHOGENESIS

The exact physiological mechanism of the reduction in blood flow in the acute compartment syndrome remains uncertain, although it is generally accepted that the effect is at the small-vessel level, either arteriolar, capillary, or venous levels. There are three main theories of how this occurs.

The critical closing pressure theory states there is a critical closing pressure in the small vessels when the transmural pressure (the difference between intravascular pressure and tissue pressure) drops. Transmural pressure (TM) is balanced by a constricting force (TC) consisting of active and elastic tension derived from smooth muscle action in the vessel walls. The equilibrium between expanding and contracting forces is expressed in a derivation of Laplace's law:

$$TM = TC \div r \quad \text{where r is the radius of the vessel}$$

If because of increasing tissue pressure the transmural pressure drops to a level such that elastic fibers in the vessel wall are no longer stretched and therefore cannot contribute any elastic tension, then there will be no further automatic decrease in the radius. $TC \div r$ then becomes greater than TM, and active closure of the vessel occurs. This concept has been verified in both animal and human local vascular beds. Critics of this theory doubt the possibility of maintaining arteriolar closure in the presence of ischemia, which is a strong local stimulus for vasodilatation.

A second theory is the arteriovenous (AV) gradient theory. According to this theory, the increases in local tissue pressure reduce the local AV pressure gradient and thus reduce blood flow. When flow diminishes to less than the metabolic demands of the tissues (not necessarily to zero), functional abnormalities result. The relationship between AV gradient and the local blood flow (LBF) is summarized in this equation:

$$LBF = (Pa - Pv) \div R$$

where Pa is the local arterial pressure, Pv is the local venous pressure, and R is the local vascular resistance. Veins are collapsible tubes, and the pressure within them can never be less than the local tissue pressure. If tissue pressure rises as it does in the acute compartment syndrome, the Pv must rise also, thus reducing the AV gradient (Pa − Pv) and therefore the local blood flow. The arteriovenous gradient is also reduced by elevation of the limb in the presence of raised tissue pressure.

A third theory, the microvascular occlusion theory, postulates that capillary occlusion is the main mechanism reducing blood flow in acute compartment syndrome. Capillary pressure in the presence of normal tissue pressures is 25 mm Hg, and a tissue pressure of similar value should be sufficient to reduce capillary blood flow. Resultant muscle ischemia leads to increased capillary membrane permeability to plasma proteins, increasing edema and obstruction of lymphatic channels by the raised tissue pressure.

Effects of Raised Tissue Pressure on Muscle

Regardless of the mechanism of vessel closure, reduction in blood flow in the acute compartment syndrome has a profound effect on muscle tissue. Skeletal muscle is the tissue in the extremities most vulnerable to ischemia and therefore the most important tissue to be considered in acute compartment syndrome. Both the magnitude and duration of pressure elevation have been shown to be important influences in the extent of muscle damage.

The importance of perfusion pressure in the reduction of muscle blood flow is now generally acknowledged. Experimental evidence supports the concept that the critical pressure threshold for muscle ischemia is 10 to 20 mm Hg below diastolic blood pressure or 25 to 30 mm Hg below mean blood pressure, with increased vulnerability in previously traumatized or ischemic muscle.

The ultimate result of reduced blood flow to skeletal muscle is ischemia followed by necrosis, with general agreement that increasing periods of complete ischemia produce increasing irreversible changes. Muscle necrosis is present in its greatest extent in the central position of the muscle, and therefore external evaluation of the degree of muscle necrosis is unreliable. The duration of muscle ischemia dictates the amount of necrosis, although some muscle fibers are more vulnerable than others to ischemia. For example, the muscles of the anterior compartment of the leg contain type 1 fibers, or red slow twitch fibers, and the gastrocnemius contains mainly type 2, or white fast twitch fibers. Type 1 fibers depend on oxidative metabolism of triglycerides for their energy source and are more vulnerable to oxygen depletion than type 2 fibers whose metabolism is primarily anerobic. This may explain the particular vulnerability of the anterior compartment to raised intracompartmental pressure.

Effects of Raised Tissue Pressure on Nerve

There is little dispute about the effects of raised tissue pressure on neurological function. Loss of neuromuscular function occurs with raised tissue pressures but at varying pressure thresholds and duration. The mechanism of damage to nerve is as yet uncertain and could result from ischemia, ischemia plus compression, toxic effects, or the effects of acidosis.

Effects of Raised Tissue Pressure on Bone

Nonunion is now recognized as a complication of acute compartment syndrome. It was first suggested over 60 years ago that "Volkmann's disease" caused obliteration of the "musculodiaphyseal" vessels and caused frequent pseudarthrosis. More recent experimental work has shown a reduction in bone blood flow and bone union in rabbit tibiae after an experimentally induced acute compartment syndrome. It is likely that muscle ischemia reduces the capacity for development of the extraosseous blood supply on which long bones depend for healing.

Reperfusion Injury

The reperfusion syndrome is a group of complications following reestablishment of blood flow to the ischemic tissues and can occur after fasciotomy and restoration of muscle blood flow in the acute compartment syndrome. Reperfusion is followed by an inflammatory response in the ischemic tissue that can cause further tissue damage. The trigger for the inflammatory response is probably the breakdown products of muscle. Some breakdown products are procoagulants that activate the intrinsic clotting system. This results in increasing microvascular thrombosis, which in turn increases the extent of muscle damage.

If there is a large amount of muscle involved in the ischemic process, the inflammatory response may become systemic. In acute compartment syndrome, this is most likely to occur in the crush syndrome. Procoagulants escape into the systemic circulation and produce systemic coagulopathy with parallel activation of inflammatory mediators. These then damage vascular endothelium leading to increased permeability and subsequent multiple organ failure. Systemic clotting and the breakdown products of dead and dying cells also lead to activation of white blood cells with the release of additional inflammatory mediators such as histamine, interleukin, oxygen free radicals, thromboxane, and many others. This is the basis for the use of agents such as antioxidants, antithromboxanes, antileucotrines, and antiplatelet activating factors that modify the inflammatory process. Some of these agents have been shown capable of reducing muscle injury in the laboratory.

DIAGNOSIS

Prompt diagnosis of acute compartment syndrome is the key to a successful outcome. Delay in diagnosis may occur because of inexperience and lack of awareness of the possibility of acute compartment syndrome, an indefinite and confusing clinical presentation, or to anesthetic or analgesic techniques that mask the clinical signs and have long been recognized as the single most common cause of failure to treat acute compartment syndrome. The factors associated with a late diagnosis of compartment syndrome are listed in Box 38-4.

Delay in treatment of the acute compartment syndrome can be catastrophic, leading to serious complications such as permanent sensory and motor deficits, contractures, infection, and, at times, amputation of the limb. In serious cases there may be systemic injury from the reperfusion syndrome. A clear understanding of the clinical techniques necessary to make an early diagnosis is therefore essential to any physician treating acute compartment syndrome.

History and Physical Examination

- The clinical symptoms and signs of acute compartment syndrome are detailed in Box 38-5.

- Pain, considered the first symptom of acute compartment syndrome, is usually severe and out of proportion to the clinical situation.
  - Pain can be very variable in its intensity, may be absent in acute compartment syndrome associated with nerve injury, or minimal in the deep posterior or foot compartment syndrome.
  - Pain is present in most cases because of the index injury but cannot be elicited in the unconscious patient and is difficult to evaluate in children.
  - Increasing analgesic requirements should raise the suspicion of the presence of an acute compartment syndrome.
  - Pain has been shown to have a sensitivity of only 19% and a specificity of 97% in the diagnosis of acute compartment syndrome (i.e., a high proportion of false-negative or missed cases but a low proportion of false-positive cases).
- Pain with passive stretch of the muscles involved is recognized as a symptom of acute compartment syndrome.
  - Pain is increased, for example, in an anterior compartment syndrome when the toes or foot are plantarflexed.
  - The sensitivity and specificity of pain on passive stretch are similar to those for rest pain.
- Paraesthesia and hypoesthesia may occur in the territory of the nerves traversing the affected compartment and are usually the first sign of nerve ischemia.
  - Sensory abnormality may be caused by concomitant nerve injury.
  - Sensory changes have a sensitivity of 13% and specificity of 98% in acute compartment syndrome, an unacceptably high false-negative rate.
- Paralysis of muscle groups affected by the acute compartment syndrome is recognized as a late sign.
  - This sign has an equally low sensitivity as others in predicting the presence of acute compartment syndrome, probably because of the difficulty of interpreting the underlying cause of the weakness.
  - This could be inhibition by pain, direct injury to muscle, or associated nerve injury.
  - It is recognized that if a motor deficit develops, full recovery is rare.
- Palpable swelling in the compartment affected can be a further sign of compartment syndrome.
  - The degree of swelling is difficult to assess accurately and may be obscured by casts or dressings.
  - Some compartments such as the deep posterior compartment of the leg are completely buried under other muscle compartments, obscuring any swelling.

■ Peripheral pulses and capillary return are always intact in acute compartment syndrome unless there is major arterial injury or disease or in the very late stages of acute compartment syndrome when amputation is inevitable.

   ■ If acute compartment syndrome is suspected and pulses are absent, arteriography is indicated.

   ■ Conversely, it is dangerous to exclude the diagnosis of acute compartment syndrome because distal pulses are present.

■ Using a combination of clinical symptoms and signs increases their sensitivity as diagnostic tools.

■ To achieve a probability of over 90% of acute compartment syndrome being present, three clinical findings must be noted.

■ The third clinical finding is paresis; thus to achieve an accurate clinical diagnosis of acute compartment syndrome, the condition has to be allowed to progress until a late stage.

   ■ This is clearly unacceptable and has led to a search for earlier, more reliable methods of diagnosis.

Compartment Pressure Monitoring

■ Intracompartmental pressure (ICP) can be measured using a number of techniques. The advantages and disadvantages of each are shown in Table 38-12.

■ Because raised tissue pressure is the primary event in acute compartment syndrome, changes in ICP precede the clinical symptoms and signs.

■ ICP is usually monitored in the anterior compartment because it is most commonly involved in acute compartment syndrome and easily accessible.

   ■ There is then a risk of missing an acute compartment syndrome in the deep posterior compartment, but measuring two compartments is much more cumbersome.

■ If the anterior compartment alone is monitored, the surgeon must be aware of the small chance of deep posterior acute compartment syndrome and measure the deep posterior compartment pressures if there are unexplained symptoms in the presence of anterior compartment pressures with a safe differential pressure (ΔP).

■ It is important to measure the peak pressure within the limb, which usually occurs within 5 cm of the level of the fracture.

Threshold for Decompression

There has been much debate about the critical pressure threshold beyond which decompression of acute compartment syndrome is required. The debate initially centered around the use of tissue pressure alone as the indication for decompression. Tissue pressures believed critical ranged from 30 mm Hg to 50 mm Hg. Use of an ICP of 30 mm Hg as a threshold for decompression has been shown to result in an unacceptably high (29%) rate of fasciotomy in tibial fractures.

It is now recognized that apparent variation among individuals in their tolerance of raised ICP is due to variations in systemic blood pressure. This is expressed by measuring the ΔP between the diastolic blood pressure and the tissue pressure or between the mean blood pressure and the tissue pressure. There is good experimental evidence demonstrating inadequate perfusion and relative ischemia in muscle when the tissue pressure rises to within 20 to 30 mm Hg of the diastolic pressure or to within 30 to 40 mm Hg of the mean blood pressure.

Several clinical studies have been performed to test this hypothesis, concluding that a ΔP of 30 mm Hg, using the diastolic pressure, is a safe threshold for compartment decompression. This threshold may differ for children who have a low diastolic pressure and are therefore more likely to have a ΔP less than 30 mm Hg. In these circumstances, the use of the mean arterial pressure rather than the diastolic pressure is likely to be more accurate.

ICP monitoring in patients at risk of acute compartment syndrome reduces the delay to fasciotomy and permanent sequelae. It is important to consider the trend of the ΔP and the ICP and the duration of pressure elevation. For example, if the ΔP is at a critical level but the ICP is

TABLE 38-12 DIFFERENT METHODS OF ICP MEASUREMENT

	Advantages	Disadvantages	Accuracy
Slit catheter	Simple No infusion Inexpensive	Possible blockage by air bubbles	+++
Wick catheter	Simple No infusion Inexpensive	Possible blockage by air or blood clot	+++
Needle manometer	Inexpensive	Cumbersome Requires infusion Easily blocked	+
Solid state transducer intracompartmental catheter (STIC)	Simple	Requires infusion for continuous measurement Intermittent measurement labor intensive	+++
Electronic transducer-tipped catheter	Simple No infusion	Expensive Difficult to sterilize	+++

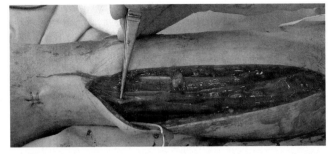

Figure 38-4   Anterior and lateral fasciotomy showing the superficial peroneal nerve.

dropping and the ΔP rising, it is safe to observe the patient in anticipation of the ΔP returning within a short time to safe levels. Fasciotomy should not be performed based on a single pressure reading except in extreme cases.

TREATMENT

- The single effective treatment for acute compartment syndrome is fasciotomy, which if delayed can cause devastating complications.
- Other preliminary measures should be taken in cases of impending acute compartment syndrome (Box 38-6).

Fasciotomy

- The basic principle of fasciotomy of any compartment is full, adequate, and prompt decompression.
- Skin incisions must be made along the full length of the affected compartment.
  - There is no place for limited or subcutaneous fasciotomy in acute compartment syndrome.
- It is essential to visualize all contained muscles in their entirety (Fig. 38-3) in order to assess their viability, and any muscle necrosis must be thoroughly debrided to avoid infection.
- In the leg, all four compartments should be released.
- One of the most commonly used techniques is the double-incision four-compartment fasciotomy.
- The anterior and lateral compartments are released through a lateral skin incision over the intermuscular septum between the compartments.

- The skin may then be retracted to allow fascial incisions over both compartments.
- Care must be taken not to injure the superficial peroneal nerve that pierces the fascia and lies superficial to it in the distal third of the leg (Fig. 38-4).
- There is considerable variation in its course, with approximately three quarters of nerves remaining in the lateral compartment prior to its exit through the deep fascia and one quarter passing into the anterior compartment.
- The two posterior compartments are accessed through a skin incision 2 cm from the medial edge of the tibia, allowing a generous skin bridge to the lateral incision but anterior to the posterior tibial artery, especially in open fractures, to protect perforating vessels that supply local fasciocutaneous flaps.
  - The superficial posterior compartment is easily exposed by skin retraction.
  - The deep posterior compartment is exposed by posterior retraction of the superficial compartment and most easily identified in the distal third of the leg (Fig. 38-5).
  - It is sometimes necessary to elevate the superficial compartment muscles from the tibia for a short distance to allow release of the deep posterior compartment along its length.
  - Care must be taken to protect the saphenous vein and nerve in this area and to protect the posterior tibial vessels and nerves.
- Single-incision four-compartment fasciotomy can be performed through a lateral incision, which affords easy

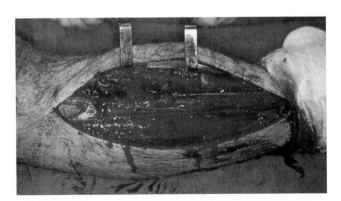

Figure 38-3   A fasciotomy showing a wide decompression.

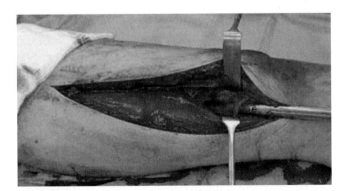

Figure 38-5   Decompression of the deep posterior compartment in the leg.

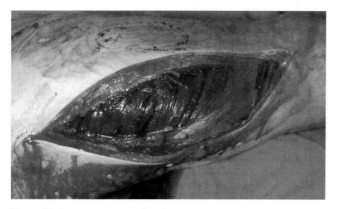

Figure 38-6 Decompression of the thigh through a single lateral incision.

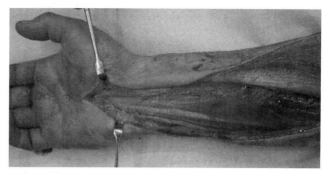

Figure 38-7 Fasciotomy of the forearm.

access to the anterior and lateral compartments, but access to the posterior compartments is more difficult with poorer visualization of the muscles than in the double-incision technique.

- In the thigh and gluteal regions, decompression is simple and the compartments easily visualized.
    - Both thigh compartments can be approached through a single lateral skin incision (Fig. 38-6), although a medial incision can be used over the adductors if considered necessary.
- In the foot there are a number of compartments to decompress, and a sound knowledge of the anatomy is essential.
    - Dorsal incisions overlying the second and fourth metacarpals allow sufficient access to the interosseous compartments and the central compartment that lies deep to the interosseous compartments (see Fig. 38-1).
    - The medial and lateral compartments can be accessed around the deep surfaces of the first and fifth metatarsal, respectively.
    - Such a decompression is usually sufficient in cases of forefoot injury, but when a hindfoot injury, especially a calcaneal fracture, is present, a separate medial incision may be required to decompress the calcaneal compartment.
- Fasciotomy of the arm is performed through anterior and posterior incisions when the compartments are easily visualized.
    - On rare occasions, the deltoid muscle should also be decompressed.
    - In the forearm, both volar and dorsal fasciotomies may be performed.
    - In most cases, the volar compartment is approached first through an incision extending from the biceps tendon at the elbow to the palm of the hand to allow carpal tunnel decompression, which is usually necessary (Fig. 38-7).
    - The deep flexors must be carefully inspected after fascial incision.
    - It may be necessary to expose and decompress pronator quadratus separately.
    - Often volar fasciotomy is sufficient to decompress the forearm, but if the ICP remains elevated in the dorsal compartment perioperatively, dorsal compression is easily performed through a straight dorsal incision.

- Decompression of the hand can usually be adequately achieved using two dorsal incisions, which allow access to the interosseous compartments (see Fig. 38-2).
    - This may often be sufficient but if there is clinical suspicion or raised ICP on measurement, incisions may be made over the thenar and hypothenar eminences, allowing fasciotomy of these compartments.

Fasciotomy Wounds

- Fasciotomy incisions must never be closed, primarily because this may result in persistent elevation of ICP.
- The wounds should be left open and dressed, and at approximately 48 hours after fasciotomy a second-look procedure should be undertaken to ensure viability of all muscle groups.
- The wounds may then be closed by delayed primary closure if possible, although this must be without tension on the skin edges.
    - In the leg commonly this technique is possible in the medial but not the lateral wound.
- If delayed primary closure cannot be achieved, the wound may be closed using either dermatotraction techniques or split skin grafting.
- Dermatotraction or gradual closure techniques have the advantage of avoiding the cosmetic problems of split skin grafting but may cause skin edge necrosis.
- A further disadvantage is the prolonged time required to achieve closure, which may be up to 10 days.
- Split skin grafting, although offering immediate skin cover, has the disadvantage of a high rate of long-term morbidity.
- The recent introduction of vacuum-assisted closure (VAC) systems is likely to be a significant advantage in this area and may reduce the need for split skin grafting with a low complication rate.

Associated Fractures

- It is now generally accepted that fractures, especially of the long bones, should be stabilized in the presence of acute compartment syndrome treated by fasciotomy.
- In reality, the treatment of the fracture should not be altered by the presence of an acute compartment syndrome, although cast management of a tibial fracture is contraindicated in the presence of acute compartment syndrome.

- Fasciotomy should be performed prior to fracture stabilization in order to eliminate any unnecessary delay in decompression.
- Stabilization of the fracture allows easy access to the soft tissues and protects the soft tissues, allowing them to heal.
- Reamed intramedullary nailing of the tibia confers excellent stabilization of a diaphyseal fracture and is now probably the treatment of choice in most centers for tibial diaphyseal fracture.
  - Reaming was implicated as a possible cause of acute compartment syndrome but has now been refuted by several studies.
- Several factors may raise ICP during stabilization of tibial fractures, including excessive traction, poor positioning of the thigh bar for countertraction, and the 90—90 position of leg elevation.
  - These should be avoided in patients at risk of acute compartment syndrome.

COMPLICATIONS

- Complications of acute compartment syndrome are unusual if the condition has been treated expeditiously.
  - Delay in diagnosis has been cited as the single reason for failure in the management of acute compartment syndrome.
  - Delay to fasciotomy of more than 6 hours is likely to cause significant sequelae, including muscle contractures, muscle weakness, sensory loss, infection, and nonunion of fractures.
- In severe cases, amputation may be necessary because of infection or lack of function.
- There is some debate about the place of decompression when the diagnosis is made late, and muscle necrosis is inevitable whether because of a missed acute compartment syndrome or a crush syndrome.
  - There seems little to be gained in exploring a closed crush syndrome when complete muscle necrosis is inevitable.
  - Increased sepsis rates with potentially serious consequences have been reported when these cases have been explored.
- If partial muscle necrosis is suspected and compartment monitoring reveals pressures above the threshold for decompression, there may be an indication for fasciotomy to salvage remaining viable muscle.
  - In these circumstances, debridement of necrotic muscle must be thorough to reduce the chances of infection.
- In rare cases, the ICP may be high enough to occlude major vessels, which is a further indication for fasciotomy to salvage the distal part of the limb.

SUGGESTED READING

Mars M, Hadley GP. Raised compartmental pressure in children: a basis for management. Injury 1998;29:183–185.

McQueen MM, Christie J, Court-Brown CM. Acute compartment syndrome in tibial diaphyseal fractures. J Bone Joint Surg (Br) 1996;78:95–98.

McQueen MM, Court-Brown CM. Compartment monitoring in tibial fractures. The pressure threshold for decompression. J Bone Joint Surg 1986;78:99–104.

McQueen MM, Gaston P, Court-Brown CM. Acute compartment syndrome: who is at risk? J Bone Joint Surg (Br) 2000;82:200–203.

Tornetta P, Templeman D. Compartment syndrome associated with tibial fracture. J Bone Joint Surg(Am) 1996;78:1438–1444.

Ulmer T. The clinical diagnosis of compartment syndrome of the lower leg: are clinical findings predictive of the disorder? J Orthop Trauma 2002;16:572–577.

NONUNIONS AND BONE DEFECTS

Nonunion is the term given to a fracture that does not unite. It is surprisingly difficult to define, and surgeons frequently apply an arbitrary time period to fractures beyond which they state that a nonunion has occurred. This approach has advantages and disadvantages. The use of a finite time limit encourages surgeons to consider early reconstructive treatment of the nonunion, thereby accelerating the patient's recovery. The concept that all fractures should unite in a fixed time period is naïve, however, because the speed of fracture union is determined by many factors including the degree of soft tissue injury, the extent of bone damage, the location of the fracture, the gap between the bone ends, the method of treatment, and the age and general health of the patient. Thus fractures can be expected to unite at different times. This fact is particularly important when considering delayed union. Union can be delayed by iatrogenic factors such as poor surgical technique with excessive soft tissue stripping or by distraction of the bone ends, but most fractures unite at a time appropriate for their severity. The term *delayed union* should probably be discarded because it is essentially meaningless.

Bone defects, by definition, lead to nonunion and require active treatment. They usually occur for two reasons. They either result from debridement of devitalized bone fragments in open long bone fragments or they are caused by bone resection during the treatment of osteomyelitis. The treatment of bone defects is similar no matter how they are caused.

DEFINITION

There is no definition of nonunion that encompasses all fractures. The accepted definition of diaphyseal nonunion is a fracture in which union has not occurred by 9 months, with no visible sign of progression of union for 3 months. This rule cannot apply to all fractures, and there are no good definitions for nonunion in metaphyseal or intra-articular fractures or following fractures of the shorter bones such as the clavicle or bones of the hand or foot. The definition of diaphyseal nonunion is reasonable in that few closed or Gustilo I through IIIa fractures will not have united by 9 months, and those Gustilo IIIb fractures that have not will show progressive signs of union. To wait 9 months to diagnose nonunion and instigate treatment would be unreasonable, however.

CLASSIFICATION

Nonunions traditionally are defined as infected or aseptic or as hypertrophic (Fig. 39-1) or atrophic (Fig. 39-2). A hypertrophic nonunion is one where there has been an attempt at union with radiological appearances of new

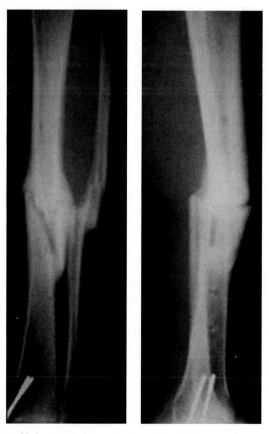

Figure 39-1 A-P and lateral radiographs of a hypertrophic nonunion of the tibia.

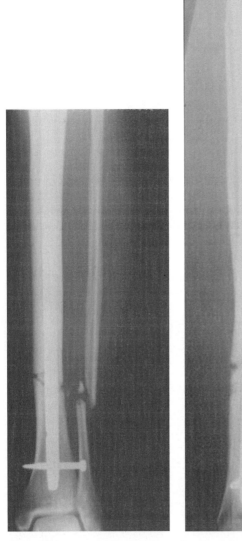

Figure 39-2   A-P and lateral radiographs of atrophic nonunions of the tibia and fibula.

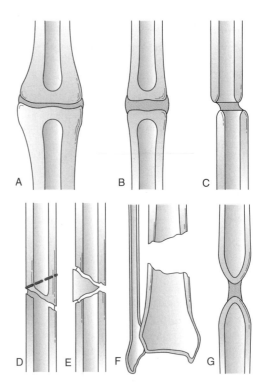

Figure 39-3   The Weber and Cech (1976) classification of nonunion. See text for explanation.

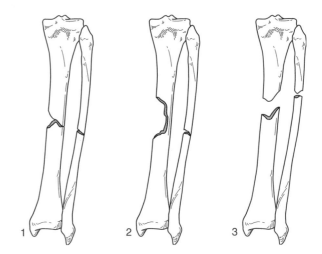

Figure 39-4   The OTA (AO) classification of bone defects.

bone formation. The assumption is usually made that the bone ends are vascularized but the stability of the fracture is inappropriate. An atrophic nonunion shows no signs of union, and it is usually assumed the bone ends are avascular. These are somewhat simplistic views because hypertrophic nonunions may occur with adequate bone stabilization, and animal and clinical studies have shown that many atrophic nonunions are in fact vascularized. There is probably a spectrum of nonunion with true hypertrophic and atrophic nonunion at each end.

The recognized classification is that of Weber and Cech (1976) (Fig. 39-3). It recognizes both hypertrophic (Fig. 39-3A) and atrophic (Fig. 39-3C) nonunions as well as oligotrophic (Fig. 39-3B) nonunions where hypertrophic new bone is present but diminished by the effect of fixation. It also recognizes the importance of butterfly

or wedge fragments (Fig. 39-3D and E) and bone defects (Fig. 39-3F) in the establishment of nonunion. The term *pseudarthrosis* (Fig. 39-3G) is sometimes used to describe a nonunion. It means "false joint," a condition that actually never occurs, although some fluid is occasionally found in a mobile nonunion. Bone defects are best classified using the OTA (AO) classification (Fig. 39-4).

Etiology

The causes of nonunion are listed in Box 39-1. Many nonunions are caused by soft tissue damage, fracture site avascularity and instability, and infection. Many other causes of nonunion are possible, however, and it is likely

BOX 39-1 FACTORS IMPLICATED IN NONUNIONS

- Infection
- Soft tissue avascularity
- Fracture site instability
- Fracture gap
- Soft tissue interposition
- Age
- Peripheral vascular disease
- Compartment syndrome
- Poor diet
- Anemia
- Diabetes mellitus
- Growth hormone deficiency
- Smoking
- Radiation
- Drugs
  - Corticosteroids
  - Anticoagulants
  - NSAIDs
  - Antibiotics
  - Cytotoxics

that in some patients the cause of nonunion is multifactorial and associated with age, general health, smoking, and medication. Age may contribute to nonunion in several ways. As people age, the incidence of diseases such as diabetes rise and the effects of social activities such as smoking are more severe. In addition, older patients are likely to be on more medication and the periosteum becomes thinner with age. Fracture gap is also important. A recent study has shown that in nailed tibial fractures, the odds of delaying union increased 12-fold with a gap of more than 3 mm. Compartment pressure is also important, and there is definitely an increased incidence of nonunion in patients who have compartment syndrome.

EPIDEMIOLOGY

The incidence of nonunion is very difficult to determine accurately. In common fractures with a relatively high incidence of nonunion such as those of the diaphyses of the humerus, forearm, femur, and tibia, accurate figures are known. In rare fractures with a low incidence of nonunion, however, little information exists. Thus data relating to nonunions of the scapula, hindfoot, tarsus, and metatarsus are scarce. In fractures of the tibial plateau, distal radius, and proximal radius, the incidence of nonunion is so low that many surgeons never encounter the problem. The last problem is that many studies come from specialist centers who accumulate problem fractures and nonunions but have no knowledge of the incidence of less severe fractures in their population. Tables 39-1 to 39-3 show the incidences of nonunion for different fractures. Each table shows the range of incidences published in the literature, together with an estimated incidence derived from examination of the literature and results of other previously unpublished prospective studies. They show that the incidence of nonunion varies widely depending on the fracture type and its treatment.

DIAGNOSIS

- Most nonunions are diagnosed on standard anteroposterior and lateral radiographs (Fig. 39-5), but not infrequently the diagnosis is difficult because of the three-dimensional orientation of the fracture and the presence of new bone.
- Oblique radiographs in the plane of the fracture are particularly useful in oblique or spiral fractures, and the use of fluoroscopy allows the surgeon to examine the nonunion in all planes and to see if it is mobile.
- Tomography or CT scanning may be useful, but even these radiological techniques are not uniformly diagnostic of the presence of a nonunion, usually because of the discrepancy between the angle of the nonunion and the radiographic cuts of the CT scan.
- Ultrasound has been used but is often difficult to interpret.
- Appropriate radiographs and imaging should be obtained, but the diagnosis of nonunion is often based on a combination of clinical suspicion and imaging.
- It is important to try to exclude infection as a cause of the nonunion, and radioisotope bone scanning and MRI scans may be useful.

TREATMENT

ASEPTIC NONUNION

- The treatment of aseptic nonunion depends on whether it is hypertrophic or atrophic and on the type of initial management.
- With increasing interest in operative fracture management in the last 20 to 25 years, many nonunions now present in aligned bones that have been previously nailed, plated, or externally fixed.
- An aligned nonunion is usually easier to treat than a malaligned nonunion that has followed nonoperative management.
- Essentially, hypertrophic aseptic nonunions are treated by alteration of the biomechanical environment and atrophic nonunions by bone grafting with a change of fracture fixation where it is indicated.
- The commonly used methods of treating nonunion and bone defects are listed in Box 39-2.

Bone Grafting

- Corticocancellous bone grafting remains the most important method of treating nonunion.
- Bone grafting is also used for filling bone defects usually after open or comminuted fractures, and specifically shaped bone grafts may be of use in preserving height or length in spinal fractures, metaphyseal fractures, or in fractures of the carpus or tarsus.
- Autografts are the most common grafts used in trauma. These are taken from the patient and several sites can be used.

TABLE 39-1 QUOTED AND ESTIMATED PREVALENCES OF NONUNION FOR DIFFERENT FRACTURES IN THE UPPER LIMB

Fracture	Prevalence (%)		Notes
	Quoted	Estimated	
Clavicle		<1	
Medial	0		
Diaphyseal	0–15	3–6	See Table 10-3
Lateral	0–46	0–22	See Table 10-4
Scapula			
Acromion	Unknown	<1	
Coracoid	Unknown	<1	
Glenoid/body	Unknown	<1	
Proximal humerus	0–7	1	8% if metaphyseal comminution present
Humeral diaphysis			
Nonoperative	3–13	4	See Table 12-3
Plate	2–8	4	See Table 12-3
Intramedullary nail	0–23	5–12	See Table 12-4
Distal humerus (type C)	0–8	5	See Table 13-4
Olecranon	3–11	4	See table 14-8
Proximal radius	0–5	1	Higher in neck than head fractures
Radius and ulna (plates)	0–7	4	See Table 15-4
Ulna (plate)	0–7	4	See Table 15-4
Radius (plate)	0–7	4	See Table 15-4
Distal radius	Unknown	0.1	Prospective study of 4,000 cases
Scaphoid			
Waist (cast)	5–15	8	See Table 17.1-5
Waist (screw)	0–11	3	See Table 17.1-5
Proximal pole (cast)	18–67	40	See Table 17.1-5
Metacarpals	0–18	<1	See Table 17.2-5
Phalanges			
Proximal and middle	0–11	<1	
Distal	25–70	30–36	Usually asymptomatic

- Small amounts of cancellous graft can be obtained from the distal radius, proximal femur, or the proximal and distal tibia.

BOX 39-2 METHODS OF TREATING NONUNIONS AND BONE DEFECTS

- Nonstructural autograft (usually corticocancellous grafts)
- Structural autograft
- Nonstructural allograft
- Structural allograft
- Vascularized grafts
- Bone transport
- Primary bone shortening and secondary lengthening
- Bone morphogenic proteins
- Exchange nailing
- Other methods
  - Electrical stimulation
  - Bone marrow injection
  - Shock-wave therapy
  - Ultrasound

- The amount obtainable is comparatively little, however, and these sites are generally only used for small local operations.
- Most corticocancellous or cancellous grafts are taken from the anterior or posterior iliac crests.
- A description of the use, results, and complications of autogenous bone grafting is given in Box 39-3.

Anterior Iliac Crest Grafting

- Anterior iliac crest grafting is a straightforward technique that produces sufficient bone graft for most operative procedures. It is summarized here.
- If a specifically shaped structural graft is required, the iliac crest must be exposed fully and the correct graft shape removed with osteotomes.
- If purely cancellous graft is needed, a 2- to 3-cm length of the iliac crest can be elevated with osteotomes and a gouge used to remove cancellous bone from between the inner and outer tables.
- In most cases of nonunion, corticocancellous grafts are used.
- The operative technique for harvesting corticocancellous grafts from the inner table of the ilium is straightforward.

TABLE 39-2 QUOTED AND ESTIMATED PREVALENCES OF NONUNION FOR DIFFERENT FRACTURES IN THE LOWER LIMB

Fracture	Prevalence (%)		Notes
	Quoted	Estimated	
Femoral head	Unknown	<1	Very rare fracture; no data
Subcapital			
Undisplaced (nonoperative))	8–14	13	See Table 21.2-6
Undisplaced (screws)	0–4	3	See Table 21.2-6
Displaced (nonoperative)	30–70	>50	Nonoperative management rarely used
Displaced (screws)	4–30	30	See Table 21.2-8
Intertrochanteric	0–2	<1	See Table 21.2-15
Subtrochanteric	0–20	3–10	See Tables 22-2–22-6
Femoral diaphysis			
Antegrade reamed	0–14	2	See Table 23-4
Antegrade unreamed	0–39	6	See Table 23-4
Retrograde reamed	0–8	5	See Table 23-6
Retrograde unreamed	13–20	8	See Table 23-6
Distal femur			
Plate	0–9	3–5	See Tables 24-3–24-5
Nail	0–10	3–6	See Tables 24-6–24-7
External fixation	0–6	3	See Table 2-8
Patella	0–2	1	<1% with ORIF. See Table 25-3
Tibial plateau (ORIF)	0	0	See Table 26-8
Tibial plateau (external fixation)	0–4	0–2	See Table 26-9
Tibial diaphysis (nonoperative)	0–24	8–10	Old data
Closed fractures			
Reamed IM nails	0–4	2	See Table 27-3
Unreamed IM nails	11–27	16	See Table 27-3
Plates	0–54	9	Open and closed fractures. See Table 27-9
Open fractures			
Reamed nails	8–36	14	See Table 27-4
Unreamed nails	4–48	21	See Table 27-4
Plates	0–54	9	Open and closed fractures. See Table 27-9
External fixation	6–41	9–18	See Table 27-6
Gustilo IIIb fractures			
Reamed nails	17–69	36	See Table 27-5
Unreamed nails	18–80	31	See Table 27-5
External fixation	14–60	27	See Table 27-7
Tibial plafond (ex fix))	0–22	2–10	See Table 28-4
Tibial plafond (plate)	0–17	1–7	See Table 28-3
Ankle	0–3	<1	See Table 29-6
Talus			
Neck	0–6	4	See Table 30-4
Lateral process	22–61	20–30	Rare injury; poor data
Osteochondral dome	56–90	25–50	Rare injury; poor data
Calcaneus			
Intra-articular	0–1	<1	
Anterior process	3–22	10–20	Rare injury; poor data
Other tarsal bones	Unknown	<1	Poor data
Fifth metatarsal			
Proximal avulsion	Unknown	<1	Rare
Proximal diaphysis	30–35	7–10	Poor data
Other metatarsal	Unknown	<1	Poor data

TABLE 39-3　QUOTED AND ESTIMATED PREVALENCES OF NONUNION IN THE SPINE AND PELVIS

	Prevalence (%)		
Fracture	**Quoted**	**Estimated**	**Notes**
Spine			
Odontoid			
Type II fractures	15–85	10–12	Lower with screw fixation (about 7%)
Type III	9–13	9–13	
C1-C2 fusion	3–15	4	
Thoracolumbar spine	0–7	0.2–4	Lower with posterior instrumentation
Pelvis	2–5	3	
Acetabulum	0–1	0.7	Prospective study of 1,000 cases

■ Palpate the anterior superior iliac spine (ASIS).
■ Make a 4- to 5-cm skin incision starting 1 to 2 cm behind the ASIS.
■ Use sharp dissection to expose the iliac crest.
■ Reflect soft tissue off the inner aspect of the crest.
■ Reflect iliacus off the inner table of the ilium.
■ Use gouge to remove corticocancellous strips from the ilium.
■ When sufficient bone has been harvested, close wound in layers.

Posterior Iliac Crest Grafting

■ More bone graft can be harvested from the posterior crest than from the anterior iliac crest.
■ The technique is slightly more difficult, and unless the graft is being used for spinal surgery, the position of the patient may require to be altered perioperatively.

■ Posterior bone graft harvesting may be used if bone graft has already been harvested from the anterior iliac crests.
■ The posterior iliac crest is palpated and a curved 8- to 10-cm incision made over the crest.
■ Sharp dissection is used to expose the posterior iliac crest, and the gluteal muscles are elevated from the ileum.
■ Corticocancellous grafts can be harvested with a gouge or larger grafts can be removed with an osteotome.
■ Closure is in layers over a suction drain.
■ The complications associated with bone grafting are listed in Box 39-3.

Other Bone Grafting Techniques

■ Other grafting techniques may be used (see Box 39-2).
■ Allograft bone is commonly used but is not as effective as autograft.

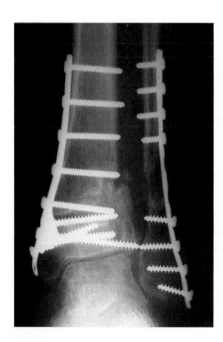
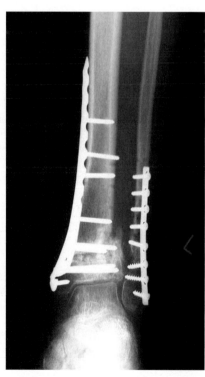

Figure 39-5　A nonunion of an extra-articular plafond fracture. The plate has bent because of the nonunion. This case was treated by replating and bone grafting using a locking distal tibial plate.

BOX 39-3 AUTOGENOUS BONE GRAFT IN NONUNIONS AND BONE DEFECTS

Use
- Usually obtained from iliac crest, distal femur, greater trochanter, proximal tibia, or distal radius
- May be structural or nonstructural
- Usually applied as nonstructural corticocancellous strips
- Survival depends on vascularization from surrounding tissues (3 weeks for small graft)
- Cancellous iliac bone graft supplies osteogenic cells and marrow
- Cortical bone graft has minimal osteogenic potential but useful for structural support

Advantages
- Applicable to most nonunions
- Success rate high in aseptic nonunion (>90%)
- May be mixed with allograft bone for larger defects
- Technically straightforward

Disadvantages
- Appropriate for smaller bone defects
- If bone defect >4 cm, two grafting procedures are often necessary
- Iliac crest donor site morbidity: local pain, hematoma, lateral cutaneous nerve damage, infection

---

- Nonstructural allograft may be mixed with autograft to fill larger bone defects (Fig. 39-6A).
- Structural allografts can be used to reconstruct diaphyseal defects (Fig. 39-6B), but union is problematic and late fracture may occur.
- A summary of the use of allografts is given in Box 39-4.
- Vascularized grafting, bone transport, or primary shortening and secondary lengthening are therefore preferred in the management of traumatic defects.
- Vascularized grafts can be used in a number of locations.
- These originally were confined to locations where the vascular pedicle was long enough to permit bone transplantation, such as filling a tibial gap with a section of fibula.
- With the advent of microsurgery, vascular grafts can be moved considerable distances, and combined bone and soft tissue grafts can also be used.
  - One example is the osteocutaneous graft from the anterior pelvis.
- Most vascularized grafts have been used to fill defects in the tibia, femur, and humerus, and usually a fibular graft has been used.

BOX 39-4 ALLOGRAFT IN NONUNIONS AND BONE DEFECTS

Use
- Widely available as nonstructural or structural grafts
- Induces inflammatory response, which impairs fracture union, therefore is frozen or freeze-dried prior to use
- More useful for tumor and arthroplasty work than in fracture treatment

Advantages
- Avoids harvesting from iliac crest
- Often used in combination with autograft, particularly for larger defects (see Fig. 39-6)
- Structural allograft may be used for large defects such as the femoral diaphysis (see Fig. 39-6)

Disadvantages
- Essential to check donor for HIV, hepatitis, and other blood-borne disease
- Nonstructural allograft less effective than autograft
- Fracture union less certain than with autograft
- Fracture of structural grafts may occur

- Up to 25 cm of fibula can be harvested.
- If the fibula is simply rotated and used to fill an ipsilateral tibial defect, the literature suggests the union rate is about 80% with a refracture rate of 8% to 10%.
- Fibular hypertrophy starts 4 to 6 months after transplantation and continues for at least 3 years.
- The use of free vascularized fibular grafts is associated with a union rate of 80% to 85%, but the incidence of vascular thrombosis is about 15%, and about 15% of patients have a stress fracture of the graft.
- Both techniques are associated with superficial peroneal palsy and ankle stiffness.

Bone Transport

- Bone transport is used mainly in diaphyseal fractures where there is a bone defect (Fig. 39-7).
- Usually it is undertaken with a small wire fixator such as an Ilizarov device, although a unilateral external fixator can be used. The principle is straightforward.
- A corticotomy is undertaken through normal bone and the bone segment is left for 7 to 14 days, after which it is moved slowly until it unites with the distal fragment.
  - The rate of transport is usually 1 mm per day divided into four movements of 0.25 mm.
- As the bone segment moves, regenerate bone is formed behind it, and eventually the regenerate bone matures into mechanically adequate bone.
- Once the segment "docks" or meets the distal fragment, union ideally occurs, although sometimes a conventional bone graft is required to facilitate union.
  - Using this technique, large bone defects can be filled.
- The technique is usually used for tibial and femoral defects. An analysis of the advantages and disadvantages of the method is listed in Box 39-5.
- The results of bone transport for tibial defects are given in Table 39-4.

Primary Bone Shortening and Secondary Lengthening

- A modification of the standard lengthening technique involves shortening the fracture primarily, achieving union, and then lengthening the bone secondarily.

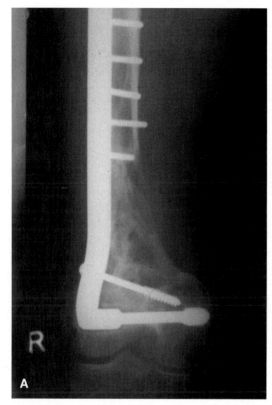
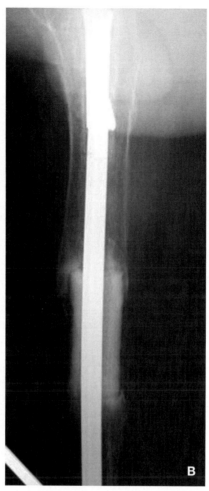

Figure 39-6 (A) Allograft bone may be combined with autograft. This is the fracture shown in Figures 24-3 and 24-5. (B) The use of structural allograft in an infected femoral nonunion.

■ As yet there is little information available about this technique, but early results are promising.
■ The results of a series of primary shortening and secondary lengthening are summarized in Table 39-4.

BOX 39-5 BONE TRANSPORT IN NONUNIONS AND BONE DEFECTS

Use
■ External fixator applied (usually a fine-wire circular frame)
■ Corticotomy performed
■ Bone segment moved
■ Regenerate tube of bone forms behind bone segment

Advantages
■ No bone graft required
■ Useful for larger bone defects (>4 cm)

Disadvantages
■ Length of treatment process
■ Muscle contracture and joint subluxation
■ Neurological and vascular damage
■ Pin site infection, refracture, and joint stiffness
■ Psychological problems

■ It can be used for defects up to 3 cm in length.
■ Longer defects should be shortened at 2 mm per day to minimize vascular and neurological problems.
■ Table 39-4 suggests that it is quicker than standard bone lengthening and the requirement for flap cover is reduced.
■ Many of the complications associated with bone lengthening still occur, however.

Bone Morphogenic Proteins

■ Bone morphogenic proteins (BMPs) are members of the TGF-beta superfamily and one of the groups of growth and differentiation factors responsible for communication among osteogenic cells that produce bone repair and remodeling.
■ Most of their use has been in animal work, but the initial clinical multicenter studies have shown promising results.
■ In one study of 124 tibial nonunions, the results of the use of BMP was equivalent to bone grafting despite a higher incidence of atrophic nonunions and smokers in the BMP group.
■ Studies of the use of BMPs in recalcitrant nonunions have also indicated a high success rate with no adverse affect.
■ It is likely that although both bone grafting and bone morphogenic proteins will continue to be used to treat

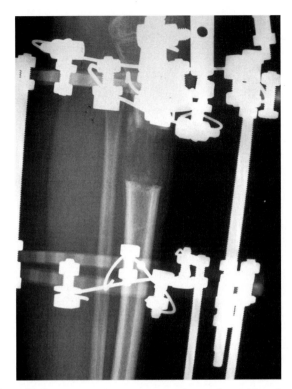

Figure 39-7 Bone lengthening using an Ilizarov device. Note the regenerate bone following distraction of a corticotomy.

nonunions, the use of bone morphogenic proteins will probably increase in the future.

- Surgeons who wish to use BMPs should remember they are naturally occurring proteins and require an adequate blood supply and osteogenic cells to allow union to occur.
  - They also require adequate stabilization and soft tissue cover.
- Thus, even if BMPs are used in preference to bone graft, the same basic principles of treatment must be followed.

Exchange Nailing

- With increased interest in intramedullary nailing, surgeons are seeing more diaphyseal nonunions in fractures

---

BOX 39-6 EXCHANGE NAILING IN NONUNIONS AND BONE DEFECTS

- Particularly useful in tibial fractures—90% success rate
- Tibial hypertrophic nonunions unite in an average of 10 to 12 weeks
- Tibial atrophic nonunions can be successfully treated
  - May take two exchange nailing procedures with the first converting the nonunion from atrophic to hypertrophic
- Will unite fracture gaps of less than 2 cm and 50% bone circumference
- Useful in OTA (AO) 1 and OTA (AO) 2 bone defects
- Does not work in OTA (AO) 3 defects, infected bone, and in diaphysis reconstructed from bone graft
- 70% to 90% success rate in femoral nonunions
- Only 40% to 45% success rate in humeral nonunions; probably relates to vascularity

---

that have been primarily treated with a reamed or unreamed nail.

- The mainstay of treating these nonunions is exchange nailing (Fig. 39-8).
- This involves removing the intramedullary nail, reaming an extra 1 to 2 mm, and inserting an appropriately sized larger intramedullary nail.
  - In about 90% of cases, cross screws are not required because the combination of the nail and fibrous union stabilizes the fracture.
- If stability is inadequate, cross screws should be inserted.
- The use of exchange nailing is covered in Box 39-6.
- The technique is very effective in tibial and femoral fractures, but it is much less effective in the treatment of humeral nonunion.
  - The reason for this is unknown but may relate to the vascularity of the humerus.
  - This may also account for the relatively high incidence of atrophic humeral nonunions.
- There is no information about exchange nailing of radius or ulnar nonunions.
- There are three possible reasons why exchange nailing is successful.

TABLE 39-4 RESULTS OF BONE TRANSPORT AND PRIMARY BONE SHORTENING AND SECONDARY LENGTHENING (COMPRESSION-DISTRACTION) IN THE TIBIA

	Bone Transport		Compression-Distraction[a]
	Range	Average	Average
Bone loss (cm)	4–10	6	5
External fixator time (mo)	8–17	10.8	7.1
Complications (per patient)	1.4–3.5	2.4	2.1
Additional surgeries (per patient)	0.5–3.5	1.6	0.4
Lengthening (mo/cm)	1.6–2.5	1.9	1.4
Success rate (%)	71–100	81	100

[a]Results from Sen C, Kocaoglu M, Eralp L, et al. Bifocal compression-distraction in the treatment of grade III open fractures with bone and soft-tissue loss: a report of 24 cases. J Orthop Trauma 2004;18:150–157.

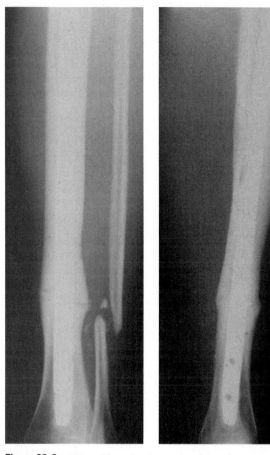

Figure 39-8 A-P and lateral radiographs of the nonunion shown in Figure 39-2 treated by exchange nailing. The persistent fibular nonunion was asymptomatic.

- It may increase the rigidity of fracture fixation, or alternatively, it may provide bone graft to the nonunion site.
- A third explanation is that, as with all reaming, there is stimulation of the periosteal vasculature and therefore periosteal new bone formation.
  - Evidence indicates that it is the latter process that is most important, although the products of intramedullary reaming have been shown to be osteogenic.

Other Treatment Methods

Electrical Stimulation
- Electrical stimulation of tissue repair has been in use for over 200 years.
- In the last 20 to 25 years, considerable interest has been expressed in the use of electrical stimulation to promote bone union.
- Success rates of 62% to 87% have been reported for the treatment of diaphyseal nonunions, but it is difficult to separate the results of electrical stimulation from the surgery undertaken to stimulate union.
- Thus, although there is no doubt that electrical stimulation does alter bone repair at a cellular level, controversy still exists regarding its clinical usefulness.

- Recent work has suggested that any benefit of electrical stimulation is mediated through stimulation of TGF-beta 1.

Bone Marrow Injection
- Injection of bone marrow containing osteoprogenitor cells has been reported to cause new bone formation in nonunions.
- The technique has been reported to cause union in up to 90% of tibial nonunions, but, as with electrical stimulation, it is impossible to separate the effect of the bone marrow from the surgery undertaken to treat the nonunions.

Shock-Wave Therapy
- Following the successful use of lithotripsy to treat renal calculi, surgeons have used shock-wave therapy to treat nonunions.
  - Although high extracorporeal shock-wave energy can fracture bones, lower energy levels can stimulate osteogenesis.
- It is stated that the healing rate of nonunions following shock-wave therapy is between 62% and 83%, and hypertrophic nonunions do better than atrophic nonunions.

Ultrasound
- Ultrasound has been shown to be useful in the treatment of nonunions in animal experiments and some clinical studies have reported good results, but as with other treatment modalities it is often difficult to separate the response to ultrasound from the reconstructive surgery that is usually undertaken at the same time.
- Further work is required to identify the role of ultrasound.

Specific Nonunion Types

Clavicle
- Table 39-1 shows that nonunions of the clavicle are likely to be either mid-diaphyseal or at the lateral end of the bone.
- Mid-diaphyseal nonunions are usually oligotrophic and require being taken down and plated.
- Intermediate loose fragments are usually removed, resulting in a bone defect that requires grafting.
- If there is overlap of the ends of the clavicular nonunion (Fig. 39-9A), it is usually difficult to regain length.
- Under these circumstances, the ends of the clavicle can be sometimes be cut and reduction obtained prior to plating (Fig. 39-9B).
  - If this is possible, grafting is not required.
  - If any defect exists, however, bone grafting must be used.
- Virtually all lateral clavicular nonunions follow Neer type II (Robinson 3B1 and 3B2) fractures with rupture of the coracoclavicular ligaments (see Table 10-4 in Chapter 10).
- The clavicle is displaced superiorly but also pulled backward posteriorly by the action of the trapezius.
- The treatment of lateral clavicular nonunion is discussed in Chapter 10.

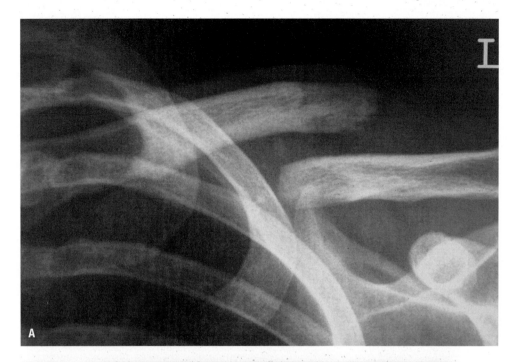

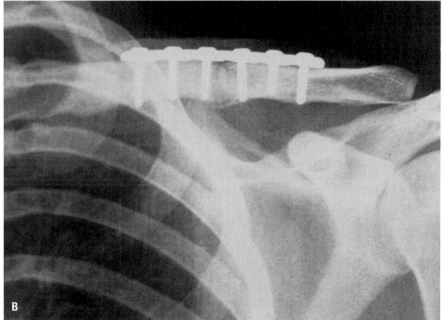

Figure 39-9   A clavicular nonunion treated by resection of the ends of the bone and plating. There was no defect and bone graft was not used, unlike Figure 10-9.

- Medial clavicular nonunions are rare and if they occur are best treated by bone grafting and plating.

Scapula
- Scapular nonunions are very rare.
- Nonunions of the acromion, glenoid, and body of the scapula require appropriate stabilization and grafting.
- Acromial stabilization is very difficult and may involve screw fixation or a plate placed across the acromioclavicular joint onto the clavicle.
  - Acromial excision leads to considerable morbidity and should be avoided.

- Coracoid nonunions are frequently asymptomatic, but if this is not the case, screw fixation or excision of the fragment with refixation of the attached muscles should be undertaken.

Proximal Humerus
- Proximal humeral nonunions are rare.
  - They are more common in the elderly and very rare under the age of 65 years.
- If symptomatic they should be treated by plating and grafting or by hemiarthroplasty.
- Their treatment is discussed in Chapter 11.

Humeral Diaphysis

- Many humeral diaphyseal fractures are treated nonoperatively, and therefore nonunions are frequently malaligned.
  - These nonunions require open reduction and internal fixation, usually with supplementary bone grafting.
- The results of the different treatment methods are given in Table 12-7 in Chapter 12.
- Humeral nonunions usually occur in older patients, and locked plates give good results (see Fig. 12-11 in Chapter 12).

Distal Humerus

- Surgeons encounter distal humeral nonunions in two circumstances.
- A small number of intra-articular distal humeral fractures fail to unite and require refixation and grafting.
- In addition, the transcondylar distal humeral fracture in the elderly patient may present with a nonunion.
  - This may be difficult to treat, and if symptoms are minor in a very elderly patient the nonunion may be left.
- In symptomatic patients, plating and grafting or secondary elbow arthroplasty may be undertaken.
- The results of these two techniques are given in Table 13-7 in Chapter 13.

Olecranon

- Olecranon nonunions are often asymptomatic.
- If symptomatic they can be treated in two ways.
  - The nonunion usually follows inadequate initial stabilization and therefore should be restabilized with a plate or with K-wires and cerclage wiring.
- Any bone defects should be filled by bone graft.
- Alternatively, in the elderly, the proximal olecranon fragment can be excised and the triceps reattached distally.

- This technique should be reserved for the elderly and infirm.

Radial Head and Neck

- Radial head nonunion is very rare indeed, but there are sporadic reports of radial neck nonunions.
- This is an atrophic nonunion, and plating and grafting are obviously very difficult.
- If symptomatic, the best treatment is either radial head excision or radial head replacement with a metal prosthesis.

Radius and Ulna

- Most displaced radius and ulna fractures are plated.
- If a nonunion occurs, the optimal treatment is replating and grafting.
- This also applies to isolated radius and ulna fractures, although a number of ulna diaphyseal fractures will have been treated nonoperatively primarily.
  - These require open reduction, plating, and grafting.

Distal Radius and Ulna

- Distal radial nonunions are very rare, and most surgeons never encounter one.
- In a prospective study of 4,000 consecutive distal radial fractures, the incidence of nonunion was 0.01%.
- Treatment is by reduction, plating, and bone grafting.
- If the distal fragment is very small, it may be difficult to gain stability with a plate.
  - Under these circumstances, the surgeon should consider a wrist arthrodesis.

Scaphoid

- Scaphoid nonunion (Fig. 39-10) is relatively common, especially in the proximal pole (see Table 17-1-5 in

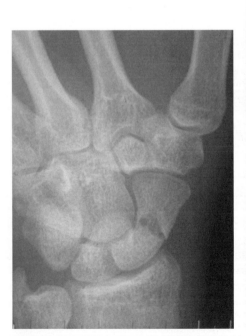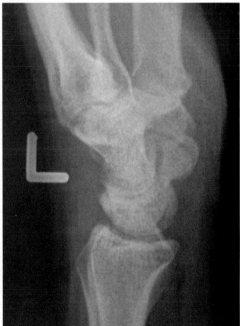

Figure 39-10   A-P and lateral radiographs of a scaphoid nonunion. Note the slight dorsiflexion of the lunate on the lateral view indicating some carpal collapse.

Chapter 17), because of the vascular supply of the scaphoid entering the bone distally and passing proximally.

■ There seems little doubt that primary percutaneous screw fixation has reduced the incidence of scaphoid nonunion from the 5% to 15% listed in Table 39-1.

■ Most scaphoid fractures continue to be treated nonoperatively, and surgeons therefore must continue to treat the problem of nonunion.

■ Scaphoid nonunions are best treated by screw fixation and supplementary bone grafting.
  ■ If this fails, consideration should be given to the use of a vascularized bone graft, localized intercarpal fusion, or wrist fusion.

Metacarpus and Phalanges

■ Nonunions of the metacarpus and the proximal and middle phalanges are unusual, with the highest incidences noted in Table 39-1 occurring in severe open fractures.

■ There seems no doubt that the incidence of metacarpal and phalangeal nonunions is higher following treatment with external fixation or K-wires where the surgeon has not reduced the fracture adequately and has left a gap between the bone ends.

■ Treatment of metacarpal and phalangeal nonunions is by plating and grafting.

Distal Phalanges

■ Distal phalangeal nonunions are relatively common.

■ There are two principal types of fractures in which nonunion may occur.

■ In open transverse fractures of the proximal end of the distal phalanx, the nail bed may become trapped in the fracture site and nonunion may ensue.
  ■ This condition should be treated primarily, but if a nonunion ensues the soft tissue should be cleared from the nonunion, which is then stabilized with K-wires and grafted.

■ The other distal phalangeal fracture in which there is a relatively high incidence of nonunion is the tuft fracture, in which nonunions of 30% to 36% at 6 months have been reported.
  ■ These are usually asymptomatic and rarely require treatment.

Femoral Head

■ The incidence of femoral head nonunion is unknown.

■ The fracture is rare and virtually always treated operatively.

■ If a nonunion occurs, it is likely to be accompanied by avascular necrosis and osteoarthritic change in the hip.

■ Treatment will inevitably be hip arthroplasty.

Proximal Femur

■ The incidence of nonunion after displaced femoral neck fracture is relatively high with the incidence rising with age (see Table 39-2).

■ Today few femoral neck fractures are treated nonoperatively, but a recent multicenter prospective analysis of femoral neck fractures has indicated a 30% nonunion rate in displaced fractures treated by cancellous screw fixation.

■ Most nonunions under these circumstances are treated by hemiarthroplasty, bipolar arthroplasty, or total hip arthroplasty with the decision of which implant usually depending on the age and general health of the patient.

■ Fit elderly patients should be treated with total hip arthroplasty, but the surgeon may elect to use a hemiarthroplasty or bipolar arthroplasty in less fit patients.

■ In younger patients, the femoral head should be preserved if possible.

■ Refixation and grafting should be undertaken together with a valgizing subtrochanteric osteotomy if the head is in varus.
  ■ This is undertaken to realign the fracture plane perpendicular to the joint reaction force.

■ In comparison with femoral neck fractures, nonunion after intertrochanteric fracture is rare, occurring in fewer than 1% of patients.

■ The intertrochanteric fracture occurs in well-vascularized cancellous bone, and nonunion usually occurs in unstable fracture patterns without an adequate posteromedial bone buttress.
  ■ They are also associated with poor surgical fixation with varus collapse of the head and cutout of the implant.

■ Treatment is by refixation combined with a valgizing osteotomy of the proximal femur, and bone grafting as required (Fig. 39-11).

■ In older patients, a hip prosthesis can be used.

Subtrochanteric

■ With the introduction of locked reconstruction nails with a side arm placed in the femoral neck and head, the incidence of subtrochanteric nonunion has declined to about 3% from the 8% to 10% associated with the use of blade plates and hip screw plate systems.

■ A nonunion in a previously nailed fracture should be treated by exchange nailing with reaming and the insertion of a larger nail.

■ If a plated subtrochanteric nonunion is well aligned, the plate should be removed and an antegrade reamed intramedullary nail or reamed reconstruction nail used, depending on whether the lesser trochanter has united.

■ If the lesser trochanter has united, adequate stability is usually achieved with a conventional antegrade femoral nail.

■ Bone grafting should be used for any defects related to the nonunion.

Femur

■ Table 39-2 shows that nonunions following femoral diaphyseal fractures are uncommon, averaging only 2% if antegrade reamed nails are used to treat the primary fracture.

■ Very few femoral fractures today are not treated with intramedullary nails.
  ■ As a result, most aseptic nonunions are likely to occur in an aligned femur, and exchange nailing is the treatment of choice.

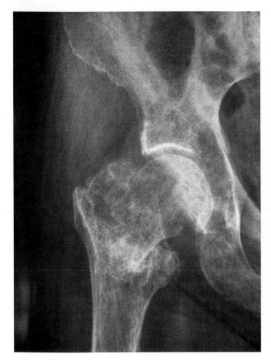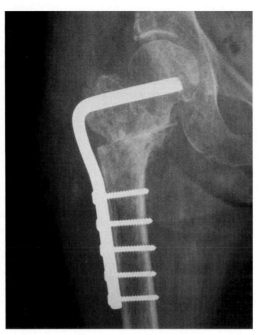

Figure 39-11   A valgizing osteotomy of an intertrochanteric nonunion. It has been fixed with a blade plate.

■ This is successful in 70% to 90% of cases (see Box 39-6), and where it fails, open bone grafting should be undertaken.

■ If the femoral fracture was initially plated, the plate should be removed and a reamed nail used.

■ If the fracture was treated nonoperatively, it is likely the femoral diaphysis will be malaligned, and it will be necessary to take down the nonunion prior to nailing.

■ Bone grafting should be used to fill any residual defects.

■ In open femoral fractures there may be a bone defect after initial debridement and stabilization.

■ This will usually have been treated earlier, but a residual defect may exist at a later stage.

■ OTA (AO) 1 and many OTA (AO) 2 defects can be successfully treated by exchange nailing, but OTA (AO) 3 defects require either bone grafting or bone transport.

■ Where possible, grafting is preferred because prolonged thigh external fixation leads to joint stiffness.

Distal Femur

■ The incidence of distal femoral nonunion is relatively low and, as with other lower limb metaphyseal nonunions, the nonunion site is often at the junction of metaphysis and diaphysis, the metaphyseal fracture having united.

■ Treatment is by fracture stabilization using a distal femoral plate or retrograde nail.

■ Bone grafting should be used.

■ In older patients with a nonunion of a low supracondylar or intercondylar femoral fracture, consideration

should be given to knee arthroplasty if knee function is reasonable.

Patella

■ Patellar nonunions are relatively uncommon.

■ Treatment is by stabilization and bone grafting if necessary.

■ Nonunion of lower pole fractures may be treated by excision of the lower pole and reattachment of the patellar tendon.

■ In older patients the nonunion may be asymptomatic.

Tibial Plateau

■ Proximal tibial metaphyseal fractures have an extremely low incidence of nonunion.

■ If it occurs, the nonunion should be treated by refixation and bone grafting.

■ In older patients, consideration should be given to total knee replacement should the fracture configuration be appropriate.

Tibia

■ Table 39-2 shows that aseptic nonunion of the tibial diaphysis is relatively common, particularly in severe open fractures.

■ In recent years, the popularity of tibial nailing has made the management of hypertrophic nonunion after closed fracture much easier because exchange nailing with a larger reamed nail (see Fig. 39-8) is effective in 90% of cases (see Box 39-6).

■ Atrophic nonunions also respond to exchange nailing, although sometimes two exchange nailing procedures are required, the first exchange nailing procedure converting the hypertrophic nonunion to an atrophic nonunion.

■ Exchange nailing failures are treated by bone grafting.

■ Surgeons frequently encounter tibial nonunion after nonoperative management.

■ In hypertrophic, cast-managed tibial nonunions, partial fibulectomy with excision of 1 to 2 cm of fibula resulted in union in about 75% of cases.

■ The technique is less commonly used now.

■ Nonoperatively managed nonunions are usually malaligned and should be taken down prior to internal fixation.

■ It is preferable to use a reamed intramedullary nail to stabilize these nonunions, with supplementary bone grafting used to fill any defects.

■ If the nonunion has been previously plated, the plate should be removed and a reamed intramedullary nail inserted.

■ Unlike the femur, external fixation remains popular for the primary management of open tibial fractures.

■ If an aligned nonunion occurs after external fixation, the fixator should be removed and the tibia nailed.

■ Secondary nailing should not be undertaken in the presence of discharging pin tracks, however.

■ Surgeons should wait until the pin tracks have granulated before nailing.

■ This may only require a delay of 1 to 2 days, during which time the nonunion can be supported in a cast or brace.

■ If malalignment has occurred with the external fixator, the fracture should be taken down and stabilized, usually with an intramedullary nail.

■ Bone defects can be treated with corticocancellous grafting or bone transport depending on their size.

■ All OTA (AO) type 1 and most type 2 bone defects can be treated by exchange nailing.

■ OTA (AO) type 3 defects should be treated by grafting up to 4 cm in length, with bone transport used for larger defects.

■ Primary shortening and secondary lengthening may be used for the treatment of bone defects in open tibial fractures.

Tibial Plafond

■ The most common site for nonunion following plafond fractures is at the junction of the metaphysis and diaphysis, the metaphyseal component of the fracture having already united.

■ This complication has become more important in recent years with increased use of external fixation to treat plafond fractures.

■ If the external fixator is removed soon after metaphyseal union, it is unlikely the diaphyseal component of the fracture will have united.

■ Treatment is usually stabilization with a plate with supplementary bone grafting (see Fig. 39-5).

■ Alternatively, a reamed nail can be used to treat a diaphyseal fracture once the external fixator has been removed.

■ As with tibial diaphyseal fractures, surgeons should be aware of the possibility of infection if primary external fixation and secondary intramedullary nailing is used.

■ Type B partial articular fractures have a low incidence of nonunion, but if one occurs it should be treated by stabilization and bone grafting.

Ankle

■ Nonunion of ankle fractures is uncommon but does occur more frequently in older patients.

■ It is more common in medial malleolar fractures.

■ Treatment is by restabilization using screws or a plate and bone grafting.

Talus

■ Nonunions of the talar body, neck, head, and posterior process are relatively unusual (Fig. 39-12).

■ They are treated by stabilization, and bone grafting as required.

■ The two areas of the talus where nonunion is more common are the lateral process and the dome where osteochondral fractures frequently fail to unite.

■ Nonunion of the lateral process can be treated by fixation if the fragment is large enough or by excision of smaller fragments.

■ The incidence of osteochondral nonunion is difficult to determine, but it is clear that type III and IV lesions (see Fig. 30-11 in Chapter 30) often fail to unite, although the patient may not be symptomatic.

■ If they are symptomatic, treatment should be by fixation of larger osteochondral fragments or, more commonly, excision of smaller fragments.

Calcaneus

■ Most calcaneal fractures unite without difficulty.

■ The rare intra-articular fracture nonunion is treated by operative stabilization with grafting as required.

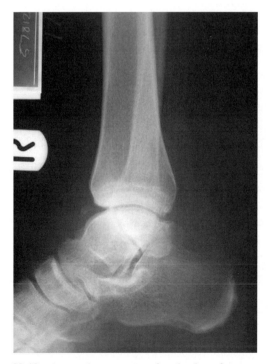

Figure 39-12 An atrophic nonunion of a talar dome fracture.

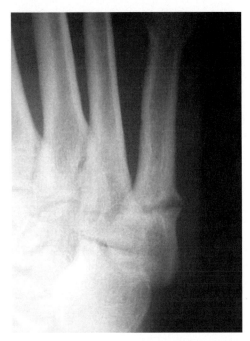

Figure 39-13 An oligotrophic nonunion of a zone 2 (Jones) fracture.

■ Fractures of the anterior process of the calcaneus are associated with a higher incidence of nonunion.
  ■ These fractures are rare but probably underdiagnosed.
■ Many anterior process fractures eventually become asymptomatic but if this does not occur, surgical treatment may be required.
■ Smaller fragments should be excised with internal fixation and grafting reserved for larger bone fragments.

Tarsus and Metatarsus

■ Tarsal nonunions are virtually unknown.
  ■ If encountered, treatment would involve internal fixation and grafting, although an option is a limited intertarsal fusion.
■ Metatarsal nonunions are also unusual, except for the fifth metatarsal where nonunions are more encountered in two areas.
■ Zone 1 (see Fig. 30-28 in Chapter 30) avulsion fractures are occasionally associated with nonunion, although most are not symptomatic.
■ Screw fixation or excision of a small fragment occasionally may be required.
■ Zone 2 (Jones) fractures (Fig. 39-13) have a higher incidence of nonunion (see Table 39-2).
  ■ These can be treated by the use of a cancellous screw passed proximally through the base of the metatarsal under fluoroscopic control.
  ■ Alternatively, plating and grafting may be used.
■ Other metatarsal nonunions are very uncommon and can be treated by internal fixation and grafting.

INFECTED NONUNION

■ Bone infections should be treated before the fracture becomes a nonunion. (The treatment of infection is discussed in Chapter 40.)

■ The earlier infection is treated, the better.
■ Surgeons do encounter infected nonunions, and these should be treated by aggressive debridement of all infected or avascular bone and soft tissues followed by reconstruction of the soft tissues using flap cover if required.
  ■ Bone reconstruction using bone grafting or bone transport is then required.
■ It is in the management of infected nonunions that bone transport is best utilized because a considerable length of bone may have to be resected to ensure all infected or avascular tissue is removed.
■ If an infected nonunion is treated in good time, debridement, soft tissue cover, and later bone grafting is all that is required.
■ Most of the literature deals with the treatment of infected tibial nonunion, and results indicate a success rate of about 90% ,with an average union time of about 26 weeks.
■ If there is a larger defect, bone transport is usually used (see Table 39-4).

SUGGESTED READING

Barquet A, Mayora G, Fregeiro J, et al. The treatment of subtrochanteric nonunions with the long gamma nail: twenty-six patients with a minimum 2-year follow up. J Orthop Trauma 2004; 18:346–353.

Biedermann R, Martin A, Handle G, et al. Extracorporeal shock waves in the treatment of nonunions. J Trauma 2003;54: 936–942.

Brighton CT, Shaman P, Heppenstall RB, et al. Tibial nonunion treated with direct current, capacitive coupling, or bone graft. Clin Orthop 1995;321:223–234.

Court-Brown CM, Keating JF, Christie J, et al. Exchange intramedullary nailing. Its use in aseptic tibial nonunion. J Bone Joint Surg (Br) 1995;77:407–411.

Court-Brown CM, McQueen MM. Compartment syndrome delays tibial union. Acta Orthop Scand 1987;12:308–312.

De Lee JC, Heckman JD, Lewis AG. Partial fibulectomy for ununited fractures of the tibia. J Bone Joint Surg (Am) 1981;63: 1390–1395.

Enneking WF, Mankin HJ. Immunologic responses in human recipients of osseous and osteochondral allografts. Clin Orthop 1996;326:107–114.

Friedlaender GE, Perry CR, Cole JD, et al. Osteogenic protein-1 (bone morphogenetic protein-7) in the treatment of tibial nonunions. J Bone Joint Surg (Am) 2001;83(Suppl Pt2):S151–158.

Gaebler C, Berger U, Schandelmaier P, et al. Rates and odds ratios for complications in closed and open tibial fractures treated with unreamed, small diameter tibial nails: a multicenter analysis of 467 cases. J Orthop Trauma 2001;15:415–423.

Ikeda T, Tomita K, Hasimoto F, et al. Long-term follow-up of vascularized bone grafts for the reconstruction of tibial nonunion: Evaluation with computed tomographic scanning. J Trauma 1992;32: 693–697.

Munk B, Larsen CF. Bone grafting the scaphoid nonunion. Acta Orthop Scand 2004;75:618–629.

Paley D. Treatment of tibial nonunion and bone loss with the Ilizarov technique. Instr Course Lect 1990;39:185–197.

Pugh GM, McKee MD. Advances in the management of humeral nonunion. J Am Acad Orthop Surg 2003;11:48–59.

Ring D, Kloen P, Kadzielski J, et al. Locking compression plates for osteoporotic nonunions of the diaphyseal humerus. Clin Orthop 2004;425:50–54.

Robinson, CM, Court-Brown CM, McQueen MM, et al. Estimating the risk of nonunion following nonoperative treatment of a clavicular fracture. J Bone Joint Surg (Am) 2004;8:1359–1365.

Sen C, Kocaoglu M, Eralp L, et al. Bifocal compression-distraction in the treatment of grade III open fractures with bone and soft-tissue loss: a report of 24 cases. J Orthop Trauma 2004;18: 150–157.

Strong DM, Friedlaender GE, Tomford WW, et al. Low-intensity pulsed ultrasound in the treatment of nonunions. J Trauma 2001;51:693–702.

Taylor JC. Delayed union and nonunion of fractures. In: Crenshaw AH, ed. Campbell's operative orthopaedics, 8th ed. St. Louis: CV Mosby, 1992.

Tiedeman JJ, Connolly JF, Strates BS, et al. Treatment of nonunion by percutaneous injection of bone marrow and demineralized bone matrix: an experimental study in dogs. Clin Orthop 1991;268: 294–302.

Weber BG, Cech O. Pseudarthrosis. Bern: Hans Huber, 1976.

INFECTION

OSTEOMYELITIS

The term *osteomyelitis* refers to infection in bone. It may be hematogenous, which is more commonly encountered in children. In adults, osteomyelitis is usually posttraumatic with organisms seeded in bone following an open fracture. Severe open fractures are frequently associated with significant damage to both bone and soft tissues, and although the fracture is ideally dealt with by an adequate debridement, total excision of all potentially devitalized tissue is difficult, and osteomyelitis can occur in any bone.

EPIDEMIOLOGY

The spectrum of osteomyelitis is very difficult to define. Much of the literature dealing with the incidence of osteomyelitis is now 25 to 30 years old and comes from an era when surgeons were extending the role of internal fixation without having the benefits of modern plastic and reconstructive surgery. Thus infection represented a significant problem for them. Together with the difficulty of defining deep as opposed to superficial infection, this has led to a wide range of infection rates being quoted. Tables 40-1 to 40-3 list the incidences of infection from the literature, but it should be remembered that in recent years the incidence of infection has decreased with improved orthopaedic techniques, improved plastic surgery, antibiotic use, and an awareness of the importance of early aggressive treatment. The infection rate following the closed management of fractures obviously is virtually zero, but nowadays many fractures are treated by internal or external fixation. In closed fractures treated by internal fixation, most authorities quote an infection rate of less than 2%. In open fractures, the incidence of infection varies with the severity of the soft tissue injury, and there is a direct

TABLE 40-1 RANGES AND AVERAGE VALUES OF OSTEOMYELITIS OF UPPER LIMB FRACTURES

Fracture	Repair Method	Range (%)	Average (%)	Table[a]
Clavicle	Plate	0.4–5.2	2.1	10-3
Lateral clavicle	K-wires	0–38.5	8.6	10-4
	Coracoclavicular stabilization	0–9.1	2	10-4
	Hook plate	0	0	10-4
Proximal humerus	K-wire	0	0	11-4
	Plate	0–50	4.5	11-4
	Nailing	0	0	11-5
Humeral diaphysis	Plate	0–6.5	3.4	12-3
	Antegrade nailing	0–6.7	1.8	12-4
	Retrograde nailing	0	0	12-4
Distal humerus (type C)	Plate	0–13	5.7	13-4
Olecranon	Tension band wiring	2.1–10.5	3.2	14-8
	Plate	0–15.4	3.3	14-8
Radius/ulna closed	Plate	0–7.4	2.5	15-4
Radius/ulna open	Plate	4.3–5.9	4.7	15-6
Distal radius		0–1	<1	

[a]Refers to the appropriate tables in different chapters.

TABLE 40-2 RANGES AND AVERAGE VALUES OF OSTEOMYELITIS OF PELVIS, HIP, AND THIGH FRACTURES

Fracture	Repair Method	Range (%)	Average (%)	Table[a]
Pelvis				
Anterior ring	Plate	2–5	2	
Posterior ring	Screws/plates	4–25	4	
Open pelvis				
Anterior thigh	Plates	5	5	
Perineum	External fixation/plates	10–50	20–40	
Femoral neck				
Young patients	Screws	0–3.4	2.0	21.2-7
Older patients	Screws	0–15	3.5	21.2-8
	Hemiarthroplasty	0–5.2	2.3	21.2-8
	Hip replacement	1.1–4	2.5	21.2-8
Intertrochanteric	Recon nail	0–4.1	1.3	21.2-15
	DHS	0–3.2	0.9	21.2-15
Subtrochanteric	95-degree blade plate	0–7.5	6.2	22-2
	DHS	0–2.1	2.0	22-4
	Nailing	0	0	22-6
Femoral diaphysis	Antegrade reamed nail	0–2.4	0.4	23-4
	Antegrade unreamed nail	0–2.9	0.8	23-4
	Retrograde reamed nail	0	0	23-6
	Retrograde unreamed nail	0	0	23-6
Femoral diaphysis (open)	Antegrade nailing	0–4.8	2.4	23-7
	Plate	0–10	4	23-9
Distal femur	95-degree blade plate	0–4.7	2.3	24-3
	DCS	0–4.3	1.4	24-4
	LISS plate	3–3.4	3.2	24-5
	Antegrade nailing	0–4.2	1.4	24-6
	Retrograde nailing	0–3.2	1.2	24-7
	External fixation	0–7.1	3.2	24-8
Patella	Tension band wiring	0–2	<1	25-3
	Partial patellectomy	0–1.5	<1	25-4

[a]Refers to the appropriate tables in different chapters.

relationship between the Gustilo grade and the incidence of osteomyelitis in most fractures. The highest incidence of infection is found where there is severe crushing injury and tissue devascularization. Generally speaking, the incidence of infection is higher in older patients and in patients who are immune compromised as a result of coexisting disease. Thus higher infection rates occur in patients with rheumatoid arthritis, diabetes, liver disease, and other medical conditions as well as in patients who smoke or who are taking corticosteroids or other drugs.

CLASSIFICATION

The classification most commonly used is the Cierny-Mader (1985) classification. This is the only classification that takes into account the host as well as the disease process, and it seems likely that future fracture classifications will have to do this if they are to be prognostic. The system is based on four factors: the degree of osseous involvement, the site of involvement, the degree of impairment caused by the disease, and the condition of the patient. The classification is summarized in Table 40-4, with the four different types of osseous involvement illustrated in Figure 40-1.

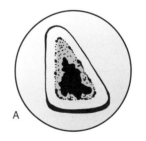
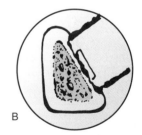
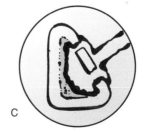
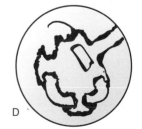

Figure 40-1 The Cierny-Mader classification of osteomyelitis. (**A**) Stage 1, medullary osteomyelitis. (**B**) Stage 2, superficial cortical osteomyelitis. (**C**) Stage 3, localized osteomyelitis. (**D**) Stage 4, diffuse osteomyelitis.

TABLE 40-3   RANGES AND AVERAGE VALUES OF OSTEOMYELITIS OF LEG AND FOOT FRACTURES TAKEN FROM THE LITERATURE

Fracture	Repair Method	Range (%)	Average (%)	Table[a]
Proximal tibia	Plate	0–4.2	3.2	26-8
	Assisted plate	0–3.9	2.3	26-8
	Bone substitutes	0–2.1	1.3	26-8
	External fixation (ring)	0–8.8	4.0	26-9
	External fixation (hybrid)	0–13.6	4.5	26-9
	External fixation (unilateral)	9.5–12.5	10.3	26-9
Tibia				
Closed	Reamed nail	0–2	1.4	27-3
	Unreamed nail	0–5.2	1.7	27-3
Open	Reamed nail	5.4–9.7	6.5	27-4
	Unreamed nail	2.4–12	6.2	27-4
Mixed	External fixation	0–11.4	5.4	27-6
	Plate	1–19	4.8	27-9
Type IIIb	Reamed nail	11–23.1	15.1	27-5
	Unreamed nail	5.9–25	15.4	27-5
	External fixation	11.1–38	16.1	27-7
Tibial plafond	Plate (open)	5.9–33.3	12.1	28-3
	Plate (minimal)	0–25	14.6	28-3
	Plate (delayed)	0–12.5	5.2	28-3
	External fixation (unilateral)	0–4.5	1.9	28-4
	External fixation (articulated)	0–8.3	1.6	28-4
	External fixation (hybrid)	0–8.1	5.2	28-4
	External fixation (ring)	0	0	28-4
Ankle	Internal fixation	0–4.9	1.8	29-6
Talus (neck)	Screws	0–10	3.3	30-4
Calcaneus (intra-articular)	K-wires	0–2.6	1.7	30-11
	Lateral plate	1–5	1.9	30-11
	Calcaneal plate	0–39	3.3	30-11

[a]Refers to the appropriate tables in different chapters.

Stage 1 is intramedullary osteomyelitis, which has assumed greater importance in the last decade because of the increased interest in the use of intramedullary nailing for femoral and tibial fractures. Stage 2 osteomyelitis is superficial and confined to the surface of the cortex. Stage 3 is full-thickness cortical osteomyelitis but confined to a specific area, and type 4 is osteomyelitis that involves the full circumference of the cortex. Table 40-4 shows the three different types of hosts. Class A hosts have normal systemic defenses, metabolism, and vascular supply. Class B hosts have systemic (Bs) or local (Bl) problems causing impaired healing. Systemic and local problems commonly coexist. Class C hosts are those in whom the treatment is worse than the presenting condition.

ETIOLOGY

Osteomyelitis is caused by bacterial contamination, which by itself is not usually sufficient to cause infection. Studies have shown that 60% to 70% of open fractures are contaminated, but Tables 40-1 to 40-3 show that the incidence of osteomyelitis is much less. For infection to occur, a number of situations must exist. The bacterial inoculum must be larger than can be dealt with, the host defense mecha-nisms are impaired, and traumatized tissue is present or there is a foreign body present in the wound.

Traumatized tissue, with an impaired blood supply, is an excellent bacterial culture medium. Dead or devitalized bone acts as a foreign body, and bacteria adhere to its surface. Bacterial adhesion depends on the physical characteristics of the bacteria, the fluid interface, and the substrate on which the bacteria are lying. The interaction between the bacteria and the substrate allows cross-linkages to form. The bacteria proliferate, and their biofilm is formed by bacterial extracapsular exopolysaccharides that bind to the substrate and participate in cell-to-cell aggregation. The biofilm enhances bacterial resistance. Devitalized bone without a normal periosteum is a good substrate for bacteria as are stainless steel, chromium-cobalt, and titanium implants. The use of implants improves stability, however, and instability is also a risk factor for bone infection.

Once a focus of infection occurs, it spreads relatively quickly. The presence of traumatized tissues adjacent to the infected focus accelerates the infection. Trauma is a stimulus for the systemic inflammatory response syndrome (SIRS) discussed in Chapter 41, and not only may this result in adult respiratory distress syndrome (ARDS) or multiple organ dysfunction (MOF) syndrome, but the host's ability to deal with the infection is compromised.

TABLE 40-4 THE CIERNY-MADER CLASSIFICATION

Stage	Anatomical Type
1	Medullary osteomyelitis
2	Superficial cortical osteomyelitis
3	Localized osteomyelitis
4	Diffuse osteomyelitis

Host type	Physiologic Class
A host	Normal
B host	Systemic (Bs) or local (Bl) compromise
C host	Treatment worse than disease

Types of host compromise
  Systemic (Bs)
  Malnutrition
  Renal, hepatic failure
  Diabetes mellitus
  Chronic hypoxia
  Immune disease
  Malignancy
  Old age
  Immunosuppression

  Local (Bl)
  Chronic lymphedema
  Venous stasis
  Vascular disease
  Extensive scarring
  Neuropathy
  Smoking

Adapted from Cierny G, Mader JT, Pennick H. A clinical staging system of adult osteomyelitis. Contemp Orthop 1985;10:17–37.

TABLE 40-5 DISTRIBUTION OF PATHOGENS IN OSTEOMYELITIS[a]

Pathogen	Prevalence (%)
Gram-positive cocci and bacilli	
Coagulase-positive *Staphylococcus*	33.6
Coagulase-negative *Staphylococcus*	11.6
Beta-hemolytic *Streptococcus*	7.5
Viridans *Streptococcus*	1.7
Enterococcus	4.6
Corynebacterium	1.7
Bacillus	1.7
Gram-negative bacilli	
Pseudomonas aeruginosa	8.7
Enterobacter	4.6
Escherichia coli	3.3
Serratia	2.9
Proteus	2.9
Acinetobacter	2.5
Klebsiella	1.2
Morganella	1.2
Aeromonas	0.8
Achromobacter	0.4
Pasteurella	0.4
Hemophilus	0.4
Anaerobes	
Bacteroides	1.2
Peptostreptococcus	3.7
Clostridium	0.8
Other	1.2
Miscellaneous	
Mycobacterium	0.4
Candida	0.8

[a]Information from Hennepin County Medical Center, 1986–1991. Adapted from Tsukayama DT, Gustilo RB. Microbiology of open fractures. In: Court-Brown CM, McQueen MM, Quaba AA, eds. Management of open fractures. London: Martin Dunitz, 1996.

The inflammatory response is diminished and the immune system depressed. Without treatment the infected focus enlarges, so any delay in treatment necessitates a more aggressive surgical excision of the infected tissues.

Bacteria

There is some regional variation in the pathogens that cause osteomyelitis, but the literature indicates reasonable uniformity with coagulase-positive staphylococci accounting for 20% to 35% of infection and gram-negative pathogens for 30% to 45%. A list of pathogens responsible for osteomyelitis in a major North American trauma center is given in Table 40-5.

DIAGNOSIS

History and Physical Examination

- Posttraumatic osteomyelitis may present with a history of a previous fracture treated by surgical fixation.
- Within a few days of treatment there is increased pain, swelling, local warmth, and erythema.

- There may be active drainage from the wound, although in the early stages it may seem that only a superficial infection is present.
- The wound is increasingly tender on palpation, and there may be restricted motion in adjacent joints.
- Alternatively, the infection may present later after the surgical wound or flap has healed.
  - Again the patient may present with local and systemic signs of sepsis, but it may be that failure of union with radiological changes suggestive of infection are the only clues to the diagnosis.
- The two most common areas of diagnostic difficulty are therefore deciding if an early infection is superficial or deep and whether a late nonunion is related to infection.

Laboratory Tests

- Laboratory investigations should include a white blood cell count and an assessment of the ratio of polymorphonuclear leucocytes to other white cells.
- An erythrocyte sedimentation rate (ESR) and a C-reactive protein (CRP) should be done.

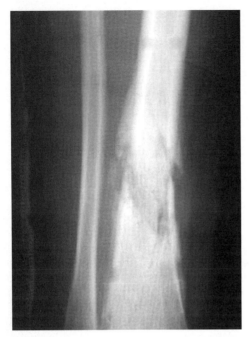

Figure 40-2 Osteomyelitis in a tibial fracture. Note the demineralization, cortical thinning, and trabecular loss. There is evidence of attempted union.

- The ESR may initially be normal but may rise to above 100 mm/hr.
- The sensitivity of the CRP has been shown to be 82% in the acute situation and 43% in chronic osteomyelitis.
- Blood cultures are positive in 50% to 75% of cases.

Radiologic Examination

Radiographs
- The earliest sign of infection on radiographs is demineralization, which may occur in the first 2 weeks.
- As the disease progresses, cortical thinning and trabecular loss become evident.
- The body attempts to unite the fracture despite the infection, and later radiographs may show signs of attempted union with periosteal new bone formation, callus formation, and significant bone sclerosis (Fig. 40-2).
- A classic involucrum and sequestrum may form, although this is much less common today with improved detection and treatment of osteomyelitis.

Bone Scanning
- Until the advent of MRI scans, isotope bone scanning was the main imaging modality used in the diagnosis of osteomyelitis.
- An area of osteomyelitis appears as a region of increased blood flow and should be "hot" in all phases of the scan.
- Technetium-99 bone scanning is reported to have a sensitivity of 32% to 100% and specificity of 0% to 100%.
- Results have been improved by the addition of gallium-67, but any process causing reactive new bone formation appear "hot" if a gallium scan is used.
- The reported sensitivity and specificity is similar to technetium, but it is particularly useful in the diagnosis of chronic soft tissue infection.

- Indium-111-labeled leucocytes can be used, and indium scans have been reported to be 97% sensitive and 82% specific for osteomyelitis.

MRI
- MRI scanning is particularly useful in that it shows both the area of osteomyelitis and the state of the soft tissues and localizes any abscess cavities (Fig. 40-3).
- Active osteomyelitis characteristically shows a decreased signal on T1-weighted images and enhanced-signal T2-weighted images.
- MRI is 92% to 100% sensitive and 89% to 100% specific for osteomyelitis.

CT Scanning
- CT scans have generally been replaced by MRI scanning but remain useful in diagnosing cortical irregularities such as sequestra.

Biopsy
- Bone biopsy is the best diagnostic procedure for chronic osteomyelitis.

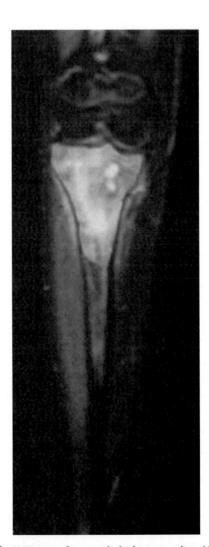

Figure 40-3 MRI scan of proximal tibial osteomyelitis. Note the edema, periosteal involvement, and abscess cavity.

- For maximum sensitivity it is important to send specimens of the bone for both bacteriological culture and histological examination.
- The procedure can usually be undertaken using fluoroscopy, but open surgery may be required.
- If a culture is taken from the discharging sinus, it does not always show the infecting organism.
- If there is concern about the presence of a septic arthritis, aspiration and bacteriological culture is mandatory.

TREATMENT

- Treatment of osteomyelitis is very similar to the treatment of an open fracture, namely aggressive debridement (see Chapter 4), antibiotic administration, fracture stabilization (see Chapters 10–30), soft tissue cover (see Chapter 4), and bone reconstruction (see Chapter 39).
- Exact treatment depends on the circumstances, with more aggressive treatment required for established osteomyelitis associated with considerable bone involvement.
- There are three basic stages at which patients present (Box 40-1).

Antibiotics

- It is important to select an appropriate antibiotic for the treatment of osteomyelitis. It is beyond the scope of this book to discuss the pharmacology of antibiotics, but in recent years surgeons have been faced with an increasing problem of methicillin-resistant *Staphylococcus aureus* (MRSA).
- Vancomycin is used extensively for this bacteria, but increasing antibiotic resistance to other bacteria is

likely to become a major problem in the next few decades.
- Some surgeons favor the use of antibiotic-impregnated (PMMA) beads.
- These are in fact very useful in stage 3 osteomyelitis.
- They provide a high local concentration of antibiotics, although if adequate bone and soft tissue clearance has been performed, it may not be particularly important.
- They do provide a "filler" for the bone defects that stops the encroachment of soft tissues into the defect and facilitates later bone grafting.
- Most of the studies of antibiotic-impregnated PMMA beads have been undertaken in open fracture management, where there is evidence they help reduce the incidence of infection.
- Evidence also indicates that the use of antibiotic-impregnated PMMA beads may reduce the length of intravenous antibiotic therapy and thereby reduce the complications associated with the prolonged use of intravenous antibiotics.
- They should not be used as a substitute for a thorough surgical debridement, however.

NECROTIZING FASCIITIS

Necrotizing fasciitis is a rapidly progressive infection localized between the superficial and deep fasciae. It may arise spontaneously such as in Fournier's disease of the scrotum, but not infrequently there is a history of trauma. Infection spreads very quickly along the fascial planes and, unless rapidly treated, may prove fatal.

BOX 40-1 THREE STAGES OF PRESENTATION OF BONE INFECTION, WITH TREATMENT REGIMENS

Stage 1
- Patients present within 2 weeks of fracture treatment.
- Ultrasound/MRI scan used to determine if pyogenic collection present.
- If no collection, maintain high-dose antibiotics for 4 to 6 weeks. If collection present, treat as for stage 2.
- Maintain fracture fixation.
- Monitor patient's progress clinically, hematologically, and radiologically.
- Fracture usually unites in appropriate time.

Stage 2
- Patients usually present 2 to 6 weeks after initial treatment.
- Ultrasound/MRI scan shows a pyogenic collection.
- Surgical decompression of pyogenic collection, culture of infected material, and appropriate antibiotic administration.
- Intramedullary canal of long bones should be reamed to remove pyogenic material.
- If primary nailing used, exchange nailing should be undertaken.
- Maintain fracture stability; restabilize if necessary.
- Remove all devitalized tissue.

- Administer appropriate antibiotics for 4 to 6 weeks.
- Monitor patient's progress clinically, hematologically, and radiologically.
- Fractures usually unite but union time prolonged.

Stage 3[a]
- Patients present late.
- There is a discharging sinus together with devitalized infected bone and poor soft tissues around the nonunion site and sinus.
- Aggressive debridement of all dead and devitalized soft tissues.
- Appropriate fracture stabilization. Usually intramedullary nailing or external fixation for long bones.
- Flap cover for soft tissue defect.
- Later osseous reconstruction. Usually grafting or bone transport.
- Appropriate long-term antibiotics.
- Amputation occasionally required.

[a]In stage 3a patients, the fracture remains ununited. In stage 3b patients, the fracture has united. The treatment is the same for both types.

ETIOLOGY

The condition is caused by a number of bacteria that occur either singly or in combination. Group A *streptococcus* and *Staphylococcus* aureus are usually the causative organisms and frequently act synergistically. Other aerobic and anaerobic organisms may be present, including *Bacteroides, Clostridia, Peptostreptococcus, Enterobacteriaceae, Coliforms, Proteus, Pseudomonas,* and *Klebsiella*. The condition can also be caused by marine *Vibrios* following a puncture wound, abrasion, or bite exposed to sea water.

Group A *streptococci* secrete exotoxins, which in turn produce the systemic inflammatory response syndrome (SIRS) detailed in Chapter 41. This may in turn may cause adult distress syndrome (ARDS) and multiple organ dysfunction syndrome (MODS).

DIAGNOSIS

History and Physical Examination

- The early clinical findings are local pain, swelling, and erythema, which may be adjacent to a wound.
- The findings mimic cellulitis, but the clinical progress is very rapid and the patient quickly becomes septic, with ARDS and MODS occurring often within 48 hours.
- Examination initially shows a cellulitis, but as the subcutaneous fat becomes involved, there is thrombosis of the subcutaneous vascular supply, resulting in skin devascularization and necrosis (Fig. 40-4).
- The condition is more common in patients with impaired immune systems and comorbidities such as diabetes, alcoholism, and drug abuse.
- If untreated, death occurs very quickly.
- The rapid spread of the disease process means the patient is usually very ill when the diagnosis is made.
- Thus a full hematological workup is essential, together with arterial blood gases and blood cultures.
- The main differential diagnosis is myonecrosis, but surgeons should be aware that because necrotizing fasciitis does not affect muscle initially, creatinine kinase levels may be low.

Radiologic Examination

- Plain radiographs show subcutaneous gas in 24% to 73% of cases.
- MRI scanning may be useful, but in reality the diagnosis is a clinical one based on the rapid progress of the disease and the clinical findings.

TREATMENT

- Because the diagnosis is usually made late, the patient typically requires intensive care and frequently needs ventilation.
- The patient usually shows signs of septic shock, ARDS, and MODS.
- The definitive treatment of the underlying condition is surgical debridement of all affected tissues, and because the fasciitis usually involves a greater area than is clinically apparent, segmental debridements with excision of all affected soft tissues are usually necessary.

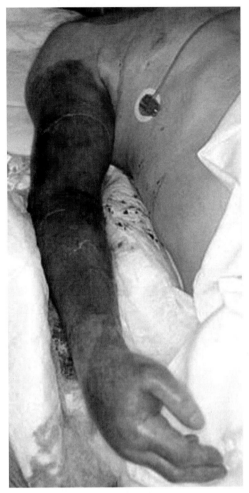

Figure 40-4   Necrotizing fasciitis in the arm of a 72-year-old man. Disarticulation was performed.

- If the patient's condition is poor, amputation may be life saving.
- Intravenous antibiotics are essential.
- A Gram stain may help detail which antibiotics should be used.
- Penicillin or clindamycin together with antistaphylococcal agents such as ceftriaxone or vancomycin should be used with a broad-spectrum antibiotic used for gram-negative organisms.
- Considerable literature deals with the use of hyperbaric oxygen in the treatment of necrotizing fasciitis; little evidence indicates it is useful, however, and in most cases it is not practical to consider using hyperbaric oxygen.
- The correct treatment is surgical debridement.

RESULTS

- In the past, the mortality following necrotizing fasciitis has been considerable, with 28% to 75% mortality reported.
- A recent study of 150 necrotizing soft tissue infections in San Francisco documented a mortality of 9.3%.
- The condition is often difficult to diagnose, and good results depend on prompt treatment.

GAS GANGRENE

Gas gangrene is a rapid myonecrosis produced by *clostridia* species. *Clostridia* are anaerobic gram-positive bacteria commonly found in the gut and in soil. Gas gangrene follows the contamination of large wounds and is typically seen in farmyard accidents or following fecal contamination of large operative wounds. It is relatively uncommon, with 900 to 1,000 cases reported each year in the United States.

ETIOLOGY

Gas gangrene is caused by exotoxins produced by *clostridial* species, of which *Clostridium perfringens* and *Clostridium septicum* are the most common. The exotoxins cause muscle destruction and create an aerobic environment conducive to further bacterial growth. Products of tissue breakdown, such as creatinine phosphokinase, myoglobin, and potassium, cause secondary toxicity. The toxins stimulate the systemic inflammatory response syndrome (SIRS) and very rapidly cause ARDS and MODS (see Chapter 41).

DIAGNOSIS

History and Physical Examination

- The initial clinical findings may well be similar to cellulitis with pain and swelling around the wound, but the pain is out of proportion to the clinical findings.
- There may be serosanguineous discharge, local edema, cutaneous bullae, and local skin discoloration.
- Muscle involvement is extensive, and the patient's clinical condition rapidly deteriorates with shock, ARDS, and multiple organ failure becoming evident.
- The patients tend to be immune compromised, and the disease is more common in diabetics, drug abusers, and alcoholics.
- It is also associated with hematological and gastrointestinal malignancies.

Laboratory Tests

- The diagnosis is frequently made late, and a full hematological workup is essential.
- This should include arterial blood gas, blood cultures, and assessment of liver function, coagulopathy, and renal function.
- Myoglobinemia and myoglobinuria will be present.
- Radiographs may show gas in the soft tissues.

TREATMENT

- The rapid progress of the disease means the patient usually presents in septic shock and requires intensive care and resuscitation.
- Amputation is usually required to the level that all disease tissue is removed.
- Muscle resection without amputation may be adequate theoretically, but this is rare and the patient and family should be warned that amputation may well be required to prevent death.
- Penicillin G is used, although clindamycin, ceftriaxone, chloramphenicol, and other antibiotics can be used.
- As with necrotizing fasciitis, surgeons often discuss the use of hyperbaric oxygen, but there is little proof of its usefulness, and the relatively short time available to the surgeon prior to treatment means hyperbaric oxygen is impractical.
- The mortality of traumatic gas gangrene is more than 25% in most series, with the mortality for nontraumatic gas gangrene much higher probably because of the late presentation.

SUGGESTED READING

Cierny G. Infected tibial nonunions (1981–1995): the evolution of change. Clin Orthop 1999;360:97.

Cierny G, Mader JT, Penninck JJ. A clinical staging system for adult osteomyelitis. Clin Orthop 2003;414:7–24.

Cierny G, Zorn KE. Segmental tibial defects. Comparing conventional and Ilizarov methodologies. Cin Orthop 1994;301:18–123.

Court-Brown CM, Keating JF, McQueen MM. Infection after intramedullary nailing of the tibia. Incidence and protocol for management. J Bone Joint Surg (Br) 1992;74:770–774.

Dirschl DR, Dahners LE. The mangled extremity: when should it be amputated? J Am Acad Orthop Surg 1998;12:460–463.

Fontes RA, Ogilvie CM, Miclau T. Necrotizing soft-tissue infections. J Am Acad Orthop Surg 2000;8:151–158.

Klemm K. Antibiotic bead chains. Clin Orthop 1993;295:63–76 .

Lazzarini L, Conti E, Ditri L, et al. Clostridial orthopedic infections: case reports and review of the literature. J Chemother 2004;16: 94–97.

Patzakis MJ, Harrey JP, Ivler D. The role of antibiotics in the management of open fractures. J Bone Joint Surg (Am) 1974:56:532–541.

Perry BN, Floyd WE. Gas gangrene and necrotizing fasciitis in the upper extremity. J Surg Orthop Adv 2004;13:57–68.

Tetsworth K, Cierny G. Osteomyelitis debridement techniques. Clin Orthop 1999;360:87–96.

Tsai YH, HSU RW, Huang KC, et al. Systemic Vibrio infection presenting as necrotizing fasciitis and sepsis. A series of thirteen cases. J Bone Joint Surg (Am) 2004;86:2497–2502.

Tsukayama DT, Gustilo RB. Microbiology of open fractures. In: Court-Brown CM, McQueen MM, Quaba AA, eds. Management of open fractures. London: Martin Dunitz, 1996.

Zalavras CG, Patzakis MJ, Holtom P. Local antibiotic therapy in the treatment of open fractures and osteomyelitis. Clin Orthop 2004;427:86–93.

41 OTHER COMPLICATIONS

DEEP VENOUS THROMBOSIS

Deep venous thrombosis (DVT) is a common condition that affects about 1 person per 1,000 population per year. It is associated with many medical conditions but is a relatively common complication of trauma. Autopsy studies of injured patients have shown that 58% to 63% show evidence of DVT, although less than 2% of patients display clinical manifestations of the condition. About 20% of multiply injured patients die as a result of a DVT. Venography has shown that approximately 50% of patients with tibial diaphyseal fractures, approximately 34% of patients with subcapital fractures, and 75% of patients with peritrochanteric fractures have a DVT. Between 3% and 13% of patients with a hip fracture are symptomatic, and a fatal pulmonary embolus occurs in 1% to 7% of patients.

The risk of DVT is associated with a number of factors, shown in Box 41-1. A prospective study of the risk factors associated with DVT in multiply injured patients showed that increasing age, the requirement for blood transfusion, the need for surgery, the presence of a femoral or tibial fracture, and spinal cord injury were all independent predictors of DVT. The risk of DVT increased by five times in patients with femoral or tibial diaphyseal fractures. In elective hip surgery the use of regional anesthesia reduced the incidence of proximal vein DVT from 73% to 23% compared with

BOX 41-1 RISK FACTORS ASSOCIATED WITH DEEP VENOUS THROMBOSIS

- Increasing age
- Extent and duration of surgical procedures
- Type of anesthesia
- Duration of immobilization
- Coexisting systemic disease
- Blood transfusions
- Presence of femoral or tibial fracture
- Spinal cord injury

general anesthesia. Pulmonary embolus (PE) has been estimated to occur in about 5,000/10,000 people/year. About 10% of patients with pulmonary emboli die of the condition.

ETIOLOGY

Venous thrombi are mainly composed of fibrin and erythrocytes together with platelets and leucocytes. They usually form in venous sinuses in the deep veins of the calf and in veins damaged by trauma. Damage to the endothelium of the veins leads to platelet adhesion, leucocyte accumulation, and the activation of the intrinsic and extrinsic pathways. Cytokines and tumor necrosis factor may be released, causing distant venous damage leading to coagulation. Venous stasis during surgery or as a result of trauma may contribute by slowing the clearance of coagulative factors. This is particularly important in lower limb surgery because the normal pumping action of the calf muscles may be slowed or abolished.

There is a clear association between DVT and PE. About 50% of patients with a proven DVT develop PE, and about 70% of patients with confirmed PE have asymptomatic DVTs. Pulmonary emboli can take the form of multiple small emboli or a single large, often fatal embolus. Most significant PEs arise from the proximal veins.

DIAGNOSIS

- The clinical signs of DVT include leg pain and swelling, edema, altered temperature, dilated superficial veins, and erythema.
- Tests include assessment of leg circumference and Homan's sign, which is calf pain caused by forced dorsiflexion of the ankle with the knee flexed.
- Comparison with venography has shown that these clinical signs and tests are inaccurate, and the diagnosis of DVT requires the use of venography, ultrasound, or impedance plethysmography.
- Venography remains the standard investigation.
    - Contrast material is injected into the superficial veins of the foot and x-rays are used to delineate areas of inadequate venous filling.

TABLE 41-1 AVERAGE RESULTS OF RCTS COMPARING ANTIPLATELET MEDICATION (USUALLY ASPIRIN) WITH UNFRACTIONATED HEPARIN AND LOW-MOLECULAR-WEIGHT HEPARIN

Medication	Asymptomatic DVT (%)		Asymptomatic PE (%)		Fatal PE (%)	
	Active	Control	Active	Control	Active	Control
Antiplatelet medication	35.9	41.9	0.8	1.6	0.4	0.8
Unfractionated heparin	27.7	49.9	3.7	3.1	2	3.1
Low-molecular-weight heparin	25	48	0.6	1.2	0	0.6

Results from SIGN Guidelines (http://sign.ac.uk).

■ It requires expert radiological assessment and is inconvenient if multiple studies are required.

■ Ultrasound is particularly useful for visualization of proximal vein DVT and is less effective for calf vein DVT.

■ An alternative technique is impedance plethysmography, which has been shown to have a high accuracy in the diagnosis of thigh DVT in particular.

■ These tests remain the standard diagnostic tests for proving the presence of a DVT.

■ The diagnosis of PE is also difficult if the surgeon relies on the clinical criteria of chest pain and breathlessness because these symptoms are caused by many different medical conditions.

■ Diagnosis is best undertaken by angiography or by a perfusion lung scan.

■ Investigations should also include an ECG to exclude cardiac problems, a chest x-ray, and arterial blood gases.

TREATMENT

■ The treatment of DVT is anticoagulation.

■ It is beyond the scope of this book to discuss treatment in detail, but usually heparin is administered to provide initial anticoagulation.

■ Warfarin is then introduced, and the dose adjusted according to the international normalized ratio (INR), which should be within the range of 2.0 to 3.0.

  ■ Warfarin treatment is continued for at least 3 months.

Prophylaxis

■ Given the high incidence of both DVT and PE and the obvious association with surgery and trauma, it is important to try and minimize the risk of both conditions.

■ There are a number of ways of doing this, of which the most commonly used are mechanical methods, antiplatelet medication, and heparin.

■ Mechanical methods of DVT prophylaxis include graduated elastic compression stockings (GECS), intermittent pneumatic compression, and mechanical foot pumps.

■ An analysis of the meta-analyses of DVT prophylaxis has shown that the use of GECS results in asymptomatic DVTs being found in 8.6% of patients compared with 27% of controls.

■ The combination of GECS with pharmacological prophylaxis is more effective than pharmacological prophylaxis alone.

■ Studies have also shown that intermittent pneumatic compression and mechanical foot pumps are effective in the prophylaxis of asymptomatic DVT.

■ An analysis of the results of randomized control trials of antiplatelet therapy (usually aspirin), unfractionated heparin (UFH), and low-molecular-weight heparin (LMWH) is given in Table 41-1.

  ■ All these treatments reduce the incidence of asymptomatic DVT and fatal PE, with aspirin and LMWH also reducing the incidence of asymptomatic PE.

  ■ Aspirin also increases the risk of perioperative bleeding.

■ In trauma patients, pharmacological prophylaxis should be used unless there are specific contraindications (Box 41-2).

■ Aspirin and LMWH are about equally effective, but aspirin is associated with greater perioperative and postoperative hemorrhage, and for this reason the use of LMWH is preferred by many surgeons.

  ■ If a patient is already taking prophylactic aspirin, supplementary LMWH is not required.

■ North American guidelines advocate the use of LMWH rather than aspirin.

BOX 41-2 CONTRAINDICATIONS TO PHARMACOLOGIC DVT PROPHYLAXIS

■ Uncorrected bleeding disorders
■ Major hemorrhage
  ■ Intracranial bleed
  ■ Pelvic hemorrhage
  ■ Esophageal varices
  ■ Peptic ulcer
  ■ Spinal cord injury
■ Anemia
■ Allergy
■ Heparin-associated thrombocytopenia
■ Aspirin-induced asthma
■ Severe liver impairment
■ Severe renal impairment

FAT EMBOLUS SYNDROME

Fat embolus syndrome (FES) is the term given to the occurrence of hypoxia, confusion, and a petechial rash soon after long-bone fracture, usually in young adults. First described in 1862 by Zenker, until relatively recently it was thought to be caused by a fat embolus arising in the bone marrow and traveling to the lungs. This may well be a cause of FES, but it has become clear that FES is part of a larger problem: adult respiratory distress syndrome (ARDS). The exact definitions of FES and ARDS are imprecise, and there is no doubt the two conditions share some clinical features and both may be produced by both traumatic and nontraumatic causes.

Good evidence indicates that fat embolization plays a key role in the development of posttraumatic respiratory compromise. Fat can be detected in the lungs soon after fracture and may pass to the systemic circulation through pulmonary capillaries and shunts or through a patent foramen ovale to produce the features of systemic embolization. Fat embolism occurs in more than 90% of patients after major trauma, but only about 1% to 5% develop FES, although it has been reported to occur in almost 10% of multiply injured patients who have unstable pelvic injuries. Animal experiments have shown that intravascular fat appears to produce a negligible inflammatory response, but presumably fat embolism is a trigger for posttraumatic respiratory insufficiency in some situations.

ETIOLOGY

The original theory of the cause of FES was mechanical and suggested that free fat globules left the marrow space and entered the venous circulation. This theory is obviously based on the proven fact that the marrow cavity is the source of the embolic fat seen in the lungs after trauma. Animal experiments have shown that the pulmonary vessels narrow after embolic showers and the transpulmonary route is a source of systemic fat embolization. It seems likely that the etiology of FES is more complex and involves the stimulation of severe inflammatory changes associated with endothelial damage, inactivation of lung surfactant, and increased capillary permeability. It has been suggested that the inflammatory reaction may be mediated through the action of toxic-free fatty acids caused by the action of lung lipase on neutral fat.

It is also likely that the inflammatory changes may be caused by other factors explaining why a number of different conditions may have pulmonary compromise as a final common pathway. Thromboplastin is released from the long bones after fracture, which activates the complement system and the extrinsic coagulation cascade through activation of factor VII. Thus the inflammatory response is activated. It seems likely that FES is a result of an increased inflammatory state that initially targets the lungs. As the condition worsens, other organs are affected, and multiple organ dysfunction syndrome (MODS) may occur.

DIAGNOSIS

- The classical signs of FES are pulmonary, cerebral, and cutaneous.
- The condition usually occurs in the second or third decades but may occur at any age.
- The pulmonary symptoms are tachypnea, dyspnea, and cyanosis, and the cerebral signs are usually headache, irritability, convulsion, delirium, and coma.
- By the second or third day, about 50% of patients develop a petechial rash on the chest, anterior axillary folds, and conjunctiva.
- Gurd and Wilson suggested the original criteria for diagnosis of FES, but these were later modified to include objective measurements of respiratory rate, PaO_2, $PacO_2$ and PH (Box 41-3).
- Laboratory investigations include arterial blood gases, chest x-ray, ECG, and a CT or MRI scan of the brain.

TREATMENT

- Treatment of FES is essentially respiratory support using oxygen therapy or mechanical ventilation.
- Long-bone fractures should be stabilized.
- The mortality rate associated with FES is between 5% and 15% but may reach 36% in patients who require mechanical ventilation.

BOX 41-3 CRITERIA FOR DIAGNOSING FAT EMBOLUS SYNDROME

Gurd and Wilson[a] (1974)
Major features
  Respiratory insufficiency
  Cardiac signs
  Petechial rash
Minor features
  Pyrexia
  Tachycardia
  Retinal involvement
  Jaundice
  Renal involvement
  Fat macroglobulinemia

Lindeque et al. (1987)
Sustained Pao_2 <8.0 kPa
Sustained $Paco_2$ <7.5 kPa
PH <7.3
Respiratory rate >35/min

[a]If Gurd and Wilson's clinical criteria are used, there should be one major and four minor features present.

ADULT RESPIRATORY DISTRESS SYNDROME

As already indicated, ARDS is a syndrome that results from a number of etiological factors such as FES. Injury causes an inflammatory reaction often referred to as systemic inflammatory response syndrome (SIRS), which may also be caused by nontraumatic stimuli such as burns or pancreatitis. The lung is targeted in the early stages of the syndrome, but if the patient survives there are often features of cardiac, gastrointestinal, renal, hepatic, hematological, and cerebral dysfunction as part of the syndrome of multiple organ dysfunction syndrome (MODS). Evidence of MODS is commonly found at autopsy in patients who die from ARDS after 72 hours.

EPIDEMIOLOGY

The incidence of ARDS was estimated to be $75/10^5$/year in the general population in 1972, and it has been suggested that 5% to 8% of major trauma patients show signs of the condition. A recent analysis of ARDS in a population of 7,192 consecutive trauma admissions has provided modern epidemiological information (Table 41-2). It has a type C distribution (see Chapter 1) affecting mainly young patients. A number of associations can aid prediction of ARDS, listed in Box 41-4. Patients generally present after high-energy trauma with a femoral fracture, injuries in more than one body system, and compromised physiological function.

ETIOLOGY

Current knowledge about the cause of the inflammatory events that stimulate ARDS is limited. The release of cytokines, interaction between platelets and circulating leucocytes with vascular endothelial cells, the extravasation and degranulation of neutrophils to produce toxic products, and the activation of neuroendocrine, complement, coagulative, or fibrinolytic pathways are involved. Once a process has commenced, it is hypothesized that secondary hits such as fracture fixation may enhance the inflammatory process, worsening the clinical situation. Other secondary hits may be hypoxia, hypovolemia, blood transfusion, and sepsis.

TABLE 41-2 EPIDEMIOLOGY OF ARDS

Incidence following traumatic injury	0.5%
Incidence in population	$0.8/10^5$/y
Men/women	55%/45%
Average age	29 y
Distribution	Type C
Blunt trauma	97%

Data from White TO, Jenkins PJ, Smith RD, et al. The epidemiology of posttraumatic adult respiratory distress syndrome. J Bone Joint Surg (Am) 2004;86:2366–2376.

BOX 41-4 PREDICTIVE CRITERIA FOR ARDS

- High-energy trauma
- Glasgow Coma Scale score <8
- Revised Trauma Score <12
- Injury Severity Score >25
- Systolic blood pressure <90 mm Hg
- Respiratory rate <10/min
- Femoral fracture
- Initial requirement for laparotomy
- Injury in more than one body system

From White TO, Jenkins PJ, Smith RD, et al. The epidemiology of posttraumatic adult respiratory distress syndrome. J Bone Joint Surg (Am) 2004;86:2366–2376.

DIAGNOSIS

- The clinical features of ARDS are pulmonary with patients initially complaining of dyspnea and tachypnea.
- Investigation includes arterial blood gases and chest radiography.

TREATMENT

- As with FES, the treatment of ARDS is mainly ventilatory support, usually with mechanical ventilation with appropriate pharmacological treatment.
- Care should be taken to monitor and treat sepsis because a combination of sepsis and ARDS influences the prognosis significantly.
- MODS may occur and require treatment.
- The mortality of ARDS has been reported to be as high as 50%.

Fracture Treatment

- The concepts of early total care and damage control surgery are discussed in Chapter 3.
- It is recommended that patients with signs of ARDS are treated using the principles of damage control surgery shown in Box 3-3 in Chapter 3.

SHOCK

Shock is inadequate tissue profusion resulting in a failure to provide the nutritional requirements of cells and to remove the products of metabolism. There are four basic types.

- Hypovolemic shock is caused by loss of fluid, usually as a result of hemorrhage.
- Cardiogenic shock arises from a reduction in cardiac output secondary to cardiac pathology.
- Neurogenic shock is caused by a failure of arterial resistance, which results in pooling of blood in the periphery and a low blood pressure. This may be seen after spinal injury.

TABLE 41-3 DEFINITION OF HYPOVOLEMIC SHOCK (AMERICAN COLLEGE OF SURGEONS)

Parameter	Class I	Class II	Class III	Class IV
Blood loss (mL)	Up to 750	750–1,500	1,500–2,000	>2,000
Blood loss (% bv)	Up to 15	15–30	30–40	>40
Pulse rate (beats/min)	<100	>100	>120	>140
Blood pressure	Normal	Normal	Decreased	Decreased
Pulse pressure	Normal or increased	Decreased	Decreased	Decreased
Respiratory rate (breaths/min)	14–20	20–30	30–40	>35
Urine output (mL/hr)	>30	20–30	5–15	Negligible
CNS/mental status	Slightly anxious	Mildly anxious	Anxious and confused	Confused and lethargic

■ Septic shock is a syndrome not dissimilar to ARDS. Endotoxins stimulate cytokine release, which in turn causes endothelial damage. This results in increased capillary permeability and an ARDS-like state that might lead to multiple organ dysfunction syndrome (MODS). Patients may have high-output or low-output septic shock. In high-output septic shock, there is decreased peripheral vascular resistance and increased cardiac output. This is the early manifestation of severe septic conditions such as necrotizing fasciitis, gangrene, and other severe infections. Untreated sepsis results in a low-output state similar to hypovolemic shock.

CLASSIFICATION

Hypovolemic shock has been usefully classified by the American College of Surgeons (Table 41-3). They have divided the clinical signs and symptoms into four categories based on their severity. Class I shock is associated with minimal symptoms. Class II shock shows increasing symptomatology, but classes III and IV show the classic signs of shock-tachycardia, tachypnea, changes in mental status, and a fall in the systolic blood pressure. Class IV is a life-threatening condition associated with a very low systolic blood pressure, an immeasurable diastolic blood pressure, and virtually no urine output.

TRAUMA PATIENTS

Hypovolemic shock is unusual in patients who have isolated fractures. There may be significant blood loss from an isolated femoral fracture, but a recent analysis of isolated femoral fractures has shown that no patient presented with class III or IV shock. Multiply injured patients may well present with hypovolemic shock, however, particularly if they have a pelvic fracture. Hemorrhage has been shown to be responsible for up to 18% of deaths after pelvic fracture.

Septic shock may be encountered with severe soft tissue infection such as necrotizing fasciitis and gas gangrene (see Chapter 40). Neurogenic shock may complicate spinal cord injuries, and although cardiogenic shock is not caused primarily by trauma, many patients have medical comorbidities, and thus the pattern of shock may be complicated by preexisting cardiac pathology.

TREATMENT

■ The treatment of shock is beyond the scope of this book because it is now frequently undertaken by intensivists, but the underlying principles must be understood.
■ Hypovolemic shock is treated by fluid resuscitation using crystalloids, colloids, and blood.
■ In cardiac, neurogenic, and septic shock, the appropriate pharmacological agents are required.

COMPLEX REGIONAL PAIN SYNDROMES

These conditions manifest themselves by the continuation of pain and other symptoms after injury. There are two types of complex regional pain syndrome (CRPS). CRPS I is still mainly referred to as reflex sympathetic dystrophy, Sudeck's atrophy, or algodystrophy. It occurs without any demonstrable nerve damage. In CRPS II, also known as causalgia, there is nerve damage usually caused by a crushing injury, gunshot wounds, or nerve laceration.

EPIDEMIOLOGY

CRPS usually affects the extremities and has been reported to occur in up to 5% of patients with peripheral nerve injuries and 30% of patients with distal radial and tibial diaphyseal fractures. It must be emphasized that most of these cases are relatively minor and present no real clinical problems. There may be an association between external fixation and CRPS, with some studies of tibial diaphyseal fractures showing a high incidence of CRPS with external fixation, although other studies do not. A higher incidence has also been reported with transarticular external fixation compared with periarticular external fixation in distal radial fractures.

PATHOPHYSIOLOGY

There is debate about the cause of CRPS. In 1916 Leriche proposed that CRPS was mediated by the sympathetic

TABLE 41-4 CLASSIFICATION OF CHRONIC REGIONAL PAIN SYNDROME

Stage	Description
I	■ Patients present with mild symptoms usually within a few weeks of the injury. ■ Burning pain, swelling, dysesthesia, and dysfunction are present and localized to the injured area. ■ The symptoms are worse than would be expected from the injury itself.
II	■ There is increasing severity of pain, dysfunction, and hypersensitivity. ■ Increased autonomic dysfunction is characterized by involvement of more distal areas of the limb, and the limb is increasingly moist, cold, and edematous with more skin mottling. ■ Joint stiffness increases with time.
III	■ The chronic autonomic dysfunction leads to dystrophic changes in skin, muscle, and bone. ■ Nail and hair growth slows and may stop. ■ The muscles atrophy, and X-rays show regional osteoporosis.

nervous system because sympathectomy improved the symptoms. This still remains the most widely accepted explanation. But it has been pointed out that if the sympathetic nervous system is involved, it would be expected that metabolites of the sympathetic nervous system would be high in CRPS I, which is not the case. Many other theories also remain unproven. These include a hypersensitivity to sympathetic nervous system neurotransmitters, abnormal synapses between the sympathetic nervous system and sensory nerves, opioid abnormalities, exaggerated immune or inflammatory responses to injury, and psychiatric abnormalities.

CLASSIFICATION

There can be increasing severity of symptoms with time. The condition has been divided into stages I through III (Table 41-4).

The problem about classifying a disease such as CRPS is that the classification implies that stage I progresses to the later stages, which frequently is not the case. The condition is often self-limiting and never proceeds beyond stages I or II. Progress from stage I varies and may depend on other factors such as the patient's psychological profile. Very few patients have irreversible stage III changes, with most patients presenting with treatable stage I or occasionally stage II changes.

DIAGNOSIS

The classic signs and symptoms of CRPS are pain, vasomotor changes, and atrophic changes in the affected areas (Box 41-5).

■ To make a diagnosis of CRPS, there should be no other cause of pain and dysfunction.

■ The symptoms tend to arise 3 weeks to 6 months after the initial injury.

■ CRPS I or reflex sympathetic dystrophy is more commonly seen by orthopaedic surgeons, and there is usually a history of trauma, but the condition may follow a burn, vascular disease, infection, or myocardial infarction.

■ CRPS II usually follows a crush injury or direct nerve damage.

■ Radiological osteopenia is a late sign, and a surgeon usually relies on increasing pain, hypersensitivity, joint stiffness, and temperature difference to make the diagnosis.

■ Triple-phase bone scans have been used because generally the bone scan is hot in stage I disease, although the results vary in stages II and III.

■ Bone scanning may be useful but does not replace clinical examination.

■ Neural blockade has been used in an attempt to distinguish between CRPS and the normal symptoms that follow injury.

■ Procaine hydrochloride usually is injected with saline used as a placebo.

■ The placebo effect of saline may be considerable! Guanethidine and phentolamine blockade have also been used to diagnose CRPS.

Psychological Assessment

■ There is a widespread belief that some patients who present with CRPS are either fabricating their symptoms or have an underlying psychological or psychiatric condition.

■ Some evidence indicates that patients with CRPS have a higher incidence of depression and anxiety, but the

BOX 41-5 SIGNS OF COMPLEX REGIONAL PAIN SYNDROME

Autonomic signs
Temperature difference
Skin discoloration
Peripheral edema

Sensory signs
Increased sensitivity to pinprick, touch, and temperature
Muscle tenderness

Motor signs
Muscle atrophy and weakness
Muscle contracture
Joint stiffness

Radiologic signs
Osteopenia

literature does not confirm other psychological or psychiatric problems.

TREATMENT

■ The primary treatment of CRPS is aggressive physical therapy combined with treatments designed to reduce pain.

■ The prognosis is better if treatment is instituted early in the disease process.

■ If a response is not evident within a few weeks, second-line management techniques should be considered including sympathetic blocks, chemical or surgical sympathectomy, intravenous or intra-arterial infusion of ganglion blocking agents, such as guanethidine, and transcutaneous electrical stimulation.

■ Antidepressants can be used if necessary.

PERIPHERAL NERVE INJURIES

Peripheral nerve injuries commonly occur in association with certain fractures or dislocations. Obviously any nerve can be damaged, and high-energy injuries, gunshot wounds, or lacerations may be associated with significant nerve damage. Peripheral nerve lesions are also found with low-energy injuries and closed fractures and dislocations, however. The incidence of a particular peripheral nerve injury is often difficult to calculate. Generally speaking, where EMG studies are used to investigate nerve injuries, the incidence is relatively high, although frequently the clinical manifestation is slight and the prognosis excellent.

EPIDEMIOLOGY

Table 41-5 gives the prevalence of peripheral nerve injuries in some of the common fractures and dislocations, and the wide variation mainly represents the difference in investigative techniques. Thus although 45% of shoulder dislocations and proximal humeral fractures probably do have a degree of nerve involvement, the prevalence of clinically important lesions is considerably less.

Table 41-5 illustrates the difference in prevalence of peripheral nerve lesions in different areas. Dislocations obviously are associated with a relatively high prevalence of nerve damage, and there is a higher prevalence of nerve damage in association with upper limb fractures than in lower limb fractures. The other obvious connection is that proximal limb injuries tend to be associated with a high prevalence of nerve damage. Table 41-5 includes informa-

TABLE 41-5 PREVALENCE OF PERIPHERAL NERVE DAMAGE ASSOCIATED WITH COMMON FRACTURES AND DISLOCATIONS[a]

Injury Location	Prevalence*	Affected Nerves
Clavicle	Rare	Brachial plexus (posterior or medial cords) Suprascapular
Proximal humerus/ shoulder dislocation	5%–45%	Axillary, suprascapular, musculocutaneous radial, ulnar
Humeral diaphysis	6%–18%	Radial
Nailing	*2%–3%*	Radial
Distal humerus	0%–15%	Ulnar (postoperative), radial
Olecranon	0%–10%	Ulnar
Elbow dislocation	<2%	Median, ulnar, anterior interosseous, radial
Forearm diaphyses (Monteggia)	Up to 45%	Posterior interosseous, ulnar, median
Distal radius	8%–17%	Median
Pelvis	10%–15%	L5, S1, sciatic, femoral
Acetabulum	Up to 35%	Sciatic, femoral, superior gluteal
	3%–18%	Operative nerve damage
Hip dislocation	8%–19%	Sciatic
Femoral diaphysis	0%–1%	Peroneal
Nailing	*2%–3%*	Pudendal (traction on post)
	<1%	Sciatic
	0%–0.8%	Peroneal
Knee dislocation	14%–35%	Peroneal (usually an axonotmesis)
Tibial dislocation	0%–10%	Peroneal, posterior tibia (open fractures)
Nailing	*0%–2%*	Saphenous and sural nerves (distal locking)
	0%–19%	Peroneal (traction and proximal screw)
Calcaneus	0%–14%	Sural (iatrogenic)

[a]The prevalence of nerve damage associated with humeral, femoral, and tibial nailing are shown in italics.

TABLE 41-6 CLASSIFICATION OF NERVE INJURIES

Type	Description
Neuropraxia	Reversible condition characterized by local ischemia and selective demyelinization of the axon sheath
Axonotmesis	More severe injury with disruption of the axons and myelin sheath but with an intact epineurium
Neurotmesis	Complete nerve division with disruption of the epineurium

tion about nerve damage relating to nailing. Plating and external fixation can also cause nerve damage, but the prevalence is not as well documented as that of nailing.

CLASSIFICATION

Seddon classified peripheral nerve injuries into three groups: neuropraxia, axonotmesis, and neurotmesis (Table 41-6). The prognosis of peripheral nerve lesions varies directly with the extent of nerve damage, with neuropraxias having a good prognosis and neurotmeses a poor prognosis.

DIAGNOSIS

- Most nerve lesions are detected clinically, but electromyographical studies and nerve conduction studies can be used to detect nerve lesions and to monitor their progress.

TREATMENT

- Nerve lesions associated with closed fractures need not be explored on the grounds that they are likely to be spontaneously resolving neuropraxias.
- If the fracture is treated operatively, the nerve can be explored, but this will not improve the prognosis except where the nerve is transected, which is very rare.
- If the nerve does not show signs of recovery by 3 months, it is recommended that it be explored to see if it is a surgically treatable lesion.
  - Frequently this does not result in an improved prognosis.
- In open fractures and dislocations, there is a high incidence of nerve transaction.
  - If this is found, the nerve can be directly repaired or grafted.
  - In many incidences the prognosis remains poor.

RESULTS

- The prognosis for nerve lesions associated with gunshot wounds depends on the location of damage and the type of projectile.

- In general, low-velocity and high-velocity gunshot wounds both have about a 70% incidence of recovery, and shotgun wounds have a 45% incidence of recovery.
- Proximal extremity nerve injuries are associated with a poorer prognosis than distal nerve injury.
- Most of the nerve lesions detailed in Table 41-5 are neuropraxias and have a good prognosis.
- About 90% of all peripheral nerve lesions can be expected to improve spontaneously, although recovery can take several months.
- The prognosis for nerve lesions associated with open fractures is worse than that of closed fractures, and the prognosis for nerve injury associated with dislocations is worse than with fractures.
- Many nerve lesions associated with dislocations are axonotmeses.

VASCULAR INJURIES

Until relatively recently, significant vascular injuries usually resulted in death if a proximal artery was involved or amputation if the damage was more distal. A number of the standard vascular reconstruction procedures were described before the First World War I, but it was during the Second World War that vascular repair became popular, although the unavoidable delay in transportation and the high infection rates meant the results were frequently poor.

Since the Second World War, there has been an increase in civilian vascular injuries in both penetrating and blunt trauma, which, combined with continuing warfare, has allowed surgeons to develop improved investigative and treatment methods for vascular injuries.

ETIOLOGY

The spectrum of vascular damage following gunshot injuries and blunt trauma is very different. Gunshot injuries can affect virtually any artery, and in low-velocity gunshot injuries the associated soft tissue damage may be relatively minor and the fracture morphology straightforward. In blunt trauma, high-velocity gunshot injuries, and explosive injuries, the soft tissue damage may be considerable and the fracture morphology very complex. Although blunt trauma may theoretically be associated with damage to a number of arteries, in practical terms it is vascular injuries associated with femoral and tibial diaphyseal fractures that may need reconstruction.

An analysis of the 960 open fractures discussed in Chapter 4 shows that only 25 (2.6%) were Gustilo type IIIc in severity (see Table 4-2 in Chapter 4) and therefore might require vascular reconstruction. Four of these fractures occurred in the fingers and five in the foot. All were severe crush injuries and treated by amputation. One IIIc forearm fracture was initially reconstructed but later required an amputation. Thus the requirement for reconstructive surgery was confined to 15 type C femoral and tibial fractures. The other traumatic injury associated with arterial damage is knee dislocation, where the incidence of popliteal artery damage requiring reconstruction is between 16% and 19%. Significant damage to the brachial artery following elbow dislocation is rare.

DIAGNOSIS

■ The classic signs of arterial damage are those of ischemia; absent or reduced pulses, pallor, paresthesia, pain, and paralysis or diminished movement.
■ There may be obvious arterial blood loss or a palpable thrill or audible bruit over a hematoma.
■ If the site of the arterial damage is obvious, immediate surgery can be undertaken.
■ Alternatively, further information may be gained from a Doppler or duplex ultrasound study or from an angiogram.
■ Surgeons should remember that any penetrating injury may cause vascular damage.
■ If there is any evidence of a significant hematoma, abnormal bruising, dysesthesia, or muscle weakness, the possibility of vascular damage should be considered even if the peripheral pulses are palpable.
■ Almost 30% of patients with gunshot wounds and a normal clinical examination have been shown to have vascular injury, although over 80% of these are minor and do not require surgery.
■ Arterial damage is investigated using Doppler ultrasound, duplex or color-duplex ultrastenography, or arteriography.
■ Arteriography remains the most commonly used diagnostic technique and may be done in the emergency department, in the operating room, or in a radiology suite.

TREATMENT

■ In general, arterial repair is undertaken using an end-to-end anastomosis or an interpositional vein graft.
■ Fasciotomy may be undertaken postoperatively, particularly if there has been a delay prior to surgery.
■ There is often debate about whether the fracture should be "quickly" stabilized before arterial repair or the artery should be reconstructed first.
  ■ Evidence suggests the latter because the requirement for fasciotomy is less.

■ An alternative is the use of a temporary vascular stent prior to fracture fixation.

RESULTS

■ The results of vascular repair in gunshot fractures are very good in experienced hands with an average success of 85% to 90% reported.
■ The prognosis is much worse if the warm ischemia time exceeds 6 hours prior to vascular repair or if there is a secondary infection.
■ In blunt trauma the success rate is much less because of associated soft tissue injury and more extensive vascular problems.
■ The amputation rate after a Gustilo type IIIc tibial diaphyseal fracture is reported to vary between 21% and 85%.
■ The incidence of secondary amputation increases with time. Amputations are discussed in Chapter 37.

MALUNION

It would seem logical that malunion should be avoided to allow correct load transmission across the joints. Malunion is often difficult to avoid, however, particularly when nonoperative management techniques are used, and surgeons have attempted to define acceptable ranges of fracture malunion that are not associated with loss of function. Surgeons have understood for many years that fracture malposition and consequent malunion creates more problems in some fractures than in others. It was accepted that the humerus could heal with more angular deformity or rotation than the tibia because of the spherical nature of the glenohumeral joint. With the increasing use of internal fixation techniques, the criteria for malunion have contracted. Whereas surgeons managing complex tibial fractures nonoperatively used to accept 1 inch of shortening, 10 degrees of varus angulation, and up to 15 degrees of external rotation, this is no longer acceptable, and most surgeons would now accept 5 degrees of angular or rotational deformity and 1 cm of shortening.

The same is true for the distal radius. When cast management was the routine method of treatment, up to 10 degrees of dorsal malalignment was often accepted because it was difficult to improve on this position. Recent work has shown that maintenance of volar angulation of the distal radius enhances function, and clearly, where possible, near anatomical reduction should be achieved.

In intra-articular fractures it is important to strive for accurate reduction and rigid internal fixation, but surgeons often accept 1 to 2 mm of articular malalignment if they feel the disadvantage of surgical intervention may outweigh the theoretical advantages of absolute reduction. This is particularly true of intra-articular fractures in the elderly.

There is considerable debate about the effect of diaphyseal malunion on adjacent joints. Very little evidence indicates that diaphyseal malunion causes significant

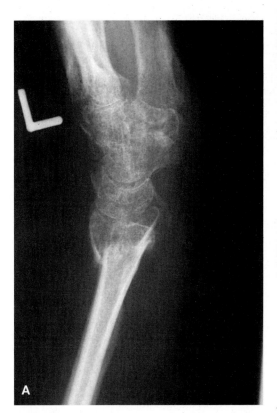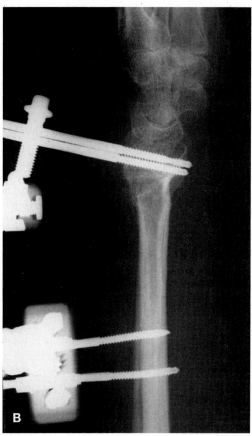

Figure 41-1 A distal radial osteotomy. Note the wedge of bone graft in B.

posttraumatic osteoarthritis in the upper limb, although a number of authors have shown that tibial malunion is associated with knee osteoarthritis. The degree of malunion is not defined, however, and the studies were all retrospective. It does seem reasonable to suggest that malunion should be avoided where possible and diaphyseal fractures treated so that angular or rotational deformity does not exceed 5 degrees and shortening is less than 1 cm. Intra-articular fractures should be completely reduced where possible to minimize postoperative osteoarthritis.

If a symptomatic malunion does occur, it should be treated by osteotomy and fixation with any defects filled by bone grafts. Both closing and opening wedge osteotomies can be undertaken in diaphyseal fractures. One of the most common osteotomies undertaken is the opening wedge distal radial osteotomy performed to correct persistent dorsal malalignment after nonoperative management of a distal radial fracture. An example is shown in Figure 41-1. An alternative to diaphyseal osteotomy is the use of distraction osteogenesis with a small wire fixator (see Chapter 39).

POSTTRAUMATIC OSTEOARTHRITIS

Whether or not malunion causes posttraumatic osteoarthritis, it is certainly a relatively common complication of

fractures, particularly if they are intra-articular. Articular cartilage damage is associated with intra-articular fractures and with abnormal loading of a joint, usually by a compressive force. Dislocation also causes posttraumatic osteoarthritis by direct articular damage during the dislocation. The incidence of posttraumatic osteoarthritis varies considerably, and it is difficult to determine in any meaningful way. It is likely that every intra-articular fracture is associated with a degree of secondary osteoarthritis, but often no treatment needs to be instituted. Treatment depends on the degree of symptomatology, but if the symptoms warrant treatment, arthroplasty or arthrodesis is undertaken depending on the involved joint and the age and general condition of the patient.

SUGGESTED READING

Anglen JO, Bagby C, George R. A randomized comparison of sequential gradient calf compression with intermittent plantar compression for prevention of venous thrombosis in orthopaedic trauma patients: preliminary results. Am J Orthop 1998;27:53–58.

Geerts WH, Jay RM, Code KI, et al. A comparison of low-dose heparin with low-molecular-weight heparin as prophylaxis against venous thromboembolism after major trauma. N Engl J Med 1996;335:701–707.

Gurd AR, Wilson RI. The fat embolism syndrome. J Bone Joint Surg (Br) 1974;56:408–416.

Lindeque BG, Schoeman HS, Dommisse GF, et al. Fat embolism and the fat embolism syndrome. A double-blind therapeutic study. J Bone Joint Surg (Br) 1987;69:128–131.

Pell AC, Christie J, Keating JF, et al. The detection of fat embolism by transoaesophageal echocardiography during reamed intramedullary nailing. A study of 24 patients with femoral and tibial fractures. J Bone Joint Surg (Br) 1993;75:921–925.

Ring D, Chin K, Jupiter JB. Radial nerve palsy associated with high-energy humeral shaft fractures. J Hand Surg (Am) 2004; 29:144–147.

Robinson CM. Current concepts of respiratory insufficiency syndromes after fracture. J Bone Joint Surg (Br) 2001;83:781–791.

Schemitsch EH, Bhandari M. Complications. In: Buchholz RW, Heckman JD, eds. Rockwood and Green's fractures in adults, 5th ed. Philadelphia: Lippincott Williams & Wilkins, 2001.

Topp R, Hayda R, Benedetti G, et al. The incidence of neurovascular injury during external fixator placement without radiographic assistance for lower extremity diaphyseal fractures: a cadaveric study. J Trauma 2003;55:955–958.

Turen CH, Dube MA, Lecroy CM. Approach to the polytraumatized patient with musculoskeletal injuries. J Am Acad Orthop Surg 1999;7:154–165.

Visser CP, Coene LN, Brand R, et al. Nerve lesions in proximal humeral fractures. J Shoulder Elbow Surg 2001;10:421–427.

White TO, Jenkins PJ, Smith RD, et al. The epidemiology of posttraumatic adult respiratory distress syndrome. J Bone Joint Surg (Am) 2004;86:2366–2376.

Wolinsky PR, Banit D, Parker RE, et al. Reamed intramedullary femoral nailing after induction of an "ARDS-like" state in sheep: effect on clinically applicable markers of pulmonary function. J Orthop Trauma 1998;12:169–175.

INDEX

References are to pages. Pages followed by "f" indicate figures; "t," tables; "b," boxes.

A

Above-elbow amputations, 486
Above-knee amputations, 490
Acetabular fractures, 238, 249
  associated injuries, 251
  avascular necrosis, 257–258
  both-column fractures, 256
  classification, 250
  complications, 257–258
  deep venous thrombosis, 258
  diagnosis, 251
  displaced fractures except both
       column, 252–255
  elderly patients, 256
  epidemiology, 238t, 251
  heterotopic ossification, 257
  history, 251
  infection, 257
  nerve injury, 257
  nonsurgical treatment, 256–257
  osteoarthritis, 257
  periprosthetic fractures, 47–48
  physical examination, 251
  plating, 435–436
  posterior wall fractures, 255–256
  pulmonary embolism, 258
  radiological examination, 251, 252f,
       253f
  surgical anatomy, 249–250
  surgical indications, 252–253
  surgical treatment, 253–255
  treatment, 251–257
Acromioclavicular dislocation, 83–84
Acromion fractures, 80
Acute carpal ligament injury, 181–184
Acute compartment syndrome, 492
  arm, 493, 495t
  associated fractures, 501–502
  compartment pressure monitoring,
      499
  complications, 502
  decompression, threshold for,
      499–500
  diagnosis, 498–500
  epidemiology, 495–496
  fasciotomy, 500–501
  foot, 492, 493f, 493t
  forearm, 493, 494t
  hand, 493, 494t, 495f
  history, 498–499
  leg, 492, 493t
  pathogenesis, 497–498
  physical examination, 498–499
  raised tissue pressure
    on bone, effects of, 497

    on muscle, effects of, 497
    on nerve, effects of, 497
  reperfusion injury, 497–498
  surgical anatomy, 492–493, 494t
  thigh, 492
  treatment, 500–502
Adult respiratory distress syndrome,
    531
Alendronate for osteoporotic fractures,
    57
Aminoglycosides for open fractures, 24
Amputations, 482
  above-elbow amputations, 486
  above-knee amputations, 490
  ankle disarticulation, 488, 489f
  below-knee amputations, 488–489,
    490f
  classification, 482
  digital amputations, 483–485
  distal phalangeal amputations,
    483–484
  elbow disarticulation, 486
  forearm amputations, 486
  goals, 483
  hip disarticulation, 490
  knee disarticulation, 489
  lower limb amputations, 486–490
  middle phalangeal amputations, 484
  midfoot amputations, 488
  multiple digital amputations, 485
  proximal phalangeal amputations,
    484
  ray amputations, 484–485
  toe amputations, 487–488
  transcarpal amputations, 486
  upper limb amputations, 483–486
  wrist disarticulation, 486
Ankle disarticulation, 488, 489f
Ankle fractures, 366
  ankle dislocation, 382
  associated injuries, 371
  bimalleolar fractures, 375, 378f
  classification, 367–368, 369f
  complications, 380–381
  diabetics, 381
  diagnosis, 371–372
  displaced fractures, 373
  distal tibiofibular dislocation, 382
  elderly patients, 381
  epidemiology, 369–371
  fracture-dislocations, 377
  history, 371
  intact deltoid ligament, 373, 374f,
    375t
  internal fixation, 375, 376f

  interosseous membrane, 369
  Kirschner wires, 457
  lateral ligament injuries, 381
  lateral malleolar fractures, 373
  medial malleolar fracture, 375, 377f
  metallic or absorbable screws, 375
  nonsurgical treatment, 372–373,
    374f
  nonunion, 517
  pathogenesis, 368–369, 370f, 371f
  physical examination, 371
  plating, 438
  postoperative mobilization, 380
  radiologic examination, 371–372
  ruptured deltoid ligament, 373, 374f
  screws
    fixation, 463–464
    metallic or absorbable, 375
  suprasyndesmotic fractures, 379–380
  surgical anatomy, 366–367
  surgical treatment, 375–380
  treatment, 372–380
  trimalleolar fractures, 375–377,
    378f, 379f
  undisplaced fractures, 372–373
Ankle replacement, 52
Ankylosing spondylitis in cervical spine
    fractures, 224
Anterior iliac crest grafting, 506–508
Anterior posterior compression (APC)
    injuries, 240, 242f
Anterior tension band injuries, 223
Antibiotics
  gunshot injuries, 30
  open fractures, 24
  osteomyelitis, 525
Antiglide plating, 432
Arthroplasty, 475
  elbow arthroplasty, 122t, 479–480
  hip arthroplasty. *See* Hip arthroplasty
  knee replacement, 49–51, 311f,
    477–478
  proximal radial arthroplasty,
    131–132, 480
  shoulder replacement, 51, 99–100,
    478–479
Aspirin for deep venous thrombosis, 529

B

Bacteria, 523
Ballistics, 27
Bandages, 424–425
Basicervical fractures, 278
Below-knee amputations, 488–489, 490f
Below-knee casts, 419–420

Bennett's fracture
  Kirschner wires, 455
  metacarpal base fractures, 193–195
Bifocal fractures, tibia, 353
Biological or bridge plating, 432, 433f
Bipolar arthroplasty, 476–477
Bipolar fracture dislocation, 150
Bisphosphonates for osteoporotic
    fractures, 57, 58
Blade plates, 429–430
Bone
  biomechanics of intact bone, 10
  cancellous bone, 10
  damage from gunshot injuries, 27–28
  grafting, 505–506, 508–509, 510f
  mass in osteoporotic fractures,
      54–55
  morphogenic proteins, 510–511
Bone tissue, 7
Bone transport, 509, 510b, 511f, 511t
Braces, 420–424
Brachial plexus lesion, 76, 534t
Bridge plating, 432, 433f
Bruner casts, 419
Buttress or antiglide plating, 432

C

Calcaneus, fractures of, 392
  epidemiology, 393–394
  extra-articular calcaneal fractures.
      See Extra-articular calcaneal
      fractures
  intra-articular calcaneal fractures.
      See Intra-articular calcaneal
      fractures
  nonunion, 517–518
  plating, 438
  screw fixation, 465
  stress fractures, 39
  surgical anatomy, 393
Calcitonin for osteoporotic fractures,
    57–58
Calcium for osteoporotic fractures, 57
Cancellous bone, 10
Capitate fractures, 181
Carpal injuries, 174
  acute carpal ligament injury,
      181–184
  anatomy, 170–171
  dislocations of the carpus, 184–186
  Kirschner wires, 453–455
  nonscaphoid carpal fractures,
      180–181
  radiocarpal fracture-dislocation, 165,
      166f
  scaphoid fractures. *See* Scaphoid
      fractures
  transcarpal amputation, 486
Carpometacarpal fracture-dislocations
    and Kirschner wires, 454–455
Carpometacarpal joint of the thumb,
    205–206
Casts, 416–417
  application, 418–419
  below-knee casts, 419–420
  Bruner casts, 419
  Colles cast, 419

forearm casts, 419
hanging casts, 419
long-arm casts, 419
long-leg casts, 420
patellar tendon-bearing casts, 420
scaphoid casts, 419
types, 419–420
use, 417–418
U-slabs, 419
Causes of fractures, 4–5
Ceftriaxone for necrotizing fasciitis,
    526
Cephalosporin
  gunshot injuries, 30
  open fractures, 24
Cerclage wires, 460–461
Cervical braces, 422–423
Cervical spine fractures, 208
  ankylosing spondylitis, 224
  anterior surgery, 218
  anterior tension band injuries, 223
  associated injuries, 213
  atlantoaxial junction, 218
  burst fractures, 220
  classification, 210–212
  clinical history and examination,
      213–214
  complications, 224
  compression fractures, 219–221
  computed tomography, 215, 216
  deep venous thrombosis, 224
  descriptive classification, 212
  diagnosis, 213–217
  diffuse idiopathic skeletal hyperosto-
      sis, 224
  dural tears, 224
  epidemiology, 212–213
  facet fractures without dislocation,
      221–222
  facet subluxation/dislocations, 222
  flexion-type teardrop fractures,
      220–221
  hangman fractures, 211–212
  hospital resuscitation, 217
  infection, 224
  initial management, 217
  magnetic resonance imaging, 215,
      216–218
  methylprednisolone, 217
  mortality, 224
  nonsurgical treatment, 217, 219–223
  nonunion, 224
  occipital condyles, 210, 211f
  occipitocervical instability, 210, 211f
  occipitocervical junction, 218
  odontoid fractures, 210, 211f
  odontoid screw fixation, 218
  pedicle and lamina fractures,
      222–223
  plain radiographs, 215, 216
  posterior surgery, 218–219
  prereduction MRI for facet disloca-
      tions, 217
  radiological examination, 214–217
  spinal canal, 210
  spinal cord, 210
  spinal cord injuries, 224

spinal cord injuries without instabil-
    ity in the spondylotic spine,
    224–225
steroids, 217
stress fractures, 41
subaxial cervical spine, 215–217
subaxial fractures, 212, 213f,
    219–221
subaxial spine, 218
surgical anatomy, 208–210
surgical treatment, 217–223
tears, 224
transverse process fractures, 225
traumatic spondylolisthesis of the
    axis, 211–212
treatment, 217–223
unrecognized tears, 224
upper cervical fractures, 219
upper cervical spine, 214–215, 218
Circular frames, 469–470, 471f
Clavicle fractures
  associated injuries, 71
  brachial plexus lesions, 76
  classification, 69
  clinical history and examination, 71
  complications, 75–76
  coracoclavicular stabilization, 74
  diagnosis, 71–72
  distal physeal fractures, 75
  epidemiology and etiology, 69–71
  hook plate, 74–75
  intramedullary pinning, 73
  Kirschner wires, 74
  lateral clavicle fractures, 74–75
  malunion, 76
  medial third clavicle fractures, 72
  middle third clavicle fractures, 72–73
  nonunion, 75–76, 512–513
  plating, 73, 433
  radiological examination, 71–72
  thoracic outlet syndrome, 76
  treatment, 72–75
Clindamycin
  necrotizing fasciitis, 526
  open fractures, 24
Colles casts, 419
Combined mechanical injuries (CMI)
    and pelvic fractures, 240
Compartment syndrome
  acute compartment syndrome. *See*
      Acute compartment syndrome
  forearm diaphysis, fractures of, 151
  intra-articular calcaneal fractures,
      399
  tibia and fibula diaphyseal fractures,
      350
  tibial plafond fractures, 363
  tibial plateau fractures, 334–335
Complex regional pain syndromes,
    532
  classification, 533
  diagnosis, 533–534
  distal radius, 167
  epidemiology, 532
  pathophysiology, 532–533
  psychological assessment, 533–534
  treatment, 534

Coracoclavicular stabilization, 74
Coracoid fractures, 80
Coronoid fractures, 135–136
Cortical bone, 10
Cranial tongs, 415

D

Damage control surgery in multiply injured patients, 15–16
Deep venous thrombosis (DVT), 528
    acetabular fractures, 258
    aspirin, 529
    cervical spine fractures, 224
    diagnosis, 528–529
    etiology, 528
    heparin, 529
    pelvic fractures, 249
    prophylaxis, 529
    treatment, 529
    warfarin, 529
Delayed union, 9, 503
Deltoid ligaments
    intact, 373, 374f, 375t
    ruptured, 373, 374f
Diffuse idiopathic skeletal hyperostosis, 224
Digital amputation, 483–485
Displaced proximal humeral fractures, 93–100
Distal femoral fractures, 303
    associated injuries, 305
    classification, 303–304, 305f
    complications, 312
    condylar buttress plates, 309
    diagnosis, 305–306
    epidemiology, 304–305, 306t
    external fixation, 310–311
    history, 305
    intramedullary nailing, 310
    knee arthroplasty, 311
    LISS plates, 309–310
    95-degree blade plates, 307, 308f, 309t
    95-degree dynamic condylar screw plates, 307, 308f
    nonsurgical management, 311
    nonunion, 516
    physical examination, 305
    plating, 307, 437
    radiological examination, 306
    stress fractures, 37
    surgical anatomy, 303
    surgical treatment, 306–311
    treatment, 306–311, 312t
Distal humeral fractures, 115
    associated injuries, 117
    classification, 115–116
    clinical history and examination, 117
    complications, 123
    diagnosis, 117–119
    elderly, fractures in, 122
    epidemiology, 117
    malunion, 123
    nerve damage, 123
    nonunion, 123, 514
    plating, 434–435

radiological examination, 118–119
    screw fixation, 462
    surgical anatomy, 115
    treatment, 119–123
    type A fractures, 119
    type B fractures, 119–121
    type C fractures, 121–122
Distal interphalangeal joint dislocation, 205
Distal phalangeal amputation, 483–484
Distal phalanges, nonunion of, 515
Distal phalanx fractures, 201–202, 204t
Distal physeal fractures, 75
Distal radial fixation, transarticular, 472
Distal radioulnar joint dislocation, 168–169
Distal radioulnar joint pain, 169
Distal radius fractures, 153
    bone substitutes, 162–163, 164t
    classification, 154, 155f–156f, 155t
    complex regional pain syndrome type 1, 167
    complications, 166–167
    diagnosis, 156–157
    dorsal displacement, 158–163, 435
    epidemiology, 155–156
    external fixation, 160–161, 471–472
    extra-articular and minimal articular fractures, 157–164
    Frykman classification, 155t
    history and physical examination, 157
    infection, 167
    instability of the distal radius, 157, 158f
    intra-articular fractures of the distal radius, 164–165
    joint pain, 167
    Kirschner wires, 453, 454f
    malunion, 166
    nerve compression or injury, 166–167
    nonsurgical treatment, 158–159
    nonunion, 167, 514
    percutaneous wiring, 161–162
    physical examinations, 157
    plating, 162, 163f, 435
    posttraumatic osteoarthrosis, 167
    radiocarpal fracture-dislocation, 165, 166f
    radiological examination, 156–157
    relation of anatomy to function, 157
    screw fixation, 462
    surgical anatomy, 153
    surgical treatment, 160
    tendon rupture, 167
    treatment, 157–167
    undisplaced fractures, 157–158
    volar displacement, 164
Distal tibial fractures, 351
    external fixation, 473
    plating, 438
    screw fixation, 463
Distal tibiofibular dislocation, 382
DVT. See Deep venous thrombosis (DVT)
Dynamic compression plates, 428

E

Early total care in multiply injured patients, 15
Elbow, floating, 111–113
Elbow amputations, 486
Elbow arthroplasty, 479–480
Elbow disarticulation, 486
Elbow dislocation, 136
    clinical history and examination, 136–137
    complications, 138
    diagnosis, 136–137
    radiological examination, 137
    treatment, 137–138
    type I dislocations, 137–138
    type II dislocations, 138
    type III dislocations, 138, 139f
    type IV dislocations, 138, 139f
Elbow replacement, 52, 479–480
Elderly patients
    acetabular fractures, 256
    ankle fractures, 381
    distal humeral fractures, 122
    femoral diaphyseal fractures, 298
    intra-articular calcaneal fractures, 399–400
    multiply injured patients, 17, 18b
    tibial plateau fractures, 335–337
Estrogen in osteoporotic fractures, 57, 58
Etidronate in osteoporotic fractures, 57
Exchange nailing, 511–512
External fixation, 467
    applications, 471–473
    circular frames, 469–470, 471f
    complications, 473
    design, 467–470
    distal radius, 471–472
    distal tibial external fixation, 473
    femoral external fixation, 472
    fine wires, 470–471
    half pins, 470
    multiplanar frames, 468–469, 470f
    pelvic external fixation, 472
    periarticular distal radial fixation, 471–472
    pins, 470–471
    proximal tibial external fixation, 473
    tibial external fixation, 472–473
    transarticular distal radial fixation, 472
    uniplanar frames, 467–468, 469f
Extra-articular calcaneal fractures, 400
    anterior process fractures, 400–401
    calcaneal body fractures, 401
    calcaneal dislocations, 402
    diagnosis, 400
    epidemiology, 400
    history and physical examinations, 400
    lateral process fractures, 401
    medial process fractures, 401
    radiologic examinations, 400
    treatment, 400–402
    tuberosity fractures, 401–402

F

Fall prevention and protection, 57
Fasciotomy, 500–501

Fat embolus syndrome, 530
Fatigue fractures, 33, 34–35
Femoral diaphyseal fractures, 290
  adolescent patients, 298
  antegrade intramedullary nailing,
    293–297
  associated injuries, 292–293
  bilateral femoral fractures, 299
  classification, 291–292
  complications, 295–296, 297, 301
  diagnosis, 293
  elderly patients, 298
  epidemiology, 292–293
  external fixation, 299
  floating knee, 298–299
  gunshot fractures, 298
  history and physical examination,
    293
  ipsilateral femoral diaphyseal and hip
    fractures, 299–301
  multiple injuries, 297–298
  nonsurgical management, 299
  open fractures, 297
  pathological fractures, 298
  plating, 299, 300f, 436–437
  radiological examination, 293, 294f
  retrograde femoral nailing, 296–297
  stress fractures, 36–37
  surgical anatomy, 290–291
  surgical treatment, 293–299
  treatment, 293–301
Femoral external fixation, 472
Femoral fractures, distal. *See* Distal
    femoral fractures
Femoral fractures, proximal. *See* Proxi-
    mal femoral fractures
Femoral head fractures, 264–265
  classification, 265, 266f–268f, 269f
  complications, 268–269
  diagnosis, 265–266
  history and physical examination,
    265–266
  nonunion, 515
  radiological examination, 266
  stress fractures, 36
  treatment, 267–268
Femoral nailing, 440, 441f
  antegrade nailing, 441–444
  avascular necrosis, 443
  complications, 443–444, 445
  cross screw insertion, 443
  external rotation deformity, 444
  femoral neck fracture, 443
  heterotopic ossification, 443–444
  nail and cross screw breakage, 444
  neurological damage, 444
  proximal femoral comminution, 443
  reconstruction nails, 445–446
  retrograde nailing, 444–445
  surgical technique, 441–443,
    444–445
Femoral neck fractures, 269, 270f, 271f
  avascular necrosis, 277
  classification, 269–270, 272f
  complications, 277
  death, 277
  diagnosis, 272–273

displaced femoral neck fractures,
    273–275, 276t
  epidemiology, 270–272
  femoral nailing, 443
  history and physical examination, 272
  infection, 277
  nonunion, 277
  radiological examination, 273
  refracture, 277–278
  stress fractures, 36, 37f
  treatment, 273
  undisplaced femoral neck fractures,
    273
Femoral nonunion, 515–516
Femoral pathological fractures, 65–66
Femoral stress fractures, 35
Fibula
  diaphyseal fractures. *See* Tibia and
    fibula diaphyseal fractures
  isolated fractures, 353
  stress fractures, 38
  tibiofibular dislocation, distal, 382
Fifth metatarsal fractures, 408–409
Fine wires, 470–471
Finger dislocations, 204–206
Floating elbow, 111–113
Floating shoulder, 81
Foot fractures and dislocations, 383
  calcaneus, fractures of. *See* Calca-
    neus, fractures of
  forefoot dislocations, 411
  Kirschner wires, 457–458
  Lisfranc dislocation, 405–406, 458
  metatarsal fractures. *See* Metatarsal
    fractures
  midfoot amputations, 488
  midfoot dislocations, 405
  midfoot fractures. *See* Midfoot frac-
    tures
  phalangeal fractures, 410–411
  sesamoid fractures, 409–410
  talar body fractures. *See* Talar body
    fractures
  talar neck fractures. *See* Talar neck
    fractures
  talus, fractures of. *See* Talus, frac-
    tures of
Forearm amputation, 486
Forearm casts, 419
Forearm diaphysis, fractures of, 141
  associated injuries, 144
  bipolar fracture dislocation, 150
  classification, 142, 143f
  clinical history and examination, 144
  compartment syndrome, 151
  complications, 150–152
  diagnosis, 144–145
  epidemiology, 142–144
  external fixation, 147
  Galeazzi fracture dislocation,
    149–150
  intramedullary nailing, 147, 148f
  isolated radial fractures, 149
  isolated ulnar fractures, 147–149
  malunion, 151
  Monteggia fracture dislocations, 149,
    150f

nerve damage, 151
  nonunion, 151
  plate removal, 150–151
  proximal radioulnar synostosis, 152
  radiological examination, 144–145
  radius and ulna fractures, 145–147
  surgical anatomy, 141–142
  treatment, 145–150
Forearm fractures, proximal. *See* Proxi-
    mal forearm fractures
Forearm nailing, 450
Forefoot dislocations, 411
Fracture compression, 427
Frykman classification of distal radius
    fractures, 155t

G
Galeazzi fracture dislocation, 149–150
Gas gangrene, 527
Gentamycin for open fractures, 24
Glasgow coma scale in the multiply
    injured patient, 13t
Glenohumeral dislocation, 84–87
Glenoid fractures, 51, 80
Grafting, bone, 505–506, 508–509,
    510f
Greater trochanter fractures, 282–283
Greater tuberosity fractures, 93–94
Gunshot injuries, 27, 30, 31b
  antibiotics, role of, 30
  ballistics, 27
  bone damage, 27–28
  cephalosporin, 30
  debridement of low-energy wounds,
    29–30
  joint injuries, 30–31
  neurological damage, 28–29
  spinal gunshot wounds, 31
  treatment, 29–31
  vascular damage, 28
Gustilo classification, 19, 20t

H
Half pins, 470
Halo-body fixation, 415–416
Halo ring traction, 415
Hamate fractures, 181
Hand fractures and dislocations, 170
  anatomy, 170–173
  carpal injuries. *See* Carpal injuries
  epidemiology, 173
  finger dislocations, 204–206
  metacarpal injuries. *See* Metacarpal
    injuries
  muscles and tendons, 172t, 173
  nerves, 173
  phalangeal injuries. *See* Phalangeal
    injuries
  stress fractures, 40
Hanging casts, 419
Hangman fractures, 211–212
Head injuries in the multiply injured
    patient, 16
Healing, 7
  biomechanics, 10–11
  bone tissue, 7
  delayed union, 9

fracture repair, 8
fractures, stabilized, 8–9
fracture union, factors that affect, 9
intramedullary nailing, 9
stages of, 10–11
woven and lamellar bone, characteristics of, 7t
Hemiarthroplasty, 475–476
Heparin for deep venous thrombosis, 529
Hip arthroplasty
anterolateral approach, 476
bipolar arthroplasty, 476–477
complications, 476, 477
hemiarthroplasty, 475–476
hip replacement, 477
posterolateral approach, 476
surgical technique, 475
Hip disarticulation, 490
Hip dislocation
anterior dislocation, 261–262, 262
avascular necrosis, 263
classification, 261–262
complications, 263–264
diagnosis, 262
epidemiology, 260–261
heterotopic ossification, 263
history and physical examination,
262
nerve damage, 263–264
osteoarthritis, 263
posterior dislocation, 260–261, 261,
262, 262t
radiological examination, 262
surgical anatomy, 259, 260f
treatment, 262–263
Hip replacement, 45–49, 275t, 477
Hook plates, 74–75
Humeral diaphyseal fractures, 103
antegrade interlocking nailing,
108–110
associated injuries, 105
classification, 104
clinical history and examination, 106
complications, 112–114
diagnosis, 106
epidemiology, 105
external fixation, 110
flexible retrograde nailing, 108
floating elbow, 111–112
indications for operative treatment,
110–112
intramedullary nailing, 108–110
malunion, 114
nerve damage, 112–113
nonsurgical treatment, 106
nonunion, 113–114, 514
operative treatment, 106–112
pathological fractures, 111
plating, 106–108, 434
radiological examination, 106
retrograde locked nailing, 110
surgical anatomy, 103
treatment, 106–112
Humeral fractures, distal. See Distal
humeral fractures
Humeral fractures, proximal. See Proximal humeral fractures

Humeral fractures and shoulder replacement, 51
Humeral nailing, 448
complications, 449
neurological damage, 449
shoulder dysfunction, 449
surgical technique, 448–449
vascular damage, 449
Humeral stress fractures, 40

I
Incidence of fractures, 1–3, 4t
Infection
cervical spine fractures, 224
gas gangrene, 527
necrotizing fasciitis, 525–526
nonunion and, 518
osteomyelitis. See Osteomyelitis
thoracolumbar fractures and dislocations, 237
Insufficiency fractures, 34, 35
Interphalangeal joint dislocation, distal,
205
Interphalangeal joint dislocation, proximal, 205
Intertrochanteric fractures, 278, 279f
classification, 278–279
complications, 282–283
diagnosis, 280
dynamic hip screw or reconstruction
nail, 281–282
epidemiology, 279
greater trochanter fractures,
282–283
history and physical examination,
280
lesser trochanter fractures, 283
nonsurgical treatment, 282
radiological examination, 280
surgical treatment, 282
treatment, 280–281, 283f
Intra-articular calcaneal fractures, 394
adolescents, 399
arthrodesis, 398–399
associated injuries, 395
classification, 394, 395f
compartment syndrome, 399
complications, 398–399
diagnosis, 395–396
elderly patients, 399–400
epidemiology, 394–395
heel pain, 399
history and physical examination,
395–396
malunion, 399
nerve damage, 399
open fractures, 399
osteomyelitis, 398
primary arthrodesis, 399
radiologic examination, 396, 397f
subtalar stiffness, 398
tendon impingement, 399
treatment, 396–398
wound infection, 398
Intramedullary nailing, 9, 440
femoral nailing. See Femoral nailing
forearm nailing, 450

humeral nailing. See Humeral nailing
nail design, 440
nail removal, 450
reaming, 440
retrograde nailing. See Retrograde
nailing
tibial nailing. See Tibial nailing
Intramedullary pinning, clavicle, 73
Isolated fibular fractures, 353
Isolated radial fractures, 149
Isolated tibial fractures, 351–353
Isolated ulnar fractures, 147–149

J
Joint injuries and gunshot injuries,
30–31
Jones fractures, 409

K
Kirschner wires, 74, 452
ankle fractures, 457
Bennett's fracture, 455
carpal injuries, 453–454
carpometacarpal fracture-
dislocations, 454–455
definitive fracture fixation, 452
distal radius, 453, 454f
foot fractures and dislocations,
457–458
Lisfranc fracture-dislocation, 458
lower limb, 457–458
metacarpal and phalangeal fractures,
455–457
metacarpal diaphyseal fractures,
455–456
metacarpal neck fractures, 456–457
metatarsal fractures, 458
phalangeal fractures, 455–457, 458
proximal humerus, 452–453
Rolando's fracture, 455
temporary fracture fixation, 452
upper limb, 452–457
Knee, 322
above-knee amputations, 490
dislocations. See Knee dislocations
proximal tibiofibular dislocation, 325
tibial plateau fractures. See Tibial
plateau fractures
Knee disarticulation, 489
Knee dislocations, 322–323
associated injuries, 323–324
classification, 323
diagnosis, 324
history and physical examination, 324
ligamentous injuries, 323–324
nerve damage, 324
nonligamentous complications, 324,
325t
radiological examination, 324, 325f
treatment, 325
Knee replacement, 49–51, 311,
477–478
K-wire migration, 459–460

L
Lamina fractures, 222–223
Lateral clavicle fractures, 74–75

Lateral compression (LC) injuries in pelvic fractures, 240, 242f
Lateral malleolar fractures, 373–374
Lesser trochanter fractures, 65, 283
Lesser tuberosity fractures, 97
Limb braces, 420–422
Lisfranc fracture-dislocation, 405–406, 458
Location-specific plates, 430–431
Locking compression plates, 428–429, 430f
Long-arm casts, 419
Long-leg casts, 420
Lower limb stress fractures, 35–39
Lumbar braces, 423–424
Lumbar spine stress fractures, 40–41
Lunatotriquetral dissociation, 186

M
Mallet injuries, 202–203
Malunion, 536–537
  clavicle fractures, 76
  distal humeral fractures, 123
  distal radius, fractures of, 166
  forearm diaphysis, fractures of, 151
  humeral diaphyseal fractures, 114
  intra-articular calcaneal fractures, 399
  pelvic fractures, 249
  proximal humeral fractures, 101
Mason I fractures, 128, 129t
Mason II fractures, 128–129
Mason III fractures, 129–132
Medial malleolar fracture, 375, 377f
Medial malleolus stress fractures, 39
Medial third clavicle fractures, 72
Metacarpal injuries
  anatomy, 171–172
  associated injuries, 187
  Bennett's fracture, 193–195
  classification, 187
  diagnosis, 187–188
  epidemiology, 187
  fractures of the metacarpal bases, 192–195
  history, 187
  Kirschner wires, 454–457
  metacarpal head fractures, 189
  metacarpal neck fractures, 189–190, 456–457
  metacarpal shaft fractures, 190–192
  multiple metacarpal fractures, 192
  nonunion, 515
  physical examination, 187
  plating, 435
  radiologic examination, 187–189
  Rolando's fracture, 195
  screw fixation, 462–463
  treatment, 189–195, 196t
Metacarpophalangeal joint dislocation, 205
Metacarpophalangeal joint of the thumb, 206
Metatarsal fractures, 406
  associated injuries, 407
  classification, 406–407
  complications, 408

diagnosis, 407–408
epidemiology, 407
fifth metatarsal fractures, 408–409
history and physical examination, 407–408
Jones fractures, 409
Kirschner wires, 458
nonunion, 518
plating, 439
radiologic examination, 408
stress fractures, 39, 409
surgical anatomy, 406
treatment, 408
zone 1 fractures, 409, 518
zone 2 fractures, 409, 518
zone 3 fractures, 409
zone 4 fractures, 409
Methylprednisolone for cervical spine fractures, 217
Metronidazole for open fractures, 24
Middle phalangeal amputations, 484
Middle phalanx fractures, 200–201, 204t
Middle third clavicle fractures, 72–73
Midfoot amputations, 488
Midfoot dislocations, 405
Midfoot fractures, 402
  associated injuries, 403
  classification, 402, 403f
  complications, 404–405
  diagnosis, 403–404
  epidemiology, 402–403
  history and physical examination, 403–404
  radiologic examination, 404
  stress fractures, 39
  surgical anatomy, 402
  treatment, 404, 405t
Minimally displaced fractures, 92
Monteggia fracture dislocation, 149, 150f
Multiplanar frames, 468–469, 470f
Multiply injured patients, 12
  assessment, 13–14
  damage control surgery, 15–16
  early total care, 15
  elderly patients, 17, 18b
  epidemiology, 12, 13f
  fracture treatment, 15–16
  Glasgow coma scale, 13t
  head injury, 16
  musculoskeletal abbreviated injury score, 13t
  outcome, 16
  resuscitation, 14–15
  revised trauma score, 14t
  spinal fractures, 16
  suggested treatment, 16–17, 18b
  top 12 "killers," 12t
  Triss score, 14t
Musculoskeletal abbreviated injury score (AIS), 13t

N
Nailing, intramedullary. *See* Intramedullary nailing
Nail removal, 450

Necrotizing fasciitis, 525–526
Neurological damage in gunshot injuries, 28–29
Neutralization plates, 428
Nonoperative management, 412, 413t
  bandages, 424–425
  below-knee casts, 419–420
  braces, 420–424
  Bruner casts, 419
  casts, 416–420
  cervical braces, 422–423
  Colles casts, 419
  cranial tongs, 415
  forearm casts, 419
  halo-body fixation, 415–416
  halo ring traction, 415
  hanging casts, 419
  limb braces, 420–422
  long-arm casts, 419
  long-leg casts, 420
  patellar tendon-bearing casts, 420
  scaphoid casts, 419
  skeletal traction, 412–414
  slings, 424–425
  spinal braces, 422–424
  splints, 425–426
  support strapping, 424–425
  thoracic and lumbar braces, 423–424
  thoracolumbar fractures, 416
  traction, 412–416
  U-slabs, 419
Nonscaphoid carpal fractures, 180–181
Nonunion, 503
  ankle, 517
  anterior iliac crest grafting, 506–508
  aseptic nonunion, 505–518
  bone grafting, 505–506
  bone grafting techniques, 508–509, 510f
  bone marrow injection, 512
  bone morphogenic proteins, 510–511
  bone transport, 509, 510b, 511f, 511t
  calcaneus, 517–518
  classification, 503–505
  clavicle, 512–513
  definition, 503
  diagnosis, 505
  distal femur, 516
  distal humerus, 514
  distal phalanges, 515
  distal radius, 514
  electrical stimulation, 512
  epidemiology, 505, 506t, 507t, 508t
  etiology, 504–505
  exchange nailing, 511–512
  femoral head, 515
  femur, 515–516
  humeral diaphysis, 514
  infected nonunion, 518
  metacarpus, 515
  metatarsus, 518
  olecranon, 514
  patella, 516
  phalanges, 515
  posterior iliac crest grafting, 508, 509b

primary bone shortening and secondary lengthening, 509–510
proximal femur, 515, 516f
proximal humerus, 513
radius, 514
scaphoid, 514–515
scapula, 513
shock-wave therapy, 512
specific nonunion types, 512–518
subtrochanteric, 515
talus, 517
tarsus, 518
tibia, 516–517
tibial plafond, 517
tibial plateau, 516
treatment, 505–518
ulna, 514
ultrasound, 512

O

Occipital condyles, 210, 211f
Occipitocervical instability, 210, 211f
Odontoid fractures, 210, 211f
Olecranon fractures, 133–135
Olecranon nonunion, 514
Open fractures, 19
    aminoglycoside, 24
    antibiotic prophylaxis, 24
    cephalosporin, 24
    classification, 19, 20t
    clindamycin, 24
    debridement, 23–24
    epidemiology, 19–21
    examination of the open wound, 21–22
    fracture stabilization, 24–25
    gentamycin, 24
    Gustilo classification, 19, 20t
    lavage, 24
    metronidazole, 24
    penicillin, 24
    polymethylmethacrylate beads, 24
    preoperative assessment, 21–22
    radiological examination, 22
    secondary debridement, 25
    soft tissue cover, 25, 26t
    tobramycin, 24
    treatment, 22–25, 26t
    wound closure, 24
Osteoarthritis
    acetabular fractures, 257
    hip dislocation, 263
    posttraumatic osteoarthritis, 537
    talar neck fractures, 388
    tibial plafond fractures, 363, 364f
    tibial plateau fractures, 335
Osteomyelitis, 520
    antibiotics, 525
    bacteria, 523
    biopsy, 524–525
    bone scanning, 524
    classification, 521–522, 523t
    CT scanning, 524
    diagnosis, 523–525
    epidemiology, 520–521, 522t
    etiology, 522–523
    history and physical examination,

523
    laboratory tests, 523–524
    MRI, 524
    radiographs, 524
    radiologic examination, 524
    treatment, 525
    vancomycin, 525
Osteoporotic fractures, 3–4, 5t, 53–54
    alendronate, 57
    bisphosphonates, 57, 58
    bone mass, 54–55
    calcitonin, 57–58
    calcium, 57
    causes of osteoporosis, 55
    definition, 54
    diagnosis, 55–56
    estrogen, 57, 58
    etidronate, 57
    fall prevention and protection, 57
    prevention, 56–58
    radiological examination, 55–56
    risedronate, 57
    risk assessments, 56
    sodium fluoride, 58
    testosterone, 57
    vitamin D, 57

P

Paget's disease, 41
Patellar dislocation, 313–314
Patellar fractures, 314
    associated injuries, 315
    classification, 314, 315f–316f
    complications, 320–321
    diagnosis, 315–317
    epidemiology, 314–315, 317f
    history and physical examination, 315–316
    nonsurgical treatment, 318
    nonunion, 516
    partial patellectomy, 319–320
    periprosthetic, 51
    radiological examination, 316, 317f
    stress fractures, 37
    surgical treatment, 318–320
    total patellectomy, 320
    treatment, 316–320
Patellar tendon-bearing casts, 420
Pathological fractures, 59
    benign tumors, 67
    classification of bone metastases, 61
    common tumors associated with pathological fracture, 60b
    diagnosis, 61–63
    etiology, 59–61
    femur, 65–66
    history and physical examination, 61
    metastases, 59–61
    nonoperative treatment, 63–64
    pelvis, 65
    prediction of fracture, 63
    primary tumors, 67
    radiological examination, 61–62, 63f
    spine, 66–67
    surgical treatment, 64–67
    treatment, 63–67
    tumor spread, 60

upper limb, 64–65
Pedicle and lamina fractures, 222–223
Pelvic fractures, 238
    anterior posterior compression injuries, 240, 242f
    associated injuries, 241–242
    classification, 239–240, 241f
    combined mechanical injuries, 240
    complications, 248–249
    deep venous thrombosis, 249
    diagnosis, 242–243
    epidemiology, 240–242
    external fixation, 472
    history and physical examination, 242–243
    infection, 248–249
    lateral compression injuries, 240, 242f
    malunion, 249
    nerve injury, 248
    nonsurgical treatment, 247–248
    nonunion, 249
    pathological fractures, 65
    plating, 435–436
    pulmonary embolus, 249
    radiological examination, 243
    stress fractures, 41
    surgical anatomy, 238–239
    surgical treatment, 243–247, 248f
    treatment, 243–248
    vertical shear injuries, 240, 242f
Penicillin
    gas gangrene, 527
    necrotizing fasciitis, 526
    open fractures, 24
Periarticular distal radial fixation, 471–472
Perilunate dislocations, 185–186
Peripheral nerve injuries, 534–535
Periprosthetic fractures, 43
    acetabular fractures, 47–48
    ankle replacement, 52
    elbow replacement, 52
    epidemiology, 43–44
    glenoid fractures, 51
    hip replacement, 45–49
    humeral fractures, 51
    intraoperative fractures, 43
    knee replacement, 49–51
    patellar fractures, periprosthetic, 51
    postoperative fractures, 43–44, 45t
    proximal femoral fracture fixation, 48–49
    proximal tibial periprosthetic fractures, 51
    risk factors, 44–45
    shoulder replacement, 51
    type A fractures, 45–46
    type B fractures, 46–47
    type C fractures, 47
Phalangeal amputation, distal, 483–484
Phalangeal amputation, proximal, 484
Phalangeal injuries, 204t, 410–411
    anatomy, 172
    associated injuries, 196, 197t
    distal phalanx, 201–202, 204t
    epidemiology, 196

Phalangeal injuries (*contd*)
Kirschner wires, 455–458
mallet injuries, 202–203
middle phalangeal amputations, 484
middle phalanx, 200–201, 204t
nonunion, 515
proximal phalanx. *See* Proximal
phalanx
screw fixation, 462–463
Phalanx fractures
distal phalanx, 201–202, 204t
middle phalanx fractures, 200–201,
204t
proximal phalanx. *See* Proximal
phalanx
Physeal fractures, distal, 75
Pins, 470–471
Pisiform fractures, 181
Plating, 73, 427
acetabular plating, 435–436
ankle fractures, 438
application, 431
biological or bridge plating, 432,
433f
blade plates, 429–430
buttress or antiglide plating, 432
calcaneal fractures, 438
clavicle fractures, 73, 433
design of plate, 428–431
distal femoral plating, 307, 437
distal humeral plating, 434–435
distal radial plating, 162, 163f, 435
distal tibial plating, 438
dorsally displaced distal radial fractures, 435
dynamic compression plates, 428
femoral diaphyseal fractures, 299,
300f, 436–437
fibular fractures, 348
fracture compression, 427
fracture reduction, 431
humeral diaphyseal plating,
106–108, 434
location-specific plates, 430–431
locking compression plates,
428–429, 430f
metacarpal plating, 435
metatarsal plating, 439
neutralization plates, 428
number of screws, 431
pelvic plating, 435–436
phalangeal plating, 435
plate contouring, 431
proximal femoral plating, 436
proximal humeral plating, 95, 98, 434
proximal radial plating, 435
proximal tibial plating, 437
proximal ulnar plating, 435
radial and ulnar diaphyseal plating,
435
reconstruction plates, 428, 429f
selection of plate type, 431
soft tissue mobilization, 431
specific fractures, 433–439
spinal plating, 436
subcutaneous plating, 433
subtrochanteric fractures, 286

techniques, 431–433
tension band plating, 431–432
tibial diaphyseal plating, 348,
437–438
tibial plafond fractures, 359
ulnar diaphyseal plating, 435
volar displaced distal radial fractures,
435
wave plating, 432–433
Polymethylmethacrylate beads for open
fractures, 24
Posterior iliac crest grafting, 508, 509b
Posttraumatic osteoarthritis, 388, 537
Posttraumatic osteoarthrosis, 167
Primary bone shortening and secondary
lengthening, 509–510
Proximal diaphyseal fractures, tibia,
350–351, 352f
Proximal femoral fractures, 264
basicervical fractures, 278
femoral head fractures. *See* Femoral
head fractures
femoral neck fractures. *See* Femoral
neck fractures
fixation, periprosthetic fractures,
48–49
intertrochanteric fractures. *See* Intertrochanteric fractures
nonunion, 515, 516f
plating, 436
screw fixation, 463
Proximal forearm fractures, 124
associated injuries, 127
classification, 124–126
clinical history and examination, 127
coronoid fractures, 135–136
diagnosis, 127
elbow dislocation. *See* Elbow dislocation
epidemiology, 126–127
management, 140
olecranon fractures, 133–135
radial head fractures. *See* Radial
head fractures
radial neck fractures, 132
radiological examination, 127
radioulnar dissociation, 138–139
surgical anatomy, 124, 125f
Proximal humeral fractures, 89
antegrade intramedullary nailing, 96
avascular necrosis, 101
axillary artery damage, 101
classification, 90–91
complications, 100–101
diagnosis, 91–92
displaced fractures, 93–100
epidemiology, 91
fracture dislocations and head-splitting fractures, 100
greater tuberosity fractures, 93–94
hemiarthroplasty, 99–100
heterotopic ossification, 101
intramedullary nailing, 98
Kirschner wires, 452–453
K-wires and tension banding, 98
lesser tuberosity fractures, 97
malunion, 101

minimally displaced fractures, 92
neurological damage, 101
nonoperative treatment, 98
nonunion, 100–101, 513
percutaneous K-wire fixation, 95
percutaneous screw fixation, 98, 99f
plating, 95, 98, 434
radiological examination, 92
retrograde intramedullary nailing, 96
screw fixation, 461–462
surgical anatomy, 89–90
surgical neck fractures, 94
surgical treatment, 95–96, 98
suture-cerclage wire, 98
three- and four-part fractures, 97–100
two-part fractures, 93–97
two-part varus impacted fractures,
96–97
valgus impacted fractures, 100
Proximal interphalangeal joint dislocation, 205
Proximal phalangeal amputation, 484
Proximal phalanx, 204t
basal fractures, 196–198
condylar fractures, 199–200
extra-articular fractures, 196–197
intra-articular fractures, 197–198
neck fractures, 199
shaft fractures, 198–199
Proximal radial arthroplasty, 480
Proximal radial plating, 435
Proximal radioulnar synostosis, 152
Proximal radius screw fixation, 462
Proximal tibia, 322
external fixation, 473
knee dislocations. *See* Knee dislocations
periprosthetic fractures, 51
plating, 437
proximal tibiofibular dislocation, 325
screw fixation, 463
tibial plateau fractures. *See* Tibial
plateau fractures
Proximal tibiofibular dislocation, 325
Proximal ulnar plating, 435

R
Radial arthroplasty, proximal, 131–132,
480
Radial fractures, 145–147
diaphyseal plating, 435
distal radius. *See* Distal radius
fractures
head fractures. *See* Radial head
fractures
isolated radial fractures, 149
neck fractures, 132, 514
nonunion, 514
proximal radial plating, 435
proximal radioulnar synostosis, 152
proximal radius screw fixation, 462
stress fractures, 40
Radial head fractures, 127
complications, 132
Mason I fractures, 128, 129t
Mason II fractures, 128–129
Mason III fractures, 129–132

nonunion, 514
radial head excision, 129–131
radial head replacement, 131–132, 480
treatment, 128–132
type IV fractures, 132
Radiocarpal fracture-dislocation, 165, 166f
Radioulnar dissociation, 138–139
Radioulnar joint dislocation, distal, 168–169
Radioulnar joint pain, distal, 169
Ray amputation, 484–485
Reconstruction plates, 428, 429f
Resuscitation of multiply injured patients, 14–15
Retrograde nailing, 449
complications, 450
surgical technique, 449–450
Reverse Segond fracture, 338
Revised trauma score for multiply injured patients, 14t
Rib stress fractures, 40
Risedronate for osteoporotic fractures, 57
Rolando's fracture, 195, 455

S
Scaphoid casts, 419
Scaphoid fractures
classification, 174
diagnosis, 174–177
epidemiology, 174
fractures of the scaphoid distal pole, 179
fractures of the scaphoid proximal pole, 178–179
fractures of the scaphoid wrist, 177–178
history, 174
nonunion, 514–515
physical examination, 174
radiologic examination, 174–177
screw fixation, 462
treatment, 177–179
Scapholunate dissociation, 184–185
Scapular fractures, 76
acromion fractures, 80
associated injuries, 78–79
classification, 76–77, 78f
clinical history and examination, 79
complications, 80
coracoid fractures, 80
diagnosis, 79
epidemiology, 77–79
fractures of the scapular body, 79–80
glenoid fractures, 80
neck fractures, 80
nonunion, 513
radiological examination, 79
spine fractures, 80
treatment, 79–80
Scapulothoracic dissociation
classification, 82t
diagnosis, 81
epidemiology and etiology, 81
treatment, 82

Screw fixation, 461, 465
ankle, 375, 463–464
calcaneus, 465
distal humerus, 462
distal radius, 462
distal tibia, 463
metacarpal and phalangeal fractures, 462–463
proximal femoral fractures, 463
proximal humerus, 461–462
proximal radius, 462
proximal tibia, 463
scaphoid, 462
syndesmosis screws, 463–464
talar body fractures, 464–465
talar neck fractures, 464, 465f
talus, 464–465
Segond fracture, 337, 338f
Sesamoid fractures, 409–410
Shock, 531–532
Shock-wave therapy, 512
Shoulder, floating, 81
Shoulder girdle, 68
clavicle fractures. See Clavicle fractures
floating shoulder, 81
scapular fractures. See Scapular fractures
scapulothoracic dissociation. See Scapulothoracic dissociation
shoulder girdle dislocations. See Shoulder girdle dislocations
stress fractures, 39–40
surgical anatomy, 68–69
Shoulder girdle dislocations, 82
acromioclavicular dislocation, 83–84
glenohumeral dislocation, 84–87
sternoclavicular and acromioclavicular dislocations, 84
sternoclavicular dislocation, 82–83
Shoulder replacement, 51, 478–479
Skeletal traction, 412–414
Slings, 424–425
Sodium fluoride in osteoporotic fractures, 58
Spinal braces, 422–424
Spinal fractures
cervical spine fractures. See Cervical spine fractures
lumbar spine stress fractures, 40–41
multiply injured patients, 16
pathological fractures, 66–67
plating, 436
stress fractures, 40–41
Spinal gunshot wounds, 31
Splints, 425–426
Stabilized fractures, 8–9
Sternoclavicular and acromioclavicular dislocations, 84
Sternoclavicular dislocation, 82–83
Sternum stress fractures, 40
Steroids for cervical spine fractures, 217
Stress fractures, 32, 33f
calcaneus, 39
cervical spine, 41
delayed menarche, 33

diagnosis, 35
distal femur, 37
epidemiology, 34–35
etiology, 33–34
exercise regimens, 34
fatigue fractures, 33, 34–35
femoral diaphysis, 36–37
femoral head, 36
femoral neck, 36, 37f
femur, 35
fibula, 38
foot type, 34
gender, 33
hand, 40
humerus, 40
insufficiency fractures, 34, 35
joint mobility, 34
lower limb, 35–39
lumbar spine, 40–41
medial malleolus, 39
metatarsus, 39
midfoot, 39
nutrition, 33
Paget's disease, 41
patella, 37
pelvis, 41
physical conditioning, 33
radiological examination, 35, 36f
radius, 40
ribs, 40
shoe wear, 34
shoulder girdle, 39–40
spine, 40–41
sternum, 40
tarsus, 39
tibial diaphysis, 37–38
types of stress fractures, 35–41
ulna, 40
upper limb, 39–40
Subaxial fractures, 219–221
Subcutaneous plating, 433
Subtrochanteric fractures, 284
associated injuries, 285–286
classification, 284–285
complications, 289
diagnosis, 286
epidemiology, 285–286
external fixation, 288
history and physical examination, 286
intramedullary nailing, 287, 288f
95-degree blade plate, 286
95-degree dynamic condylar screw plate, 286, 287f
nonsurgical treatment, 289
nonunion, 515
135-degree dynamic hip screw, 286–287
pathological fractures, 288
plating, 286
radiological examination, 286
reconstruction nails, 288
surgical anatomy, 284
surgical treatment, 286–288
treatment, 286–289
Support strapping, 424–425
Suture anchors, 465
Syndesmosis screws, 463–464

T

Talar body fractures, 388
  epidemiology, 388
  lateral process fractures, 389–390
  osteochondral fractures, 390, 391f
  posterior process fractures, 389
  screw fixation, 464–465
  shear and crush fractures, 388–389
  subtalar dislocation, 391–392
  talar dislocations, 391–392
  talar head fractures, 391
  total talar dislocation, 392
  treatment, 388–392
Talar neck fractures, 386
  avascular necrosis, 388
  complications, 388
  epidemiology, 386
  nonsurgical treatment, 386–387
  posttraumatic osteoarthritis, 388
  screw fixation, 464, 465f
  surgical treatment, 387
  treatment, 386–388
Talus, fractures of, 383
  associated injuries, 385
  body fractures. See Talar body frac-
    tures
  classification, 384–385
  diagnosis, 385–386
  epidemiology, 385
  history and physical examination,
    385
  neck fractures. See Talar neck
    fractures
  nonunion, 517
  radiologic examination, 385–386
  screw fixation, 464–465
  surgical anatomy, 383–384
Tarsus
  nonunion, 518
  stress fractures, 39
Tension band plating, 431–432
Tension band wiring, 458–459
  cerclage wires, 460–461
  K-wire migration, 459–460
Testosterone in osteoporotic fractures,
  57
Thoracic and lumbar braces, 423–424
Thoracic outlet syndrome, 76
Thoracolumbar fractures and disloca-
    tions, 226
  anterior surgery, 235
  associated injuries, 229
  burst and compression fractures,
    231–236
  classification, 226–228, 229f
  clinical history and examination,
    229, 230t
  combined anterior and posterior
    surgery, 235
  complications, 236–237
  computed tomography, 230
  diagnosis, 229–231
  dural tears, 237
  epidemiology, 228–229
  flexion-distraction injuries, 235–236
  fracture-dislocations, 236
  infection, 237

instrument failure, 237
  late deformity, 237
  magnetic resonance imaging,
    230–231
  neurological outcomes and canal
    compromise, 235
  nonoperative management, 416
  nonsurgical management, 231–232
  nonsurgical versus surgical treatment
    of burst fractures, 232
  nonunion, 237
  posterior surgery, 233–234
  radiological examination, 229–231
  surgical anatomy, 226
  surgical timing, 236
  surgical treatment, 232
  treatment, 231–236
Thumb, carpometacarpal joint of,
  205–206
Tibia
  diaphyseal fractures. See Tibia and
    fibula diaphyseal fractures
  distal fractures. See Tibial fractures,
    distal
  external fixation, 472–473
  nailing. See Tibial nailing
  nonunion, 516–517
  plafond fractures. See Tibial plafond
    fractures
  plateau fractures. See Tibial plateau
    fractures
  proximal. See Proximal tibia
Tibia and fibula diaphyseal fractures,
  339
  amputations, 350
  associated injuries, 342
  bifocal fractures, 353
  classification, 340, 341f
  compartment syndrome, 350
  complications, 349–350
  diagnosis, 342–344
  distal tibial fractures, 351
  epidemiology, 341–342
  external fixation, 345–348
  history and physical examination,
    342–343
  intramedullary nailing, 344–345,
    346t
  isolated fibular fractures, 353
  isolated tibial fractures, 351–353
  nonsurgical treatment, 348–349
  plating, 348, 437–438
  proximal diaphyseal fractures,
    350–351, 352f
  radiological examination, 343–344
  reflex sympathetic dystrophy, 350
  stress fractures, 37–38
  surgical anatomy, 339–340
  surgical treatment, 344–348
  treatment, 344–349
Tibial fractures, distal, 351
  external fixation, 473
  plating, 438
  screw fixation, 463
Tibial nailing, 446
  bone damage, 448
  complications, 447–448

hardware breakage, 448
  knee pain, 447
  neurological damage, 447–448
  surgical technique, 446–447
  thermal necrosis, 448
  vascular damage, 448
Tibial plafond fractures, 354
  associated injuries, 356
  classification, 354–355, 356f
  combined tibial diaphyseal and
    plafond fractures, 363
  compartment syndrome, 363
  complications, 363
  diagnosis, 357
  epidemiology, 356
  external fixation, 359–362
  history and physical examination,
    357
  intramedullary nailing, 362
  nonsurgical treatment, 358
  nonunion, 517
  osteoarthritis, 363, 364f
  plating, 359
  radiological examination, 357, 358f
  surgical anatomy, 354
  surgical treatment, 359–362
  treatment, 357–362
  unreconstructable plafond fractures,
    364f, 365
Tibial plateau fractures
  associated injuries, 327–329
  bicondylar fractures, 333, 334f
  classification, 325–326, 327f
  compartment syndrome, 334–335
  complications, 334–335
  diagnosis, 329
  elderly patients, 335–337
  epidemiology, 326–329
  history and physical examination,
    329
  medial plateau fractures, 333–334
  meniscal and ligament injuries, 338
  nonunion, 516
  osteoarthritis, 335
  osteochondral defects, 335
  radiological examination, 329, 330f
  reverse Segond fracture, 338
  Segond fracture, 337, 338f
  tibial eminence fractures, 337
  treatment, 329–334, 335t
Tibiofibular dislocation, distal, 382
Tobramycin for open fractures, 24
Toe amputations, 487–488
Traction, 412–416
Transarticular distal radial fixation, 472
Transcarpal amputation, 486
Transverse process fractures, 225
Trapezium fractures, 181
Trapezoid fractures, 181
Traumatic spondylolisthesis of the axis
  (hangman fractures), 211–212
Triangular fibrocartilage complex,
  injuries to, 169
Trimalleolar fractures, 375–377, 378f,
  379f
Triss score for multiply injured patients,
  14t

U

Ulnar fractures, 145–149
classification, 154, 155f–156f
distal radioulnar joint dislocation, 168–169
distal radioulnar joint pain, 169
isolated ulnar fractures, 147–149
nonunion, 514
plating, 435
proximal radioulnar synostosis, 152
proximal ulnar plating, 435
radioulnar dissociation, 138–139
stress fractures, 40
surgical anatomy, 153
Uniplanar frames, 467–468, 469f

Upper cervical fractures, 219
Upper limb pathological fractures, 64–65
Upper limb stress fractures, 39–40
U-slabs, 419

V

Valgus impacted fractures, proximal humerus, 100
Vancomycin
necrotizing fasciitis, 526
osteomyelitis, 525
Vascular injuries, 535–536
gunshot injuries, 28
humeral nailing, 449
tibial nailing, 448

Vertical shear (VS) injuries, 240, 242f
Vitamin D for osteoporotic fractures, 57
Volar displaced distal radial fracture plating, 435

W

Warfarin for deep venous thrombosis, 529
Wave plating, 432–433
Woven and lamellar bone, characteristics of, 7t
Wrist disarticulation, 486

Z

Zones 1–4, fifth metatarsal, 409